TEACHING NURSING

Developing a Student-Centered Learning Environment

TEACHING NURSING

Developing a Student-Centered Learning Environment

Lynne E. Young, PhD, RN
Associate Professor
University of Victoria
Vancouver, British Columbia

Barbara L. Paterson, PhD, RN
Professor and Tier 1 Canada Research Chair
University of New Brunswick
Fredericton, New Brunswick

Lippincott Williams & Wilkins
a Wolters Kluwer business
Philadelphia • Baltimore • New York • London
Buenos Aires • Hong Kong • Sydney • Tokyo

Senior Acquisitions Editor: Elizabeth Nieginski
Senior Managing Editor: Helen Kogut
Editorial Assistant: Marivette Torres
Production Project Manager: Cynthia Rudy
Director of Nursing Production: Helen Ewan
Senior Managing Editor / Production: Erika Kors
Art Director: Joan Wendt
Manufacturing Coordinator: Karin Duffield
Production Services / Compositor: Schawk, Inc.
Printer: Donnelley–Crawfordsville

9 8 7 6 5 4 3 2

Library of Congress Cataloging-in-Publication Data
Teaching nursing: developing a student-centered learning environment /
[edited by] Lynne E. Young, Barbara L. Paterson.
p. ; cm.
Includes bibliographical references and index.
ISBN 13: 978-0-7817-5772-0
ISBN 10: 0-7817-5772-X (alk. paper)
1. Nursing—Study and teaching. 2. Student-centered learning. I. Young, Lynne E. II. Paterson, Barbara L.
[DNLM: 1. Education, Nursing. 2. Learning. 3. Teaching—methods. WY 18 T2523 2006]
RT71.T343 2006
610.73071—dc22

2005032488

LWW.com

To our students

Who teach us

How to teach

And to embrace learning

And our teachers

Who instilled in us

A passion

To learn

New ways

Of teaching.

"The academy is not paradise. But learning is a place where paradise can be created. The classroom, with all its limitations, remains a location of possibility. In that field of possibility we have the opportunity to labor for freedom, to demand of ourselves and our comrades an openness of mind and heart that allows us to face reality even as we begin to move beyond boundaries, to transgress."

hooks, b. (1994). *Teaching to transgress: Education as the practice of freedom* (p. 207). New York: Routledge.

Contributors

M. Kathleen Brewer, PhD, RN
Associate Professor
Georgia Baptist College of Nursing
Mercer University
Atlanta, Georgia
Chapter 14

Helen Brown, PhD (Cand.), MSN, RN
School of Nursing
University of Victoria
Victoria, British Columbia
Chapters 5 and 7

Anne Bruce, PhD, RN
Assistant Professor
School of Nursing
University of Victoria
Victoria, British Columbia
Chapter 19

W. Dean Care, EdD, MEd, BN
Associate Professor
Faculty of Nursing
University of Manitoba
Winnipeg, Manitoba
Chapters 6, 13, and 22

JoEllen Dattilo, PhD, RN
Associate Dean for Undergraduate Program
Georgia Baptist College of Nursing
Mercer University
Marietta, Georgia
Chapter 14

Rene A. Day, PhD, RN
Professor and Associate Dean, Executive and Partnership Development
Faculty of Nursing
University of Alberta
Edmonton, Alberta
Chapter 10

Gweneth Hartrick Doane, PhD
Associate Professor
School of Nursing
University of Victoria
Victoria, British Columbia
Chapter 5

David M. Gregory, PhD, MN, BScN, RN
Professor
Faculty of Nursing
University of Manitoba
Winnipeg, Manitoba
Chapter 22

Margaret Thorman Hartig, PhD, APRN, BC
Associate Professor and Chair
Department of Primary Care and Public Health
College of Nursing
University of Tennessee Health Science Center
Memphis, Tennessee
Chapters 6, 13, and 22

Susan Jacob, PhD, RN
Executive Associate Dean and Professor
Department of Primary Care and Public Health
College of Nursing
University of Tennessee Health Science Center
Memphis, Tennessee
Chapter 13

Carol Jillings, PhD, RN
Professor
School of Nursing
University of British Columbia
Vancouver, British Columbia
Chapters 17 and 21

Carol Lockhart, PhD, RN
Associate Professor
Department of Primary Care and Public Health
College of Nursing
University of Tennessee Health Science Center
Memphis, Tennessee
Chapter 13

Bruce Maxwell, PhD (Cand.), MA
Researcher and Lecturer
Institution for General Studies in Education
University of Münster
Münster, Germany
Chapters 1 and 2

Janice McCormick, PhD, BSN
Assistant Professor
School of Nursing
University of Victoria
Vancouver, British Columbia
Chapter 20

Victoria S. Murrell, PhD
Director of Instructional Technology
University of Tennessee
Memphis, Tennessee
Chapters 6, 13, and 22

Sarah Mynatt, EdD, MS
Center for Health Evaluation and Lifestyle Promotion (HELP)
College of Nursing
University of Tennessee Health Science Center
Memphis, Tennessee
Chapter 13

Florence Myrick, PhD, RN, CPsych
Professor and Associate Dean
Faculty of Graduate Studies and Research and Faculty of Nursing
University of Alberta
Edmonton, Alberta
Chapter 18

Marilyn H. Oermann, PhD, FAAN
Professor
College of Nursing
Wayne State University
Detroit, Michigan
Chapter 12

Kathy O'Flynn-Magee, MSN, RN
Lecturer
School of Nursing
University of British Columbia
Vancouver, British Columbia
Chapter 17

Daniel D. Pratt, PhD
Professor
Department of Educational Studies
University of British Columbia
Vancouver, British Columbia
Chapters 3 and 4

James M. Pruett, PhD, MS, BS
Professor and Assistant Dean for Student Affairs
University of Tennessee Health Science Center
Memphis, Tennessee
Chapter 13

Catherine Pugnaire-Gros, MSN, RN
Faculty Lecturer
School of Nursing
McGill University
Montreal, Quebec
Chapter 9

Mary Ellen Purkis, PhD, RN
Associate Professor and Dean
Human and Social Development
University of British Columbia
Victoria, British Columbia
Chapter 16

Patricia Rodney, PhD, RN
Associate Professor
School of Nursing
University of Victoria
Vancouver, British Columbia
Chapter 7

Cynthia K. Russell, PhD, APN
Associate Professor and Associate Dean for Distributive Programs
College of Nursing
University of Tennessee
Memphis, Tennessee
Chapters 6, 13, and 22

Cheryl Cummings Stegbauer, PhD
University of Tennessee Health Science Center
Memphis, Tennessee
Chapter 13

Janet L. Storch, PhD, RN
Professor
School of Nursing
University of Victoria
Victoria, British Columbia
Chapter 24

Carol Thompson, PhD, MSN
University of Tennessee Health Science Center
Veterans Administration
Memphis, Tennessee
Chapter 13

Sally Thorne, PhD, RN
Professor and Director
School of Nursing
University of British Columbia
Vancouver, British Columbia
Chapter 15

Colleen Varcoe, PhD, RN
Associate Professor
School of Nursing
University of British Columbia
Vancouver, British Columbia
Chapter 20

Beverly Williams, PhD, RN
Assistant Professor
Faculty of Nursing
University of Alberta
Edmonton, Alberta
Chapters 10 and 23

Angela Wolff, PhD (Cand.), MSN, RN
School of Nursing
University of British Columbia
Vancouver, British Columbia
Chapters 2 and 11

Olive J. Yonge, PhD, RN
Professor
Faculty of Nursing
University of Alberta
Edmonton, Alberta
Chapter 18

Reviewers

Gail Armstrong, ND, RN
Assistant Professor
University of Colorado Health Sciences Center
School of Nursing
Denver, Colorado

Michele A. Baqi-Aziz, MS, CNS, FNP, RN
Clinical Lecturer and Course Coordinator
University of Pennsylvania School of Nursing
Philadelphia, Pennsylvania

Mary D. Bondmass, PhD, RN
Assistant Professor
University of Nevada Las Vegas
Las Vegas, Nevada

Debbie Ciesielka, EdD, MSN, CRNP
Assistant Professor
Clarion University of Pennsylvania
Pittsburgh, Pennsylvania

Cynthia F. Corbett, PhD, RN
Associate Professor
Intercollegiate College of Nursing
Washington State University
Spokane, Washington

Catherine Dearman, PhD, RN
Chair, Maternal Child Health
Director, Nurse Educator Program
University of South Alabama
Mobile, Alabama

Jeffrey A. Eaton, PhD (Cand.), MS, MA, ARNP
Clinical Associate Professor
University of New Hampshire
Durham, New Hampshire

Joan Ellis, PhD, CNS, RNC
Chair, Graduate Nursing Programs
Our Lady of the Lake College
School of Nursing
Baton Rouge, Louisiana

Linda Foley, PhD, MSN, RN
Associate Chairperson and Professor
Nebraska Methodist College
Omaha, Nebraska

Carroll L. Iwasiw, EdD, MScN
Professor
University of Western Ontario
London, Ontario

Sarah B. Keating, EdD, RN, FAAN
Professor
University of Nevada Reno
Orvis School of Nursing
El Dorado Hills, California

Jane Koeckeritz, PhD, ANP, RN
Professor of Nursing
Technology Coach for College of Health and Human Sciences
University of Northern Colorado
Greeley, Colorado

Marylou K. McHugh, EdD, RN
Adjunct Faculty
Drexel and Temple Universities
Holland, Pennsylvania

Deana L. Molinari, PhD, CNS, RN
Assistant Professor
Washington State University
Spokane, Washington

Virginia Nehring, PhD, RN
Associate Professor
Wright State University
Dayton, Ohio

Rosemary Plank, PhD, RN
Academic Coordinator and Associate Clinical Professor, Physiological Nursing
University of California, San Francisco School of Nursing
San Francisco, California

Barbara Powell, PhD, RNC
Retired Adjunct Faculty
Delta State University
Cleveland, Mississippi

Kerry S. Risco, MSN, CRNP
Assistant Professor of Nursing
Slippery Rock University
Slippery Rock, Pennsylvania

Karen Moore Schaefer, DNSc, RN
Director, Undergraduate Program, College of Health Professions
Department of Nursing
Temple University
Philadelphia, Pennsylvania

Nancy Shirley, PhD, MSN, BS, RN
Associate Professor, Program Chair, LEAP (RN Completion Program)
Creighton University
Omaha, Nebraska

Carol K. Starling, PhD, RN
Clinical Assistant Professor
University of Kansas, School of Nursing
Kansas City, Kansas

Karen Gahan Tarnow, PhD, RN
Clinical Assistant Professor
University of Kansas
Kansas City, Kansas

Jean C. Toliver
Assistant Professor
Bowie State University
Reston, Virginia

Scott Weber, EdD, RN, FACHE, FHIMSS
Assistant Professor and Coordinator
Nursing Education Program
University of Pittsburgh
Pittsburgh, Pennsylvania

Yu Xu, PhD, MSN, MEd, BA
Associate Professor
University of Connecticut
Vernon, Connecticut

Foreword

This book, among the first in the 21st century to focus on the science and art of teaching, ushers in a new era through its forward-looking and innovative approaches. Provocatively presented, it provides a useful addition to the scholarly literature on higher education and teaching in nursing. Through reflections on their own personal experiences, the contributors to *Teaching Nursing: Developing a Student-Centered Learning Environment* share ways to empower students, thus modeling the goals of both student-centered learning and client-centered nursing practice. This knowledge helps faculty tackle the task of providing a multidiverse student population with the skills necessary to be creative, critical, and cooperative problem solvers.

For years nursing education has included as its major objectives the development of problem-solving skills, critical thinking, and group process facilitation. It has nevertheless continued to focus on the teacher, who determines what will be taught, with students considered as the passive recipients of information. Behaving as though students are "empty vessels" to fill or "blank slates" on which the teacher writes his or her knowledge, nursing educators concentrate more on the subject than on the students. Such a model leaves little or no room for students to critically appraise what is presented. By contrast, in student-centered teaching, the shift moves away from the content and the teacher toward the learner.

There has never been a more compelling reason for faculty to learn new ways to foster learning. The pace of change continues at an amazing rate. The promise of technology and its potential for changing the world is increasing at probably the most rapid rate we have ever known, both in our practice and our education. The reasons for changing the learning environment are crystal clear, and yet change in nursing education has been slow to arrive. Possibly the most powerful reason for this inertia in universities, in addition to the reward system, is that many faculty simply do not know how to go about making these changes. This book will help teachers make the conceptual shift toward being facilitators of learning who will engage students in relational, generative learning experiences. Through the use of examples and exercises, its authors, committed nurse educators and leaders, demonstrate a prototype of student-centered teaching. They confidently take the novice and experienced teacher by the hand and guide them toward understanding true student needs and building learning partnerships by providing the skillful interweaving of theory with practical advice on how to achieve the goals of student-centered learning. This provides nurse educators with a rare opportunity to trace the past, consider the present, and envision the future of student-centered teaching.

The issues that are discussed in *Teaching Nursing: Developing a Student-Centered Learning Environment* are much the same as they were several decades ago. We must redefine the activities that comprise learning and not continue to base so much of what transpires in the classroom on the outdated transmission model of teaching and learning. We must allow students to reconstruct information themselves through the processes of making sense of it. This is not an easy task, owing to the constraints in higher education and to the fact that teachers tend to teach as they were taught. The authors of this text show the way for faculty who are willing to give up the control of being keepers of knowledge to instead foster an environment of trust and reward by being facilitators and coaches for learning. This is teaching scholarship at its best, and it will make a significant difference in nursing education.

Rheba de Tornyay, EdD, FAAN
Dean & Professor Emeritus, School of Nursing
University of Washington, Seattle
Editor Emeritus, *Journal of Nursing Education*

Preface

As the editors of *Teaching Nursing: Developing a Student-Centered Learning Environment,* we had different reasons for believing in the need for a book like this one. Lynne entered the academy to study nursing at the baccalaureate level after several years of professional practice. She was shocked that the academy and its practitioners, in pursuit of "teaching," did not draw on and develop the practical knowledge base of those like her—using dialogue about learning and nursing and the relationship between the two as a resource to further thinking about nursing. Such a process, she reasoned at the time, had potential to develop and deepen the intellects of not only the students but also of the nursing academics. Therein lay the seeds of her curiosity about, and commitment to, student-centered learning. Through scholarship aimed at clarifying health-promoting nursing practice, Lynne came to appreciate the salience of client-centeredness in nursing and concomitantly appreciated the potential that student-centered teaching held to teach students the core principles of client-centered care through modeling. Thus, Lynne was convinced that current and future nurse educators could benefit from a state-of-the art text about this important topic.

Barbara's passion for student-centered teaching arose when she discovered in her work as an administrator of a tertiary care hospital and in her doctoral research about clinical teaching that the traditional teacher-centered approaches resulted in graduates who learned how to be students more than they learned how to respond creatively to the ever changing needs of patients and to the complex and highly political world of nursing practice. She questioned whether students who had been taught with teacher-centered approaches would ever be truly equipped to nurse in a patient-centered and family-centered way. She saw the incorporation of student-centered teaching in nursing education as an effective alternate. Recently Barbara completed a 3-year stint as an in-house scholar in a tertiary care hospital medical unit. There, through a partnership process, Barbara and the nursing staff developed a creative, enthusiastic, and welcoming nursing team who provided competent and compassionate care to patients and families and embraced both learning and learners. This experience convinced her that student-centered teaching is not only beneficial to nursing students, but it is crucial to the growth and continued development of nurses, teachers, and the profession.

As converts to this way of teaching, we each sought to learn how to teach as student-centered nurse educators. We read the relevant literature. We asked colleagues.

We went to scholarly conferences that promised to enlighten us. What we learned over the years was that many nurse educators were successfully teaching in a student-centered way, but they were not necessarily sharing what they did or what they had learned with others.

This book represents our attempt to bring together expert nurse educators to contribute to the current knowledge about student-centered teaching in nursing education, while at the same time identifying the gaps and contradictions in this body of knowledge and suggesting avenues for future discussion and study. It corresponds to the history of student-centered teaching as an important social movement in nursing education. For several years, individual educators have been integrating student-centered teaching while working in institutions that do not effectively support or reward such teaching. It is time now to move beyond functioning as individuals who are isolated from each other. We need to publicly share our approaches and challenges in student-centered teaching so that we may receive feedback and critique, and so that we can sustain the vision of the student-centered teaching movement. This book enables the achievement of such a goal.

Featured in each chapter are opening scenarios, learning activities, and resources for educators.

- **Opening Scenarios:** Each chapter begins with a story of a lived experience of the chapter author that is designed to draw the learner into the world of the author in a way that bridges the theory of teaching nursing with the practice of teaching nursing.
- **Learning Activities**, found at the end of each chapter, are designed to engage students in exercises that foster further learning about the main ideas presented in each chapter. Collectively, the learning activities challenge students to apply a range of ways of knowing in their learning; for example, theoretical, empirical, esthetic, affective, and critical knowing.
- **Resources for Educators** are presented in two subsections: *Planning the Teaching/Learning Experience* and *Evaluating the Teaching/Learning Experience.* Each subsection addresses one or more of the following topics:

  Planning the Teaching/Learning Experience

  Questions to Support a Thoughtful Reading

  Questions in this subsection are designed to challenge readers to consider the ideas presented in the chapter in light of the readers' experiences and beliefs.

  Instructions for Educators

  Instructions in this subsection provide guidance for incorporating the main ideas presented in the chapter into teaching practice.

  Tips for Developing a Student-Centered Learning Environment

  In this subsection, authors provide readers with practical ideas for fostering student-centered learning.

Evaluating the Teaching/Learning Experience

Questions to Elicit Feedback From Students on Their Learning

Evaluating students' learning by eliciting feedback from them relative to the goals of the teaching/learning session allows educators to assess the effectiveness of the educational process. In this subsection, questions that have potential to draw out learners' understanding of the main ideas of the chapter are offered.

Reflective Questions for the Educator

Through reflection, one develops self-knowledge. Thus, in this subsection, we offer questions to prompt educators' reflections on their teaching to inspire a value for self-development.

Sample Evaluation Strategies and Tools

Strategies and tools that can be used by educators for evaluating learning are offered in this subsection.

In this book, we hope to entice you to challenge the "traditional" in nursing education. To that end, we provide you with theoretical grounding, ideas for implementation, and arguments about some arising issues. We present student-centered teaching as paradoxical—in order for you to embrace the power of student-centered teaching, you must be prepared to give up the power that is traditionally allocated to teachers. If you are new to the notion of student-centered teaching and engage the chapters of this book, you will question at least some of your assumptions about teaching and learning, as well as the traditional socialization to independence and autonomy as a teacher. Although this will be assuredly difficult at times, we promise that it will also prove to be extremely liberating. We invite you to enter into a way of teaching that not only yields student achievement but will draw you into a community of scholarship in which both teacher and student thrive because of the learning and interdependence they share. If you are well-versed in the tenets of student-centered teaching, you will find that the book will provoke you to new insights and questions about teaching in this way. You will find solace and support in your commitment to student-centered teaching, as well.

Whether you are new to student-centered teaching or familiar with it, we hope that you become as committed as we are to centering your teaching on the needs, gifts, and interests of students. We assure you that if you have the courage to invite students to center their learning on their abilities, needs, goals, experience, and interests, both you and the students you learn with will experience many blessings.

Lynne E. Young
Barbara L. Paterson

Acknowledgments

We acknowledge Dr. Rheba de Tornyay for writing the Foreword to this book. Dr. de Tornyay is a nurse, educator, and person we greatly admire for her lifetime of contributions to advancing nursing in general and nursing education in particular. Dr. de Tornyay lives the values essential to building a vibrant nursing community—authenticity, commitment to excellence, and humility—and in that we find Dr. Rheba de Tornyay a most inspiring person.

We also acknowledge the support and contributions of the chapter authors and the publisher, particularly Helen Kogut. Her continued patience and her conviction that this book was significant to nursing education have made the editing of the book a rewarding experience.

Finally, we acknowledge the many students and teachers in our experience as nurse educators who challenged and engaged us by the questions they raised and the examples they modeled. They sometimes caused us to feel uncomfortable—even at times irritated—but they, more than any others, have refined and shaped our understanding of student-centered teaching, including the gaps and the areas of confusion that exist in the field. Our learning from what they taught us convinced us that a book such as this was critically important to our profession and to nurse educators in general. We thank you.

LEY
BLP

Contents

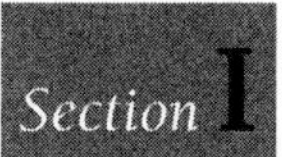

Section I TEACHING NURSING: THEORIES AND CONCEPTS, 1

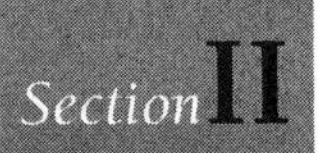

METHODS AND APPROACHES TO STUDENT-CENTERED LEARNING IN NURSING, 139

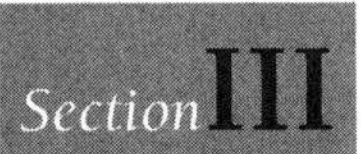

CONSTRUCTING NURSING CURRICULA: CHALLENGES AND ISSUES, 323

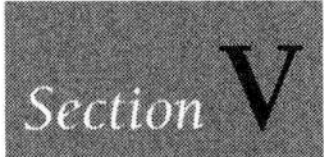

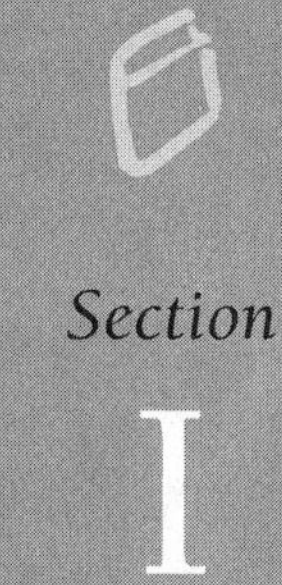

Section

I

TEACHING NURSING: THEORIES AND CONCEPTS

Chapter 1

Student-Centered Teaching in Nursing: From Rote to Active Learning

Lynne E. Young
Bruce Maxwell

As the instructor for upper level baccalaureate students, I[1] designed a case analysis learning activity that was student centered. The goal of the case was for students to identify knowledge gaps and address them while practicing problem solving, group process, and lifelong learning skills. A further goal was to provide students with an opportunity to practice group facilitation skills. Students were group members for four cases and a group facilitator for one case. In the spirit of student-centered learning, students submitted a self-assessment of their performance as group facilitator after the completion of this assignment.

In her self-assessment, one student wrote: "During previous case story analyses in which I was a participant, the facilitator provided group members with articles to use to help them with their learning issues. In preparing for my assignment as group facilitator, I reflected on this and decided that I would not provide research articles to my group members for several reasons. First, I realized that it would be nearly impossible to get information on every possible learning issue embedded in the case story. Instead, I decided, it would be much more beneficial to spend some time ensuring that everyone felt comfortable obtaining the information they needed. I spent time reviewing how to access library and Internet resources so that I could share this information with group participants. Then, I made sure that every group member had my phone number and e-mail address if they needed help finding resources for their learning issues between classes. In retrospect, I am glad that I did not hand out articles which I had researched in advance as I did not find this approach conducive to the facilitation of my learning when I was in the role of group member."—*Julie Ward*

After reading Julie's self-assessment, it struck me that Julie reflected on not only how she developed as a group facilitator but also how she became more aware of her preferred style of learning through this activity.

[1] The first-person "I" in this section is that of author Lynne Young.

INTENT

Nursing education that is student-centered is consistent with main philosophical tenets of client-centered nursing practice. Student-centered teaching designed to develop cutting-edge professional skills in students, such as problem solving, group process and facilitation, and lifelong learning skills, while engaging students in a relational, generative process model is what nurse educators hold to be essential for client-centered nursing practice. This chapter explicates the links between student-centered teaching and client-centered nursing. Then because the constructivist view of learning is an important overarching worldview that underpins conceptual tools and strategies of **student-centered learning**, the idea of constructivism is introduced and builds a theoretical foundation for what follows in subsequent chapters. To this end, selected writings of John Locke, Immanuel Kant, Jean Piaget, and John Dewey are presented as background to the notion of constructivist views on learning. Constructivism informs a number of theoretical perspectives on teaching and learning with two main theories in this genre highlighted, cognitive constructivism and social constructivism. Further, since the biomedical sciences are so important in the world in which nurses practice, we discuss tensions arising between the constructivist view and empiricism, particularly as this relates to the highly critical stance taken by constructivism toward natural sciences' claim to objectivity. This chapter a provides theoretical framework for the chapters that follow.

OVERVIEW

INTRODUCTION

Nursing education is dominated by theories, methods, and systems that are generally adopted and applied with little attention to bridging the gaps between nursing education, nursing practice, and knowledge development. Traditionally, educators in institutes of higher learning have assumed an active role of "sage-on-the-stage," with students assuming the complementary role of passive learner, "soaking up" the wisdom of the sage. Currently, educators in professional practice schools such as education, law, business, medicine, and nursing question the appropriateness of a passive role for learners for a number of reasons (Antepohl & Herzig, 1999; Barnes, Christensen, & Hansen, 1994; Rideout, 2001; Wasserman, 1996; Williams, 1992). Such traditional approaches tend to elicit rote learning, the product of which may soon be forgotten or outdated in this world of rapidly changing information (Barrows, 1994). Further, fostering rote learning is a missed opportunity for developing students' capacities for professional problem solving and lifelong learning. Thus, educators of professionals in a wide range of disciplines are shifting the center of teaching from the teacher to the student by adopting pedagogies and androgogies that bear labels such as **student-directed learning**, **process-oriented learning**, **experiential learning**, **situated learning**, **learning collaboratory**, **narrative pedagogy**, and **relational pedagogy**. What is common to these approaches is that educators actively engage learners; this in contrast to conventional modes of teaching in which the teacher is the content expert who controls the learning experience using a sage-on–the-stage approach. Active engagement of learners goes some way toward fostering: lifelong learning, problem solving, **critical thinking**, group process skills, creativity, **information literacy**, student success, and empowerment, depending on the model (Barrows; Bevis & Watson, 1989; Diekelmann, 2001; O'Shea, 2003; Knowles, 1975; McLellan, 1995). Approaches such as these are based on the tenets of constructivism in which learning is assumed to be best facilitated by providing learners with opportunities to *construct* knowledge in the context of social environments, not simply facilitating them to *obtain* it (Brooks & Brooks, 1993).

What Is Student-Centered Teaching?

Student-centered teaching is an approach to teaching that contrasts with the traditional content-centered and teacher-centered approaches that most of us experienced as students. Content-centered teaching focuses on mastery of specific material designated by the curriculum that is implemented by the instructor. In such teaching, there is little or no flexibility to shape the content to the needs of the learners or to the styles of the teachers and learners. Such an approach is closely aligned with instructor-centered teaching in which the teacher is the expert on the content and the delivery method. Here it is the teacher who determines what will be taught with students as passive recipients of information. The students are "empty vessels" to fill or "blank slates" upon which the teacher writes his or her knowledge. In such models, there is often little or no room for students to critically appraise what is presented. By contrast, in student-centered teaching, the shift moves away from the content and the teacher to the learner. The teacher asks: Who are the learners? What do they bring to the learning situation? How might their learning needs be met? How might their learning styles be accommodated? This does not mean that the teacher must meet everyone's needs; rather, the boundaries of the content and modes of teaching expand to better accommodate learners (Piccinin, 1997).

Why Student-Centered Teaching in Nursing?

In nursing, a shift to a student-centered approach to teaching not only provides nurse educators with a new vision for teaching, but also parallels a paradigm shift in nursing practice from nurse-centered to client-centered nursing practice (Bevis & Watson, 1989; Engebretson & Littleton, 2001). In client-centered nursing, the nurse begins by understanding the lived experience of the client or patient rather than with the nurses' understanding; the nurse collaborates with the patient or client rather than "doing for" or "doing to" the patient (Young, 2002). Similarly, in student-centered teaching,[2] the educator begins with the experience of the student and together they build knowledge, skills, and competencies for professional practice (Bergum, 2003; Bevis & Watson; Demarco, Hayward, & Lynch, 2002; Doane, 2002; Nehls, 1995). Nurse educators who embrace student-centered teaching not only prepare student nurses with the substantive knowledge necessary for competent practice, but also create an environment in which students learn to think critically, practice reflectively, work effectively in groups, and access and use new information to support their practice, while modeling respect for meanings of lived experiences, learning, and collaborative processes (Bevis & Watson; Diekelmann, 2001; Johns, 2002). However, such a shift in what has been traditionally revered in nursing education creates tensions and challenges such as: students' resistance to new methods, classroom management issues, curriculum issues, evaluation quandaries and dilemmas, time constraints, role confusion, and challenges and resistance from traditional colleagues (Biley, 1999; Diekelmann, 2001; Hewitt-Taylor, 2001; Knowlton & Sharp, 2003; Woods, 1994). If the nurse educator is not the sage-on-the-stage, what is he or she? If he or she is not lecturing, is he or she teaching?

Nursing, as we envision it, is a dynamic, interpersonal, generative, and caring practice (Bergum, 2003; Bevis & Watson, 1989; Young, 2002). To be consistent with this view of nursing, teaching nursing should be a relational, generative practice that occurs formally and informally: between the learner and the educator; the learner and the patient or client; the learner and colleagues; the learner and peers; and the learner and professionals from other disciplines (Bevis & Watson). Such learning occurs in diverse settings including the classroom, lab, and clinical areas; that is, hospitals as well as community sites. Teaching nursing requires facilitating a thoughtful engagement between the learner and learning materials to ensure that learners acquire the skills and knowledge for a relational practice that often occurs in highly scientific, technological, and political environments that are characterized by rapidly changing, complex knowledge bases and organizational systems, and often disturbing, and sometimes vicious, compe-

[2] In this book we use the term *student-centered* teaching to refer to approaches to teaching that actively engage the learner. Such approaches encompass self-directed learning, process-oriented learning, and experiential learning to name a few. Our purpose in selecting the term student-centered as an overriding qualifier for active approaches to teaching best fits with the language of client-centeredness of nursing, an approach to nursing that we hold is foundational to health-promoting nursing practice.

tition for resources (Diekelmann, 2001; Koerner, 2003; O'Shea, 2003; Rodney, et al., 2002). Such a practice environment requires the nurse to have sophisticated interpersonal, problem solving, group process, communication, clinical and moral decision making, caring, and select technical skills as well as knowledge grounded in a range of disciplines including nursing, the biomedical and related sciences, social and psychological sciences, critical perspectives, ethics, and health care organization.

Facilitating learners' acquisition of this broad range of skills and knowledge is not easy to design or execute. Teaching nursing in such a way calls nurse educators to move from the comfortable position of "teaching the way we were taught" to the "edge of the safe zone" where students acquire disciplinary knowledge while developing sophisticated interpersonal, caring, political, interpretive, and technical skills. An important first step is for nurse educators to identify new approaches to teaching practice. We suggest that student-centered teaching has potential to support such a shift while educating knowledgeable, personable, creative, ethical, and compassionate nurses who live what they learn.

Relationship Between Student-Centered Teaching and Teaching Nursing

Student-centered teaching has a number of features that fit well with how nursing is envisioned in this part of the 21st century, and nurse educators play a vital role in preparing students for the "new nursing" (Morris & Turnbull, 2004; O'Shea, 2003). First, student-centered teaching is conceptually aligned with client-centered or patient-centered nursing, both approaches that are relational and generative. Nurses who practice client-centered care begin with respect for the lived experience of the patient or client (Doane, 2002; Hardy, Garbett, Titchen, & Manley, 2002; Young, 2002); the nurse educator practicing student-centered teaching begins with the experience of the learners. Second, student-centered teaching fosters professionalism by developing students' capacities for lifelong learning which is envisioned as the ongoing acquisition of knowledge and skills necessary for practice as a professional (Candy, 1991; Jerlock, Falk, & Severinson, 2003; Koerner, 2003). In the past two decades information across practice disciplines, including nursing, has exploded beyond what is imaginable. Thus, knowledge for practice expands exponentially such that a fact that is learned in nursing school has an extremely short half-life. Skills for lifelong learning include the capacities for problem solving, reflection, decision making, use of technology, information literacy, and the ability to use deductive and inductive reasoning (Jacobs, Rosenfeld, & Haber, 2003; Jerlock, et al., 2003; Johns, 2002). Third, student-centered teaching fosters professional responsibility shifting the center of the evaluation of learning from the teacher to the learner, a process that supports the development of students' capacities for competence by fostering enhanced self-awareness through reflection (Bandura, 1986; Lepp, Zorn, Duffy, & Dickson, 2003). Finally, most student-centered approaches provide opportunities for students to learn from each other, processes that support and underscore the centrality of colearning in nursing practice (MacIntosh, MacKay, Mallet-Boucher, & Wiggins, 2002).

Student-centered teaching interpreted literally, however, may not be successful for a variety of reasons. Students may come to learning experiences expecting nurse educators to teach in traditional ways (MacIntosh, et al., 2003). Such students may experience dissonance and distress when asked to be active rather than passive learners. For example, one educator recounts a situation in which foreign students were enrolled in a student-centered curriculum and they launched a formal complaint arguing that since they had paid high tuition fees, why did the work of learning fall to them and not to the teachers? Further, some students' learning styles may not be well suited to the self-assessments or group work central to student-centered classrooms. Regarding self-assessments, students who are linear concrete thinkers may have difficulty sorting out what they know, from what they do not know, about a particular topic making the self-assessment process an individual-level barrier to student-centered learning. Regarding learning during group work, students who perceive learning to best occur as an individual-level enterprise are not well positioned to value colearning in groups and may therefore be disruptive or nonparticipants during group work.

Student-centered learning is a break from the traditions of teaching in institutions of higher learning and therefore poses challenges. However, its possibilities for bridging the gaps between education, practice, and knowledge development in professional schools such as nursing are promising. Locating teaching within the constructivist view opens possibilities for nursing education to close these gaps by transforming nursing education from a teacher-centered activity to a learner-centered activity. Thus, we introduce the constructivist view of learning in the following sections.

CONSTRUCTIVISM: A THEORETICAL GUIDE FOR NURSE EDUCATORS

Constructivism is a theoretical position that holds the view that knowledge is socially constructed, which is a position that is gaining favor among educators in many corners of the world and in a variety of disciplines. However, educators in all fields eventually come to learn that teaching fads come and go. Given this, adopting a position of cautious conservatism with regards to proposals for new pedagogies, in particular when they seem to be a radical departure from accepted practice, is certainly a responsible thing to do. For some, adopting a student-centered pedagogical orientation would constitute a discontinuity in their teaching practice. Further, many experienced educators could point to cases of injudicious learning activities and approaches adopted in the name of student-centered teaching. The application of a theory is sometimes just as difficult as developing it and as such, it is important not to judge a general theory on the basis of the particular ways in which it is applied. With this in mind, this section aims at no more than to convince the reader of the soundness of the broad theoretical underpinning of student-centered learning—a theory of learning known as "constructivism."

Constructivism, as it will be understood here, refers to a descriptive theory of the process of learning based on widely uncontroversial tenets of developmental psychology to teaching practice (Alexander & Murphy, 1998).[3] In contrast with the traditional **transmission model of learning**, which holds that whatever knowledge students bring

[3] Constructivism shares several components with social learning theory and self-efficacy (Bandura, 1986).

to a learning situation has little or no direct relevance to the learning process, the constructivist model of learning regards students' prior knowledge as foundational to the learning process. Constructivism holds that learning is a process of meaning making or knowledge building in which learners integrate new knowledge into a pre-existing network of understanding. The main weakness of the traditional model of teaching, then, is that it seems to work against the way students actually learn rather than with it. If the constructivist theory of learning is correct, teaching strategies will be more successful if they shift the focus of teaching from the material to be taught to the *relationship* between that material and what students already know. In more specific terms, constructivist teaching is not as much a matter of straightforwardly introducing students to new information and concepts as it is of placing students in learning situations that raise a challenge to their current understandings. This way, it is hoped, students will learn—that is, they will become actively engaged in the adjustment of, addition to, and straightening out of their conceptions of the way the world is. The challenge for the educator is how to best use these structural relationships to the profit of student learning in day-to-day teaching. The following section provides a sketch of the conceptual foundations of constructivism in support of this goal; nurse educators who understand the philosophical and theoretical underpinnings of the constructivist view of learning are better placed to not only apply it faithfully in their own teaching but also to assess whether a particular pedagogical technique, device, or approach which claims legitimacy in virtue of being constructivist or progressive is indeed consistent with the underlying principles of this general pedagogical orientation.

Foundational Thought of Constructivist Views

Contemporary constructivism in education—indeed contemporary developmental psychology as a whole—goes back to the Enlightenment philosopher **Immanuel Kant**. *Critique of Pure Reason* was Kant's (1929) main work, and it hinged on one central insight: all meaningful experience, or "understanding" as he called it, was the result of interaction between the world and certain innate structures of the mind. For anyone with even the most cursory acquaintance with cognitive psychology, this idea will seem trivial but at the end of the 18th century it was nothing short of revolutionary. What made it so important was that it completely overturned the dominant and common sense view that our meaningful perceptions of the world, even the most basic among them, could be rightly considered to derive their meaning from the actual characteristics of the world as it is understood independently of the perceiver. This view is most often referred to as **empiricism**. Thus, Kant helped to develop the idea that learning was an interactive meaning-making process.

In the 18th century, empiricism provided the generally accepted answer to the main question of **epistemology**—namely, where does knowledge come from? The English philosopher, **John Locke**, was at the time (and remains today) its most pre-eminent proponent. Locke is best known for his description of the mind as a blank slate or ***tabula rasa***. What this metaphor was principally meant to capture was Locke's idea that all ideas that human beings have, even their most abstract ideas, are ultimately derived from sense experience. Hence, before a person begins to accumulate ideas through sense experience—at birth—the mind is blank or empty. To get a sense of what this means, take the idea of a snowball. Locke analyzed the process of coming to have an idea of a thing into two steps. First, the perceiver receives through the senses what Locke called "simple ideas"—ideas like white, hard, cold, and round. Next, these simple ideas are combined or assembled in the mind to form "complex ideas." The idea of snowball, then, is a sort of composition of the simple conceptual elements.

The main weakness that Kant saw in the empiricist model of epistemology is quite simple. According to Locke's (1959) empiricism, the simple properties of objects are, for all intents and purposes, identical to the simple ideas of those properties reflected in the mind. Kant viewed Locke's idea that the mind passively receives simple ideas as implausible. Unless the mind actively imposed some kind of order on raw sense experience, Kant argued, experience would be a meaningless perceptive jumble. In order to give substance to this idea, Kant posited that the mind is hard-wired with certain innate structures that play an indispensable role in creating our ideas of the world. He labelled these capacities the **categories**, and they included such concepts as quantity, absence, and existence.[4] As Kant saw it, the ordinary properties objects have—indeed, the perception of them as existing in relation to a spatiotemporal framework—are not mind-independent properties of the world we discover. Instead, we perceive these properties only because our minds are so structured as to impose a framework for understanding them.

Cognitive Constructivism

Jumping ahead almost two centuries, it was the Swiss psychologist **Jean Piaget** who refined Kant's important insights into the basic shape of contemporary cognitive constructivism. Kant rejected empiricism insofar as he held that experience emerges from the interaction of certain innate structures of the mind with experience of the world. For Piaget, however, Kant's criticism of empiricism did not go far enough. Kant considered the categories to be cognitive structures that were both static and given from birth. In other words, there is no qualitative difference between the mental processes of adults and children; children know less than adults do only because they have less accumulated experience. As Piaget tried to show in his seminal research on cognitive development, children's cognitive capacities become increasingly differentiated as they mature following a set sequence of developmental stages. For example, the acquisition of the idea of class inclusion is acquired between the ages of about 2 and 6, a competency Piaget considered to be representative of operational (i.e., logical or abstract) thought. A preoperational child, if asked "Are there more people than girls or girls than people," he or she will characteristically respond that there is the same number of people as there are girls because he or she focuses on the most salient characteristic of the situation—namely, personhood. But he or she fails to consider the hierarchical aspect of the problem. The principal way in which Piaget's work improved Kant's was to show that the basic conceptual

[4]See Immanuel Kant's *Critique of Pure Reason*, esp. Transcendental Doctrine of Elements, First Part and First Division, Book I, Chapter 1, Section 3.

tools with which human beings come to understand the world are not fixed and given at birth but develop in early childhood through interaction with problems (Piaget, 1970, 1971a, & 1971b). Piaget's own term of choice for this theory was "genetic epistemology" but the idea is more commonly known as constructivism.[5] Although the fine print of constructivism is rife with controversy and of a highly technical nature, the basic principles of constructivism as are today not a subject of dispute in cognitive psychology. The critical question from an educator's point of view, then, is not *whether* learning is a constructive activity but rather, *if* learning is a constructive process then what, if anything, does this mean for the development of effective teaching practices?

Before Piaget's most influential works were published in the 1970s, the idea that classroom learning can be improved by getting students to be more actively engaged in their own learning had been in the air for some time. It was a staple of the **liberal progressive movement** of the late 19th and early 20th centuries[6] and the advantages of more active learning—and the disadvantages of the formalism, verbalism, and authoritarianism of traditional schooling—were also themes in the work of the influential American philosopher of education **John Dewey**.[7] Be that as it may, inspired by Piaget a distinction between **developmental** and **rote** learning emerged in educational circles. Many educators associate constructivist or developmental methods with learning that is "active and making a lasting difference in how students approach problems and new situations" and rote learning and teaching that follows the traditional transmission model with learning that is "passive, temporary, and useless for further learning" (Noddings, 1998, p. 115). However, such a characterization of the constructivist model is really of little help in trying to determine what cognitive constructivism means for teaching. Simply equating constructivist methods with active, solid, and lasting learning and traditional methods with passive, temporary, and superficial learning contains a conceptual error that obscures what, from a constructivist point of view, would be the best reasons for rejecting the traditional model. If *all* learning is active, as constructivism holds it is, then the learning that does occur in a rote learning situation is clearly active too. Conversely, activity in a learning setting in and of itself is of course no guarantee that learning will occur at all, much less solid and lasting learning. If the transmission model of teaching is a poor one, it is not first and foremost because it leads to ersatz understanding, but it tends to lead to ersatz understanding because it is ill-suited to the way human beings actually learn. Thus, in order to find out what constructivism means for pedagogy, we need to ask what kind of learning situations are propitious to developmental (or generative) learning and how these learning situations differ from traditional ones. For our purposes, suffice it to make a few careful generalizations about how constructivism gives the lie to some of the central suppositions of the traditional transmission model of pedagogy and what constructivism suggests in terms of alternative approaches.

The transmission model of teaching is often criticized for presenting new material to students as if it were assimilable in isolation from students' existing knowledge. New

[5] It is also sometimes referred to as "interactionism."

[6] See Vadeboncoeur, 1997, pp. 18–19. See also Gutek (1997) on Progressivism in *Philosophical and Ideological Perspectives on Education* (2nd ed.).

[7] See Dewey's central educational text, *Democracy and Education* (1916).

knowledge and understanding, constructivism claims, is not cognitively isolated but exists in relation to, and is built on, a pre-existing knowledge base. The structures or links that learners build between their prior understandings and new experiences and information take a variety of forms. These include, but are not limited to, adding to, modifying, or reorganizing existing knowledge or skills. The triggering mechanism of learning, as both Piaget and Dewey argue, is the human tendency to be ill at ease with contradictions and inconsistencies in knowledge structures. As Piaget believed, the development of all knowledge consists in the attempt to resolve such conflicts via a process he called "equilibration." Equilibration consists of two complementary elements, **assimilation and accommodation**. Assimilation involves making sense of some new information in terms of an existing body of knowledge—for example, bringing the previously unknown concept of metatarsus, under the higher level concept of bone. Accommodation, for its part, involves modifying an existing concept in order to accommodate a new inconsistent example as, for instance, when studying one-celled organisms one learns that it is the way an organism metabolizes that determines whether an organism is a plant or animal not having or lacking roots, stems, and leafy structures.

From the Piagetan perspective, then, the first and most general challenge of constructivist teaching is to trigger the equilibration process by creating an atmosphere that challenges students' concepts and ways of thinking. Second, and more specifically, constructivist education should engage students in tasks that lead to a reorganization of their existing cognitive maps (Richardson, 1997). These general guidelines for how to translate cognitive constructivism into teaching practice can be interpreted in a variety of ways. The constructivist educator could resort to such techniques as concept mapping, thematic organization, or categorizing in order to connect new material with prior understandings and help students build a conceptual framework in which to locate new material. Another approach that constructivism seems to entail is the adoption of a dialectic approach to problem solving. As the students attempt to find a solution to the problem, the teacher prompts them to articulate their strategy and follows up with challenges, variations on the problem, questions about the appropriateness of the methods the students have chosen to solve it, and other forms of questioning that dig deeply into students' beliefs. In this way, the educator creates an atmosphere in which those beliefs may be examined.[8]

Problem-based learning, the favored pedagogical method of John Dewey, seems also to be consistent with constructivist principles. As Dewey argued, through confronting students with meaningful real life problems, those students are likely to encounter in their future professional lives or which affect them as members of a given community, the development of creative intelligence is fostered (Dewey, 1916, 1963/1938). Further, by favoring the development of the capacity to solve problems rather than the mastery of solutions to existing problems, such activities are indispensable to education for rapidly changing professional contexts. In many cases, the problems that future professionals will face years or decades further on in their careers do not exist. In others, they are even inconceivable from a contemporary viewpoint.

[8] See discussions of the application of cognitive constructivism to classroom practices in Davis, Mather, & Noddings (1990) and Richardson (1997).

A second but related principal criticism of the traditional model of teaching stems from the passive metaphors that it inspires. The notion that education aims to shape, mold, make, or model students is inconsistent with the constructivist claim that the creation of links between prior and new understandings that characterizes learning is not something that can be done to a student by a teacher (or anyone else for that matter) but must be done by the student himself or herself. This "meaning-making process," as Richardson (1997, p. 5) puts it, can be facilitated through **collaborative learning**, or the direct involvement of students in the learning process by engaging students in such activities as researching course material and working together with the instructor. Box 1.1 presents an example of one such activity.

Whichever way the aim of promoting interaction between students' prior and new understandings is pursued, constructivism seeks to replace the traditional passive imagery with a set of guiding metaphors that more accurately express the nature of the

BOX 1.1 COLLABORATIVE LEARNING

While teaching upper level nursing students in both classroom and clinical settings, an opportunity for collaborative learning surfaced during a clinical visit. A student told me about a man in her care who on Day 1 following surgery reported pain levels of 8 that were not responding to treatment. The student, her preceptor, and I explored possible courses of action. When I spoke with the student the next day, she reported that the patient was much more comfortable on Day 2 in response to a newly developed care plan. Then, to my surprise and delight, the student offered to present this challenging case to students in my theory class. Together, we took the bare bones of the case and wrote a case story that we subsequently used in a case story analysis exercise. Through this process, it was not only Jane and the students who learned something about system-level influences on pain management, but I was inspired to begin a collaborative process with nurse leaders in our community to address system-level influences on pain management. As a constructivist educator, I wonder if student-centered approaches such as this contribute to the development of learning communities.

MIKE'S PAINFUL JOURNEY: JANE'S STORY

It was my first day on the neuro unit after being in school for over a year. I certainly learned something about how system-level influences contribute to patient suffering this first shift.

Mike was assigned to George, my preceptor, and me. Mike was a 42-year-old lute maker who suffered from pain and numbness in his left arm for a prolonged period of time. Against his doctor's advice he drove with his partner Glenn to a distant city for a lute makers' conference. Upon returning home he presented to emergency with excruciating pain in his left shoulder and arm. He was booked for surgery and came to the unit following a discectomy at the C5/6 level.

We were caring for Mike (and his partner) postoperatively on Day 1. Our pain assessment indicated that his pain level was 8. He was on Morphine IV 1mg/hr and his mobility orders were confusing. Should he be supine or up? Glenn was livid that the pain was still a problem as they had been reassured that the surgery would take away the pain . . . and now this. George asked me to spend time with Glenn. Glenn and Mike insisted that Mike be allowed to take his own pain medication which I learned was cyclobenzaprine.

education. Metaphors such as education as "growth" (Dewey) and "evolution" (Piaget) shift the source of the changes that occur in the learner during the education process from the teacher to the learner himself or herself and suggest that the proper role of the educator is not primarily that of transmitting of knowledge but rather that of creating environments propitious to students' growth, development, and evolution.[9]

Cognitive constructivism, as we have seen, maintains that learning is best understood as a process of individual meaning making or knowledge building. The transmission model, which is generally held to suppose that the understanding—or perhaps better put, the *lack* of understanding—that students bring to a learning situation is precisely what is pushed out of the way or replaced when learning occurs, cognitive constructivism views prior knowledge as foundational to learning. And this is because the constructivist's view is that learners actively integrate new knowledge into a pre-existing network of understanding. Thus, learning is best construed not as a matter of supplanting the understandings that students bring to the classroom with new ones, as much as it is of adjusting, adding to, straightening out, or even completely reconstructing them. The typical strategy of the constructivist teacher is to place students in situations in which they undergo a certain degree of cognitive conflict or dissonance with the hope, of course, that students will become engaged in the activity of restructuring their own cognitive maps.

Social Constructivism

As is the case with all highly influential theories, cognitive or strict Piagetan constructivism is the subject of enormous critical attention ranging from outright rejection to conditional acceptance. The objection most often raised to it from among educational thinkers who are generally in concurrence with Piagetan constructivism is that it is excessively individualistic. Concentrating, as it does, on indicators of development in individuals' behavior and cognitive processes, it is claimed, Piagetan constructivism overlooks the inexorable social dimensions of learning. The broad theoretical approach that rejects individual-oriented cognitive constructivism yet remains focused on the psychological aspects of learning is generally referred to as **social constructivism** or sociocognitive constructivism. Although many forms of sociocognitive constructivists have been developed,[10] what social constructivist approaches tend to have in common is the influence of interpretations of the work of the Russian psychologist, **L. S. Vygotsky**. For our purposes, this section will briefly examine what is generally held to be the main difference between the work of Vygotsky and Piaget and then consider the lesson that an educator might draw from the Piaget–Vygotsky antinomy.

Like Piaget, Vygotsky used empirical research to understand human cognitive development. But whereas Piaget was led to the conclusion that knowledge is constructed through individual interaction with the world—according to Piaget, the stages of devel-

---

[9] Recommended texts on the application of constructivist principles in classroom teaching: Davis, Mather, & Noddings (1990), Steffe & Thompson (2000), Brooks & Brodes (1993), and Fosnot (1996).

[10] See Richardson (1997) for an enumeration and explanation of at least four variations of social constructivism. On the difficulty of defining social constructivism see Matthews (1999).

opment could in effect be read off the way children solve problems involving the manipulation of objects—Vygotsky found that development was primarily social in origin.

Vygotsky distinguished between **intermental** and **intramental** psychological abilities. The first term refers to functions that one is able to perform in a social setting or in interaction with others and the latter to those one is able to perform independently. Vygotsky believed that each step or stage in a child's development occurs first in the course of social interaction; only once a competency has been performed intermentally can it begin to be called upon and performed independently, or intramentally. To understand this idea, consider how a child comes to behave according to social expectations. At first, parents attempt to control the child's behavior by saying "no" to socially inappropriate behavior; the child acts in response to the parents' disapproval. As the child develops a greater sense of what is, and what is not, socially acceptable, he or she appropriates some of this control and begins to approve and disapprove of his or her own desires and to act accordingly. According to Piaget, all learning originated in the process of equilibration; in Vygotsky's view ultimately all of what he termed the "higher mental functions", those capacities which enable human beings to solve problems and to act deliberately, and which include voluntary attention, logical memory, and the formulation of concepts, originate in relations between human individuals.[11] One might summarize the difference between the Piagetan and the Vygotskian approaches, then, by saying that while for the Piagetan the mind is psychogenetic—an individual's development occurs via interactions with the world—the Vygotskian sees the individual's development as passing by way of social interactions. For Vygotskians the mind is, in other words, sociogenetic (Vygotsky, 1978).

How might the insights of social constructivism be applied to teaching? As Noddings (1998, p. 132) pointed out, one form of the widely popular educational movement known as cooperative learning draws inspiration from social constructivism. Advocates of social constructivist cooperative learning argue that:

> *Through interaction with others, we learn the basic questions of reflective inquiry: How did I arrive at this result? Does it work? What is it useful for? How can I be sure? How can I explain it to others? Are there viable alternatives? As others put such questions and challenges to us, we internalize their questions and develop the habit of asking them of ourselves. Further, we can complete many tasks with the help of others that we are, at first, unable to complete on our own.* (Noddings, 1998, p. 116)

In this statement we can see a clear reflection of Vygotsky's ideas on development. The underlying idea here is that when students work through problems in situations of social interaction—groups—they are able to call on problem-solving capacities (Vygotsky's higher mental functions) that they would likely be unable to evoke if working on

---

[11] Offered here is the customary interpretation of the decisive differences between Piaget and Vygotsky, but there is some disagreement as to whether this is the best one. Cole and Wertsch (1996), for instance, argue that it places too narrow an emphasis on the question of whether the mind is psychogenetic or sociogenetic while ignoring the core difference between them; namely, the importance of culture on development. See Moll (1990) and Davydov (1995) on the question of how this interpretation of Vygotsky might be applied to educational problems.

BOX 1.2 PEDAGOGICAL GUIDELINES FOR APPLYING CONSTRUCTIVISM

- Provide students with activities and situations that actively engage them by presenting challenges to their current understandings. The first step toward doing this effectively is becoming familiar with a group of students' particular preconceptions and thinking patterns. Where appropriate, an informal essay assignment on the course theme in the first week of the semester might be instructive in this regard.
- Use a diversity of such learning activities (e.g., concept mapping, Socratic dialogues, problem-based learning, collaborative learning, etc.). Learning styles differ and no two students come to a learning situation with exactly the same prior understandings.
- Take advantage of the classroom as a social setting. For many students social interaction facilitates the learning process. Group discussions and learning activities support these students' learning style.

the same problem independently. Only when learners have developed habits of employing such capacities intermentally will they then be able to go on to using them autonomously. At the end of the day, social constructivism may simply be a psychological explanation for what teachers have known all along—namely, that attempting to articulate what one believes to others and to understand what other people are saying is the best way to learn: *docendo discimus.*[12] Box 1.2 provides a set of guidelines for how the main implications of constructivism discussed in this section might assist the development of effective teaching strategies.

Sociological Constructionism

This chapter has focused mainly on one of two broad sets of educational concerns to which the term constructivism usually refers. In the first sense, constructivism is a widely accepted psychological theory of learning whose methods are discussed in this book and represented in many of its exercises. What is also clearly present in this volume is another pedagogical theme or mood. At the core of this second form of constructivism is a highly critical stance toward natural science's claim to **objectivity**. The main claim of constructivism in this sense is that established knowledge is not value-free and objective, but instead it inescapably reflects the social context in which it is developed. In terms of teaching practices, this idea is reflected in activities and material that demonstrate the fallibility of scientific authority or which involve or encourage the exploration of ways of knowing that are offered as alternatives to scientific methods. We will call this form of constructivism, **sociological constructionism** on the grounds that construct*ion*ism suggests better than construct*iv*ism the notion of knowledge as a social artifact and because "sociological" recognizes the doctrine's origins in the field of sociology.

Science began to be confronted with a set of objections from sociological quarters in the 1960s. A great deal of the related literature is highly technical and difficult. The most

[12] Latin saying: We learn by teaching.

accessible approach to understanding these ideas is to look at the way that case studies of scientific research can show that social factors clearly inform the results of scientific research. This case-study approach goes back to at least the 19th century German economist and political theorist Karl Marx.[13] Marx's work focused on the influence of class on knowledge production, with contemporary critiques drawing on a wider range of sociological data including gender bias, the influence of individual prestige and reputation within scientific communities, as well as economics, race, and class. Typically, research in the sociology of scientific knowledge analyzes the process by which the scientific community arrives at agreement on one question or another and shows that the weight of social power and authority, considerations which should be irrelevant in these negotiations, have shaped their outcomes. Especially in recent years, feminist thinkers have led this research and the search for alternative ways of knowing.

The optimistic response to such analyses might be to say that the influence of illegitimate social factors tend to be weeded out as knowledge of a subject of research improves. One widely cited example illustrating this is that of Chandrasekhar, the first scientist to provide evidence for black holes. When Chandrasekar first put forward his calculations, a leading authority in the field, Sir Arthur Eddington, dismissed his findings as absurd. The scientific community accepted Eddington's judgment even though he was in the wrong. It took two generations of research for the astronomical community to come around to consensus on the existence of black holes. The general lesson the optimist would draw from this example, then, is that in order to overcome biases, what researchers need to do is to persist in applying the scientific method (i.e., continue to scrutinize and check their theories against the empirical data) and nature would decide the issues in the end. However, in face of mounting evidence in the form of particular case studies of male bias in knowledge production (Box 1.3), the optimistic hypothesis appeared in the eyes of many feminist thinkers to have little credibility, leading some to wonder whether the methods that science employs, and on which scientific knowledge ultimately rests, were not themselves infected with gender bias.

The case supporting the claim that the scientific method itself can be seen as a manifestation of male ideology has been made by a number of pre-eminent feminist thinkers. Central to this argument is that reflected clearly in the scientific method are patriarchal society's image of so-called normal male–female social relations, relations that have historically been imposed on women and helped maintain their social subordination. The treatment of nature as foreign and essentially different from the investigating subject, the tendency to feminize nature and treat her as a mystery reluctant to disclose her secrets, the aim of scientific knowledge being in order to predict, control, and thereby dominate have all been adduced for the fact that science, far from being the supreme ideal of knowledge acquisition, is actually a characteristically patriarchal approach to knowledge and nature. In this light, science is not just alien to women. If it is male social dominance in disguise then women would appear to have good reason to suspect that it is also potentially hostile to their interests.[14] To make matters worse,

---

[13] See Maxwell (1997).

[14] For analyses along these lines see Longino, 1990; Bleier, 1988; Keller, 1985; Tuana, 1989; Nelson & Nelson, 1996; Keller & Longino, 1996; Harding, 1986; and Lennon & Whitford, 1994.

BOX 1.3

The critical spirit of sociological constructionism is illustrated in the opening lines of Emily Martin's (1991) "The Egg and the Sperm: How Science Has Constructed a Romance Based on Stereotypical Male–Female Roles":

> *As an anthropologist, I am intrigued by the possibility that culture shapes how biological scientists describe what they discover about the natural world. If this were so, we would be learning about more than the natural world in high school biology class; we would be learning about cultural beliefs and practices as if they were part of nature. In the course of my research I realized that the picture of egg and sperm drawn in popular as well as scientific accounts of reproductive biology relies on stereotypes central to our cultural definitions of male and female. The stereotypes imply not only that female biological processes are less worthy than their male counterparts, but also that women are less worthy than men. Part of my goal in writing this article is to shine a bright light on the gender stereotypes hidden within the scientific language of biology. Exposed in such a light, I hope they will lose much of their power to harm us. (p. 485)*

Martin, E. (1991). The egg and the sperm: how science has constructed a romance based on stereotypical male–female roles. *Signs, Journal of Women in Culture and* Society, *16,* 485–501.

the scientific notion of knowledge is not restricted to the confines of the scientific community but has, as it is sometimes argued, become the standard for what constitutes genuine knowledge in the broader culture. If masculinist ideology dominates society and the objectivist ideal of knowing is a masculine approach to knowledge, small wonder, then, that the objectivist ideal is the predominant view of knowledge. Faced with this, some feminist thinkers argue that the dominance of masculinist epistemological standards needs to be resisted. By the same token, they promote the exploration of **feminist epistemologies**, sources of knowledge that have been badly underrepresented, neglected, or repressed. These areas include interpersonal knowledge such as that which develops out of ethical or emotional experience, through hearing and telling narratives or stories, the experience of embodiment, and aesthetic experience. From this standpoint, the scientific method, far from being the one, monolithic, universal standard of all human knowledge properly so called, is one among a plurality of ways of getting at knowledge.[15] Thus, nurse educators who teach in a highly scientific biomedical context must be skilled in reading, critiquing, and interpreting knowledge generated by traditional scientific methods while being aware of alternate forms of knowledge and ways of knowing.

[15] See Code, 1991 and 1995; Jaggar, 1996; Lugones, 1996; Williams, 1991; Goldberger, et al., 1996.

SUMMARY

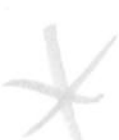

In recent years, nursing has evolved from a largely nurse-centered activity in which the nurse is expert actor to a relational, generative, client-centered practice—the new nursing. Nurse educators play a central role in transforming nursing through educational processes that parallel or mirror this shift. Constructivism, as an orienting framework for teaching nursing, provides the foundation for a conceptual shift from the teacher as "sage-on-the-stage" and student as rote learner, to teacher as facilitator of learning, one who engages students in relational, generative learning experiences. Constructivism, a world view that holds that knowledge is socially constructed, has generated a number of theoretical perspectives on teaching and learning with two primary theories featured in this chapter, cognitive constructivism and social constructivism. Cognitive constructivism maintains that learning is best understood as a process of individual meaning-making or knowledge-building. Here, the educator designs learning experiences that surface students' knowledge to foster knowledge or skill acquisition using generative or developmental educative processes. Social constructivism extends the ideas of cognitive contructivism by articulating that since knowledge is socially constructed, social processes are central to knowledge acquisition. Teaching and learning from a social constructivist perspective is therefore held to be a relational process. Since we hold that nursing is a relational practice, social constructivism has particular relevance for nursing education. Constructivism is a world view that opens up possibilities for envisioning teaching nursing as a generative, relational practice that draws on multiple ways of knowing, a practice that resonates with the new nursing. Thus, nurse educators who practice within the constructivist view create educational climates wherein what is taught resonates with how it is taught.

LEARNING ACTIVITY

CRITICAL KNOWING EXERCISE: DETECTING BIAS

T. B. Maxwell with L. E. Young

Bias may be defined as a predisposition or prejudice in favor of, or against, a particular statement, belief, claim, or interpretation. Contrary to popular belief, most often bias is not the intentional manipulation of others through false representation; rather, it tends to occur unconsciously.

People are particularly subject to bias in cases in which they have a strong emotional attachment to the idea that a particular claim or statement is true. Because self-evaluation is an emotionally charged issue, identifying and then working knowingly with bias in one's self-presentation is an important challenge when preparing a teaching portfolio. As nurse educators interested in preparing a teaching portfolio that represents one's work in a convincing manner (i.e., positioning one's work in a point of view from which claims may be judged impartially or, in a nonbiased way) it is in our interest to be aware of some of the signs of bias in writing.

Detecting bias involves first and foremost the exercise of good judgment. As good judgment is complex and improves with experience, there is no easy formula or set of instructions for how to decisively identify bias in a piece. There are, however, some techniques that authors often unconsciously employ that are clear indicators of bias in reporting:

The use of loaded language—A loaded term is any term with a clear descriptive meaning and a positive or negative evaluative meaning that is used in an attempt to persuade us to accept the evaluation conveyed by the term (e.g., terrorists, freedom fighters, and militia).

The use of false confidence—An attempt to persuade a reader to accept a claim by presenting it with great confidence (e.g., I certainly don't want to suggest that all adopted children are miserable, but the fact is that the majority of adopted children do suffer from a serious problem of self-identify, and that the problem is most serious during their teenage years).

Poor use of evidence—Controversial claims that are not supported by evidence such as a direct quote or the citation of a credible report or study should be viewed with suspicion. The proper documentation of sources is also a sign, but by no means a guarantee of, unbiased reporting.

Selective attention—Selective attention involves taking into consideration only evidence that confirms one's hypothesis while ignoring evidence that speaks against it. A common instance of selective attention is reasoning from a single example or a few isolated examples to a generalization (e.g., Do you see the way you're talking to me? You never treat me fairly).

Inconsistency—Inconsistency occurs when there is a logical inconsistency of claims (e.g., A nurse educator claims to be student centered, yet, the course materials indicate that she exclusively employs didactic lecturing. A nurse educator claims that his subject must be taught in a didactic manner (physiology) despite noting that experiential learning theories are foundational to the curriculum within which his course is located.)

Instructions

The articles that accompany this assignment are:

1. Johnson, M. (1999). Observations on positivism and pseudoscience in qualitative nursing research. *Journal of Advanced Nursing,* 30, 67–73.
2. Straneva, J. A. (2002). Therapeutic touch coming of age. *Holistic Nursing Practice,* 1493, 1–13.
3. Davis, M., Johnston S. R., DiMicco, W., et al. (1996). The case for a student honor code and beyond. *Journal of Professional Nursing, 12,* 24–30.

What is common to these three articles is that they address controversial areas of concern and debate for nurses in research, practice, and education respectively. Your assignment is to read all three articles critically then select one article as the focus of a short essay of approximately 500 words in which you will answer the following question: Does this article present a balanced view?

In developing your response, consider the following questions: Does the author use loaded language or false confidence? How does the author use supporting evidence for his or her claims and how well is that evidence documented? Is the author guilty of selective attention or inconsistency? Are there any other ways that the text seems to be biased besides the ones listed? Please justify and explain your impressions

Before proceeding to assess the relative credibility of the articles, state in your own words the main claim of each article. Make sure to justify your answer using specific examples from the text.

Evaluation Criteria

1. Appropriateness of use of terms studied in class, organization and coherence of ideas, and adequate justification of point of view. (/10)
2. Quality of formal English and clarity of style. (/5)
3. Proper use of APA style (in-text citations and list of works cited). (/5)

RESOURCES FOR EDUCATORS

PLANNING THE TEACHING/LEARNING EXPERIENCE

Questions to Support a Thoughtful Reading

1. Before reading this chapter, think about a time when you loved learning and therefore learned easily. What helped you learn?
2. Think about a time when you were in a formal learning situation and resisted learning by acting out or being bored. What was it about this learning experience that put you off?
3. Think about a time when you were in a formal learning situation and began by feeling frustrated but, in the end, you discovered that you learned many things that you did not expect that now have great value for you.
4. Think about what best helps you deepen your understanding of nursing practice. What way or ways of knowing best support your developing understanding?
5. Do you think of nursing as a relational practice? If yes, why? If not, why not?
6. How do your views on teaching and learning fit with the tenets of constructivism?

Instructions for Educators

In-Class Activity:

Prior to assigning this chapter for reading, have students write a paragraph or two that describes "What is nursing" that is submitted to you. At the end of the class in which this activity takes place, assign Chapter 1 as the reading for the next class. Between classes analyze their submissions for main themes and relationships. Begin the next class offering your reflection on the similarities and differences between the students' views on nursing and those of the authors of the chapter, inviting comments and questions upon completing your reflections.

Online Activity:

For online teaching, adapt this activity by asking students to post a paragraph or two that describes "What is nursing" that is prepared prior to reading Chapter 1. Then instruct students to read Chapter 1 following which they will post a reflection that addresses the impact of the chapter on their perception of nursing. As an instructor, read the posted comments and summarize main points and questions arising.

Tips for Developing a Student-Centered Learning Environment

Student-centered learning generally draws heavily on group work, thus participation of students in the learning activities is essential to ensure an environment that is conducive to learning for all involved. Therefore, when preparing the course outline one strategy that will foster participation is to assign marks for students' contributions to the collective. When assigning marks for participation make it clear what counts as an activity or contribution that will be rewarded.

EVALUATING THE TEACHING/LEARNING EXPERIENCE

Questions to Elicit Feedback from Students on Their Learning

1. In your own words, describe the relationship between client-centered nursing and student-centered teaching.
2. What is the difference between cognitive constructivism and social constructivism?
3. The authors speak of the tension between the constructivist view and empiricism. In your own words, what is that tension?

Reflective Questions for Educators

1. Preparing for this class, what tensions or challenges did you experience when considering how you would design the learning experience in class to be consistent with the tenets of the constructivist view of learning?
2. What challenges or tensions emerged from the students during the class? Can you postulate why these tensions or challenges occurred? What did you do to manage the tensions? What might you do differently next time?
3. What did you learn from the students in class today?

Sample Evaluation Strategy

Hardy et al. (2002) write that "expertise . . . can be regarded as an ability to use multiple forms of knowledge and self in an apparently seamless way" (p. 201). Write a story from your teaching practice that exemplifies your expertise as defined by Hardy et al. In your story make sure that the readers understand how you drew on at least two ways of knowing in your expert practice.

References

Alexander, P. A., & Murphy, P. K. (1998). The research base for APA's learner-centered principles. In N. M. Lambert & B. L. McCombs (Eds.). *Issues in school reform: A sampler of psychological perspectives on learner-centered school* (pp. 25–60). Washington, DC: The American Psychological Association.

Antepohl, W., & Herzig, S. (1999). Problem-based learning versus lecture-based learning in a course of basic pharmacology: A controlled, randomized study. *Medical Education, 33,* 106–113.

Bandura, A. (1986). *Social foundations of thought and action: A social cognitive theory*. Englewood Cliffs, NJ: Prentice-Hall.

Barnes, L. B., Christensen, C. R., & Hansen, A. J. (1994). *Teaching and the case method.* (3rd ed.). Boston: Harvard Business School Publishing Division.

Barrows, H. S. (1994). *Practice-based learning: Problem-based learning applied to medical education.* Springfield, IL: Southern Illinois University School of Medicine.

Bergum, V. (2003). Relational pedagogy. Embodiment, improvisation, and interdependence. *Nursing Philosophy, 4,* 121–128.

Bevis, E. O., & Watson, J. (1989). *Toward a new curriculum: A new pedagogy for nursing.* New York: NLN.

Biley, F. (1999). Creating tension: Undergraduate student nurses' responses to a problem-based curriculum. *Nurse Education Today, 19,* 586–591.

Bleier, R. (Ed.) (1986). *Feminist approaches to science.* New York: Pergamon.

Brooks, J. G., & Brooks, M. G. (1993). *In search of understanding: The case for constructivist classrooms.* Alexandria, VA: Association for Supervision and Curriculum.

Candy, P. (1991). *Self-direction for life-long learning.* San Francisco: Jossey-Bass.

Code, L. (1991). *What can she know: Feminist theory and the construction of knowledge.* Ithaca, NY: Cornell University Press.

Cole, M., & Wertsch, J. V. (1996). Beyond the individual-social antimony in discussions of Piaget and Vygotsky. *Human Development, 39,* 250–256.

Davis, R. B., Mather, C., & Noddings, N. (Eds.). (1990). Constructivist views on the teaching and learning of mathematics. *Journal for Research in Mathematics Education Monograph Series,* No. 4. Reston, VA: National Council of Teachers of Mathematics.

Demarco, R., Hayward, L., & Lynch, M. (2002). Nursing students' experiences with and strategic approaches to case-based instruction: A replication and comparison study between two disciplines. *Journal of Nursing Education, 41,* 165–174.

Dewey, J. (1916). *Democracy and education.* New York: Macmillan.

Dewey, J. (1963/1938). *Experience and education.* New York: Collier Books.

Davydov, V. V. (1995). The influence of L.A. Vygotsky on educational theory, research and practice. *Educational Researcher, 24,* 12–21.

Diekelmann, N. (2001). Narrative pedagogy: Heideggerian hermeneutical analysis of lived experiences of students, teachers, and clinicians. *Advances in Nursing Science, 23,* 53–71.

Doane, G. (2002). Beyond behavioral skills to human-involved processes: relational nursing practice and interpretive pedagogy. *Journal of Nursing Education, 41,* 400–404.

Engebretson, J., & Littleton, L. Y. (2001). Cultural negotiation: A constructivist-based model for nursing practice. *Nursing Outlook, 49,* 223–230.

Fosnot, C. T. (Ed.). (1996). *Constructivism: Theory, perspectives, and practice.* New York: Teachers College Press.

Goldberger, N., Tarule, J., Clinchy, B., & Blenky, M. (Eds.) (1996). *Knowledge, difference, and power: Essays inspired by "women's ways of knowing".* New York: Basic Books.

Gutek, G. L. (1997). *Philosophical and ideological perspectives in education* (2nd ed.). Boston: Allyn and Bacon.

Harding, S. (1986). *The science question in feminism.* Ithaca, NY: Cornell University Press.

Hardy, S., Garbett, R., Titchen, A., et al. (2002). Exploring nursing expertise: Nurses talk nursing. *Nursing Inquiry, 9,* 196–202.

Hewitt-Taylor, J. (2001). Self-directed learning: Views of teachers and students. *Journal of Advanced Nursing, 36,* 496–504.

Jacobs, S. K., Rosenfeld, P., & Haber, J. (2003). Information literacy as the foundation for evidence-based practice in graduate nursing education: A curriculum-integrated approach. *Journal of Professional Nursing, 19,* 320–328.

Jaggar, A. (1996). Love and knowledge: Emotion in feminist epistemology. In A. Garry & M. Pearsall (Eds.), *Women, knowledge, and reality.* (2nd ed., pp. 166–90). London: Routledge.

Jerlock, M., Falk, K., & Severinsson, E. (2003). Academic nursing education guidelines: Tools for bridging the gap between theory, research and practice. *Nursing and Health Sciences, 5,* 219–228.

Johns, C. (2002). *Guided reflection: Advancing practice.* Oxford: Blackwell Science.

Kant, I. (1929). *Critique of pure reason.* Trans. Norman Kemp Smith. London: MacMillan.

Keller, E. F. (1985). *Reflections on Gender and Science.* New Haven, CT: Yale University Press.

Keller, E. F., & Longino, H. (Eds.) (1996). *Feminism and science.* Oxford: Oxford University Press.

Knowles, M. (1975). *Self-directed learning.* Chicago: Follet.

Knowlton, D. S., & Sharp, D. C. (2003). *Problem-based learning for the information age: New directions for teaching and learning #95.* Somerset, NJ: J. Wiley/Jossey-Bass.

Koerner, J. G. (2003). The virtues of the virtual world. Enhancing the technology/knowledge professional interface for life-long learning. *Nursing Administration Quarterly, 27,* 9–17.

Lennon, K., & Whitford, M. (Eds.) (1994). *Knowing the difference: Feminist perspectives in epistemology.* London: Routledge.

Lepp, M., Zorn, C. R., Duffy, P. R., & Dickson, R. J. (2003). International education and reflection: Transition of Swedish and American nursing students to authenticity. *Journal of Professional Nursing, 19,* 164–172.

Locke, J. (1959). *Essay concerning human understanding. 2 Vol.* New York: Dover.

Longino, H. (1990). *Science as social knowledge: Values and objectivity in scientific inquiry.* Princeton, NJ: Princeton University Press.

Lugones, M. (1996). Playfulness, 'word'-traveling, and loving perception. In A. Garry & M. Pearsall (Eds.), *Women, knowledge, and reality* (2nd edition, pp. 419–33). London: Routledge.

MacIntosh, J., MacKay, E., Mallet-Boucher, M., et al. (2002). Discovering co-learning with students in distance education sites. *Nurse Educator, 27,* 182–186.

Martin, E. (1991). The egg and the sperm: How science has constructed a romance based on stereotypical male-female roles. *Signs, Journal of Women in Culture and* Society, *16,* 485–501.

Matthews, M. R. (1999). *Social constructivism and mathematics education: Some comments.* In *Philosophy of Education Society Yearbook.* Retrieved October 17, 2005 from http://www.ed.uiuc.edu/EPS/PES-yearbook/1999/matthews.asp.

Maxwell, L. (1997). Foundational thought in the development of knowledge for social change. In S. E. Thorne & V. E. Hayes (Eds.). *Nursing praxis: Knowledge and action* (pp. 203–218). Thousand Oaks, CA: Sage.

McLellan, H. (1995). *Situated learning perspectives.* Englewood Cliffs, NJ: Educational Technology Publications.

Moll, L. (Ed.). (1990). *Vygotsky and education: Instructional implications and applications of sociohistorical psychology.* Cambridge: Cambridge University Press.

Morris, D., & Turnbull, P. (2004). Using student nurses as teachers in inquiry-based learning. *Journal of Advanced Nursing, 45,*136–144.

Nehls N. J (1995). Narrative pedagogy: Rethinking nursing education. *J. Nurs. Educ. 34,* 204–210.

Nelson, L. H., & Nelson, J. (Eds.). (1996). *Feminism, science, and the philosophy of science.* Dordrecht: Kluwer.

Noddings, N. (1998). *Philosophy of education.* Boulder, CO: Westview Press.

O'Shea, E. (2003). Self-directed learning in nurse education: A review of the literature. *Journal of Advanced Nursing, 43,* 62–70.

Piaget, J. (1970). *Genetic epistemology.* New York: Columbia University Press.

Piaget, J. (1971a). *Biology and knowledge.* Chicago: University of Chicago Press.

Piaget, J. (1971b). *The insights and illusions of philosophy.* New York: World.

Piccinin, S. (1997). Making our teaching more student-centered. Retrieved October 17, 2005 from http://www.uottawa.ca/academic/cut/options/Dec_97/Student_centered.htm.

Richardson, V. (1997). Constructivist teaching and teacher education. In V. Richardson (Ed.). *Constructivist teacher education* (pp. 3–14). London: Routledge Falmer.

Rideout, E. (2001). *Transforming nursing education through problem-based learning.* Toronto, ON: Jones & Bartlett Publishers.

Rodney, P., Varcoe, C., Storch, J. L., et al. (2002). Navigating towards a moral horizon: a multisite qualitative study of ethical practice in nursing. *Canadian Journal of Nursing Research, 34,* 75–102.

Steffe, L. P., & P. W. Thompson (Eds.). (2000). *Radical constructivism in action: Building on the pioneering work of Ernst von Glasersfeld.* New York: Routledge Falmer.

Tuana, N. (Ed.). (1989). *Feminism and science.* Bloomington, IN: Indiana University Press.

Vadeboncoeur, J. A. (1997). Child development and the purpose of education. In V. Richardson (Ed.). *Contructivist teacher education* (pp. 15–37). London: Routledge Falmer.

Vygotsky, L. (1978). *The mind and society.* Cambridge, MA: Harvard University Press.

Wasserman, S. (1996). *Introduction to case method teaching: A guide to the galaxy.* New York: Teacher's College Press.

Williams, P. (1991). *The alchemy of race and rights.* Cambridge, MA: Harvard University Press.

Williams, S. M. (1992). Putting case-based instruction into context: Examples from legal and medical education. *The Journal of the Learning Sciences, 2,* 367–427.

Woods, D. (1994). *Problem-based learning: How to gain the most from PBL.* Waterdown, ON: Donald R Woods.

Young, L. (2002). Transforming health promotion practice: Moving toward holistic care. In L. Young & V. Hayes (Eds.). *Transforming health promotion practice: Concepts, issues, and application* (pp. 3–21). Philadelphia: F. A. Davis.

Additional Resources

1. Narrative Pedagogy Web site. Available at: http://www.son.wisc.edu/diekelmann/research/slt/index.html. Accessed October 17, 2005.
2. Leap into student centered learning. Retrieved Oct. 17, 2005, from http://www.adelaide.edu.au/clpd/material/leapinto/stud_ctvd_lrng.pdf.

Chapter 2

Decision Making in Nursing Education: A Model to Support Student-Centered Learning

Lynne E. Young
Bruce Maxwell
Barbara L. Paterson
Angela Wolff

Recently I had an opportunity to teach in a "smart" classroom.[1] As a one who has spent considerable time considering the theoretical foundations of student-centered teaching and experimenting with its application in diverse settings, the smart classroom presented new challenges. A smart classroom is one laden with technology that provides virtual access to learning. Students can attend class either in person, by teleconference and computer, by media streaming, or they can access an archived version of the session. The educator is at a podium with the videotaped image and PowerPoint presentation beamed simultaneously to students attending virtually. Students in the classroom see the real person and the PowerPoint presentation on a screen behind the speaker. One strategy that I use to create a student-centered learning environment while lecturing is to rove around the lecture theater connecting with students. My first challenge in the smart classroom was that this option was not acceptable as I was instructed to stay behind the podium moving only a few inches from the center position to facilitate videotaping. The second challenge was to determine who was attending. With those attending in person and by teleconference, I could do a roundtable check-in to determine who was present and to learn a bit about each student. For those media-streaming into the session, there was no way to determine who was present. Thus, my teaching style in the context of the smart classroom was akin to fitting a round peg into a square hole. The experience was a marvelous opportunity for me to be exposed to cutting edge educational technology, but gave me pause to consider how technology can influence teaching decisions.

[1]The first-person "I" is that of author Lynne Young.

INTENT

In this chapter, a conceptual model to guide nurse educators' decision making as it relates specifically to student-centered learning in nursing education is introduced. The chapter begins with a description of the elements of this model. Here, we envision that decisions about teaching practice are informed by a range of ways of knowing including theoretical, empirical, critical, ethical, personal, interpersonal, technological, and aesthetic. Evaluations further shape decisions about teaching and can be formal as in program, school, course, or instructor evaluations, or informal such as episodic class or term evaluations. Informal feedback from students and peers plays a role in shaping teaching-related decisions. When making decisions, teachers face numerous barriers and facilitators that include those arising from the institution, curriculum, instructional strategies, faculty, learner, and technical and personal factors. Critical reflection and dialogue with colleagues, students, and other influential persons is salient to resolving the various influences on decision making. To illustrate the process of decision making for teaching in nursing, a case example that underscores the complexities of using evidence to support a decision to use mind mapping in teaching is provided. The chapter closes with some suggestions regarding how to move forward the agenda of student-centered teaching in nursing education.

OVERVIEW

INTRODUCTION

Teaching nursing and professional nursing practice can be guided by shared principles. For example, student-centered teaching derives from the same principles as client-centered nursing. As argued in Chapter 1, a nurse practicing client-centered nursing begins by understanding the lived experience of the client or patient rather than with the nurses' understanding; the nurse collaborates with the patient or client rather than doing for or doing to the patient (Young, 2002). Similarly, in student-centered teaching, the educator begins with the experience of the student and together they build knowledge, skills, and competencies for professional practice (Bergum, 2003; Bevis & Watson, 1989). Currently in professional nursing practice, evidence-based decision making is a much embraced idea which originates in the discourse of medicine and therefore holds much sway. **Evidence-based decision making** is a reasoning process in which clinical decisions are based on empirical evidence generated using large clinical trials. In nursing, it is widely held that clinical decision making should be robust and defensible; it should be informed not only by empirical evidence but also by a more expansive definition of knowing (Corcoran-Perry, Narayan, & Cochrane, 1999; Fawcett, Watson, Neuman, Walker, & Fitzpatrick, 2001; Kuiper & Pesut, 2004; Narayan & Corcoran-Perry, 1997). Similarly, detractors in medicine critique evidence-based discourse in medicine for its sole reliance on empirical evidence (Cohen, Stavri, & Hersh, 2004). Like clinical decision making in nursing, we posit that decision making in nursing education is a reasoned process in which defensible judgments and decisions made in support of students' learning derive from a range of ways of knowing, including empirical.

Regarding decisions about student-centered teaching, a common challenge posed relates to the question about relative effectiveness. What is often tacitly understood by this is that the onus is on the proponents of student-centered methods to provide evidence that students learn better as demonstrated by higher quality of submitted work and higher marks. From this perspective, the task of determining whether student-centered methods are indeed more effective than traditional methods ultimately comes back to a question of applying established empirical evaluative methodologies.

Some educational researchers have responded to this challenge. In medical and nursing faculties, student-centered curricula have been tested. Many of these studies find that student-centered methods are more effective than traditional ones (Baxter & Gray, 2001; Chase & Geldenhuys, 2001; Rideout, 2001). However, the most systematic research on student-centered learning was conducted several decades ago. In the 1970s, public concern was expressed that large numbers of teachers and schools were unilaterally adopting so-called progressive or student-centered teaching methods. One of the most comprehensive studies responding to the question of the pedagogical worth of student-centered methods was Neville Bennett's *Teaching Styles and Pupil Progress*. Bennett (1976) conducted a large multidimensional study of the twofold question of do differing teaching styles result in disparate pupil progress? and do different types of pupils perform better under certain styles of teaching? (p. 148). In short, he concluded that his evidence strongly favored traditional methods. He summarizes:

> *The results form a coherent pattern. The effect of teaching style is statistically and educationally significant in all attainable areas tested. In reading, pupils of*

> *formal and mixed teachers progress more than those of informal teachers, the difference being equivalent to some three to five months' difference in performance. In mathematics, formal pupils are superior to both mixed and informal pupils, the difference in progress being some four to five months. In English formal pupils again out-perform both mixed and informal pupils, the discrepancy in progress between formal and informal being approximately three to five months. (p. 152)*

As noted above, similar studies do exist that arrive at disconfirming evidence and, as Bennett cautions himself, no study is immune to methodological objections. From the perspective of nursing education the most salient methodological objection to Bennett's (1976) study is that its subjects were all children and it is quite possible that adult learners respond differently to what he labeled informal or student-centered teaching styles. Be that as it may, for Bennett and other like-minded scholars of his day (Ward & Barcher, 1975) the question of the effectiveness of traditional versus student-centered methods was a case closed.

As decisive as this might seem at first blush, from another viewpoint, Bennett's criteria of educational success—namely, students' mastery of a preset body of material over a given time period and as measured by success on formal examinations—is questionable as a general measure of the worthiness of a teaching method. One does not have to look far to see that there are other equally worthwhile or even necessary educational aims that cannot be measured this way (Carr, 2003, pp. 214–218). One perennial view of general education called **noninstrumentalism**, for example, holds that the purpose of education is to promote a broad comprehension of the world and one's place in it (Carr, 2000, pp. 174–179; Peters, 1966). John Dewey's (1916/1997) conception of the aims of education is equally difficult to square with objective measures of learning. As we saw in the last chapter, Dewey (1916/1997) assigned to the mastery of a discipline's knowledge base secondary importance on the grounds that, in rapidly changing contemporary societies, such knowledge is rapidly outdated. Far better, then, for education to concentrate on the development of more versatile second-order competencies such as problem-solving skills and learning to learn. Another similarly practical minded view of the aims of education, **instrumentalism**, considers a subject as educationally worthwhile if it can be shown to be useful in personal, social, or economic terms. Of course, professional education such as nursing is necessarily instrumentally oriented. Yet, even within the relatively rigid framework of professional preparation any attempt to reduce educational aims to the acquisition of a basic skill set or knowledge base is questionable. In addition to transmitting the field's science-derived knowledge base, professional education is also a form of **socialization** that involves the development of a set of professional attitudes. In nursing and medicine, these attitudes rally together certain social skills that define, in ethical terms, the clinician's role as a care provider. Finally, education at all levels and in all fields should aim to promote curiosity and an appetite for more learning, or student motivation. In sum, even if traditional education methods are more effective in promoting the mastery of particular units of information or quantitatively measurable cognitive skills, it is clearly a mistake, in light of the multiplicity of sometimes normative educational aims, to consider this kind of success as the gold standard for the success of all educational methods.

The fact that the effectiveness of any pedagogical method must always be gauged in reference to a range of worthwhile educational aims makes decision making for educational methods highly complex. For instance, while a collaborative learning activity in which students work together on a task such as defining scientific terms might not be preferable to a traditional method such as memorization, the traditional method lacks the advantage of promoting the worthwhile educational aim of developing collaborative skills. Although an experience with collaborative learning might be virtually superfluous from the aim of acquiring the science-derived knowledge base of a profession, such an experience might prove invaluable when viewed from the point of view of developing such skills as interacting with clients, coworkers, and comprehending the workings of health and social services (Howe, 2001). Adding further complexity to the decision-making process, there is the possibility that even if a particular method is highly effective from the vantage point of one educational aim, there may be evidence for rejecting it on moral or ethical grounds. We can see this idea at work in Robert Glew's (1994) assessment of the introduction of a fully case study, student-centered curriculum at the faculty of Medicine at the University of New Mexico where he is professor:

> *Though the medical world has yet to evaluate the New Curriculum by any set of hard data, my experience has shown me that we have at least managed to create between students and faculty a sense of community and respect that I had not seen in decades as a teacher. Regardless of future board scores or the number of primary care physicians graduated or even the quality of residency positions attained, I will regard this experiment as truly successful only when I see our students emerging from medical school caring for themselves, for each other, and most importantly, for the citizens of the communities in which they will live and practice sound medicine. (p. 743)*

To restate his point, the fact that the student-centered curriculum does not have the same dehumanizing effect as the traditional medical school curriculum is grounds enough for preferring it, even if it turns out that student success rate drops when measured in terms of standardized tests, numbers graduating, and the prestige of postgraduate positions attained. In sum, the fact that educational decisions must be made in reference to a multiplicity of sometimes mutually conflicting professional, social, ethical as well as cognitive aims means that good decision making in this area demands a great deal of practical wisdom. Far from being cause for despair, an appreciation of the complexity and the controversial nature of methodological decision making in education is an inevitable step on the path toward genuinely reflective teaching.

To this end, in the following section of this chapter, a model intended as a sketch of what is involved in the complex process of decision making in nursing education is laid out. While there are endless ways of knowing, and often a multitude of interpersonal and bureaucratic processes that inform a nurse educators' decisions about what and how to teach nursing, the model described below represents a first step toward open dialogue about decision making in nursing education.

A MODEL TO GUIDE DECISION MAKING IN NURSING EDUCATION

Practical reasoning is the process of formulating logical statements that lead to judgments that inform an action that is taken (Narayan & Corcoran-Perry, 1997). Reasoning in nursing education draws on the types of knowledge that are central to knowing in nursing: theoretical, empirical, critical, and ethical knowing as well as personal, interpersonal, and aesthetic knowing (Carper, 1978; Fahy, 2002; Fawcett, et al., 2001; Kuiper & Pesut, 2004; Lamond & Thompson, 2000; Nelms & Lane, 1999; Pierson, 1999; Ruth-Sahd, 2003; Silva, Sorrell, & Sorrell, 1995). Reflection and dialogue are intrapersonal and interpersonal processes that deepen the capacity to know by augmenting what is known with new information and expanding awareness beyond accepted assumptions.

Because of the complexities of teaching and learning, the model in Figure 2.1 appears one-dimensional; however, the model we envision is hardly that. This model is multidimensional. The types of knowledge that form the knowledge base with decisions are shaped by formal feedback generated through:

- Evaluation processes, both formal and occasional or episodic.
- Informal feedback from students, peers, and other colleagues.
- Numerous other barriers and facilitators, including institutional, curricular, instructional, technological, faculty-related, learner-related, and/or personal.

Reflection and dialogue are two crucial strategies that deepen understanding of nursing education's knowledge base and thus influence how knowledge is applied in practice.

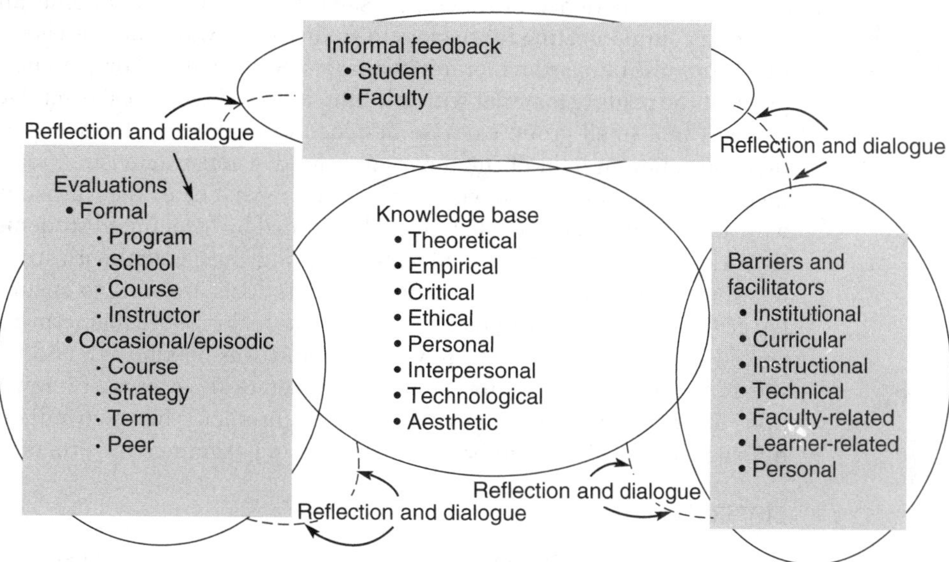

■ **FIGURE 2.1** Decision-making model for student-centered teaching in nursing.

Decision Making in Nursing Education: Patterns of Knowing

According to this model, foundational knowledge that informs decisions about teaching nursing derives from various ways of knowing: theoretical, empirical, critical, ethical, personal, interpersonal, technological, and aesthetic. In this section, these ways of knowing are defined, their role in decisions about nursing is explained, and sample strategies are offered.

THEORETICAL

Theoretical knowledge is knowledge of particular constellations of assumptions constructed to explain some phenomenon (e.g., nursing, loss, infant bonding, hypertension). Theoretical formulations draw on abstract reasoning and speculation to explain and delimit the constructs or elements of a phenomenon, their interrelationships, and boundaries (Bacharach, 1989; Weick, 1995). Theoretical knowledge for nursing education is acquired through the study of educational, nursing, and nursing-related theories, and theoretical formulations that link the two. This process can be referred to as theorizing. A nurse educator may understand the teaching and learning process to be consistent with such theories as cognitive constructivism, **social learning theory**, or the **McGill Model of Nursing**, a model that bridges between teaching/learning theory and nursing theory.

Consider, for example, the nurse educator who holds to the cognitive constructivist view of patient education. Acquiring health information will be understood by this nurse as a process of knowledge-building and meaning-making and as an active interpretive, relational process that is a social act that affects patients' and nurses' learning. Further, this nurse might ascribe to the view that learning will be influenced by factors such as the experience of illness, personality, information content, and the environment. In communicating these ideas to students in a way that **models** various aspects of the theory, the nurse educator might assign reading material on patient education, complement the reading material with a lecture followed by critical discussion, then engage students in a small group exercise designed to explore students' experiences with patient education in light of the theory of cognitive constructivism. Finally, the educator might conclude the session with a reflection on what he or she learned during the class, with a particular focus on what he or she learned by listening to students' reflections on their experiences with patient education. During engagement with students, the educator would tune into the meta-experience of students' learning to ensure that the learning environment was favorable by, for example, making sure that term assignments were spaced out, that the students' physical comfort was maximized, and that the educator was fully present to students. Thus, with theoretical patterns of knowing as a foundation, the nurse educator can develop a synchronicity between nursing practice and nursing education that can be articulated to, and examined by, others.

EMPIRICAL

Empirical patterns of knowing are linked to theoretical knowledge in that empirical knowledge is framed by a set of theoretical assumptions. Like theoretical knowledge, empirical knowledge is generated to describe, explain, and predict phenomenon

(Carper, 1978). However, whereas theoretical knowledge is, generally speaking, derived from the analysis of abstract concepts, empirical studies try to generate supporting evidence for some hypothesis by making carefully planned observations of the phenomenon that researchers are attempting to explain and describe. Empirical patterns of knowing for student-centered teaching nursing are acquired by appraising research on a particular educational topic for its value or by generating original research that contributes to the body of empirical knowledge about student-centered learning.

While there is a good deal of evidence to support evidence-based decision making in clinical nursing practice, problems exist related to using evidence to guide decision making in teaching when using a student-centered approach. With the exception of **problem-based learning** (PBL), a student-centered strategy that has been adopted throughout the world by nurse educators (Lee, Wong, & Mok, 2004), there are relatively few databased studies about the effectiveness of student-centered learning strategies. For example, reflective practice has until recently received little attention in the empirical or critical literature despite its widespread adoption in nursing education (Burnard, 2005; Hargreaves, 2004; Ruth-Sahd, 2003). Further, because there are a variety of ways to refer to student-centered teaching strategies, the literature is fragmented. Few studies explore the same phenomenon and those studies that do often use small samples. For example, **mind mapping** (also called **concept mapping**) has been discussed as an important student-centered strategy to advance critical thinking. However, only five databased articles on this topic in nursing journals were retrieved (Wheeler & Collins, 2003; Wilkes, Cooper, Lewin, & Batts, 1999) using mind mapping as a key term. Concept mapping used as a key term yielded two articles. (See the case study at the end of this chapter for a full discussion of the use of evidence to support adopting mind mapping in nursing education practice.) Thus, beyond PBL, the lack of empirical studies in this area makes an evidence-based decision about whether to adopt a particular student-centered strategy based on empirical knowledge beyond PBL a challenge.

That said, and as discussed at length in the previous chapter, it is important to bear in mind that empirical patterns of knowing are widely held to be legitimate genres of knowing that complement and are complemented by other ways of knowing. Drawing on a multiplicity of ways of knowing to guide decision making is particularly relevant in nursing because of its complexity; its problems and issues can best be addressed by nurses who can know in diverse ways and who assume accountability for using various ways of knowing to inform clinical decisions. Thus, in drawing parallels between practicing nursing and teaching nursing, we suggest that the empirical pattern of knowing is one way of knowing that is important in formulating decisions about teaching nursing using a student-centered approach. Like generating knowledge for nursing practice using empirical methods, empirical knowledge that supports decisions about nursing education must be generated by rigorous methods.

CRITICAL

Relative to theoretical and empirical knowledge, critical knowledge—knowledge about the sociopolitical contexts of health—is a newcomer to the discipline of nursing. One nurse writes "My previous educational experiences contained very little about race, culture, and health beyond a few interesting anecdotes [. . .] or the occasional frightening statistic such as the higher infant mortality rate among African Americans [. . .]. My ongoing critical examination of the last ten years of nursing periodicals and texts indicates that this is in a large part true of nursing education and research in general" (Maeda Allman, 1992, p. 36). Such knowledge is generated through systematic critique guided by **postmodern, poststructural, feminist, and postcolonial** theories that reveal what was previously hidden. For example, Bjorklund (2004) used a feminist ethics framework to examine the concept of invisibility in nursing. Critical theories are lenses through which phenomenon are examined to reveal that which is hidden from consciousness to generate new critical knowledge. Such work tends to be provocative because it challenges accepted social and political norms. Critical theories are instrumental in identifying the limitations of theoretical and empirical formulations in nursing education. For example, postmodern critiques of case-method teaching in nursing have led to new ways of thinking about how best to use cases when teaching nursing (see Chapter 7). Such theories are foundational to students' capacities to challenge limiting conventions and to resist habitual ways of knowing and doing. Application of critical theories in nursing education leads to more expansive and passionate engagements in which students reveal and challenge what is taken for granted (hooks, 1994).

Critical knowledge is developed in nursing students by ensuring that the links between such factors as race, gender, age, social status, and health are addressed in nursing classrooms and practice experiences. Nurse educators who aspire to student-centeredness will be sensitive to such issues in the classroom, and model applications of relevant principles in the classroom. Falk-Rafael, Chinn, Anderson, Laschinger, and Rubotzky (2004) have studied the effects of applying feminist pedagogical principles[2] in nursing education classrooms. They conclude that in classrooms where such principles are applied, students are empowered, a state they postulate extends beyond the classroom to personal and professional contexts. Banister and Schreiber (1999) point out that while there are many rewards of teaching in a curriculum based on critical and feminist theory, educators face new and sometimes difficult challenges when implementing these ideas in the nursing classroom.

Drawing from my experience, the following example demonstrates how critical theory was used to shed light on a case story in a nursing classroom. Students were asked to present and analyze a clinical case to the class. Following a presentation by a male student, Joel, a female student, Adrienne, approached me and expressed concern about the sexist nature of the presentation. In his presentation, Joel claimed that it was difficult to accurately assess women's pain because women are more expressive than men when in pain. Adrienne and I discussed her concerns about this statement, and her concerns about approaching Joel about the issue. Adrienne revealed that his much larger size was intimidating to her and a reason for her concern about confronting Joel about his statement. In the end, Adrienne devised a way of expressing her concerns to Joel. Through these interchanges, Adrienne not only identified a sexist bias but had an

---

[2] Feminist pedagogical principles as envisioned by P. Chinn (2001) relate to a commitment to: Praxis, defined as reflection and action to transform the world; Empowerment that fosters personal strength and arises from group solidarity; Awareness of self and others; Cooperation to group solidarity and integrity; Evolvement, defined as growth where change and transformation are conscious and deliberate.

opportunity to practice expressing her concerns about sexism to a male colleague. The exchange between Adrienne and Joel raised Joel's awareness of a bias that he holds about women and pain. As for my learning, I came to understand that I need to be more attuned to bias in students' work as I had completely missed the student's biased statement.

Finally, critical knowledge about nursing education can be developed by **deconstructing** educational phenomenon in nursing such as the culture of stress that appears to envelope nurse educators and infuse nursing education.

ETHICAL

Ethical patterns of knowing are developed through formulating moral judgments typically framed as judgments of right and wrong drawing on diverse and evolving sources of wisdom (Carper, 1978; Rodney, Pauly, & Burgess, 2004). Ethical knowledge in nursing education can be developed by using models of moral education for example, McDonald's Ethical Decision Making Framework (McPherson, Rodney, McDonald, Storch, Pauly, & Burgess, 2004) to examine research on the moral dimensions of nursing education and appraise how this knowledge fits with the structures and processes of the teaching/learning experience. For instance, in a cross-sectional Finnish study in which questionnaires were sent to 52 first-year students and 54 last-year students, Auvinen, Suominen, Leino-Kilpi, and Helkama (2004) found that students faced with ethical dilemmas in practice were more likely to demonstrate enhanced moral development than students who did not. Thus, an educator might choose clinical experiences for students that have potential to elicit ethical reasoning. Taking a student-centered approach to ethical analysis might entail asking students to reflect on ethical dilemmas arising from clinical situations in a journal or in response to discussions with peers. Further, educators who hold to student-centered learning would use everyday occurrences to model a commitment to ethical principles. For example, when confronted by marking issues this educator would be respectful of all voices and make his or her decisions transparent to all those who may be touched by the decision.

PERSONAL AND INTERPERSONAL KNOWLEDGE

Personal knowledge, or knowledge of the self, is defined by Carper (1978) as "the knowing, encountering, and actualizing of the concrete, individual self" (p. 220). Knowing the self is never absolute; one continually strives to know the self. Personal knowledge is accessed through such things as reflection and dialogue, tuning into **embodied responses**, reflecting on the meaning of personal narratives and intuitions, producing, then reflecting on artistic pursuits such as drawing or painting, and through physical/spiritual practices such as yoga or meditation. Doane (2004) links embodied knowing to ethical knowing arguing that: "Through our bodies we have an implicit sense of a situation and the intricacy of it" (p. 439). Polanyi (1962) speaks of personal knowing as an art, the contribution of the knower to his knowledge. Personal knowing according to Polanyi is an ever-sharpening intellectual capacity that involves a commitment to integrate signs and symbols in a way that supports focal attention, or tacit knowing. Personal knowing encompasses knowing the self as an individual person, as well as a transformative process through which repeated mental effort yields an increasing capacity to comprehend what before could not be seen.

Carper (1978) posits that it is through engaging in authentic relationships with oneself and with others that one comes to know the self. Thus, authenticity is a foundation of self-knowledge and in this way personal knowledge fuses with interpersonal knowledge (see Chapters 5 and 11).

For nurse educators, developing personal knowledge is far-reaching and includes such matters as sharpening one's intellectual capacity for, and skills with, the act of teaching and becoming aware of the emotions one experiences while teaching. Scholarly work, teaching practice, and reflection, for example, foster the development of personal knowledge. Questions one might ask during such reflections include: What are my physical responses to interchanges with students in clinical settings? During class? In response to questions posed by students during my lectures? Connecting with self and developing intellectual capacity are critical to personal knowledge development.

Interpersonal knowing is about self in relation to others. Like acquiring personal knowledge, acquiring interpersonal knowledge can be enhanced through reflection, dialogue, and formal and informal feedback from students, peers, and colleagues. Educators seeking interpersonal knowledge might reflect on whose voice of authority shapes their teaching decisions. For example, they might ask the following question: In teaching team meetings how do opinions of those in positions of power influence my decisions about teaching? Another kind of interpersonal knowing relates to knowing our students collectively and individually. After conducting a class evaluation, it surprised me to find that some groups of students prefer group work to individual work, while other groups prefer individual work over group work. Acquiring information about particular learning preferences of groups of students is essential to making good decisions related to the fit between preferred learning activities and particular activities offered to that group. Another important aspect of interpersonal knowing occurs when educators are open to learning from students. For example, I came to realize that students in my upper level course brought many rich stories, both personal and professional, to class that could be used to support learning about nursing. Opening spaces for students' stories became opportunities for me to learn about cultural health practices unfamiliar to me such as postnatal rituals that were part of many of the students' worlds.

Closing the loop between personal and interpersonal knowledge, hooks (1994) posits that self-actualized teachers bring excitement, freshness, and passion into a classroom that inspire students to authentic engagement with learning.

TECHNOLOGICAL

Decisions about teaching are shaped by technology-related knowledge and skills that an educator brings to the experience of teaching and learning. Technological knowledge involves knowing what technology is available to support teaching practice, knowing how to use the technology, and knowing the strengths and limitations of technical applications as they pertain to student-centered teaching. As technology develops, new applications become available. For example, a new technology formally called Web Logs (informally referred to as "**blogs**"[3]) is a commonly used Internet-based writing tool that can be adapted as an educational tool for health professionals. Although this technology is seldom used in nursing education (Maag, 2005), this technological application holds potential to support student-centered learning particularly in its focus on connecting personal thoughts to information that is in the public domain.  Simulation technology, that is technology that simulates nursing care situations, for example clinical decision making, is another technological application that has potential to contribute to student-centered learning. Simulation technology provides students with opportunities to work independently and at their own speed. Yet, even though this technology is widely available in nursing education, it is not utilized to its full potential (Medley & Horne, 2005). Acquiring knowledge and skills relative to technological tools for nursing education applications may become increasingly important for student-centered learning as technological applications improve.

AESTHETIC KNOWING

Aesthetic is defined as responsive to, or appreciative of, what is pleasurable to the senses (Merriam-Webster Online, 2005). Attention to the aesthetic has long been a part of knowing in nursing since Nightingale (1860) in *Notes on Nursing* encouraged nurses to be cognizant of the affect of their work on the senses of their patients. To that end, Nightingale encouraged nurses to be aware of the way they moved around their patients' beds and to be cognizant of the noise to which patients were exposed. In a section of *Notes on Nursing*, titled "Patient's repulsion to nurses who rustle," Nightingale writes "A nurse who rustles . . . is the horror of a patient . . . The fidget of silk and of crinoline, the rattling of keys, the creaking of stays and of shoes, will do a patient more harm than all the medicines in the world will do him good" (p. 27). Carper (1978) expands Nightingale's conception of aesthetics in nursing by speaking of aesthetics in terms of the "balance, rhythm, proportion, and unity of what is done" (p. 220). Thus, aesthetics in nursing is derived from both sense-related and the holistic definitions.

Student-centered educators drawing on aesthetic knowing may incorporate learning activities that are pleasing to the students' senses into their teaching. For example, students could be assigned projects that involve writing stories, plays, or poetry. The educator may also reflect on the aesthetic dimensions of his or her teaching practice by considering the aesthetic qualities of the teaching/learning environment.

In this model, these sources of knowledge and ways of knowing form the base for decision making in nursing education. A student-centered nurse educator will base decisions about teaching on an informed understanding of the theoretical foundations of the field, empirical evidence that validates the theoretical ideas and the use of particular teaching strategies, an ever-deepening understanding of ethical and critical knowledge that pertains to nursing practice and education, potential technological applications, and an ever-expanding understanding of the self and the self in relation to others.

---

[3] Blog: A chronological publication of personal thoughts and Web links that is generally a mixture of personal events and what is happening on the Web relative to these events. *Blogs* are also called *Web logs* or *Weblogs*. However, since Web log can also mean a server's log files, blogs is a less confusing term to use when referring to this tool. Retrieved Feb 9, 2005 http://www.marketingterms.com/dictionary/blog/.

Evaluation

Program and curriculum evaluations are organized systematic processes of acquiring and appraising information about a nursing education program and the materials and methods used in its implementation. Such evaluations are designed to determine how the program achieves its goals (Iwasiw, Goldenburg, & Adrusyszyn, 2005). Evaluation can be formal or informal, systematic or occasional, formative or summative. To ensure an accountable and ethical evaluation process, information gathered for appraisal must be transparent and represent all stakeholder groups. Thus, educational units such as schools of nursing are well advised to ensure that some faculty members are well prepared and supported in terms of release time and continuing education to provide leadership for the evaluation process.

FORMAL EVALUATION

All nursing programs conduct evaluations in order to improve effectiveness (Sing, 2004). Curriculum evaluations as part of program evaluation can be internal or external. Internal curriculum evaluations are undertaken by members of the school to surface strengths and weaknesses of the curriculum and to monitor students' learning experiences for the purpose of guiding revisions (Iwasiw, et al., 2005). External curriculum evaluations are part of a wider program evaluation and may be conducted by accreditation bodies. As constructivism underpins Guba and Lincoln's (1989) *Fourth Generation Evaluation*, this approach to program evaluation in nursing education is **ontologically**, epistemologically, and methodologically consistent with how we envision student-centered learning.

Using a *Fourth Generation Evaluation* process, the evaluator understands that:

- Truth is consensus, not something that corresponds with an objective reality.
- Facts have no meaning except in the context of a values framework.
- Accountability implicates all interacting parties equally.

Qualitative methods are used to capture contextual information, uncover what has been hidden by more conventional approaches, reveal social processes such as power relationships, help audiences understand the particulars of situations, and inform the development of quantitative evaluation instruments. Qualitative methods are used to explicate relationships identified using quantitative methods (Guba & Lincoln, 1989). Thus, the evaluator aims to generate an evaluation that all stakeholders coconstruct, that empowers stakeholders equally, that teases out local understandings, and replaces self-importance, overconfidence, and superiority with respect, consideration, and empathy.

Sing (2004) proposes a framework for nursing education program evaluation based on Stufflebeam's (2000) context, inputs, process, and products (CIPP) model. This model holds promise as a framework to be used by constructivist evaluators since it allows for formative and summative evaluation of core nursing education program components: context, inputs, process, and products. Context evaluation elicits information about the fit between the vision of the organization and the program and the capacity of the organization to meet its goals and objectives. A broad question such as, are the mission and program goals being met, guides context evaluation. Input evaluation elicits information about human and other resource allocation and cost-effectiveness. A broad question such as whether the quality and quantity of human resources meet the students' needs, guides input evaluation. Process evaluation elicits information about program implementation and is guided by questions about the extent to which program components were being implemented as planned? Product evaluation identifies and evaluates both intended and unintended program outcomes and may be guided by considering what intended and unintended impacts and outcomes have resulted from this program? A constructivist evaluator works with stakeholders to develop subquestions and related indicators as the evaluation progresses. Further, stakeholders are consulted about sources of data and the best methods for data collection. A constructivist evaluator constructs the final evaluation in consultation with stakeholders to ensure that meanings derived are consistent with the values of the school or faculty of nursing and that the findings are empowering and communicated to stakeholders in respectful ways.

Formal program evaluation undertaken by a school will entail surveys of students and alumni at multiple points and may include asking employers and colleagues of the school's graduates to evaluate student competencies. For example, the University of Washington, School of Nursing, the top-ranked School of Nursing in the United States every year since the first survey was conducted in 1984, evaluates program effectiveness on the basis of critical thinking, nursing therapeutics, and communication ability. Tools that elicit data about demographics, responses to stress, and perceived functional ability of students are administered to students who agree to complete the forms three times across the curriculum: on entry into the program, midpoint, and before graduation.

SCHOOL EVALUATIONS

Schoolwide evaluations of courses and instructors are common practice. Such evaluations elicit feedback from students, employ tools developed by the school or university, are confidential, and are used to strengthen the program. Course evaluations may inform course and curriculum revisions. Instructor evaluations may be used by deans or directors to inform discussions with specific faculty members about aspects of their teaching, and may be used by administrators to determine the best fit between an instructor and course. Course and instructor evaluations are included in a professor's teaching portfolio in institutions that require such documentation for tenure and promotion processes. Feedback derived from the tenure and promotion process is an important influence on an educator's decision making.

OCCASIONAL OR EPISODIC EVALUATIONS

To complement formal evaluations, educators may conduct occasional or episodic evaluations. These formative evaluation strategies may include, but are not limited to, class evaluation, evaluation of a particular teaching strategy, and term or semester evaluations. Class evaluations and teaching strategy evaluations may be as simple as requesting that students indicate what they liked and did not like about a particular class or teaching strategy. However simple such evaluations may be, they provide educators with a means to become better acquainted with student preferences. Term or semester evaluations may be used to better understand students' perceptions of their workload across a term or semester as well as the students' perceptions of the usefulness, relevance, and currency of course readings. Term or semester evaluations may be most useful in planning the sequencing of assignments in a term, provide valuable information about course content, and may inform curriculum design.

An educator may elicit a one-time evaluation of his or her teaching by a peer or colleague. For this kind of evaluation, forms may be available through the university; however, the questions on such forms may not be consistent with a constructivist approach to evaluation. A question that appears on a Peer Evaluation Form for Nurse Educators, available at: http://www.kent.edu/nursing/Faculty/upload/Teaching-Evaluation-Form.doc, exemplifies this. For instance, the question, "did the instructor allow students to ask questions and give opinions?" requires peer evaluators to choose one of three responses: evident, not evident, or not applicable. This kind of evaluation does not elicit the complexities and richness of classroom dynamics to inform the development of the educator. An educator and his or her peer evaluator might prefer to design the evaluation questions together to ensure that the process is empowering and the product can be used to inform decisions about competency development. Like course and instructor evaluations, peer evaluations become part of a professor's teaching portfolio and may be considered in the tenure and promotion process. Further, peer evaluations are a source of knowledge of the self, and the process of accessing a peer evaluation may be a source of interpersonal knowledge that can be used to inform decisions about teaching that an educator must make.

INFORMAL FEEDBACK

Verbal and nonverbal feedback from students and faculty colleagues are an important source of evaluation information for nurse educators. Verbal feedback from students about one's teaching style or particular teaching strategies can be solicited or unsolicited. Educators who elicit verbal feedback from students must be cognizant of the importance of creating a climate in which it is safe for students to do so honestly. While seasoned teachers may readily elicit feedback from students and colleagues about their teaching, novice educators may be too shy or anxious to elicit such feedback. Faculty mentors play an important role in encouraging novice educators to elicit feedback and in supporting them as they reflect on the feedback they have received.

Nonverbal feedback from students can be disturbing or exhilarating, but either way it can point to major factors that influence students' learning and be a bellwether for poignant interpersonal dynamics and issues in a classroom. Examples of nonverbal feedback that are informative include expressions of tension in students when discussing assignments, a student reading a newspaper in class, students acting out during a lecture, or students palpably engaged in a specific learning activity in class or seminar. In November and March, when the halls of nursing schools seem to vibrate with the anxiety of students and faculty who are overtired and overworked, I have become careful about how I use time in class during these stressful periods. For these periods I plan activities that have stress-reducing benefits for students, such as extra time in class to work on group assignments.

Informal feedback from colleagues solicited during discussions about teaching or sought to shed light on a particular issue is another vital source of information. Colleagues' perspectives on the feasibility of a particular teaching activity or strategy, information about excellent articles, books, videos, or other resources, how to best approach a particular student issue, or how to address a troublesome student dilemma or problem, may be invaluable. When discussing particular student matters with colleagues, issues of confidentiality need to be respected and protected. Faculties keen to promote such interchanges will create opportunities for teaching faculty to share ideas and information by organizing think tanks on a specific topic such as mind mapping, or holding special "brown bag" lunch sessions for discussing teaching issues.

Barriers and Facilitators

Decisions about teaching practice are shaped by a multitude of factors that can be barriers or facilitators. By way of highlighting factors at the societal level, the commitment to student-centered learning is a deliberate focus in German higher education. As evidence, German universities charge no tuition fees. This enables access to higher education regardless of a learners' economic status. Further, the credit system in German universities is such that students are empowered to be thoughtful about the choices they make about courses, assignments, and how evaluation of learning will occur. Such societal-level factors play a crucial role in shaping what kind of decisions nurse educators can make. Unfortunately, however, these factors are generally not at a level of consciousness among nurse educators.

Related to societal-level factors are barriers and facilitators that operate at the institutional, curricular, instructional, and faculty levels and which shape approaches to student-centered learning. An example of an institutional barrier is a policy that does not allow students to assign themselves a mark for their work. An example of a curricular barrier in a practice profession such as nursing is evident in the requirement of graduates to have certain professional competencies upon graduation. Thus, curricula in nursing must ensure that graduates meet professional competencies. Curricula then must be designed to serve the interest of the profession rather than the interest of particular students. Student-centered nurse educators work within the tension of meeting the needs of the profession while meeting the needs of students when making decisions about teaching. Instructional factors that play a role in shaping decisions about student-centered learning turn on the availability of resources. Is the time allotted during class adequate to engage students in this way? Are class sizes amenable to student-centered approaches? At the faculty level, decisions about student-centered learning may be affected by colleagues' opinions about such approaches. For example, one educator tells of an occasion in which she used a student-centered approach and was later chastised for doing so by a colleague on the basis that she "wasn't teaching." In contrast, if student-centered approaches are valued in a school and some faculty are champions of such approaches, novice educators may find that they are mentored and encouraged to develop expertise in the use of such methods. And technology may shape how an educator can approach teaching. Barriers and facilitators that operate at a system level are central to the type of decisions faculty make about student-centered teaching (see Chapter 21).

In addition to these factors, learners and the teacher may shape such decisions. Learners may arrive at a student-centered classroom having experienced only traditional teaching methods. Such students may find it distressing and confusing when asked to be active learners. Woods (1994), a prominent PBL scholar, cautions that students new to such methods as PBL may experience stress which could catalyze an iterative cycle of anger and so-called "trigger thoughts." When I introduce PBL to learners, I have found it useful to present to students Woods' model of stress, anger, and trigger thoughts before introducing the method as a strategy of anticipatory guidance. Decisions about how much time to spend in a class on active learning versus passive learning may be a result of an educator's perception of students' comfort level with active learning strategies. At the personal level, educators may espouse a student-centered philosophy but may use teacher-centered approaches in practice (Schaefer & Zygmont, 2003). This suggests that while some nurse educators might like to teach in student-centered ways, they lack skill and knowledge or are faced with seemingly overwhelming barriers such as institutional and departmental constraints, or unfavorable student or peer attitudes to do so.

Critical Reflection and Dialogue

As Brookfield (1995) observes, teaching is not an innocent act:

> *One of the hardest things that teachers have to learn is that the sincerity of their intentions does not guarantee purity of practice. The cultural, psychological, and political complexities of learning and the ways in which power complicates all human relationships (including those between students and teachers) mean that teaching can never be innocent. (p. 1)*

Critical reflection and dialogue as this relates to making decisions about teaching are concerned with exposing the things that are taken for granted that shape relationships of power that influence students' learning. Acquiring an awareness of how relational, emotional, and contextual factors influence teaching-related decisions complements the rational dimensions of decision making, such as those deriving from theoretical or empirical roots. Combining the relational, emotional, and contextual with the rational empowers nurse educators toward making insightful decisions that have potential to achieve the intended goal of placing students at the center of teaching, not teachers and content.

Since power relations are insidious and largely invisible, particularly for women and nurses who have historically been in power-down positions in societies, critical reflection and dialogue on such matters may be awkward at best and unproductive or not welcome at worst. For those unable or unwilling to engage in critical reflection, seeing power dynamics in nursing is like fish seeing the water in which they swim. Thus, many nurse educators may be unaware of power-related issues that influence the teaching/learning experiences in which they are engaged. Further, nurse educators may be unaware of the issue of voice that ubiquitously affects women. This leaves them unable to participate fully in reflective or dialogic strategies that involve using one's inner and outer voices.

The term critical reflection, as it is used in this chapter, involves surfacing and examining the assumptions that inform teaching decisions. Strategies for critical reflection include:

- Articulating in writing, then critiquing, a teaching philosophy.
- Journaling about a learning activity or a poignant moment with a student.
- Reflecting on the meaning of instructor, course evaluations, or peer evaluations.

- Reflecting in writing then deconstructing experiences of the institutional and curricular factors that shape teaching in a particular situation.
- Writing theoretical articles.
- Engaging in empirical research.

Such reflection has potential to deepen understandings of what lies behind the decisions we take as educators and may lead us to sharpen our teaching skills or guide us to acquire new knowledge.

While critical reflection may occur in isolation, Brookfield (1995) and others (Boys, 1999; Burbules, 1993; Friere, 1970) suggest that dialogue plays a role in surfacing and examining assumptions and finding voice. Critical dialogue may occur through engaging students' in reflections about a defining moment related to their learning at the end of a class (Boys), engaging colleagues in critical conversations (Brookfield), and organizing reflection groups in which educators come together to discuss the literature (Brookfield). Burbules, (1993, cited in Boys, 1999) suggests three principles to guide such exchanges:

- Participation is voluntary and characterized by an openness to questions and new ideas.
- Commitment to discussing difficult matters and disclosing personal perspectives.
- Reciprocity in process characterized by mutual respect and concern.

Nurse educators continually make decisions about teaching. In this section, we provided a model for decision making to guide student-centered teaching. The model integrates two divergent approaches to nursing practice and education that are often depicted as mutually exclusive; that is, scientific and reflective (Jones & Graham, 2004). Like Jones and Graham, we believe that a combination of these approaches reflects the actualities of nursing practice and education and has potential to stimulate rich and intellectually rewarding debates.

CASE STUDY: MIND MAPPING

As a graduate student, I[4] was introduced to the technique of mind mapping as a way of organizing my thinking in preparation to write a term paper. Intrigued by its possibilities, I set out to use it as an educator in a continuing education program. My journey is presented here as a case to illustrate the model described in Figure 2.2.

A mind map is a weblike diagram (Figure 2.3) that provides a visual display of an individual's ideas and thoughts about a given topic area. The intent of mind mapping is to help individuals learn, recall, organize, and make information meaningful. Mind maps are subjective because they represent how an individual interprets a particular topic, making the maps ideal for individualized learning. The emphasis of mind mapping is placed on the understanding and linking of ideas, as opposed to memorization. In the context of teaching, mind mapping is an effective strategy for visual learners to organize their ideas (e.g., note taking and studying), to engage in reflection and dialogue, to summarize their thinking (e.g., care planning or course presentation), or

[4] The first-person "I" is that of author Angela Wolff.

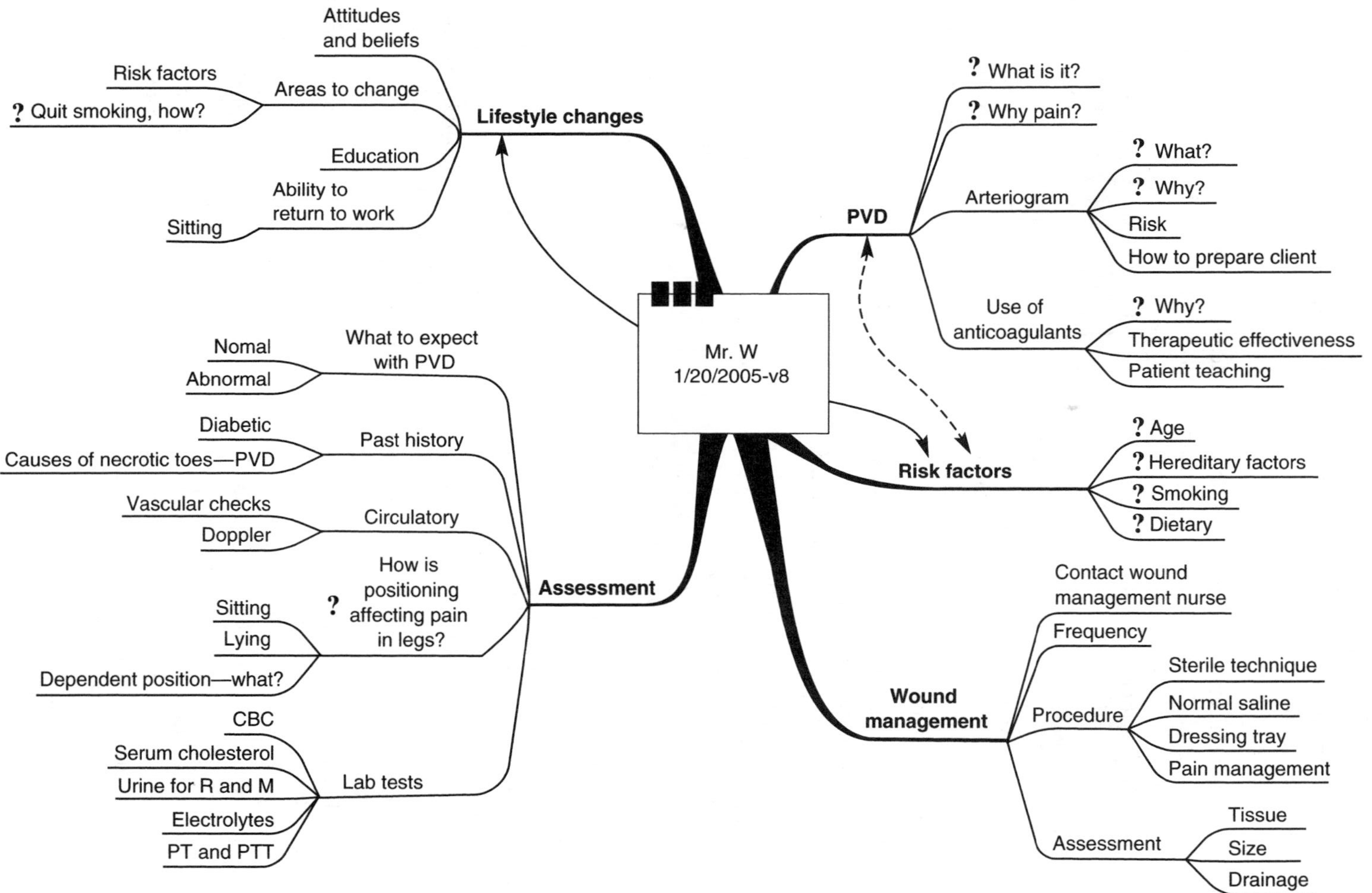

■ **FIGURE 2.2** Mind mapping model.

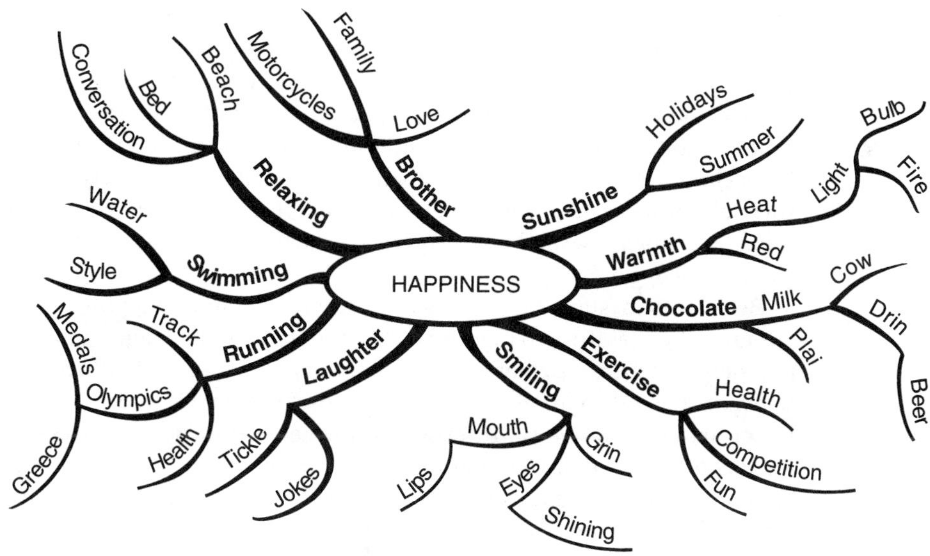

■ **FIGURE 2.3** Mind map.

brainstorm in small group learning situations (e.g., problem-based learning; for more information see Chapter 10). This technique focuses on the students' learning and builds on the prior knowledge of the learner (Buzan & Buzan, 1998). Sensing a fit between my thought process and this cognitive technique I sought to find out more. My first source of information was from the gurus of mind mapping, Tony and Barry Buzan. Reading about mind mapping heightened my understanding of this learning technique from cognitive sciences perspectives (e.g., psychology, neurophysiology, semantics, neurolinguistics, creative thinking, and information theory). While I continued to reflect upon my personal use of the technique, it was not until I was teaching a group of second-year nursing students that I incorporated mind mapping into my classroom practice as an educator. Initially I used mind mapping with this group of students to brainstorm around a case study regarding peripheral vascular disease (see Figure 2.2). Because I was familiar with the technique, I took on the role of facilitating the students' discussion and drawing the mind map on the whiteboard. On a separate piece of paper one student copied verbatim the map that I drew so that I could then photocopy the map for each group member. As the students generated hypotheses and identified issues, we created a mind map that was reflective of the students' thinking. Upon completing the map, each student identified learning gaps, prioritized their learning needs, established learning goals, and identified possible resources to utilize for self-study. I sought formal and informal feedback from the students regarding the utility of this learning technique. After successfully using this teaching strategy in my learning and with this group of students, I continued to integrate it into my teaching in different contexts using student feedback to guide implementation (e.g., students in various stages of the nursing program and in both the classroom and the clinical setting). Later on in my career, I had the opportunity to create a workshop for nurse educators about mind mapping. In preparing for this event, and in keeping with my professional standards to interpret and use current evidence to make education decisions (RNABC, 2003), I decided to move beyond the use of my episodic formal evaluations of this strategy to a more rigorous examination of the literature. Prior to this, my decisions about the use of mind mapping in teaching were shaped through the theoretical, personal, interpersonal, and aesthetic ways of knowing. In attempting to make judgments of and decisions about the use of mind mapping I revisited the theoretical knowledge and gathered the published empirical knowledge.

Because no systematic reviews exist regarding mind mapping, I sought to critically appraise the literature to identify current practices and examine theoretical ambiguity and debate. One particular area of ambiguity previously identified was the difference between a mind map and a **concept map** (Figures 2.4 and 2.5). In conducting my literature review (e.g., Internet resources, nursing databases, and education databases) more than 50 citations were located with regards to cognitive mapping techniques used in education, nursing, psychology, and other health related disciplines. To answer my questions I selected 27 of the 50 articles, which were anecdotal, descriptive, and empirical in nature. During the review process, various terms were used in reference to mapping strategies, such as mind mapping, concept mapping, cognitive mapping, creative graphing, clustering, webbing, correlation mapping, and knowledge mapping. Although the terms were similar in that they all represented some type of visual teaching strategy, no operational definition of such terms existed. In comparing and critiquing the references pertaining to the various mapping strategies two main terms emerged: mind mapping and concept mapping. While both mind mapping and concept mapping visually represent one's thinking about an idea

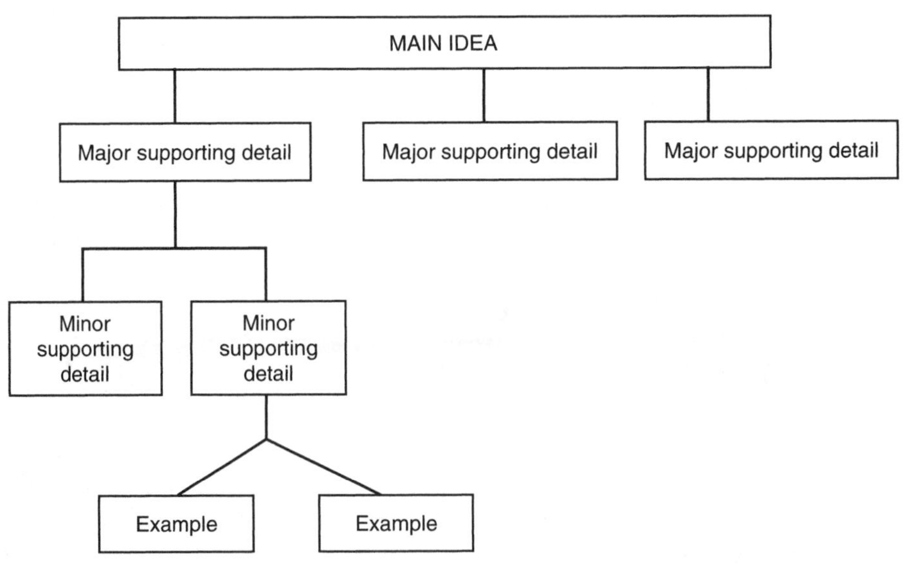

■ **FIGURE 2.4** Concept map.

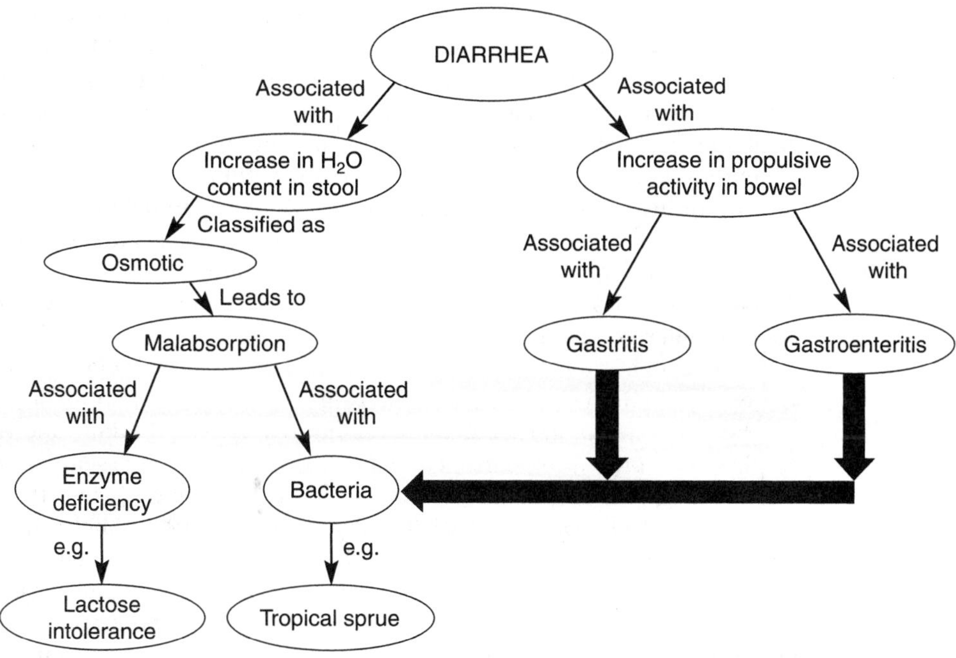

■ **FIGURE 2.5** Concept map.

or concept and share some of the same underlying assumptions, they differ in multiple ways.[5]

To determine the effectiveness of using mind mapping in nursing education I reviewed various sources of evidence generated from both empirical and interpretative modes of inquiry. The findings from five nursing studies (Caelli, 1998; Daley, 1996; Daley, Shaw, Balistrieri, Glasenapp, & Piacentine, 1999; Nortridge, Bayeux, Anderson, & Bell, 1992; Rooda, 1994) and two education studies (McCagg & Dansereau, 1991; Schmidt & Telaro, 1990) indicated that mind mapping was an effective strategy in terms of supporting the development of students' performance, conceptual thinking, critical thinking, comprehension, and overall learning. Some longitudinal studies have supported these findings. At the same time, faculty evaluations about the use of mind mapping with students report benefits in facilitating learning, improving comprehension, and assessing thinking processes.

[5] First, mind mapping is a "big picture" representation of a body of information or ideas, and not solely a particular concept as in concept mapping. Mind mapping is more reflective of brainstorming or a burst of thought with ideas coming from multiple directions. Instead of encouraging random thinking about a given situation, concept mapping provides a more top-down hierarchical and linear display of the concepts of interest. While both mapping techniques represent the learner's grasp of the information, the focus shifts from explaining a concept as opposed to encouraging divergent thinking among learners and enhancing recall and retention. Second, the mind mapping technique follows some guiding principles that are adapted to your personal style, whereas concept mapping can be more specific with clear links/associations made between concepts and propositions. Visually it is easier to distinguish between a concept map and a mind map; theoretically they both may be providing a means to the same end.

Depending on the degree to which a teacher wishes to implement this teaching strategy, the decision-making model (see Figure 2.1) depicts that different barriers or facilitators may be encountered. Implementing mind mapping into my teaching I encountered few barriers. The curriculum was flexible enough to allow for variation among faculty in teaching style and by role modeling the strategy to the student they begin to adopt the technique. As with any new teaching strategy, one should be cognizant of the time factor involved in introducing it and the students' initial hesitancy and anxiety toward new strategies. Several nurse educators have published descriptions of how to introduce mind mapping to students in ways that create a learning environment conducive to adult learning (Buzan & Buzan, 1998; Leauby & Brazing, 1998; Michelini, 2000; Mueller, Johnston, & Bligh, 2001).

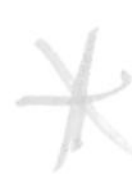

Reviewing the literature, I learned that mind mapping is an effective way to help people learn by building on the prior knowledge of the learner, to promote the natural way in which the human brain functions, to improve critical thinking and recall while deemphasizing rote learning, to encourage active learning that is self-paced, and to create a stimulating environment conducive to learning (Buzan & Buzan, 1998; Daley, 1996; Daley, et al., 1999; Dobbin, 2001; Leauby & Brazing; 1998; Michelini, 2000; Phillips, 1994). To validate these claims and to substantiate my decision about using mind mapping as a teaching strategy, both the scientific and reflective approaches to nursing education were used. On a personal level, when using mind mapping, my recall of information improved and my thinking became more critical and integrated. Informal feedback from my colleagues indicated that mind mapping was a useful way to teach and learn, to create a composite sketch of the groups' thoughts, and to evaluate student learning. In my experiences as a teacher, the learners gave positive indications toward the utility of mind mapping. Knowledge gained from these experiences, combined with the theoretical and empirical knowledge published in the literature solidified my decision to continue to use this strategy with learners. As I apply mind mapping in different contexts, gather forthcoming knowledge, and engage in reflection and dialogue I will continue to draw conclusions about the appropriateness of mind mapping as a best practice in student-centered teaching.

SUMMARY

This chapter outlines some of the complex and often overwhelming issues that relate to the evaluation of student-centered teaching and emphasizes the need to move beyond basing teaching decisions on conjecture, past experience, precedence, and personal preference to basing it on evidence and its congruence with a constructivist perspective. However, student-centered teaching has as yet a weak evidence base that does not exist within nursing education. If, as we have suggested, student-centered teaching is difficult to evaluate in a way that provides evidence to support or discount the efficacy of various student-centered teaching approaches, what are the implications of this for future directions in research about student-centered teaching and what are the implications for the future of nursing education?

The central tenet of evidence-based student-centered teaching is that educators' practices must be based on good quality evidence (Hale & Raven, 2000). Systematic reviews of published literature are one way to determine what evidence is of the appropriate quality to be applied as best practice in student-centered teaching. Unfortunately, few such published reviews exist within the nursing literature and the findings of the few evaluative studies that have been conducted in this area are not consolidated. The potential contributions of systematic reviews are illustrated in the work by Nairn, Jardy, Paramal, and Williams (2004) regarding how to assist students to become culturally sensitive in a constructivist approach. In a detailed analysis of the relevant literature, they uncovered a philosophical debate between antiracism and multiculturalism as the central tenets of such teaching in nursing education. They argue that these ethical stances represent divergent ways of conceptualizing cultural sensitivity and that the multiculturalist stance preferred by nurse educators does not sufficiently address the critical issue of racism within nursing practice. These authors point to the largely descriptive nature of research in this area and to the paucity of studies that provide definitive evaluative evidence to suggest that there needs to be research that evaluates the outcomes of student-centered teaching strategies to promote cultural sensitivity. They also suggest that there needs to be research conducted about the efficacy of specific teaching strategies to promote ethically-congruent student behaviors.

Ideally, if systematic reviews do not exist in an area of interest, we should be able to determine the evidence to support student-centered teaching through a critical appraisal of the literature to identify current practices, as well as areas of theoretical ambiguity and debate that are apparent within the field (Nairn, et al., 2004). However, as Nairn et al. illustrate, this is at times an unrewarding undertaking that only adds to the confusion about which teaching approaches work best, when, for what students, and in which settings. Because the notion of evidence-based nursing education has only recently received worldwide attention, there have been few attempts within the literature to define the body of evidence in particular areas of student-centered teaching. For example, we located only anecdotal evidence in the literature about what it means to provide a safe environment for students to participate as partners in the teaching–learning process, and even fewer that actually addressed how to facilitate such an environment. A related concern is that nurse educators often publish descriptions of student-centered strategies they have used but rarely provide formal evaluative data. In addition, there is a paucity of replication studies in nursing literature about student-centered teaching; therefore, it is difficult to determine if the strategy would be effective in another setting with another teacher and other students.

There is a need for more funding venues for research that specifically addresses the evaluation of student-centered teaching strategies, including qualitative meta-syntheses and quantitative meta-analyses. In the early years of nursing academia, research focused on nursing education. This focus has changed sharply over the years toward clinical research (Yoder-Wise, 2000). In the interim, the development of student-centered teaching has created the need for research that determines the effectiveness of specific teaching strategies.

Because most health research funding agencies have preferred clinical to education research in their funding agendas, education research within nursing has been poorly funded. Consequently, nurse researchers have tended to select topics for study that are clinically-based rather than nursing education related. Nurses must conduct more research in this area, as well as develop creative ways to disseminate the research findings across institutions and countries. However, without lobbying efforts aimed at research funding agencies to increase support for such research such evidence will not be forthcoming. Action, therefore, is needed.

As discussed above, one source of evidence for what constitutes effective student-centered teaching in nursing is the experience of other educators applied in different contexts and judged to be effective. This is difficult in the current climate of clinical nursing education where nurse educators have limited opportunities to share with and learn from one another. Although working as coteachers in a classroom setting is a common experience, in clinical teaching the norm is that clinical teachers work as part-time sessional faculty who interact with other faculty only occasionally. It seems unlikely, therefore, that there will be a comprehensive evidence base for student-centered teaching in the clinical setting if the model of educators working in isolation from each other persists.

It is readily apparent that the evidence that exists in relation to student-centered teaching is insufficient to base decisions about student-centered teaching approaches. This evidence-practice gap has many implications for nurse educators, particularly those who are beginning teachers who have not yet developed the capacity to use and generate the evidence they need to determine what teaching strategies are most efficacious, in which settings, and for what students. Nurse educators who are unable to provide the evidence for self-evaluation skills vis-à-vis their teaching practices will be tempted to embrace new teaching approaches and to discard familiar teaching practices with equal abandon.

There is a need to develop an "evaluative culture" (Thomson, Angus, & Scott, 2000, p. 164) within nursing education that establishes the evidence basis of student-centered teaching as the norm for teaching decisions. This will mean that nurse educators must learn the skills of seeking appropriate evidence to support their teaching decisions, communicate this evidence to other educators within the educational institution, and perhaps within the profession, apply it in their teaching, and assess its application and outcomes (Thomson, et al.). It will entail support for nurse educators in terms of education, as well as time and other resources, such as access to a mentor, in order for them to be able to locate, assess, apply, disseminate, and monitor evidence in their teaching. Developing an evidence base that is experiential and shared between nurse educators is only possible if educators are able to discuss their teaching practices openly and in an environment that encourages reflective thinking and critical analysis. Such reflection takes time and energy, as well as trust that one's experience and opinions will be valued. Nurse educators who work in educational programs that provide little space to reflect on one's teaching practices, and those that are characterized by competition, distrust, and negativity are often unable to engage in such reflective thought (Freshwater & Stickley, 2004).

The picture we have painted about the nature of evidence in student-centered teaching is not a bright one. There is a need for further dialogue, debate, and formal research study focused on strengthening the evidence base of student-centered teaching. However, there is a light at the end of the tunnel. Recently, there have been several articles that have addressed the evidence-practice gap in nursing education (e.g., Hale & Raven,

2000; Thomson, et al., 2000). In addition, there has been recognition in some countries such as the United Kingdom that in order for nursing education programs to demonstrate to accreditation bodies that they have evidence to support what they do well and which areas require improvement, there is a need for an evidence base in student-centered teaching (McSherry & Marland, 1999). This book represents an attempt to contribute to this goal. These new developments herald a heightened awareness for the need for evidence-based student-centered teaching and a commitment to generating, applying, and disseminating such evidence in nursing education. We await the continued developments in this area with excited anticipation.

LEARNING ACTIVITY

Identify a student-centered teaching strategy such as reflective journaling. Search for research studies that generate knowledge about the strategy you have selected.

1. Note the search engines used for your search.
2. Note the key words used.
3. Note the number of relevant articles that you identified using these strategies.
4. Select one research study from your search that stands out for you.
5. Critique the study using a framework that is relevant to the methodology of the study.
6. Delineate how this study might inform your decision to apply this strategy in your teaching practice.
7. In class time, work in pairs to review the searches, critiques and next steps. (Allow about 40 to 60 minutes of class time for this exercise.)
8. Once you have received input on your work, reflect on what you learned from sharing your work with a classmate. Write a short summary of this learning.
9. Submit your search strategy, a copy of the article selected, your critique of the research, your next steps, and the summary of what you learned during the pair/share exercise. Submit to your instructor as part of the course requirements.

RESOURCES FOR EDUCATORS

PLANNING THE TEACHING/LEARNING EXPERIENCE

Questions to Support a Thoughtful Reading

1. In your previous teaching experiences, what decision-making processes have you used?
2. How did this decision-making process resonate with your decision making in nursing practice?
3. In this chapter the authors make the claim that decision making in nursing education can be a reasoned process. Think of an occasion in which you were a learner and the reasoning process underpinning the learning experience was apparent to you.

Tips for Developing a Student-Centered Learning Environment

- Plan an active learning lecture to introduce the model for evidence-based teaching drawing on ideas about active lecturing presented in Chapter 12.
- At the conclusion of the class in which you introduce the decision-making model described in this chapter, ask the students to evaluate your teaching. At the beginning of the next class, provide an overview of the evaluative comments submitted, and indicate how you will use the students' feedback to shape your teaching.

EVALUATING THE TEACHING/LEARNING EXPERIENCE

Reflective Questions for Educators

1. How did your presentation of materials stimulate student involvement? Reflect in writing on the level of involvement of one student or one student group, then critically question what you have written.
2. Did students raise questions that inspired you to think more deeply about the model presented in this chapter?
3. Reflect on your experience with active lecturing. How would you revise the questions used? Your timing?
4. What other student-centered methods might you use to present the model?
5. What is your physical response to active lecturing?

References

Auvinen, J., Suominen, T., Leino-Kilpi, H., & Helkama, K. (2004). The development of moral judgment during nursing education in Finland. *Nurse Education Today, 24*, 538–546.

Bacharach, S. B. (1989).Organizational theories: Some criteria for evaluation. *Academy of Management Review, 14*, 496–515.

Bandura, A. (1977). *Social learning theory*. Englewood Cliffs, N.J.: Prentice-Hall.

Banister, E. M., & Schreiber, R. (1999). Teaching feminist group process within a nursing curriculum. *Journal of Nursing Education, 38*, 72–76.

Baxter, S., & Gray, C. (2001). The application of student-centered learning approaches to clinical education. *International Journal of Language and Communication Dialogue, 36*, 396–400.

Bennett, N. (1976). *Teaching styles and pupil progress*. London: Open Books.

Bergum, V. (2003). Relational pedagogy: Embodiment, improvisation, and interdependence. *Nursing Philosophy, 4*, 121–128.

Bevis, E. O., & Watson, J. (1989). *Toward a new curriculum: A new pedagogy for nursing*. New York: NLN.

Bjorklund, P. (2004). Invisibility, moral knowledge and nursing work in the writings of Joan Liaschenko and Patricia Rodney. *Nursing Ethics, 11*, 110–121.

Borgman, A. (1992). *Crossing the post-modern divide*. Chicago: The University of Chicago Press.

Boys, M. (1999). Engaged pedagogy: Dialogue and critical reflection. *Teaching Theology and Religion, 3*. Retrieved October 15, 2005, from http://www.prs-ltsn.leeds.ac.uk/relig_studies/reviews/ttr2/ttr2_3_1999_boys.html.

Brookfield, S. (1995). *Becoming a critically reflective teacher*. San Francisco: Jossey-Bass.

Burbules, N. C. (1993). *Dialogue in teaching: Theory and practice*. New York: Teachers College Press.

Burnard, P. (2005). Reflections on reflection. *Nurse Education Today, 25*, 85–86.

Buzan, T., & Buzan, B. (1998). *The mind map book*. London: BBC Books.

Caelli, K. (1998). Shared understanding: Negotiating the meaning of health via concept mapping. *Nurse Education Today, 18*, 317–321.

Carper, B. (1978). Fundamental ways of knowing in nursing. *Advances in Nursing Science, 1*, 13–23.

Carr, D. (2000). *Professionalism and ethics in teaching*. London: Taylor & Francis.

Carr, D. (2003). *Making sense of education*. London: Routledge Falmer.

Chase, C. C., & Gledenhuys, K. M. (2001). Student-centered teaching in a large heterogeneous class. *Medical Education, 35*, 1071.

Chinn, P. (2001). Peace and power: Building communities for the future, (5th ed.). Boston: Jones & Bartlett.

Cohen, A. M., Stavri, P. Z., & Hersh, W. R. (2004). A categorization and analysis of the criticisms of Evidence-Based Medicine. *International Journal of Medical Informatics, 73*, 35–43.

Corcoran-Perry, S. A., Narayan, S. M., & Cochrane, S. (1999). Coronary care nurses' clinical decision making. *Nursing & Health Sciences, 1*, 49–61.

Daley, B. J. (1996). Concept maps: Linking nursing theory to clinical nursing practice. *Journal of Continuing Education in Nursing, 27*, 17–27.

Daley, B. J., Shaw, C. R., Balistrieri, T., Glasenapp, K., & Piacentine, L. (1999). Concept maps: A strategy to teach and evaluate critical thinking. *Journal of Nursing Education, 38*, 42–47.

Dewey, J. (1916/1997). *Democracy and education*. New York: Simon & Schuster.

Doane, G. (2004). Being an ethical practitioner: The embodiment of mind, emotion, and action. In J. Storch, P. Rodney, & R. Starzomski (Eds.). *Toward a moral horizon: Nursing ethics for leadership and practice* (pp. 433–446). Toronto, ON: Prentice Hall.

Dobbin, K. R. (2001). Applying learning theories to develop teaching strategies for the critical care nurse. *Critical Care Nursing Clinics in North America, 13*, 1–11.

Fahy, K. (2002). Reflecting on practice to theorise empowerment for women: Using Foucault's concepts. *Australian Journal of Midwifery, 15*, 5–13.

Falk-Rafael, A. R., Chinn, P. L., Anderson, M. A., Laschinger, H., & Rubotzky, A. (2004). The effectiveness of feminist pedagogy in empowering a community of learners. *Journal of Nursing Education, 43*, 107–115.

Fawcett, J., Watson, J., Neuman, B., Walker, P. H., & Fitzpatrick, J. J. (2001). On nursing theories and evidence. *Journal of Nursing Scholarship, 33*, 115–119.

Freshwater, D., & Stickley, T. (2004). The heart of the art: Emotional intelligence in nurse education. *Nursing Inquiry, 11*, 91–98.

Friere, P. (1970). *Pedagogy of the oppressed.* New York: Seabury.

Gaines, C. (1999). Clearing up the "concept fog." *ABNF Journal, 10*, 52–53.

Glew, R. (1994). Student-centered curriculum teaches more than pathophysiology. *Journal of the American Medical Association, 272*(9), 743.

Guba, E. G. & Lincoln, Y. (1989). *Fourth generation evaluation*. Newbury Park,CA: Sage.

Hale, C., & Raven, K. (2000). Evidence-based education: A vision for the future? *Clinical Effectiveness in Nursing, 4*, 1–2.

Hargreaves, J. (2004). So how do you feel about that? Assessing reflective practice. *Nurse Education Today, 24*, 196–201.

hooks, b. (1994). *Teaching to transgress. Education as the practice of freedom*. New York: Routledge.

Howe, A. (2001). Patient centered medicine through student-centered teaching: a student perspective on the key impacts of community-based learning in undergraduate medical education. *Medical Education, 35*, 666–672.

Iwasiw, C., Goldenburg, D. F., & Andrusyszyn, M. A. (2005). *Curriculm development in nursing education*. Toronto, On: Jones & Bartlett.

Jones, P. C., & Graham, L. (2004). Learning and teaching for evidence-based and reflective practice. In P. Smith, T. James, M. Lorentzon, & R. Pope (Eds.). *Shaping the facts: Evidence based nursing and health care* (pp. 197–218). Toronto, ON: Churchill Livingstone.

Kuiper, R. A., & Pesut, D. J. (2004). Promoting cognitive and metacognitive reflective reasoning skills in nursing practice: Self-regulated learning theory. *Advanced Nursing, 45*, 381–391.

Lamond, D., & Thompson, C. (2000). Intuition and analysis in decision making and choice. *Journal of Nursing Scholarship, 32*, 411–414.

Leauby, B. A., & Brazing, P. (1998). Concept mapping: Potential uses in accounting education. *Journal of Accounting Education, 16*, 123–138.

Lee, W. M., Wong, F. K., & Mok, E. S. (2004). Problem-based learning: An ancient Chinese educational philosophy reflected in a modern educational methodology. *Nurse Education Today, 24*, 136–144.

Maag, M. (2005). The potential use of "blogs" in nursing education. *Computers, Informatics, Nursing, 23*, 16–24.

Maeda Allman, K. K. (1992). Race, racism, and health: Examining the "natural" facts. In J. Thompson, D. Allen, & L. Rodrigues-Fisher (Eds.). *Critique, resistance, and action: Working papers in the politics of nursing*. New York: NLN Press (Pub.No. 14-2504).

McCagg, E. C., & Dansereau, D. F. (1991). A convergent paradigm for examine knowledge mapping as a learning strategy. *Journal of Educational Research, 84*, 317–324.

McPherson, G., Rodney, P., McDonald, M., et al. (2004). Working with the landscape: Applications in health care ethics. In J. Storch, P. Rodney, & R. Starzomski (Eds.). *Toward a moral horizon: Nursing ethics for leadership and practice* (pp. 98–125). Toronto, ON: Prentice Hall.

McSherry, W., & Marland, G. (1999). Student discontinuations: Is the system failing? *Nurse Education Today, 19*, 578–585.

Medley, C. F., & Horne, C. (2005). Using simulation technology for undergraduate nursing education. *Journal of Nursing Education, 44*, 31–34.

Merriam-Webster Online Dictionary. Retrieved October 17, 2005, from http://www.m-w.com.

Michelini, C. A. (2000). Mind map: A new way to teach patients and staff. *Home Healthcare Nurse, 18*, 318–322.

Mueller, A., Johnston, M., & Bligh, D. (2001). Mind-mapped care plans: A remarkable alternative to traditional nursing care plans. *Nurse Educator, 26*, 75–80.

Nairn, S., Jardy, C., Paramal, L., et al. (2004). Multicultural or anti-racist teaching in nurse education: A critical appraisal. *Nurse Education Today, 24*, 188–195.

Narayan, S. M., & Corcoran-Perry, S. (1997). Line of reasoning as a representation of nurses' clinical decision making. *Research in Nursing & Health, 20*, 353–364.

Nelms, T. P., & Lane, E. B. (1999). Women's ways of knowing in nursing and critical thinking. *Journal of Professional Nursing, 15*, 179–186.

Nightingale, F. (1860). *Notes on nursing: What it is, and what it is not.* New York: D. Appleton and Company. [First American Edition] Retrieved October 17, 2005 from http://digital.library.upenn.edu/women/nightingale/nursing/nursing.html.

Nortridge, J. A., Bayeux, V., Anderson, S. J., et al. (1992). The use of cognitive style mapping as a predictor for academic success of first semester diploma nursing students. *Journal of Nursing Education, 31*, 352–356.

Novak, J. D., & Gowin, D. B. (1984). *Learning how to learn.* New York: Cambridge University Press.

Peters, R. (1966). *Ethics and education.* London: George Allen and Unwin.

Phillips, L. D. (1994). Teaching intravenous therapy using innovative strategies. *Journal of Intravenous Nursing, 17*, 40–50.

Pierson, W. (1999). Considering the nature of intersubjectivity within professional nursing. *Journal of Advanced Nursing*, 30, 294–302.

Polanyi, M. (1962). *Personal knowledge.* London: Routledge & Kegan Paul.

Registered Nurses Association of British Columbia [RNABC]. (2003). *Standards for registered nursing practice in British Columbia.* Vancouver, BC: Author.

Rideout, E. (2001). *Transforming nursing education through problem-based learning.* Sudbury, MA: Jones & Bartlett.

Rodney, P., Pauly, B., & Burgess, M. (2004). Our theoretical landscape: Complementary approaches to healthy care ethics. In J. Storch, P. Rodney, & R. Starzomski (Eds.). *Toward a moral horizon: Nursing ethics for leadership and practice* (pp. 77–97). Toronto, ON: Prentice Hall.

Rooda, L. A. (1994). Effects of mind mapping on student achievement in a nursing research course. *Nurse Educator, 19*(6), 25–27.

Ruth-Sahd L. A. (2003). Reflective practice: a critical analysis of data-based studies and implications for nursing education. *Journal of Nursing Education, 42*, 488–497.

Schaefer, K. M., & Zygmont, D. (2003). Analyzing the teaching style of nursing faculty. Does it promote a student-centered or teacher-centered learning environment? *Nursing Education Perspectives,* 24(5):238–245.

Schmidt, R. F., & Telaro, G. (1990). Concept mapping as an instructional strategy for high school biology. *Journal of Educational Research, 84*, 78–85.

Silva, M. C., Sorrell, J. M., & Sorrell, C. D. (1995). From Carper's patterns of knowing to ways of being: An ontological philosophical shift in nursing. *Advances in Nursing Science, 18*, 1–13.

Sing, M. D. (2004). Evaluation Framework for Nursing Education Programs: Application of the CIPP Model. *International Journal of Nursing Education Scholarship, 1*, Article 13.

Spivak, G. C. (1990). *The post-colonial critic: Interview, strategies, dialogues.* New York: Routledge.

Stufflebeam, D. L. (2000). The CIPP model for evaluation: An update, a review of the model's development, a checklist to guide implementation. Paper presented at 2003 Annual Conference Oregon Program Evaluators Network (OPEN), Portland, Oregon.

Thomson, P., Angus, N. J., & Scott, J. (2000). Building a framework for getting evidence into critical care education and practice. *Intensive and Critical Care Nursing, 16*, 164–174.

Ward, W. D., & Barcher, P. R. (1975). Reading achievement and creativity as related to open classroom experience. *Journal of Educational Psychology, 67*, 683–691.

Weick, K. E. (1995). What theory is *not*, theorizing *is*. *Administrative Science Quarterly, 40*, 385–390.

Wheeler, L. A., & Collins, S. K. (2003). The influence of concept mapping on critical thinking in baccalaureate nursing students. *Journal of Professional Nursing, 19*, 339–346.

Wilkes, L., Cooper, K., Lewin, J., & Batts, J. (1999). Concept mapping: Promoting science learning in BN learners in Australia. *Journal of Continuing Education in Nursing, 30*, 37–44.

Williams, P., & Chrisman, L. (Eds.). (1994). *Colonial discourse and post-colonial theory: A reader*. New York: Columbia University Press.

Woods, D. (1994). Problem-based learning: Helping your students to gain the most from PBL. McMaster University, ON: Woods.

Yoder-Wise, P. S. (2000). Changing practice based on evidence: Changing education too. *Journal of Continuing Education in Nursing, 31*, 198.

Young, L. (2002). Transforming health promotion practice: Moving toward holistic care. In L. Young & V. Hayes (Eds.). *Transforming health promotion practice: Concepts, issues, and applications* (pp. 3–21). Philadelphia: F. A. Davis.

Additional Resources

- Chism, N. (1999). *Peer review of teaching: A sourcebook*. Bolton, MA: Anker.
- Hutchings, P. (1996). *Making teaching community property: A menu for peer collaboration and peer review*. Washington, DC: American Association for Higher Learning.
- Millis, B. (1992). Conducting effective peer classroom observations. In D. Wulff & J. Nyquist. (Eds.), *To Improve the Academy* (pp. 189-201). Stillwater, OK: New Forums Press.
- Peer evaluation of Teaching Form. Available at http://www.temple.edu/cst/forms/peer_evaluation_form.doc. Last accessed on October 20, 2005.
- Sample nursing program evaluation. Available at: http://www.son.washington.edu/students/bsn_eval_program.asp. Last accessed October 20, 2005.

Chapter 3

Perspectives on Teaching: Discovering BIASes

Daniel D. Pratt
Barbara L. Paterson

Discussions of teaching often center around the style of teaching that is the best to effect student-centered teaching. Some nurse educators argue that the best way to teach nursing students is to nurture and "mother" them. Others believe that the most effective way is to have clearly defined expectations of skill performance and to require students to practice skills "until they get it right." Still others believe that students and teachers should be equal partners in the teaching and learning process, codeterminers of what occurs in the learning arena. Novice teachers are often confused and frustrated by such debates. They look to their more experienced colleagues for advice about teaching and are dismayed when there seems to be no consistent message.

INTENT

In this chapter, nurse educators are encouraged to consider five variations on what student-centered means in teaching through the lens of teaching **BIAS**es. Each variation is discussed in terms of **B**eliefs, **I**ntentions, **A**ctions, and **S**trategies for teaching and learning. The authors argue that nurse educators may want to reflect upon their own BIASes and, in conversation with colleagues, discuss the means by which different philosophical views of teaching can be not only student centered but also more effective across variations in personal style, philosophy, and venues for teaching and learning.

OVERVIEW

INTRODUCTION

Nursing today is increasingly pluralistic and critical in its practice and its scholarship. Effective nursing requires a critically reflective stance and an unwillingness to accept ideas or practices on authority alone or to slavishly follow the status quo. Nurses today are expected to look for the unasked questions and challenge existing patterns of thought and practice by exposing the assumptions, values, and biases that underlie them. In many ways, nursing scholarship stands as an example for other health professions in the provision of rigorous critique in order that ineffective practices and oppressive processes may be challenged and alternatives established (Holmes, 2002).

This same critical reflection is part and parcel of most nursing education programs. It is common practice across North America to have nursing students use a variety of reflective techniques as a way of deconstructing practices that are taken for granted to promote deeper understanding of the underlying theories, philosophies, and ideologies that guide their reasoning. Yet, how many teachers apply the same critical reflection to their pedagogy? Do nurse educators do what they require of their students; that is, critically reflect on the philosophical, theoretical, and political assumptions and beliefs that guide their pedagogical practices? And, more to the point, how might nurse educators reflect with a degree of critical rigor on what it means to be student centered in their teaching? Is there, for example, a dominant or predetermined view of teaching implied in the phrase student centered? Or is there more than one acceptable view of teaching that might reasonably be called student centered? These are the questions that will be addressed by this chapter as we look for defensible variations on the theme of student-centered teaching in nursing education.

UNVEILING OUR BIASES

In 1971, Gramsci observed that:

> *The starting point of critical elaboration is the consciousness of what one really is, and is "knowing thyself" as a product of the historical process to date which has deposited in you an infinity of traces without leaving any inventory.* (cited in Clark, 1999, p. 324)

The central theme of Gramsci's quote is that we must start by knowing ourselves. Not only must we know ourselves, but we must also be critically sensitive to the fact that we are a product of forces beyond our own agency. We are, in effect, a combination of things, some of which we are only marginally (if at all) aware. For example, all nurses come to the practice of teaching with certain biases. Some biases are of their own making; others have been assimilated from their training and upbringing. In any case, they teach from those biases, whether they want to or not. And, of course, some biases are more student centered than others.

For over 20 years, one of the authors has been exploring the way teachers of adults, including nurse educators, go about their work. He and his students have observed the teaching and explored the thinking of hundreds of teachers, trying to understand teaching from their point of view. They started their research in Canada, but soon expanded to include several other countries (Pratt, 1992; Pratt & Associates, 1998). Across a wide range of people, disciplines, and contexts they found that teachers vary on four dimensions that are called teaching BIASes:

B – **BELIEFS** about learners, about the process of learning, about the content or skills to be learned, and about the role and responsibilities of a teacher;

I – **INTENTIONS** as to what learners are to learn or what the person teaching them is trying to accomplish;

A – **ACTIONS** or ways in which the teacher enacts the role of teacher using techniques and methods in particular ways to help people learn;

S – **STRATEGIES** or ways in which a teacher combines beliefs, intentions, and actions into strategic thinking and decision making.

Although approaches to teaching are, in part, a unique reflection of the person, the researchers did not find hundreds of different BIASes. Instead, they found a great deal of commonality across the hundreds of teachers they studied. In all, there were only five significantly different sets of BIASes. Each set of BIASes defined a different philosophical perspective on teaching; that is, a qualitatively different set of beliefs, intentions, actions, and strategies. The five perspectives are: transmission, developmental, apprenticeship, nurturing, and social reform.

These findings are not unique; they correspond to the findings of many other researchers around the world whose work spans 20 years and several countries. In reviewing most of that research, Kember (1997) found a surprisingly high level of correspondence across time, context, and disciplines. What is important here is to recognize that no single perspective dominated in its potential for being effective teaching. This notion of a plurality of effective teaching is important for two reasons: first, because it supports a basic tenet of Gramsci's quote and of this chapter—to be an effective teacher, you must know yourself—your values, strengths, weaknesses and what you stand for; and second, because it means we must be open to a plurality of views and approaches to effective teaching—some of which are more student centered than others.

Thus, nurse educators have a responsibility, in proportion to their level of understanding, to reflect not only on their professional knowledge and skill, but also on the BIASes that guide their pedagogical practice. Reflecting on what one brings to teaching, then categorizing the reflections according to the BIAS schema is a first step in making visible the invisible inventory of which Gramsci speaks and central to a responsible teaching practice. For if we teach who we are, and if our BIASes are deeply embedded in the soul and body of our being, then it is our responsibility to unveil those BIASes and subject them to the light of critical reflection.

PERSPECTIVES ON TEACHING

A **perspective on teaching** is a lens through which we view our work as educators. We may not be aware of our own perspective because it is something we look through, rather than at, when teaching. It is a way of being in relation to the content, the learners, and the work we do as teachers. Each perspective represents a different way of thinking about adults as learners, the process of learning, the content to be learned, and the context within which learning and teaching are to take place.

Each perspective is a unique blend of BIASes; yet there is overlap between them. Similar actions, intentions, and even beliefs can be found in more than one perspective. Educators holding different perspectives may, for example, have similar beliefs about the importance of critical thinking in the preparation of learners for professional practice. To this end, all of them may espouse the use of case studies and thought-provoking questions as a means of promoting critical thinking. However, the way they use case studies, or ask questions, and the way in which they listen and respond when learners consider those cases or questions, will vary considerably across perspectives. These variations are directly related to underlying beliefs and strategies about how best to help people learn critical thinking.

What follows is a brief overview of the five perspectives and their respective BIASes. The descriptions vary in length based on how important each perspective is within nursing education and how much that view might reasonably be called student centered. Perspectives that are more relevant to nursing because of their clinical practice element (e.g., apprenticeship) are given greater detailed explanation and description.

Transmission Perspective

The transmission perspective is a common orientation to teaching in higher education and much of nursing education, including the clinical years. From a **transmission perspective**, effective teaching is dependent on thorough mastery of one's content or subject matter. From this perspective, the nurse educator's primary responsibility is to demonstrate professional skill and dispense professional knowledge accurately and efficiently. Learners, in turn, are responsible for learning a well defined corpus of skills and knowledge in its authorized form; that is, in ways that resemble the teacher's ways of knowing and doing. Box 3.1 contains a summary of underlying BIASes and common difficulties associated with a transmission perspective on teaching

For many readers, negative examples of transmission-oriented teachers might be the first to come to mind. For example, you may recall teachers who were little more than talking heads. Such teachers, whether they were teaching students or patients, taught as if their only role was to disseminate information. There is little evidence to support dissemination-only strategies if the goal is to be student centered and thereby improve professional practice. As a result, the talking-head approach to teaching has been discredited in much of nursing education, especially in clinical and community

BOX 3.1 TRANSMISSION PERSPECTIVE

KEY BELIEFS

- Content should be learned in its authorized form.
- Teachers should be experts in the content area.
- Teachers should present that content accurately and efficiently.
- The process of learning is additive, which means that teachers should take care not to overload students with too much information.
- With proper delivery by the teacher, and appropriate receptivity by the learner, knowledge can be transferred from the teacher to the learner.

PRIMARY INTENTIONS

- Cover a certain amount of content efficiently.
- Transfer professional knowledge to students.
- Present information not otherwise available.
- Clarify or elaborate on information in the text.
- Exemplify ways of talking about practices.
- Enthuse students about an aspect or area of practice.

COMMON ACTIONS

- Planning:
  - Be thoroughly prepared.
  - Specify clear objectives.
  - Organize content for presentation.
  - Schedule teaching time to cover content.
- Delivery:
  - Present in clear and organized fashion.
  - Differentiate between right and wrong ways of knowing and doing.
  - Provide clear structure and sequence of learning tasks.
  - Answer questions directly and clearly.
  - Correct errors immediately.
  - Make efficient use of instructional time.
  - Provide reviews and summaries.
- Assessment:
  - Set standards for achievement.
  - Develop objective means of assessment.
  - Provide corrective feedback early.
  - Provide summary of strengths and weaknesses.
  - Locate learner within hierarchy of knowledge or competence.

TYPICAL STRATEGIES

- Assume a common/shared starting place for a group of learners.
- Pace instruction so as to not overload learner's memory/capacity.

■ BOX 3.1 Transmission Perspective (continued)

- Gear one's teaching to the mid-to-high end of the learning group.
- Vary the pace of delivery to accommodate high and low ends of the group.
- Assess students in relation to a body of knowledge.
- Use feedback to point out errors of understanding or application.

COMMON DIFFICULTIES

- Tendencies to:
  - Equate talking (lecturing) with teaching.
  - See every student response as an opportunity to talk some more.
  - Focus feedback on what is wrong, rather than what is right or good.
- Working with people who have difficulty with the content or its logic.
- Anticipating where and why learners might have difficulty with content.
- Remembering what it was like to not know this material.
- Thinking that their way of understanding is the best way or the only way.

practice settings. At the same time, many of us have positive memories of transmission-oriented educators who were passionate about their content, animated in its delivery, and determined that we go away with respect and enthusiasm for their subject. They took us systematically through a set of tasks and procedures that led to mastery of the content. They were clear and enthusiastic about their content and conveyed that enthusiasm to their students. They also engaged us, intellectually and emotionally, challenging us to think, to defend, and to question that which they delivered with such apparent ease. They were, in many instances, virtuoso performers of their knowledge or expertise. Such individuals may have inspired us to take up a particular specialty because their deep respect and enthusiasm for what they did was infectious. It is the memory of those educators that must be preserved if we are to see transmission as a potentially legitimate perspective in the stable of student-centered approaches to nursing education.

Developmental Perspective

Many student-centered approaches to nursing education are based on a view of learning (and teaching) that is called constructivism. (See Chapter 1 for a full discussion of constructivism.) The fundamental principle of constructivism is that learning is a search for meaning based on what one already knows. Therefore, prior knowledge is a main ingredient in the processes of both learning and of teaching. The developmental perspective on teaching is deeply rooted in constructivism. From a **developmental perspective**, effective teaching must be planned and conducted from the learner's point of view. Effective teachers, therefore, must understand their learners' prior understanding of the content, entry levels of skill, and attitudinal predispositions.

The primary goal of this perspective is to help learners develop increasingly sophisticated ways of thinking and reasoning. The key to changing learners from naïve to sophisticated ways of thinking lies in a teacher's ability to:

1. Engage learners with the content through questions, problems, or cases that challenge the inadequacy of naïve reasoning and thinking.
2. Use bridging knowledge, often in the form of examples, metaphors, stories, or other easily accessible renderings of content, to help learners link their prior knowledge to new, more complex, and sophisticated forms of reasoning and problem solving.
3. Withhold answers to allow learners time to come to their own understanding.
4. Develop forms of assessment that do not undermine these strategies.

Within this perspective, a critical component of effective teaching is the adaptation of a teacher's knowledge to the students' experience and ways of understanding. In other words, cognitively speaking, the teacher goes to the learners, rather than requiring students to come to the teacher. This is in sharp contrast to the transmission perspective on teaching. Box 3.2 contains a summary of underlying BIASes and common difficulties associated with a developmental perspective on teaching.

While this may be the quintessential student-centered perspective on teaching, it is not easy to teach from this perspective, especially if one has been trained under a different perspective. For example, those who have trained within a transmission perspective and are now expected to teach from a developmental perspective may have difficulty knowing what to do with their professional knowledge when facilitating small group problem-based learning (PBL) tutorials. Within the developmental perspective teachers are to bracket; that is, withhold their experience and professional knowledge rather than answering students' questions and presenting their knowledge. Facilitators are to probe the students' reasoning and offer what if propositions. They are to reposition their professional knowledge, not as information and answers but as metaphors, examples, puzzles, problems, questions, and challenges that will guide student thinking toward better reasoning. Because one's professional identity is intimately tied to professional knowledge, this shift is even more difficult.

In a developmental orientation, learners and their teachers must be cognitively active and engaged. Students are actively engaged when they are inquiring and problem solving; teachers are actively engaged when they ask good questions, the kind of questions that require time to think and to reason before answering. And after asking a question, teachers are active when they listen patiently, bracketing their own knowledge while waiting for students to think through and to voice their understanding. Teachers are active when they listen closely to the forms of reasoning that students use as they negotiate understanding through an open discussion. In tutorial groups it is difficult to refrain from telling students what we know and shortening their path to an answer. However, doing so only puts them back into a passive cognitive role, expecting that we will give them answers, rather than letting them figure it out for themselves.

The central commitment to the learners' level of knowledge/skill as a starting point is laudable. However, the progression from espousing to enacting the developmental perspective involves much more than a repertoire of techniques for engaging learners in problems and discussion. It also means that educators must use their knowledge and

BOX 3.2 DEVELOPMENTAL PERSPECTIVE

KEY BELIEFS

- Learning is a search for meaning.
- Learners search through association.
- Prior knowledge influences the search.
- Less (coverage) can be more (understanding).
- It is the teacher's responsibility to adapt his or her professional knowledge to the learners.
- The desired outcome is more complex reasoning strategies.
- Students' perception of assessment will influence their approach to learning.

PRIMARY INTENTIONS

- Develop deeper understanding of content.
- Differentiation in problem analysis.
- Ability to solve unfamiliar problems.
- Foster better, more complex forms of reasoning.

COMMON ACTIONS

- Engage learners through use of cases, problems, or questions.
- Start with what learners already know.
- Link new material to learner's prior knowledge.
- Allow sufficient time for learners to develop understanding.
- Foster horizontal discussion exchanges between learners.
- Withhold correct answers while students explore their own reasoning and thinking.
- Challenge reasoning behind learner's responses.
- Correct misconceptions as necessary.

TYPICAL STRATEGIES

- Start with the learner's point of view.
- Activate students' prior knowledge.
- Adapt expertise/knowledge to the learners' level.
- Use bridging knowledge to link learners' knowledge with teacher's knowledge (for example, through stories, metaphors, illustrations, or real examples).
- Introduce new ways of thinking through problems or cases.
- Provide more questions than answers.
- Let students construct their own understanding.
- Challenge students' ways of understanding.
- Involve students in setting evaluation/assessment.
- Keep assessment consistent with learning tasks.

COMMON DIFFICULTIES

- Asking higher-level questions.
- Allowing time to let learners figure it out.
- Constructing helpful bridges to students' experience.
- Developing learning and assessment tasks that are congruent.

expertise in ways that do not undermine the goal of helping learners actively construct their own forms of understanding, usually in the company of other students. Indeed, from this perspective, sometimes less (telling) means more (learning).

Apprenticeship Perspective

This view of teaching is as old as nursing itself. Yet, it may be the least understood and the most easily dismissed, simply for its title. Indeed, the title may have connotations that are negative, in which case prior learning might interfere with reading about this perspective. Even though the title elicits such mixed reactions, the perspective is central to nursing education and it will be given more elaboration than other perspectives. We invite you to set prior notions of apprenticeship aside as you consider what the apprenticeship perspective on teaching means, particularly in the context of clinical teaching.

Most nurse educators have apprenticed under a range of preceptors and mentors. Some of those were marvelous teachers, modeling the best of nursing practice and allowing access to their experiential knowledge. They provided guidance as learners' progressed toward becoming competent, independent, skillful practitioners. There were others that kept students in fear and virtual servitude as they worked long hours with little appreciation, waiting for the chance to move on to a different clinical experience. It is the former we wish to describe as representative of effective **apprenticeship perspective**. As we learn more about why so little classroom instruction transfers to clinical settings, the apprenticeship perspective becomes increasingly meaningful. This perspective on teaching rejects any notion of learning that views cognition solely as "an inner realm richly populated with internal tokens that stand for external objects and states of affairs" (Clark, 1999, p. 347). Rather, this view assumes that learning is both an individual cognitive process and a collective social process. Learning, therefore, is facilitated when students work on authentic tasks in real settings of application or practice and alongside other, more experienced, practitioners.

In nursing education, this is one of the most common and important forms of training. Yet, it is fraught with difficulty because it is often misunderstood. How often have we heard someone say, "I was so busy today that I didn't have time to teach?" Embedded in this statement is an assumption that teaching is done in the time when we stop clinical practice to talk or teach. Then when the teaching is done, we return to work. This separation of work, learning, and teaching is antithetical to the apprenticeship perspective where both teaching and learning are embedded in the doing of work, not just in talking about it.

Within this perspective effective teaching is more than demonstrating and having learners observe our skillful practice. It is as well, a process of acculturating students into a set of social norms and into a professional identity. From this point of view, educators must be experienced and highly skilled practitioners of what their students are to learn. In fact, they are usually selected to teach precisely because of their expertise and experience.

However, as they make the transition from working as a skilled practitioner to teaching about skilled practice, their experience and expertise must be rendered in forms that are accessible and meaningful to novices. What they used to do without thinking, they must now do with thought as to how it is perceived and understood by those watching and/or participating. As they work, skillful clinicians must translate their work into steps and language that help learners understand not only the skill of doing, but also the inner workings of "what is going on here." In effect, they must articulate the embodied knowledge of skillful performance.

At the same time, effective apprenticeship teachers realize that the context is a powerful teacher. Even in the most hurried moments of clinical work, students are witness to the decisive movement and reasoning of experienced clinicians, filtered through the chaos of activity and coupled with the subtle negotiation of authority and privilege. As they watch, they learn. As with children in a family, they learn by example more than by words. And they leave with impressions of what it means to be a nurse in relation to a host of other workers. They learn, for example, how to deal with conflict, how to avoid difficulties, how to negotiate with different levels of authority, and how to multitask under varying conditions of stress. All of this is part of learning an identity as well as a set of competencies and much of it can only be learned in the work place. Thus, the context is a powerful teacher, whether we want it to be or not. That is precisely why we put students in clinical placements.

While students are in clinical placements, it is the teacher's responsibility to decide what they can and cannot do and how to engage them in meaningful work and learning. Vygotsky (1978) argues that much of the work of teaching is a matter of engaging learners' within their **zone of proximal development**, the learning space that falls between what they can do on their own and that which they can do with expert guidance. It is here, in the zone of proximal development, that learning and teaching become student centered, rather than teacher centered. As learners mature and become more competent, their zones of proximal development move and the teacher's role changes. Learners are still assigned tasks based on their level of maturity and skill development. But over time, apprenticeship teachers offer less direction and give more responsibility as their students progress from being dependent learners to becoming independent workers. Box 3.3 contains a brief summary of the essential BIASes and difficulties that characterize student-centered teaching from this perspective.

The apprenticeship perspective is highly congruent with clinical teaching. However, as learning shifts from classroom to clinical arena, complications abound. In clinical settings, the nature of what is to be learned and the role of the teacher are integral to the work and the context of work. More than any other venue for learning, within clinical settings, the role of the teacher must shift dramatically. As Gaberson and Oermann (1999) observe, in clinical learning, teaching is not telling, it is not dispensing information, and it is not merely demonstrating skills. Instead, if clinical teaching is to be student centered, it must involve the student as an active and legitimate participant in the work. However, this does not negate the importance of explanations, even in a busy and chaotic clinical setting.

In clinical settings, explanations are an integral part of providing health care. Nurses need to be able to explain to patients, families, peers, and others what they are going to do, why that is necessary or reasonable, and how they have arrived at these decisions. However, one explanation will not work for all situations. A patient's condition might have to be explained to colleagues, professionals from other fields, students that are just

BOX 3.3 APPRENTICESHIP PERSPECTIVE

KEY BELIEFS

- Learning is a process of socialization into a community of work.
- Knowledge is embedded in social relations (e.g., between coworkers).
- Learners know socially before they know cognitively.
- Knowledge is best learned in the contexts in which it is to be used.
- The product of learning is of two kinds:
  - Competence or skilled performance.
  - Professional identity and values.
- An authentic work context is the best teacher.

PRIMARY INTENTIONS

- Train for competent and safe practice.
- Link theory and practice.
- Model how to work in the real world.
- Bring novices into a community of work.

COMMON ACTIONS

- Orient student to work schedule and other staff members.
- Clarify performance expectations.
- Provide meaningful work/engagement from the first day.
- Ask for student's assessment and reasoning.
- Provide positive feedback as well as corrective feedback.
- Schedule time for one-on-one teaching.
- Model and demonstrate competent practice.

TYPICAL STRATEGIES

- Identify the learner's zone of proximal development.
- Provide tasks that are within their zone of proximal development.
- Fade direction and feedback based on learner's progress and maturity.
- Let students see strategic thinking and moments of uncertainty.
- Model appropriate ways of working with others.
- Use context as a teacher.
- Assess learning based on standards of the community of practice.

COMMON DIFFICULTIES

- Finding relevant and authentic tasks if doing classroom instruction.
- Matching the learner's capability with legitimate tasks.
- Putting one's craft, knowledge, or skill into words.
- Finding ways to do the work while also engaging the learner.
- Getting bogged down teaching between tasks.

beginning a clinical placement, and/or the patient and family. This range of explanatory skill is not part of professional training; it comes with time and experience.

A further complication arises when trying to explain not only how to do a procedure but how to think about it while doing it. As Donald Schön (1983) observed:

> *When we go about the spontaneous, intuitive performance of the actions of everyday life, we show ourselves to be knowledgeable in a special way. Often we cannot say what it is that we know. When we try to describe it we find ourselves at a loss, or we produce descriptions that are obviously inappropriate. Our knowing is ordinarily tacit, implicit in our patterns of actions and in our feel for the stuff with which we are dealing. It seems right to say that our knowing is in our action. (p. 49)*

Much of what experienced nurses do is performed with intuitive knowing that Schon and others call **tacit knowledge** or craft knowledge. Such knowledge is a blend of quick recognition of patterns, scripts that are familiar and well-honed patterns of response. Thus, the knowledge that students need is embedded in routines that are performed with a degree of automatic skilled execution. No longer is it necessary for the experienced nurse to be quite so deliberate as it was in earlier, novice stages of working and learning. Earlier deliberations and procedures that were foreign have become familiar, fluid, semiautomatic, and skilled performances that are embodied within a way of being as well as a way of working. That, which appears to be so seamless and done with such ease and efficiency, now needs to be taken apart, unwoven, before it can be rewoven by the newest member of the community, the learner.

Putting such embodied knowledge into words is difficult. As a result, for many nurses, the shift from nursing practice to clinical teaching is difficult. They often say, "I know what to do; but it's difficult telling others how I do it." This is most evident in nurses that have extended experience working in situations that require complex reasoning. The longer we have been doing complex tasks, the more routine the tasks become. The more routine they are, the less we need to articulate what we do; we just do it. Yet, that is precisely what learners need, namely someone who can reveal the inner workings of skilled performance.

Teaching from this perspective is also complicated by competing demands between work and learning. This issue is often framed in terms of teaching versus service, where teaching finds no place within the context of accountability. In nursing education, there will always be a tension between education and service. However, to frame it as a question of balance or of trade-off is to miss the underlying premise of this perspective; that is, education and service should be one and the same thing. There should be no separation between the pedagogical curriculum of education and the work curriculum of service. Swenson and Sims (2003) illustrate one way of not separating practice and teaching through their study of a narrative curriculum that focuses on dialogues that shape practice. They also illustrate the seamless and intimate bond that ties teaching to clinical practice when both are viewed as lived experiences in a clinical setting. From this perspective, it is a false dichotomy to assume that teaching takes place when work stops. There is no way to stop teaching because there is no way to stop students from observing us in the midst of work.

From an apprenticeship perspective, the work curriculum can teach far more than can be stated in the pedagogical curriculum. When we lose sight of this, for example when substituting simulated patients for real patients, we risk losing the context as a teacher. We seem to know this but do not quite make the best of it; this is evidenced by the extent to which we place students in contexts of work, but have them watch far too long before having them authentically engaged in the work we do. Moments of prolonged observation outside the legitimate boundaries of work are far from student centered. Thus, apprenticeship is a commonly espoused perspective, but one in which it is uncommon to find truly effective student-centered teaching.

Nurturing Perspective

The perspective that is most often associated with the caring ethic of nursing is the **nurturing perspective**. This perspective assumes that longterm, hard, and persistent efforts to achieve come from the heart, not the head. Within this view, people are motivated and become productive learners when they are working on issues or problems without fear of failure. Learners are therefore nurtured by the knowledge that:

- Achievement is within their reach.
- Achievement is a product of their own effort and ability, rather than the benevolence of an educator.
- Their efforts to learn will be supported by their teacher and their peers.

It is a guiding premise that the more there is pressure to achieve, and the more difficult the material to be learned, the more important it is that there be cognitive and emotional support for learners. Student centeredness, therefore, implies a positioning of the whole student, heart and mind, at the core of the educational enterprise.

Effective nurturing perspective teachers care deeply about their students as learners but they are also sensitive to other obligations, roles, and responsibilities that may preoccupy students. They strive to help students succeed with approaches to teaching that focus more often on relationships than on technique. Nurturing educators believe there is an important relationship between self-esteem, confidence, and learning. As a consequence, they pay close attention to effort as well as achievement when providing feedback and support.

Yet, it would be a mistake to think that effective nurturing perspective teachers are "soft" and easily manipulated by students. They make no excuses for learners. Rather, they encourage significant effort by challenging students to do the best they can. To do this, nurturing educators promote a climate of caring and trust, helping people set challenging but achievable goals, and supporting learners' efforts as well as their achievements. Effective nurturing perspective teachers provide encouragement and support, along with clear expectations and reasonable goals for all learners. Box 3.4 contains a brief summary of the essential BIASes and difficulties that characterize a nurturing perspective on student-centered teaching.

Although nurturing is the most common perspective among nurse educators, it is not unusual to find colleagues who do not value this orientation to teaching. The name,

BOX 3.4 NURTURING PERSPECTIVE

KEY BELIEFS
- Learning is both a cognitive and an affective process.
- Knowledge (knowing) and emotion (feeling) are interactive.
- When anxiety is raised too high, learning is seriously impaired.
- Threats to a learner's self-esteem interfere with learning.
- High level of demand must be matched with a high level of support.
- Teaching requires a balance between caring and challenging.

PRIMARY INTENTIONS
- Build learners' self-confidence and self-efficacy.
- Encourage learners to challenge themselves.
- Promote a supportive learning environment.
- Do not harm or reduce learners' self-esteem.
- Build confidence while guiding students through content.
- Promote success in learning.
- Challenge ideas, while caring about people.
- Foster a climate of trust and respect.

COMMON ACTIONS
- Listen and respond to emotional needs.
- Provide encouragement and support.
- Encourage expressions of feeling.
- Reinforce effort as well as achievement.

TYPICAL STRATEGIES
- Get to know people as more than students.
- Balance challenges with support.
- Encourage collaborative approaches to learning and achievement.
- Promote positive interdependence with individual accountability.
- Involve students in designing learning contracts.
- Encourage students to engage in self-evaluation.

COMMON DIFFICULTIES
- Providing feedback to those who are failing.
- Setting boundaries between teaching and counseling.
- Defending to others that nurturing is a part of teaching.
- Finding a good balance between challenge and caring.
- Wanting (too much) to be liked.

nurturing may suggest a less than rigorous approach and lower standards. Yet, for those who are most exemplary of this perspective, there is no less rigor and no lowering of standards. There is instead a matching of high standards with high support. Teachers with a nurturing perspective make reasonable demands and set high expectations for their learners, while providing an equal amount of emotional and intellectual support. Caring does not necessarily negate high expectations. For effective nurturing educators, the primary goal is helping people to achieve and to realize that their achievements are the result of their own effort and ability. These are the keys to developing student self-efficacy. From this perspective, these are also the essential attributes of student-centered teaching for lifelong learning. Because of this, these educators are never willing to sacrifice self-efficacy on the altar of academic achievement.

Some may wonder whether this is a viable student-centered perspective within the competitive world of nursing education. After all, the achievement bar is increasingly raised for entry to nursing such that those who are admitted will do well regardless of what their teachers do. This may be true, yet we know the stress and fatigue that accompanies much of nursing education and clinical experiences. Even the most advanced learners are often pushed to the limits of their ability to cope, sometimes suffering under the additional stress and fatigue of a particularly demanding clinical assignment. These stresses are made all the more potent when a student is trying to balance personal and professional obligations. In other words, these people bring to their learning needs which go beyond the intellectual and which reach into the personal and emotional realms of self. It is here that the nurturing perspective is vital. Nursing educators who exemplify a nurturing perspective take on a role that focuses on removing barriers or blocks to student learning. With a bright, highly motivated group of students, there is less need to direct learning. As a result, these teachers can focus more on removing obstacles and providing supportive and safe environments for learning. Indeed, their motto might well be: *Students may forget what you said, but they will never forget how you made them feel.* In combination with one or more of the other perspectives, this can be a powerful and effective student-centered orientation to teaching.

Social Reform Perspective

Social reform is the most difficult perspective to describe because it is rare and challenges many norms of practice that are taken for granted. In the initial research, (Pratt, 1992) researchers found social reform educators in community development, Native education, AIDS awareness, Mothers Against Drunk Driving, the civil rights movement, environmental education, women's health, labor union education, religious education, and even within such established occupations and professions as automotive repair, nursing, and medical education (Pratt & Associates, 1998). In every instance, the social reform educator was a leader, a rebel, or both. As rare as it is, when this teaching is effective, it is unforgettable and disproportionately powerful in its influence on learning. For that reason alone, it is worth drawing your attention to the BIASes and difficulties of a social reform perspective on student-centered teaching in nursing.

From a **social reform perspective**, effective teaching is intended to change nursing practice and/or society in substantive ways, while also educating students to be competent practicing nurses. However, it is the collective, rather than the individual, that is the object of social reform teaching. Thus, student centeredness here means awakening students to the values and ideologies that lie hidden in the texts and common practices in nursing. Teachers challenge the status quo and encourage students to consider the ways in which they and their patients are positioned and constructed within particular discourses and nursing practices. Texts are interrogated for what is said, what is not said, what is included and what is excluded, and how each actor is represented in the dominant discourses within nursing or within health care more broadly. The purpose of encouraging students to take this critical stance is to give them power to take social action to improve the practice of nursing. However, critical deconstruction, though central to this view, is not an end in itself. Box 3.5 contains a brief outline of the specific BIASes and difficulties that characterize this most unusual, but potentially critical perspective on student-centered teaching.

Readers may wonder whether this is a viable perspective in a book on student-centered nursing education. We would argue that it is not only viable, but essential. Nursing education both shapes and is shaped by the practices that are taught. From a social reform perspective, nurse educators either reproduce the status quo or they work to change it. But in either case, nurse educators must be critically aware of their complicity in the ongoing struggle for empowerment and social justice within nursing education and nursing practices.

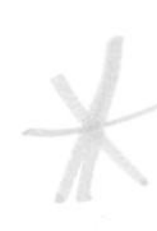

Social reform educators are student centered when they make the familiar strange and ask awkward questions. For example, Diekelmann, Ironside, and Harlow (2003) ask their readers to consider the following questions: How do teacher-centered pedagogies reproduce unproductive and unhealthy power relationships within nursing? Should caregivers have power and control over patients the way teachers have power and control over students? How does what (and how) we teach influence both the skills obtained by students and the way they think about their practice? This example, based on feminist critical theory, asks students to look carefully at taken-for-granted pedagogies and ways of practicing nursing that may reproduce inequities or inappropriate power relations. By foregrounding such issues social reform educators expose various forms of oppression in nursing education, illuminating just how the personal is political in the practice of nursing and in nursing education (McEldowney, 2003). The social reform perspective shifts the focus of intended change (through learning) away from the individual learner and redirects it toward the social and professional structures and practices in which the student will be working. This does not mean they are any less student centered, only that their focus changes to embrace professional competence and nursing identities as they are nested within larger social structures.

Nurse educators who embody the social reform perspective are few and far between. But those who do are likely to have left a lasting impression on us. We may have had an educator that caused us to question things we took for granted, about ourselves or about society-at-large. It may have been the first critical theory course we took; or a feminist educator we knew; or a spiritual leader that caused us to rethink our deepest assumptions and convictions. In any case, such teachers are usually unforgettable.

BOX 3.5 SOCIAL REFORM PERSPECTIVE

KEY BELIEFS

- The knowledge that guides professional practice is saturated with ideals and values.
- Those ideals and values must be examined and raised to question.
- Knowledge should not be adopted without critical examination of underlying values.
- Learning to think critically arises from a state of disequilibrium.
- An important aspect of training is to liberate individuals and change society. The goal of education is not just to learn about the world but to change it.

PRIMARY INTENTIONS

- Challenge students to look more deeply at that which they take for granted.
- Make the process of critical thinking transparent, rigorous, passionate and personal.
- Develop both cognitive and political insight into the nature of professional practice.
- Be consistent in representing the desired ideals, in words and actions.
- Clarify the relationship between ideology, ideals, and goals within training.
- Justify and defend desired ideals and goals against challenges.
- Look at the familiar in new ways and to give students a critical view.

COMMON ACTIONS

- Draw out what people think, believe, or know in relation to the ideals.
- Direct teaching toward the learner as a representative of social structures.
- Develop awareness of political and ideological aspects of content.
- Integrate ideals and content with the lives of the learners.
- Base assessment on moving individuals toward commitment and action.

TYPICAL STRATEGIES

- Focus on the norms and discourses rather than individual behavior.
- Deconstruct literature and professional practices that perpetuate a "wrong."
- Critique dominant values regarding power and privilege in the profession.
- Raise to question that which is familiar and taken-for-granted.
- Review current taken-for-granted practices and policies.
- Explain how such practices perpetuate a wrong.
- Link the problematic practices/policies with the desired goals or ideals.
- Have students construct solutions or courses of action to redress that which is perceived to be inappropriate or wrong.

COMMON DIFFICULTIES

- Accommodating those who just want to learn content.
- Accepting those who object to the teacher's ideals.
- Having patience with learners who assume content to be value neutral.
- Dealing with those who want to maintain the status quo.

PERSPECTIVES, TECHNIQUES, AND STYLES OF TEACHING

We must add a caution at this point: It is common for people to confuse perspectives on teaching with methods or techniques and with styles of teaching. Most books on teaching, whether in nursing or in adult and higher education generally, are about methods and techniques of teaching—the tools of teaching. Perspectives are not the same as techniques or tools. Perspectives are the philosophical orientation you bring to those tools. Your perspective influences what tools you use, how you use them, and how you reflect on the success of their use.

It is also common to hear people confuse perspectives on teaching with styles of teaching. Teaching style, as we are using it, is the personal dimension of teaching; it is the unique expression of your person in the role of teacher. If Palmer (1998) is right when he says that we teach who we are, then the first rule of teaching ought to read: be yourself. To neglect our personal style, by taking on some other role or persona, is to jeopardize our authenticity and thus our effectiveness as a teacher.

Ultimately, effective teachers seek harmony between all three—perspective, style, and technique. Harmony comes from reflection on the relationship and fit between our personal style, our philosophical perspectives, and the tools we use as teachers. When we reach the stage of expert teacher, we will have moved from scripted technical knowledge to embodied craft knowledge in how we respond to familiar and unfamiliar circumstances. Craft knowledge means the tools are no longer separate from us; they have been adapted to our personal style and have become part and parcel of our perspective on teaching.

DISCOVERING YOUR PERSPECTIVE ON TEACHING

How might you discover your perspective(s) on teaching? The Teaching Perspectives Inventory (TPI) is freely available at: www.TeachingPerspectives.com. It takes about 15 minutes to complete the inventory and submit your results. Results are then displayed in graphic form, showing how you score on each of the five perspectives. It also shows which of the perspective(s) most characterize your views of teaching. As of 2005, over 35,000 educators from more than 100 countries have taken the TPI.

Although everyone has some of each of the five perspectives within them, people do not equally value all five perspectives. Indeed, 90% of those who have taken the TPI show a single perspective as their preferred or dominant perspective and two others as backup perspectives. Holding both a dominant and one or two backup perspectives affords a measure of flexibility as people shift between venues of teaching.

IMPLICATIONS FOR NURSE EDUCATORS

Embedded within each perspective are underlying assumptions and ways of thinking about student-centered learning and instruction. The variations on the theme of student-centered teaching are based on different beliefs about means and ends, including what constitutes knowledge, effective practice, student learning, professional competence, and identity as a nurse. As with philosophies of life, different approaches to student-centered teaching are neither good nor bad; they are simply different orientations to being in relation to learners and the aims we wish to accomplish through student-centered instruction. It is important, therefore, to remember that each perspective represents a different, but legitimate view of student-centered teaching and specific purposes to be served through that teaching. Although some perspectives seem more congruent with the underlying aims of student-centered teaching, it is the plurality of views on student-centered teaching that we wish to emphasize. Collectively, they suggest how nurse educators might reflect more critically on their own views of student-centered teaching and learning.

Note that respecting a plurality of views does not mean that any and all views of student-centered teaching are acceptable or defensible. That would be neither intellectually honest nor professionally helpful. If reflection is to be rigorous we must avoid the extreme of anything goes. Equally important, if we are to acknowledge and respect a plurality of views on student-centered teaching, we must also avoid the opposite notion that one size fits all.

At the same time we must acknowledge that some views are likely to be more effective and student centered in some venues than in others. Educational venues that are largely didactic (e.g., lecture halls) are different in pace, purpose, and process from small group tutorials. And clinical venues for teaching are different yet again, because they are nested within a context of accountability that often determines when and how educators and learners can interact. Each educational venue—didactic, tutorial, and clinical—will have an influence on appropriate ways of teaching. To acknowledge that there is more than one acceptable view of student-centered teaching and that some perspectives are best suited to one venue rather than another is essential if nurse educators are to engage in authentic and critical reflection on their teaching across such varied landscapes of learning.

Although the various perspectives on teaching are informed by different orientations to the theme of student centered, they converge in their focus on improving learning and ultimately nursing practice. We believe that it is only through critical reflection that we can peer behind the veil of student-centered teaching and ask ourselves what it means, what ends are served by such a view, why those ends are justified and what variations are acceptable in pursuit of those ends. By thoughtfully revisiting assumptions and beliefs that support student-centered teaching, preconceived notions of effective teaching can be challenged as nurse educators are asked to consider effective for whom and for what? In every case, it is important to remember that any perspective on student-centered teaching can be wonderful or dreadful, depending upon the quality of its implementation and our readiness to embrace its underlying BIASes.

SUMMARY

A perspective on teaching is an interrelated set of beliefs, intentions, actions, and strategies (BIASes) that gives direction and justification to teaching. It is a personal lens through which one views teaching and learning. We may not be aware of our perspective (or our BIASes) because it is something we look through, rather than look at, when teaching.

It is common for people to confuse perspectives on teaching with methods of teaching. Indeed, some nurse educators say they use all five perspectives, at one time or another, depending on circumstances. On the surface, this seems reasonable. Similar actions can be found in more than one perspective. However looking more deeply at the underlying BIASes, one can see that perspectives are far more than methods.

Nurse educators holding different perspectives may, for example, have similar beliefs about the importance of critical reflection in clinical and classroom contexts. To this end, all may espouse the use of higher-level questions as a means of promoting critical thinking. However, the way questions are asked, and the way in which nurse educators listen and respond when students consider those questions, may vary considerably across perspectives. It is how they are used, and toward what ends, that differentiates between perspectives and thus the personal BIASes we bring to teaching.

LEARNING ACTIVITY

Interview two people whose teaching you greatly admire. Ask them to identify which of the five teaching perspectives best describes their beliefs, actions, intentions, and strategies in their teaching. (Hint: you may want to provide them with the description in this chapter of the teaching perspectives.) Ask them if their teaching perspective has changed over time and in response to the content, the setting, and the level of the student. If they indicate that their perspective has changed, ask them to elaborate how and why it changed. Also ask them to talk to you about what they see as the rewards and challenges of maintaining such a perspective.

When you have completed your interview, compare this person's answers with what you believe and understand about teaching. What perspective best describes your teaching? How does it compare with those teachers you admire? Why is your perspective different or the same as those whom you admire? What are the implications of sustaining such a teaching perspective in all teaching situations and with all students?

RESOURCES FOR EDUCATORS

PLANNING THE TEACHING/LEARNING EXPERIENCE

Questions to Support a Thoughtful Reading

1. Which set of BIASes (or teaching perspective) is most consistent with your understanding of student-centered learning and instruction? Why?
2. When teaching in clinical settings, how might you use context as a teacher?
3. What would characterize effective student-centered teaching in a clinical setting?
4. Discuss ways in which the use of one's professional knowledge or expertise would differ when moving from classroom teaching to clinical teaching.
5. What would characterize appropriate student assessment within each of the perspectives on teaching?

Instructions for Educators

In this chapter, students are not required to read the chapter as a means of remembering its content. Rather, they should be invited to read it as a means of exploring ideas, issues, or problems that teaching BIASes might help them understand.

To launch such discussions, pose a question such as "What teaching perspective do you prefer and why?" Set the question before students read the chapter. Then ask students to spend a few minutes collecting their thoughts on paper or otherwise working on the question individually before talking with each other. Ask students to share their thoughts with someone sitting nearby ("think then pair"). After a few more minutes, ask pairs to pair up ("think/pair/square"). Finally, bring the entire class together for a full discussion, starting with the ideas already discussed in the smaller venue, calling on one or two groups to report and defend their conclusions or recommendations. This is commonly called the "think/pair/square/share" technique and works equally well for classes of 20 to 200.

If an instructor asks students to take the TPi, it is important to remember that the TPi is meant to be a conversational tool, not a diagnostic tool. As such, students should be invited to discuss the extent to which it does (or does not) represent their views and approaches to teaching.

When students have little or no teaching experience, it may be more useful to have them fill out the TPi on their instructor and with the instructor leading the discussion, explore the following: (a) how consistent or inconsistent are students in their view of this instructor; (b) when there is a difference, what do students say caused them to see the instructor one way or another; and (c) how do the perceptions of the students match (or not) with the instructor's view of herself (having filled out the TPi, he or she could then show students his or her own profile).

Organizing and managing the class depends on the goals of the class, the nature of the students attending the class, and who is teaching the class. The authors do not assume a one-size-fits-all organization or management strategy for a class; organization and management strategies depend on many things, including the teacher's dominant perspective on teaching. We suggest a reflexive, iterative planning process wherein the educator applies a strategy such as think/pair/square/share with a particular class, evaluates the strategy at the end of the class, revises the strategy for subsequent use, and re-evaluates its revised application.

EVALUATING THE TEACHING/LEARNING EXPERIENCE

Sample Evaluation Strategy

The following strategy is to be used to assist students to explore their teaching perspective in a classroom setting.

During class, you were asked to engage in a think/pair/square/share exercise. Please take a minute to reflect on how this exercise supported your learning. After each of the following questions, write a sentence or two in the spaces provided:

1. What was the most effective aspect of this exercise in supporting your learning about teaching BIASes?
2. Was there anything about this exercise that interfered with your capacity to learn?
3. How might the professor improve the application of this exercise?

References

Clark, A. (1999). An embodied cognitive science? *Trends in Cognitive Sciences, 3*(9), 345–351.

Diekelmann, N. L., Ironside, P. M., & Harlow, M. (2003). Introduction. In N. L. Diekelmann (Ed.). *Teaching the practitioners of care: New pedagogies for the health professions,* pp. 3–21. Madison, WI: The University of Wisconsin Press.

Gaberson, K. B., & Oermann, M. H. (1999). *Clinical teaching strategies in nursing*, Springer Series on the Teaching of Nursing. New York: Springer Publishing Company, Inc.

Holmes, C. (2002). Academics and practitioners: Nurses as intellectuals. *Nursing Inquiry*, *9*(2), 73–83.

Kember, D. (1997). A reconceptualization of the research into university academics' conceptions of teaching. *Learning and Instruction, 7(3)*, 255–275.

McEldowney, R. A. (2003). Critical resistance pathways: overcoming oppression in nursing education. In N. L. Diekelmann (Ed.). *Teaching the practitioners of care: New pedagogies for the health professions* (pp. 194–231.) Madison, WI: The University of Wisconsin Press.

Palmer, P. J. (1998). *The courage to teach: Exploring the inner landscape of a teacher's life.* San Francisco: Jossey-Bass Publishers.

Pratt, D. D. (1992). Conceptions of teaching. *Adult Education Quarterly 42*(4), 203–220.

Pratt, D. D. & Associates. (1998). *Five perspectives on teaching in adult and higher education.* Malabar, FL: Krieger Publishing.

Schön, D. A. (1983). *The reflective practitioner: How professionals think in action.* New York: Basic Books.

Swenson, M. M., & Sims, S. I. (2003). Listening to learn: Narrative strategies and interpretive practices in clinical education. In N.L. Diekelmann (Ed.). *Teaching the practitioners of care: New pedagogies for the health professions.* Madison, WI: The University of Wisconsin Press.

Vygotsky, L. S. (1978). *Mind in society: The development of higher psychological processes.* Cambridge, MA: Harvard University Press.

Additional Resources

TPI Web site: www.TeachingPerspectives.com

Authors' Web sites:

Daniel Pratt: www.edst.educ.ubc.ca/pratt.html

Barbara Paterson: www.unb.ca/research/research_chair/paterson.htm

Chapter 4

Learning Styles: Maps, Myths, or Masks?

Barbara L. Paterson
Daniel D. Pratt

I was a clinical teacher for fourth year students on a busy medical unit in a tertiary care hospital. I had studied about learning styles in my graduate course on teaching. The theory made sense to me and I was excited to put into practice what I learned. When I met the students in my clinical group, I gave them a learning styles inventory to complete. I discovered that they were diverse as to how they liked to learn. I told them I would accommodate their learning styles in my teaching. But what I discovered was that I was so busy, often so frantic for time—between running to be with students who had to do a skill for the first time, as well as responding to crises and answering questions for eight students, the nurses on the unit, and others —I rarely thought about their learning styles. I just did what was expedient and what had worked in the past. At the conclusion of the rotation, the students rated me highly as a clinical teacher. No one seemed to notice that I hadn't delivered on my promise about learning styles. So my question is, should I just give up on the idea of learning styles because it isn't practical and no one seems to care if I do or not, or should I keep on trying to teach according to students' learning styles? In addition, is it really feasible to tailor learning based on students' learning styles on a busy clinical unit?—*Anonymous nurse educator*

INTENT This chapter focuses on learning style theory and its application in student-centered nursing education. The authors discuss how learning style theory has contributed to nursing education, but they will also identify the conundrums and areas of concern, particularly in regard to the use of learning style instruments to diagnose students' learning styles. They will conclude the discussion with some hints and illustrations as to how nurse educators could most effectively use learning style theory in clinical and classroom settings.

OVERVIEW

INTRODUCTION

Opening this chapter is a story told during an interview by an experienced clinical nurse educator who at the time was teaching in a baccalaureate nursing education program. It typifies some of the dilemmas that nurse educators encounter as they attempt to integrate learning style theory in their teaching practice. In this chapter, we will attempt to answer the teacher's question by providing an in-depth critical analysis of the benefits and challenges of applying learning style theory in student-centered nursing education. **Learning style** is defined in this chapter as cognitive, affective, and physiological behaviors that serve as indicators of how learners perceive, interact, and respond to the learning environment (O'Neill, 1990).

In this discussion, we will honor the contribution that learning style theory has made to nurse educators' understandings of how students learn. However, we will also untangle why the use of learning styles in nursing education, particularly in the assessment of students, is frequently impractical, theoretically ambiguous, lacking strong empirical evidence to support its use, and often irrelevant to the unique nature and contexts of nursing education. We will critique the common assumptions underlying the adoption of learning styles as a concept in nursing education by profiling the empirical and conceptual confusion that proliferates and guides the application of learning style theory in classroom and clinical settings. The chapter concludes with a discussion about what such an analysis of learning styles means to nurse educators who are struggling with decisions about the application of learning styles theory in their teaching.

AN OVERVIEW OF LEARNING STYLE THEORY

The debate about what learning style actually is and what constitutes learning style has existed in the academic and teaching practice communities for at least 90 years (Riding & Cheema, 1991). The various conceptualizations of learning style are extensive. They have been a source of confusion for educators and researchers alike.

Learning Style Theory

Since 1970, there has been a proliferation of learning style theories in a variety of disciplines, including nursing. Many theorists have developed learning style theories, without apparent consideration of how the constructs within the theory overlap and incorporate previously developed theories (Furnham, 1992). In 1993, Thompson indicated that there were so many learning styles theories in existence, with so many varied conceptualizations of learning style, that it was difficult to synthesize or make sense of this theoretical field. Curry (1983) attempted to resolve this problem by categorizing the vast array of learning styles theories in layers of the Onion Model of Individual Difference. The outermost layer of the onion contains the most observable differences in learning style; that is, instructional and environmental preferences. The second layer of the onion, social interaction theories, includes learning style theories that focus on the influence of sociocultural context on learning styles. The middle layer of the onion contains **information processing** theories of learning style. The final, innermost layer includes personality models or theories that describe how learners' personalities influence their preferences for learning. Although some learning styles theories incorporate more than one layer of the onion, Curry's Onion Model (Curry, 1983) has proven useful in differentiating and articulating the contributions of various learning styles theories to our understanding of learning differences. Consequently, we have chosen to profile particular learning style theories that are popular in nursing education and are representative of each layer of the onion.

The outermost layer of Curry's Onion Model (Curry, 1983) pertains to theories that emphasize instructional and environmental preferences in learning. Dunn and Dunn and others (1990; Dunn, 2000; Dunn & Griggs, 1998) developed a learning styles model that considers the influence of student preferences for social interaction and the effect of the environment in which the learning takes place. This model considers learners' general processing style (referred to as global or analytic), their preferred way of learning (kinesthetic, tactile, auditory, visual) and their need for structure and authority. The theorists identify the following preferences as significant in determining what learning strategies students select: environmental preferences such as sound, light, temperature, and size of class; emotional preferences such as motivation, the need for structure, and perceived responsibility to learn; sociological preferences for teacher-led, single, paired, peer, team, or varied learning relationships; and psychological preferences, both related to analytic mode and perceptual strategies (Dunn & Griggs, 1998).

Social interaction theories of difference in learning, the second layer of the onion, consider the influence of sociocultural context on learning style. An example of such context is gender. A study by William Perry (1970) involving male Caucasian students at Harvard University, has been the basis for much current research about the influence of gender in learning styles. Perry claims that university students can journey through nine stages of development in which they evolve from dualistic thinkers and received knowing to the integration of knowledge that has been learned from others and that occurs as a result of personal experience and reflection. Others have built on Perry's work to propose learning style differences that can be attributable to gender. For example, Belenky, Clinchy, Goldberger, and Tarule (1986) interviewed 135 American women about their ways of knowing as learners. They suggest that some learners (particularly women) learn best when they can situate new information within a context, generally a personal and relational context. They documented how institutions of learning can unwittingly silence women as learners. Their findings indicated that because educational institutions often privilege learners who are analytical, competitive, and independent in their learning, learners who learn in relational or connected ways often experience learning in these institutions as lonely and frustrating.

The third layer of the onion contains information processing theories of learning style. They are the most common learning styles theories used in nursing education. Witkin (1967) was among the first to conduct research to investigate individual differences in information-processing strategies; he termed these differences "cognitive learning style." He categorized learners as either **field dependent** or **field independent**. Field independence or dependence refers to ways in which learners use data from the context to understand and make sense of new information (Smith, 2002). Field dependent learners view new learning holistically and globally; they see the forest, rather than the trees when they learn; and they tend to favor interactive learning methods (Smith, 2002). Field independent learners, on the other hand, tend to analyze new information, learning the pieces before they view the whole; and they tend to prefer lecture and discovery methods of learning (Smith, 2002). Research about field independence–dependence among learners has demonstrated that certain disciplines appear to attract and possibly to socialize learners in particular learning styles. For example, nurses have been shown by researchers to be more field dependent in their learning, while dental, pharmacy, and fisheries students tend to be more field independent (Pithers, 2002).

One of the most popular learning styles theories was developed by David Kolb (1984); it was called the Experiential Learning Theory (ELT). Kolb studied how people perceive and process information (Jones, Reichard, & Mokhtari, 2003). He developed a learning styles theory in which he proposed that learning occurs as an **experiential learning cycle (ELC)** whereby learning occurs as a process of transformation through experience (Kolb, 1984). This theory focuses on the ways that learners prefer to grasp and transform experiences (Jensen & Kolb, 2000). Learners are classified in this theory as grasping knowledge through apprehension (concrete experience) or comprehension (abstract conceptualization). The ways that learners transform knowledge is either reflective (reflective observation) or active (active experimentation). Kolb (1976) describes learners as **divergers**, **assimilators**, **accommodators**, and **convergers**. Divergers have the ability to synthesize diverse opinions and observations. They are creative, intuitive, imaginative, and are people oriented. These same attributes sometimes obscure their ability to make decisions (Hsu). Assimilators are systematic, focused learners who use logic and inductive reasoning to organize new information. They may feel uncomfortable in situations of ambiguity and when the practical relevance of the information is not clear (Hsu). Convergers tend to be logical, highly pragmatic, and able to transform information to new ideas or solutions to problems. Their range of interests tend to be narrow and they are often accused of being close-minded and unimaginative (Hsu, 1999). Accomodators grasp new information through their feelings and are highly action oriented. They enjoy taking risks and exploring new ideas and environments. They tend to use a trial-and-error method to solve problems. They may disregard well-established procedures and theory in the process (Hsu,1999). Kolb (1984) indicates that assimilators tend to attain the highest cumulative grade point averages in universities because the predominant teaching strategy in universities is lecture, a method that best suits assimilators' analytic and inductive learning style.

The final layer of the onion contains theories that pertain to the influence of personality on learning style. Some learning theorists have focused on the association between personality and learning styles, arguing that personality type can affect the way in which people prefer to learn. For example, Myers (1978) developed the Myers-Briggs Personality Type Indicator, an instrument intended to diagnose personality types but also to identify learning styles. It sorts personalities into 16 types based on Carl Jung's typology of personality (i.e., **extrovert** versus **introvert**, **sensing** versus **intuitive**, **thinking** versus **feeling**, **judging** versus **perceiving**) (Huston & Huston, 1995). Introvert learners are energized by focusing on ideas, concepts, and abstractions. They want to understand the world, but they need time and space for reflection. They learn best by teaching others. Extrovert learners, on the other hand, find energy in interaction with others. They are action oriented and like working in groups. Sensing learners prefer facts and observations over abstract concepts. They enjoy solving problems. Intuiting learners prefer concepts and interpretations rather than facts. They like variety in their work but may become bored if there is too much detail. Thinking learners use analysis, logic, and principle to understand new information. Mr. Spock in *StarTrek* is an example of the thinking learner. Feeling learners rely on their emotions and their values to learn. Judging learners prefer to use new information in a planned and systematic way to complete the assigned task as quickly and as efficiently as possible. Perceiving learners are more likely to want to explore the various aspects of the new information, posing questions about it, and exploring alternatives. The completion of the task is not as much a concern for perceiving learners; they tend to focus on the learning itself (McClanaghan, 2000).

The Conceptualization of Learning Style

The roots of learning style theory can be traced to the studies of intelligence, perception, cognitive processes, and personality types in psychology (Curry, 1987). Most learning style theories can be categorized as arising from a particular field of psychology, such as the study of perception, cognition, mental imagery, or personality (Sadler-Smith, 2001a). In accordance with its roots in cognitive psychology, learning is generally viewed in learning styles theory as the processing of information; information is transmitted to the learner, processed, and then retrieved by the learner at will. It is not surprising, therefore, that learning style is most often reported as an aptitude–treatment interaction (Snider, 1992) in which a person's distinctive aptitude (learning style) can be matched to a particular treatment (instructional method) that results in a statistically significant interaction (a better learning outcome than could have been achieved otherwise.)

The learning theories that are based on psychological models of information processing have been sharply criticized within the past decades. Learning style is presented in such theories as a single overarching construct in which what the teacher does directly affects students' learning; this notion contradicts prevalent views in student-centered teaching that learning is constructed by the learner and not simply a product of the teacher's instruction (Kaplan & Kies, 1995). Critics of the information processing model of learning styles point out that people do not always behave in such predictable and linear ways; they do not maintain a preferred learning style nor do they respond to an instructional approach in the same way at all times (Curry, 1990; Sadler-Smith, 2001a & b). Another criticism of the psychology-based learning styles theories is that they are grounded in an assumption that learning occurs in isolation or just inside the person's head (Hansman & Wilson, 2002). Proponents of situated views of learning, however, believe that people learn as they interact with others within a community of practice as they participate in the culture, rules, and ways of being of that community (Hansman & Wilson, 2002).

The conceptual confusion that characterizes much of the learning style literature exists in part because learning style theorists have used learning style as a term synonymous with such diverse psychological concepts as cognitive style, information processing, and learning strategy (Curry, 1990; Reynolds, 1997). Kolb's (1976, 1984) learning style theory, for example, incorporates the stages of cognition (Miller, 1991; Sadler-Smith, 2001a). The relationship between constructs, such as personality and intelligence, in learning style theories is often unclear.

Some theorists conceptualize learning styles in terms of cognitive skills and instructional preferences, others incorporate constructs such as expectancy, values, affective components, self-concept, reflective ability, anxiety, and study strategies (Snow, Corno, & Jackson, 1996). The similarities, cross-references, and overlaps between learning style theories offers an explanation as to why the field is so fraught with ambiguity (Hayes & Allinson, 1996; Riding & Cheema, 1991). For example, early in the 1900s, Carl Jung proposed a theory of personality type that paired a person's perceptions with their judgment tendencies (Leonard, Scholl, & Kowalski, 1999). He typified perception as sensing, intuition, thinking, and feeling. He also defined people as extroverts or introverts. Some readers will recognize these as the categories that make up the Myers-Briggs Personality Type Indicator (Myers, 1978). Kolb identified four types of learners as divergers, assimilators, convergers, and accommodators (Kolb, 1976, 1984, 1985). These are similar in description to the Myers-Briggs dimensions of learning style.

Sadler-Smith (2001b) suggests that because the term learning style has been adopted, diluted, and over extended by researchers in various disciplines, there is an increasing lack of clarity about what learning style entails. In the 1980s, learning style theories were adopted and revised by researchers in fields other than cognitive psychology, notably education and management (Sadler-Smith, 2001a). These researchers generally adopted a traditional cognitive psychology lens; however, they also applied other, often competing, perspectives from their disciplines in developing their theories.

Learning Style Instruments

In the evolution of learning styles theories, most theorists attempted to operationalize their theories. They used their theory as a basis to develop a quantitative tool or instrument to identify students' learning style. Six learning style theorists were interviewed recently (DelahoUssaye, 2002). They concluded that learning style inventories are not intended to reveal a person's learning style with complete accuracy. They are at best tools to assist the learner and teacher to dialogue about the student's experience in learning.

The most popular learning style instruments used in nursing education are Kolb's (1984) Learning Style Inventory and the Myers-Briggs Type Indicator (Myers, 1978). One researcher (Van Wynen, 1997) investigated the learning styles of baccalaureate nursing students by using the learning style instrument developed by Dunn and Dunn, (1991, 1993) the Productivity Environmental Preference Survey, to determine if a class of nursing students were primarily global or analytic learners. Van Wynen (1997) determined that among the 35 students in the study, 24 reported needing structure, 19 said they learned best in a warm temperature, 14 indicated they learned best with peers, and 17 were auditory learners. Van Wynen used these findings to revise her own course so that students had more choices in their assignments and there was more opportunity for peer learning.

Two researchers (Snelgrove & Slater, 2003) based their investigation of the learning approaches of 300 first-year nursing students on the **presage–process–product model** developed by Biggs (1987, 1993). Biggs' model incorporated presage factors that influenced learning style; these included personal factors such as the student's intelligence, personality, and motivation, as well as contextual factors, such as the size of the classroom. Process factors in Biggs' model refer to the type of approaches that the student takes in learning; that is, surface, deep, or achieving learning approaches. **Surface** approaches entail learning only what one needs to achieve the minimum requirements; **deep** approaches involve an in-depth understanding of what is being learned; and **achieving** approaches are directed toward achieving the best possible grades (Biggs, 1995). Snelgrove and Slater (2003) conducted a factor analysis and additional psychometric testing of the questionnaire developed by Biggs to determine students' learning styles. They identified some conceptual overlap between the various approaches, as well as a concern that some of the questionnaire items conveyed that there is an ideal way to learn.

THE APPEAL OF LEARNING STYLES IN NURSING EDUCATION

Nurse educators' adoption of learning style as a central construct in their teaching practices has been widespread and generally positive (Boekarts, 1999). The notion that people prefer to learn in different ways has a strong attraction for nurse educators, particularly those who are committed to student-centered teaching and diversity. Learning style has an intuitive appeal to nurse educators, largely because learning styles provide a basis for educators to understand and make decisions in regard to the different ways students process information (O'Neill, 1990). In addition, nurse educators actually experience such differences among students in their everyday practice (Sternberg, 1997).

Inspiring Dialogue and Reflection

One of the contributions of learning styles to nursing education is that they can inspire dialogue and reflection among educators as to how curricula, educational institutional policies, and teaching and evaluation practices contribute to students developing and sustaining certain learning styles, while excluding others. University professors can be sometimes overheard complaining that all that beginning university students want is to be told what will be on the test; they report that students are not interested in conceptual integration. Some researchers suggest that this student behavior may partly arise from the socialization that they receive in high school (Boekarts, 1999). In their intensive study of Dutch students over the course of their high school education, researchers discovered that the students primarily used surface learning to reproduce their learning for an exam or an essay (i.e., read a test, reread it, memorize it) (Boekarts, 1997). Likewise, in one study, Irish nursing students demonstrated a preference for teacher-structured instruction, rather than active learning approaches (Cowman, 1995). Researchers have suggested that deep level learning is not often required in most universities for students to receive acceptable examination marks (Busato, Prins, Elshout, & Hamaker, 2000). They propose that students who are constrained by money and time are forced to adopt surface level learning styles to pass courses as quickly and as effortlessly as possible (Busato, et al., 2000).

One of the attractions of Kolb's (1976, 1984) ELT to nurse educators is that it appears to address an ongoing concern: the tendency to focus solely on the concrete in teaching nursing students the skills and knowledge they will need. The integration of Kolb's theory in nursing education curricula helps to remind nurse educators of the need to address the more abstract elements of the profession (Bolan, 2003). Another appeal of ELT is that it gives nurse educators language to assist a student to develop more effective learning processes. For example, they can use Kolb's components of a learning style to explain to students who are analytical but unreflective why they are experiencing difficulty in the more abstract elements of nursing.

Learning styles can also highlight for nurse educators that there is no one best way to learn. Students experience both advantages and disadvantages as they apply different learning styles in learning situations. For example, students who tend to learn by seeing the whole picture are often advantaged in writing essays about nursing issues because they are able to conceptualize and synthesize information, whereas students who are more analytical often experience difficulty tying the bits of information together into a cohesive whole. Students who are uncomfortable until they can see the whole picture in clinical situations often deliberate for a long time about the meaning of seemingly isolated pieces of data, such as blood pressure and lack of appetite, until they can see the whole picture, whereas those who are more comfortable with the pieces may have no trouble interpreting and responding to the discrete data.

Insights About Students' Responses

Learning style research and literature can provide insights for nurse educators as to the reason for various responses that students have to particular teaching and evaluation approaches. Such insights might be helpful to educators in planning their teaching approaches and curricula. For example, although problem-based learning (PBL) has earned resounding support from nurse educators because of its student centeredness and process orientation, students who have a learning style that relies on the expert teacher telling them what to learn will encounter considerable difficulty, and perhaps resentment, in the largely self-directed, inquiry-based learning that it characterizes

(Sadler-Smith & Smith, 2004). Nurse educators who teach in PBL courses can mediate this by including teaching and other support to assist such learners to develop new ways of learning that are congruent with PBL.

Recent learning style theorists have emphasized the importance of context in determining learning style (Chase, 2001; Curry, 1990; DiBartola, Miller, & Turley, 2001). This is a reminder to nurse educators that there are many contextual influences on nursing students' learning styles beyond the nursing education program. For example, the single mother of three small children who works a part-time job, has no family or other supports and is studying for a nursing exam will likely adopt a learning style that is efficient and time-saving. The student might adopt a more surface learning style than a student who has no other demands on his or her time and can study without significant distraction. An educator who is cognizant of the effects of context on learning style will be more likely to consider this as the reason why students behave differently in different contexts, rather than simply concluding that the student is having a bad day or has inconsistent performance.

Learning style theory can also assist nurse educators to reflect on why certain learning experiences do not result in intended learning outcomes. For example, matching a student who prefers to learn in interaction with others, together with a preceptor who has a great need for reflective space will most likely prove to be difficult for both student and preceptor unless they are helped to develop strategies to mediate their differences (Lockwood-Rayermann, 2003).

THE CHALLENGES OF APPLYING LEARNING STYLES IN NURSING EDUCATION

The idea of teaching to a student's learning style is pervasive in nursing literature largely because the notion of acknowledging and addressing student diversity has become an important goal in nursing education curricula. However, although learning style offers much to nursing educators, it also poses many challenges. There are two basic assumptions that strengthen the integration of learning styles in nursing education:

1. Learning style is a useful construct to determine how students learn.
2. Matching instructional approaches to a student's learning style produces optimal learning and achievement outcomes.

At first glance, both assumptions appear reasonable. However, there are significant concerns with each, particularly as they have been derived primarily from a body of research that has substantial limitations.

Conceptual Confusion

Although no one would deny that people are different and that they learn in different ways, the problem with the first assumption is that in order for learning style to be useful to teachers and students, both the conceptualization of learning style and the assessment of learning style must be trustworthy. The conceptual confusion that abounds in this field has already been discussed; however, this confusion translates into many of the limitations of learning style instruments. For example, researchers investigated the relationship between personality and learning style (Jackson & Lawty-Jones, 1996). They concluded that learning style is a subset of personality. They suggest that the lack of differentiation between these constructs is one of the reasons that many learning style instruments have demonstrated such poor validity and reliability.

The Limitations of Instruments

The reliability and validity of most learning style instruments has been strongly criticized (Curry, 1990; Reynolds, 1997; Sadler-Smith, 2001b; Stahl, 1999). Despite differences in terminology among various learning styles and their instruments, the research to support the use of learning style theories and their related instruments has remained the same; that is weak and inconclusive (Stahl). Some critics suggest that many learning styles theorists have not tested the reliability and validity of their instruments well enough before printing the inventory for educators' use (Curry, 1990; Stahl). Another criticism is that many learning style instruments are referenced to other instruments, blurring the distinctions between the theoretical perspectives on learning style (Curry, 1990). Several reviewers of learning style instruments conclude the user can have little confidence in the ability of many learning style instruments to identify distinctive learning styles among students (Curry, 1990; Garner, 2000; Henson & Hwang, 2002; Reynolds; Stahl).

Using learning style instruments to categorize students might privilege some students and marginalize others (Messick, 1984; Sadler-Smith, 2001b). This is particularly a concern when ideals espoused in the curriculum, such as reflective ability, are regarded by nurse educators as the preferred style and other styles that appear to be less reflective are regarded as problematic. Labeling students as nonreflective may lead to the students being excluded from learning opportunities designed to foster reflective learning styles (Reynolds, 1997).

Several nursing researchers have used learning style instruments as a means of determining why certain populations of students, mainly minority in terms of ethnicity or gender, have high attrition and failure rates in nursing education. However, because these instruments are often not culturally relevant for minority students, the results are not particularly informative. An empirical model of learning style or a learning style instrument that has been developed in a Western context and by Western theorists is often irrelevant in social and cultural contexts that differ significantly from the Western view (Sadler-Smith, 2001b). McCarty, Lynch, Wallace, and Benally (1991) illustrate this in their discussion of why an educational program, based on a typology of personalities and learning styles, failed to capture the cultural context of the students, mostly of Navajo origin. They conclude that their research findings actually reinforced the stereotypical views of Navajo students as nonverbal and analytical.

The Myth of Matching Teaching to Learning Style

The difficulty with the second assumption underlying the use of learning styles in nursing education, that matching teaching approaches to learning style produces the best educational outcomes, is that the empirical evidence to support this assumption is weak at best. Numerous reviews of this body of research have been unable to provide conclusive evidence that short term or long term learning is enhanced by matching teaching approaches to students' learning styles (Curry, 1990; Reynolds, 1997; Snider, 1992; Stahl, 1999; Thompson & Crutchlow, 1993). The correlation between students' learning style and grade point average has not been demonstrated by researchers to date (Boekarts, 1999). It may be that the instruments used by researchers to determine this correlation are not valid means of determining students' learning styles. Another explanation is that the learning style measurements require students to choose items that reflect their learning style. Some research suggests that students may be unaware of their learning style or provide answers that they think reflect the ideal student (Boekarts, 1997).

The practicalities of trying to accommodate the learning styles of all students in all situations discourages many educators from addressing learning style in their teaching. For example, if only one student in a class of 100 has a particular learning style, how feasible is it for a nurse educator to teach to that style in a 1-hour lecture? Anecdotal evidence about teachers' experience in incorporating learning style theory in their teaching is often overwhelming and discouraging. One researcher interviewed an unidentified number of reading teachers who had attended a workshop or conference on learning styles (Stahl, 1999). The teachers in this study reported learning new teaching methods, an enhanced appreciation of the diversity of ways of learning, and a renewed belief in the possibilities of teaching to the learning styles of students. In 1 year, all had abandoned the notion of matching teaching approaches to students' learning styles and did not sustain their initial enthusiasm for such a goal (Stahl, 1999).

Another difficulty with teaching to learning styles is that it is not necessarily beneficial to students to confine their learning experiences so that they never have to integrate other ways of learning. Providing holistic teaching approaches to match students' learning style may actually jeopardize their learning of basic concepts and facts, such as the learning of medical terminology and the steps of a psychomotor skill (Snider, 1992). In nursing, for example, experimentation is an appropriate learning approach if the student is attempting to discover which position causes the patient to feel most comfortable. Because of the accountability to patients and their welfare in nursing, experimentation would be inappropriate as a means of discovering how much activity the patient could tolerate before the patient had a myocardial infarction.

Teaching in ways that are mismatched to students' preferred learning style has been demonstrated to cause students to learn flexibility in ways of learning (Kowoser & Berman, 1996; Vaughn & Baker, 2001). There are clinical situations in which a nurse must gain new learning in the fastest and most direct way possible by asking questions of experienced practitioners, such as determining the appropriate procedure for sending a specimen to the laboratory when the patient is about to arrest. In other situations, reflection and dialogue over a period of time is more appropriate, such as determining the ethical response to a complex patient situation. Nurses must be aware of what learning styles are most appropriate in what situations and they must be able to adapt their preferred learning style to the contextual cues and demands of the situation. Consequently, nurse educators have a responsibility to ensure that students learn how to be flexible in their learning approaches. Such a goal is unlikely to be achieved if nurse educators only teach to the student's learning style.

IMPLICATIONS FOR NURSE EDUCATORS

It is apparent that the field of learning styles is fraught with contradictions and confusion. The challenges to its application in nursing education are equal in impact to its appeal. What does this mean to nurse educators? Should they simply announce that learning style is an outdated and poorly conceptualized notion and abandon it as a consideration in their teaching? We will argue in this section of the chapter that there is much to be learned from both the advantages and challenges of learning styles, particularly the directions for nurse educators as to how they can improve their teaching practice.

The Uniqueness of Nursing Education

One of the sources of the difficulties that arise in the application of learning style theories to nursing education is that most research that has investigated the application of learning style theory has not been conducted within organizational contexts, such as within a clinical setting (Sadler-Smith, 2001b). Nursing education has unique contextual and cultural influences that determine what learning style is most appropriate and preferred in specific situations. The implications for nurse educators in regard to learning styles are unique in comparison with many other disciplines, such as fine arts, in which accountability for the welfare of patients is not a consideration.

Nurse educators can use learning style theory to help students become aware of different approaches and stages in learning (Garner, 2000). Such an approach would make the "learning process explicit" (Garner, p. 6). This is particularly helpful in the clinical setting where certain learning styles might be disadvantageous to the patient's well-being. For example, clinical nurse educators can advise students that there are times in nursing when knowing something in-depth, reflecting on its meaning, is not feasible or appropriate, such as in times of patient crises when nurses must act quickly, often as a result of a more experienced nurse telling them what to do, in order to safeguard the patient's well-being.

Assessing Learning Style in Alternative Ways

Typically, nurse educators have relied on published learning style inventories to determine students' learning styles. However, as these are often conceptually and psychometrically flawed and at best, identify a student's learning style only at one point in time, nurse educators should consider using other means to determine how students learn. One nurse educator asks students at the beginning of a clinical rotation to describe two recent learning experiences they had that were successful; one that involved learning a skill (e.g., how to locate and print online journal articles from the library) and one that involved problem solving an unfamiliar problem (e.g., what to do when you lock your keys in the car). The educator asks them to describe in detail how they tackled the learning and what they liked about the experience. The educator speaks with each student about what he or she gleans from the student's narratives (e.g., I see that you learned the computer program over several days and by yourself. You also spent a lot of time reading the manual before you actually tried working the program). He or she encourages the student to clarify and revise these insights if she is incorrect. He or she also asks the student questions about the situation in order to clarify elements of the story and to begin to formulate ideas about how the student's learning style could be accommodated in the clinical setting (e.g., You will be able to study the procedures and policies before most of the new skills you do in this rotation but there are times when you will be in a hurry because the patient needs something done right away. How will you handle learning a new situation in these times and how can I best help you?)

Another means of identifying students' learning styles is to observe how they respond to new learning situations and to make visible for them the processes the nurse educator has observed. Two researchers identified students' preference for visual or verbal learning in multimedia instruction (Leutner & Plass, 1998). They concluded that observation proved to be a more reliable method of diagnosing students' learning styles than a questionnaire. An important component of this research was that the researchers validated their observations with the students in the study.

Providing feedback to learners about what their preferred learning style appears to be is a way that the learners can validate the educator's impressions and educators can foster a dialogue about the implications of such a learning style. This strategic approach involves helping learners to determine what learning approaches they use in particular situations and why, as well as helping them to select the approach that is most effective and accommodating their learning style when the context or situation demands it (Sadler-Smith & Riding, 1999). For example, the educator might observe, "You seem to be so preoccupied with getting the task done sometimes that you don't ask enough questions about what the patient actually needs. You seemed so focused on getting his dressing done but you didn't seem to hear the nurse when he said that the doctor wanted to see the wound and you didn't seem to notice that the patient was grimacing in pain." If the student agrees with this observation, the educator could then introduce him or her to Kolb's (1976) view of assimilators or the Myers-Briggs (Myers, 1978) introverted, sensing, thinking, and judging learner. The educator could also use Dunn and Dunn's (1990; Dunn, 2000; Dunn & Griggs, 1998) theory to illustrate the factors that might influence the student's selection of that style in particular situations (e.g., if this is the first time for changing an operative dressing in the clinical area). The educator could use this discussion as a forum to discuss the strengths and limitations of this style, as well as to generate possible ways of overcoming the limitations.

Accommodating and Encouraging Different Learning Styles

Nurse educators can accommodate various learning styles by recognizing that students in any classroom or clinical rotation will have different learning styles and by teaching with a variety of teaching modalities. For example, they can verbally present information to accommodate learners who learn best by hearing. They can also use diagrams, pictures, and PowerPoint slides to present the same content to learners who learn best by seeing. This reasoning can also be applied to the selection of evaluation methods for a course or clinical performance. For example, in a course in adult acute care nursing, students are given a choice about whether they wish to complete a mind map, (Farrand, Hussain, & Hennessy, 2002) that is a schematic representation of the links between a patient's history, sociodemographic data, diagnosis, tests and treatments, and nursing care, to write a paper about the patient's plan of care, or to present the information as a class presentation. Students demonstrate a clear preference as to which assignment best meets their learning style.

It should be noted, however, that matching teaching or evaluation strategies to students' learning styles is not always a desirable goal; it could in fact compromise students' ability to function in situations that demand alternate learning approaches. Educators should recognize that one of their objectives in student-centered teaching is to assist students to behave in flexible and different ways whenever situations demand that they move out of their psychological comfort zone (Sadler-Smith & Smith, 2004). Helping students to adapt their preferred learning style in such situations will require that the nurse educator: (a) identify learners' styles and provide feedback to the learner about them; (b) deliberately select learning opportunities to help the learner understand and appreciate the implications of learning style in particular contexts and situations; and (c) enter into agreement with learners, through the use of formal written or informal verbal contracts, about the student's goals and needs for learner support in the accommodation of learning approaches, styles and preferences (Sadler-Smith & Smith, 2004). In one such situation, a third-year nursing student discussed with the teacher that she became preoccupied with talking to the patients about their situation and therefore was often late administering medications. They entered into a discussion about both the benefits (i.e., she formed excellent rapport with patients) and the limitations (i.e., she often was delayed in providing significant aspects of the patient's care) of this learning style. They determined that the student would use some organizational reminders (e.g., a watch alarm set for medication times). In addition, the educator arranged for the student to work with a nurse who was skilled in forming interpersonal relationships with patients and their families, while at the same time, effectively organizing her care. On the first day, the nurse provided the majority of care for four patients, while the student observed. She also spoke to the student about her tricks for organizing care, placing boundaries on her time for conversation with patients, and talking to patients while you do what you have to do. On the next day, the student cared for the patients while the nurse observed and provided feedback about the students' organization. Students who focus on tasks, and miss the big picture in patient care can be encouraged to chunk pieces of information together by building a compare/contrast table, flowchart, or concept/mind map about the information. Learners who are highly introverted could be encouraged to develop extroverted skills in learning by teaching their peers or nurses about aspects of a patient's care. Students who are not particularly reflective can be assisted to reflect on their experience by posing specific questions in this regard (e.g., What would you do differently if you cared for this patient again tomorrow? Why?).

Assessment approaches are one of the most significant contextual factors that influence students' learning style (Tweed & Lehman, 2002). Certain assessment strategies, such as multiple choice examinations and intensive questioning of students in the clinical setting about facts such as the actions of medications, encourage students to adopt learning styles that permit them to memorize discrete knowledge. This occurs because the surface learning that is successful in such assessments is generally rewarded with marks and the teacher's affirmation. Some assessment strategies in nursing education should encourage and reward students for assuming more integrative and deeper learning styles. Cooperative learning, portfolios, and certain essay questions that encourage students to demonstrate integration of their learning have been shown to encourage such a learning style (Cano-Garcia & Hughes, 2000).

Teachers tend to teach in accordance with their own learning styles because they are most comfortable using the approaches they know best (Thompson & Crutchlow, 1993). The concept of learning style provides an opportunity for nurse educators to reflect on how open they have been to alternative styles in their teaching and in their own learning. Gifted musicians often challenge themselves to learn a new instrument in addition to their primary instrument because it broadens their musical talents. It also provides them with new enthusiasm and learning to bring to the playing of the primary instrument. In the same way, nurse educators can challenge themselves to move beyond the box in their teaching to incorporate new styles.

SUMMARY

As in all other attempts to capture the complex dimensions of human behavior in a single theory, no one learning style theory explicates the variations in learning style that can exist, nor is there one theory that incorporates all the contextual, personal, and mediating influences that determine why a student selects a particular style at any one time. Although the empirical evidence to support any one learning style theory and its instrumentation is not strong, there remains a pervasive sense among nurse educators that particular learning styles exist and account for variations in student performance beyond ability (Stahl, 1999). The conceptual and theoretical confusion that characterizes the field of learning styles has caused some authors to refer to learning style as a redundant concept (Reynolds, 1997).

There is no doubt that we are all different. Effective nurse educators recognize individual differences and present new information to students in a variety of ways through more than one teaching approach. They identify students' differences and their unique needs in learning through their interactions with students over time in relationship with the student. It is this dialogical feature of learning styles that offers nurse educators a beacon to guide their teaching practice in student-centered education.

LEARNING ACTIVITY

Read the following situation. Think of a situation in your own teaching practice and generate a Question of the Week.

One clinical nurse educator accomplishes the goal of encouraging deeper learning styles by posing a written Question of the Week to each student in the clinical group immediately before the students' clinical day. A nursing student had cared for two patients with multiple sclerosis (MS) over the course of 3 weeks and was assigned to care for Mrs. M., another person with MS the following day. The educator wrote, "All three patients have been diagnosed with their disease for approximately the same time but they demonstrate considerable differences in their mobility, continence, psychosocial functioning, and communication. In the next 2 days, please research the disease and the patients' charts, as well as talk to Mrs. M. this week, to determine what factors determined the trajectory and manifestations of MS in these patients. When you are satisfied that you know, tell me the answer to this question: How will you incorporate your knowledge about the determiners of the trajectory and manifestations of MS in your care of patients with MS? Remember that you can ask me for help in completing this task. As well, the MS clinic is on the first floor of the hospital as an additional resource. You can answer the question verbally or in writing (handwritten or as an e-mail message). Please answer the question before Friday at noon.

RESOURCES FOR EDUCATORS

PLANNING THE TEACHING/LEARNING EXPERIENCE

Questions to Support a Thoughtful Reading

There are no correct answers to the following questions. We offer them to you simply as a way of helping you to reflect on how you should integrate your understanding about learning styles in planning the teaching/learning experience.

1. Should a clinical nurse educator teach nursing students to adopt various learning styles that are situation appropriate and if so, how would this be achieved?
2. What student learning styles are generally embraced in nursing education? What are the implications of this for nursing education curricula and teaching practices?
3. Do people choose professions on the basis of their learning style or does the profession socialize them to particular learning styles that fit with the discipline?
4. What learning styles are problematic in nursing education and for whom?
5. What place, if any, do learning style instruments have in nursing education?

EVALUATING THE TEACHING/LEARNING EXPERIENCE

Questions to Elicit Feedback from Students on Their Learning

1. What conclusions can you make about the nature of learning styles from this review of the literature?
2. Choose one of the learning style theories that were profiled in this chapter and assess the theory's contribution to the following questions. Is learning style:
   a. A relatively stable attribute (trait) or an adaptive strategy (state) of the individual?
   b. Referencing the learner (state or trait) or the process of learning?
   c. Compatible with contemporary theories of learning?
   d. Conceptually linked to something richer than just an instrument?
   e. An empirical, theoretical, or normative construct?
   f. Culturally derived or culturally neutral?
   g. Sufficiently valid and reliable to be predictive of learning?
   h. Differentially useful in nursing education? If so, how and for what?
   i. Philosophically consistent with diversity as it informs student-centered nursing education today?

References

Ash, B. (1986). *Identifying learning styles and matching strategies for teaching and learning.* U.S. Department of Education, Office of Educational Research and Improvement. (ERIC Document Reproduction Service No. ED270142).

Belenky, M. F., Clinchy, B. M., Goldberger, N. R., Tarule, J. M. (1986). *Women's ways of knowing: The Development of self, voice, and mind.* New York: Basic Books.

Biggs, J. (1987). *Student approaches to learning and studying* Hawthorn, Victoria: Australian Council for Educational Research.

Biggs, J. (1993). What do inventories of students' learning processes really measure? A theoretical review and clarification. *British Journal of Educational Psychology, 63*(1), 3–19.

Biggs, J. B. (1995). Learning in the classroom. In J. Biggs, & D. Watkins (Eds.), *Classroom learning: Educational psychology for the Asian teacher.* (pp. 147–166). Singapore: Prentice Hall.

Boekarts, M. (1997). Self-regulated learning: A new concept embraced by researchers, policy makers, educators, teachers, and students. *Learning and Instruction, 7*(2), 161–186.

Boekarts, M. (1999). Self-regulated learning: Where are we today? *International Journal of Educational Research, 31*(6), 445–457.

Bolan, C. M. (2003). Incorporating the experiential learning theory into the instructional design of online courses. *Nurse Educator, 28*(1), 10–14.

Busato, V. V., Prins, F. J., Elshout, J. J., & Hamaker, C. (2000). Intellectual ability, learning style, personality, achievement motivation and academic success of psychology students in higher education. *Personality and Individual Differences, 29*(6), 1057–1068.

Cano-Garcia, F., & Hughes, E. H. (2000). Learning and thinking styles: An analysis of their interrelationship and influence on academic achievement. *Educational Psychology, 20*(4), 413–418.

Chase, C. R. (2001). Learning style theories: matching preceptors, learners, and teaching strategies in the perioperative setting. *Seminars in Perioperative Nursing, 10*(4), 184–187.

Cowman, S. (1995). The teaching/learning preferences of student nurses in the Republic of Ireland: background issues and a study. *International Journal of Nursing Studies, 32*(2), 126–136.

Curry, I. (1987). *Integrating concepts of cognitive or learning styles: A review with attention to psychometric standards.* Ottawa: Canadian College of Health Executives.

Curry, L. (1983). An organization of learning style theory and constructs. In Curry, L. (Ed.), *Learning style in continuing education* (pp. 115–131). Halifax: Dalhousie University.

Curry, L. (1990). A critique of the research on learning styles. *Educational Leadership, 48*(2), 50–57.

DelahoUssaye, P. (2002). The perfect learner. *Training, 39*(5), 28–36.

DiBartola, L. M., Miller, M. K., & Turley, C. L. (2001). Do learning style and learning environment affect learning outcome? *Journal of Allied Health, 30*(2), 112–115.

Dunn, R., Dunn, K., & Price, G. (1986). *Productivity environmental preference survey* Lawrence, KS: Price Systems Inc.

Dunn, R., & Dunn, K. (1990). Rita Dunn answers questions on learning styles. *Educational Leadership, 48*(2), 15–20.

Dunn, R., & Dunn, K. (1991). Teaching students through their individual learning styles: A practical approach. Reston, VA: Reston Publishing.

Dunn, R., & Dunn, K. (1993). Teaching secondary students through their individual learning style Needham Heights, MA: Allyn and Bacon.

Dunn, R., & Griggs, S. (1998). Learning styles: Link between teaching and learning. In R. Dunn, & S. Griggs, (Eds.), *Learning styles and the nursing profession.* (pp. 11–23). New York: NLN Press.

Dunn, R. (2000). Learning styles: Theory, research, and practice. *National Forum of Applied Educational Research Journal, 13*(1), 3–22.

Farrand, P., Hussain, F., & Hennessy, E. (2002). The efficacy of the "mind map" study technique. *Medical Education, 36*(5), 426–432.

Furnham, A. (1992). Personality and learning style: a study of three instruments. *Personality and Individual Differences, 13*(4), 429–483.

Garner, I. (2000). Problems and inconsistencies with Kolb's learning styles. *Educational Psychology, 20*(3), 341–349.

Hansman, C. A., & Wilson, A. L. (2002). *Situating cognition: Knowledge and power in context.* Paper presented at the Annual Meeting of the Adult Education Research Conference. Raleigh, NC.

Hayes, J., & Allinson, C. W. (1996). The implications of learning styles for training and development. *British Journal of Management, 7*(1), 63–73.

Henson, R., & Hwang, D.-Y. (2002). Variability and predictability of measurement error in Kolb's learning style inventory scores: A reliability generalization study. *Educational and Psychological Measurement, 62*(4), 712–727.

Hsu, C. H. C. (1999). Learning styles of hospitality students: Nature or nurture? *International Journal of Hospitality Management, 18*(1), 17–30.

Huston, J. L., & Huston, T. L. (1995). How learning style and personality can affect performance. *The Health Care Supervisor, 13*(4), 38–45.

Jackson, C., & Lawty-Jones, M. (1996). Explaining the overlap between personality and learning style. *Personality and Individual Differences, 20*(3), 293–300.

Jensen, P. J., & Kolb, D. A. (2000). Learning style and meaning-making in conversation. In R. J. Riding, & S. G. Rayner, (Eds.), *International perspectives on individual differences Volume 1: Cognitive styles.* Stamford, CT: Ablex Publishing Corporation.

Jones, C., Reichard, C., & Mokhtari, K. (2003). Are students' learning styles discipline specific? *Community College Journal of Research and Practice, 27*(5), 363–375.

Kaplan, E. J., & Kies, D. A. (1995). Teaching styles and learning styles: Which came first? *Journal of Instructional Psychology, 22*(1), 28–34.

Kolb, D. A. (1976). *Learning style inventory technical manual* Cambridge, MA: Sloan School of Management, MIT.

Kolb, D. A. (1984). *Experiential learning: experience as the source of learning and development.* Englewood Cliffs, NJ: Prentice Hall.

Kolb, D. A. (1985). *The learning style inventory: Technical manual.* Boston: McBer.

Kowoser, E., & Berman, N. (1996). Comparison of pediatric resident and faculty learning styles: implications for medical education. *American Journal of Medical Science, 312*(5), 214–218.

Leonard, N. H., Scholl, R. A., & Kowalski, K. A. (1999). Information processing style and decision making. *Journal of Organizational Behavior, 20*(3), 407–420.

Leutner, D., & Plass, J. L. (1998). Measuring learning styles with questionnaires versus direct observation of preferential choice behavior in preferential choice behavior in authentic learning situations: the visualizer/verbalizer behavior observation scale (VV-BOS). *Computers in Human Behavior, 14*(4), 543–557.

Lockwood-Rayermann, S. (2003). Preceptor leadership style and the nursing practicum. *Journal of Professional Nursing, 19*(1), 32–37.

McCarty, T. L., Lynch, R. L., Wallace, S., et al. (1991). Classroom inquiry and Navajo learning styles: A call for reassessment. *Anthropology and Education Quarterly, 22*(1), 42–59.

McClanaghan, M. C. (2000). A strategy for helping students learn how to learn. *Education, 120*(3), 479–486.

Messick, S. (1984). The nature of cognitive styles: Problems and promise in educational practice. *Educational Psychologist, 19*(2), 59–74.

Miller, A. (1991). Personality types, learning styles, and educational goals. *Educational Psychology: 11*(3 & 4), 217–237.

Myers, I. (1978). *Myers-Briggs Type Indicator.* Palo Alto, CA: Consulting Psychologists' Press.

O'Neill, J. (1990). Making sense of style. *Educational Leadership, 48*(2), 4–10.

Perry, W. G. (1970). *Forms of intellectual and ethical development in the college years: A scheme.* New York: Holt, Rinehart & Winston.

Pithers, R. T. (2002). Cognitive learning style: A review of the field dependent–field independent approach. *Journal of Vocational Education and Training, 54*(1), 117–132.

Reynolds, M. (1997). Learning styles: A critique. *Management Learning, 28*(2), 115–133.

Riding, R. J., & Cheema, I. (1991). Cognitive styles—an overview and integration. *Educational Psychology, 11*, 193–215.

Sadler-Smith, E., & Riding, R. J. (1999). Cognitive style and instructional preferences. *Instructional Science, 27*(5), 355–371.

Sadler-Smith, E. (2001a). A reply to Reynolds' critique of learning style. *Management Learning, 32*(3), 291–304.

Sadler-Smith, E. (2001b). Does the learning styles questionnaire measure style or process? A reply to Swailes and Senior (1999). *International Journal of Selection and Assessment*, 9(3), 207–214.

Sadler-Smith, E., & Smith, P. J. (2004). Strategies for accommodating individuals' styles and preferences in flexible learning programmes. *British Journal of Educational Technology*, *35*(4), 395–412.

Smith, J. (2002). Learning styles: Fashion fad or lever for change? The application of learning style theory to inclusive curriculum delivery. *Innovations in Education and Teaching International*, *39*(1), 63–70.

Snelgrove, S., & Slater, J. (2003). Approaches to learning: psychometric testing of a study process questionnaire. *Journal of Advanced Nursing*, 43(5), 496–505.

Snider, V. E. (1992). Learning styles and learning to read: A critique. *Remedial and Special Education, 13,* 6–18.

Snow, R. E., Corno, L., & Jackson, D. (1996). Individual differences in affective and cognitive functions. In D. C. Berliner & R. C. Calfee, (Eds.), *Handbook of educational psychology* (pp. 243–310). New York: Simon & Schuster.

Stahl, S. A. (1999). Different strokes for different folks? A critique of learning styles. *American Educator*, *23*(3), 27–31.

Sternberg, R. J. (1997). *Thinking styles* Cambridge: Cambridge University Press.

Thompson, C., & Crutchlow, E. (1993). Learning style research: A critical review of the literature and implications for nursing education. *Journal of Professional Nursing*, 9(1), 34–40.

Tweed, R. G., & Lehman, D. R. (2002). Learning considered within a cultural context: Confucian and Socratic approaches. *American Psychologist, 57*(2), 89–99.

Van Wynen, E. (1997). Information processing styles: One size doesn't fit all. *Nurse Educator* 22(5), 44–50.

Vaughn, L., & Baker, R. (2001). Teaching in the medical setting: balancing teaching styles, learning styles and teaching methods. *Medical Teacher*, 23(6), 610–612.

Witkin, H. A. (1967). A cognitive style approach to cross-cultural research. *International Journal of Psychology*, 2(4), 233–250.

Chapter 5

From Filling a Bucket to Lighting a Fire: Aligning Nursing Education and Nursing Practice

Helen Brown
Gweneth Hartrick Doane

There was so much for me[1] to learn as a new grad in the neonatal intensive care unit. Newborn pathophysiology was a complex and intimidating subject area when I was still trying to figure out basic pathophysiologic processes in adult patients. How could I feel at home in a place where I seemed to know so little? After about 6 months of practicing in the NICU, I was asked by the nurse educator to be a preceptor for a new staff person who was an experienced RN. This seemed to me like a crazy request. What did I know after being there as a new grad for 6 months? How could I have possibly accumulated enough knowledge to teach a more experienced nurse? I told the nurse educator that she had the wrong person and that she probably had me mixed up with a more senior nurse. She said she was clear that she wanted me, and she stated the reasons why. She said teaching was not about having accumulated knowledge in my head, but was about the way in which I approached learning. I was perplexed. If I was not to pass on knowledge, then what was my purpose? What was I doing in my own learning that indicated I could teach and maybe inspire another person's learning? How could the fact that my knowledge of neonatal pathophysiology was far from complete not matter? I assumed this was the basis upon which preceptors were chosen.

Years later I think I have begun to figure out why this educator thought I could make a good teacher. She said a few things like "It's more than what you know that makes for a good teacher, it's about who you are as a nurse and the way you ask questions, are satisfied or dissatisfied with answers, set to figuring out what you need to know, seek out resources for families based on what they need, and the way you acknowledge that babies and families know about, and contribute to, their own healing."

[1] The first-person "I" is that of author Helen Brown.

INTENT

Reflecting on the narrative above, how do the criteria the educator was using in selecting a preceptor compare to what you think makes a good teacher? Certainly the educator was looking for things that are different from what has traditionally been assumed to be the foundations a teacher needs. The educator seemed to be looking for a particular kind of nurse—for a person who approached nursing as an inquirer, who actively questioned his or her own knowledge and sought to know more. Rather than looking for someone who excelled in substantive knowledge and/or teaching experience, the educator was looking for someone who developed a certain kind of relationship with NICU families and with his or herself as a learner. She also sought out someone who viewed families as both teachers and learners. Overall, it seems that in her effort to find a good preceptor/teacher, the educator above was searching for a person who was a good nurse. It is this link between good nursing and good teaching that we explore in this chapter. Specifically, we focus on showing how good nursing practice provides the basis for good teaching in nursing education.

OVERVIEW

INTRODUCTION

In this chapter we are proposing that good teaching arises out of the same qualities, attitudes, and ways-of-being as does good nursing. Based on this proposition, we suggest that nursing education needs to be more intentionally aligned with, and flow out of, the practice of nursing. Rather than assuming that it is substantive knowledge and/or educative methods and strategies that lead to high quality learning/teaching we contend that similar to nursing practice, exemplary teaching lies in how educators engage with the people they are teaching and how they approach and live knowledge. The Irish poet, William Yeats, suggests that education is not filling a bucket but lighting a fire. To approach teaching in a way that lights fires is quite different than undertaking the job of filling buckets. To light fires, we believe that learning/teaching must be structured not according to substantive content and/or educational methods but in accordance with the ever changing process of nursing practice. Moreover, we believe that bequeathing educative authority to content and methods offers an insufficient foundation for nursing education and potentially hinders the learning/teaching of nursing. Therefore, in this chapter we invite you to consider how it might be possible to move beyond substantive content-based and/or method-based teaching practices to align the process of nursing education with the process of nursing practice.

A PHILOSOPHICAL BEGINNING

We begin our discussion at the philosophical level because we have found that there is a particular **philosophical perspective** that has been at the center of our own practice as nurses and at the center of our learning/teaching work (Hartrick Doane, 2003). When we speak of a philosophical perspective, it is important to emphasize that we are not referring to an abstract theoretical position. As Hadot (1995) explains, in its origin philosophy was a method for instructing people to continually live and look at the world in new ways. In this way, philosophy is viewed as the art of living—". . .it is a concrete attitude and determinate lifestyle, which engages the whole of existence" (Hadot, 1995, p. 83). Hadot describes that in contrast to today's understanding and practice of philosophy, philosophers in antiquity[2] lived their ideas. Their questions and writings were questions they were posing to themselves and living into. At the same time, as teachers, the philosophers in antiquity inspired others to live into the questions of life. Hadot explains that the written work of philosophers was "written not so much to inform the reader of a doctrinal content but to form him, to make him traverse a certain itinerary" (Hadot, p. 105).

Hadot's description of the exercises that philosophers of old took up and lived are similar to the ones that we have found ourselves living in our nursing practice and in our learning/teaching work. For example, the Stoics practiced exercises of reading, listening, research, reflecting, investigating, self-mastery, and so forth (Hadot, 1995). They intentionally and consciously put themselves into question and forced themselves

[2] The historical period of philosophy to which Hadot (1995) refers to as antiquity is the first century B.C. Within this period four schools of philosophy were prominent—Platonism, Aristotelianism, Epicureanism, and Stoicism—thereby preceding the philosophers associated with the Enlightenment period, such as Descartes, Kant, and Rousseau, among others.

to pay attention to how they were moving into life. This inquiry into everyday living meant they intentionally and consciously paid attention to what knowledge they were living and how they were enacting that knowledge. It is this way of moving into life as an inquiring person, and how one approaches and lives knowledge, that we believe is at the center of nursing work, whether that work is as a nurse in clinical practice or as a learner/teacher in an educative setting (Hartrick, 2002a, 2002b; Hartrick Doane, 2002a, 2003; Hartrick Doane & Varcoe, 2005).

Living Knowledge: A Pragmatic Perspective

As nurses/learners/teachers, we have taken a pragmatic approach to knowledge and to living our knowledge. Inspired by philosophers in the **pragmatist tradition**, including William James, John Dewey, Richard Rorty, and Barbara Thayer-Bacon, we have come to understand knowing as a relational, experiential action (Hartrick 2002a; Hartrick Doane & Varcoe, 2005). A pragmatic view of knowledge assumes the existence of multiple truths and interpretations and understands that it is impossible to obtain knowledge that is certain and/or universal. Knowledge is never certain since, as Thayer-Bacon (2003) describes, "the only truths we have access to are derived through our own error-prone . . . procedures" (p. 63). Thus, from this pragmatic perspective, all knowledge is understood to be limited and fallible and any theory or expert truth is considered to be in need of continual scrutiny. Another feature of a pragmatic approach to knowledge that has informed our nursing work is the connection of knowledge, experience and practice (Hartrick Doane & Varcoe, 2005, in press). In contrast to the **Cartesian** view that separates theoretical knowledge from practical knowledge, pragmatists do not see a deep split between theory, practice, and experience (Hartrick Doane & Varcoe). From a pragmatic perspective, all so-called theory is understood to arise from and be grounded in experiences and practices (Rorty, 1999). Subsequently, pragmatists share Berman's (2000) contention that truth is a verb; it happens to an idea. Ideas become true and are made true by events (James, 1907).

One example of this pragmatic approach to knowledge within neonatal teaching concerns newborn death and grief and loss theory. Although theories in this area offer frameworks for understanding the experience of newborn death and families' loss and grief experiences, they do not reflect the way it is for all families and rarely do they offer accurate and/or complete representations of the complex human experience of a family experiencing newborn death. Yet, in learning about newborn death, it is common for unquestioned authority to be given to the theories of, for example, Elizabeth Kübler Ross and Therese Rando. In many ways it seems that the theories are taken up in an effort to find some prescribed way to learn about and know newborn death, to be able to make sense of and still the flux, and ultimately be better able to manage the uncertainty and pain that such life experiences entail.

In contrast to the above example, from a pragmatic perspective, the value of knowledge lies in its pragmatic contribution. That is, theory is not seen as offering truths to follow and knowledge is not valued because it offers us more theoretical certainty or more ability to manage our practice. Rather, what is important is how theory and knowledge can pragmatically enable us to be more effective in the world. That is, loss and grief theory is considered true and valuable to the extent that it enhances our knowing and response to particular families in particular situations. For example, emerging theories about parental grief following the death of their infant suggests that some parents seek to live with their infant's death rather than finding ways to get back to life as it was being lived before the death. A pragmatic perspective guides us in moments of caring for a particular family to hear, and respond to, the needs of the family in living with their grief. From a pragmatic perspective we might ask how this view of grief could help us to more effectively respond to a family and perhaps help them find ways to meaningfully memorialize their infant's life. For example, rather than encouraging them to put the loss behind them and move on, we might honor and support their decision to plant a tree to create a visual and living presence to embody their infant's life.

A Pragmatic Approach to Nursing Education

Throughout the past two decades, postmodernism has challenged the Cartesian view of knowledge, including the separation of mind, body, and emotion and the distinction between objective, rational thought, and subjective experience. However, in many ways, the Cartesian view is still evident in how nursing practice and education are structured and taken up. For example, within the clinical area, many assessment and/or recording forms emphasize the physical aspects of a person's health and healing and the related objective indicators that are measurable, observable, and treatable. Unless there is some problem, the subjective aspects of a person's experience (for example, the emotional, spiritual, and social) are often not reported on and/or addressed. Similarly, in developing curricula, although there is the rhetoric of learner focused, the overriding emphasis is frequently on the external deliverables—on the content, objectives, outcomes, and measurables of learning.

In addition, models of education continue to separate knowledge, theory, and practice. For example, knowing what (theory) is often separated from knowing how (practice). Such an approach to education has been challenged extensively by writers such as Eraut (1994, 2000), Habermas, (1987), and Schön (1987) who argue that any knowledge of theory/practice is influenced by context; that is, theory arises from and is grounded in experiences of practice.

What is particularly problematic about this separating of theory and practice within nursing is that focusing on external deliverables and separating theory from practice often leads to objectification and depersonalization of the processes of both nursing practice and nursing education. For example, as teachers we have recurring requests from students to give them all the knowledge they need to practice nursing and/or tell them what they need to know and do to get an A. It is assumed that knowledge is a thing to be obtained and learning is about receiving that thing—it is about obtaining "it" so they as students/nurses can deliver it to teachers and/or to the people they care for. Of course this assumption is not really surprising given the traditions that have dominated nursing education. All too often, the educative process has mirrored Freire's (1988) notion of the banking form of education. Learning has been viewed as a conscious, objective, and rational process, while teaching has involved an all-knowing teacher making deposits of knowledge into unknowing students. Although the curriculum revolution of the 1980s inspired the move away from this banking approach and also fostered the development of more learner-centered living educative approaches (Bevis & Watson, 1989; Moccia, 1988), our educational systems and methods are, in many ways, still reflective of this banking education. For example, content still dominates curriculum development and course delivery, and many teachers still default to a search for methods to deposit the content into students. One way this occurs is figuring out the best ways to present the content to students, assuming that if I teach it, it is learned.

Unfortunately, when nursing practice and/or teaching is reduced to finding the right method and students are viewed as repositories of knowledge, learning and knowledge development is constrained. The overriding commitment to quantification, method, rationality, and prescriptive techniques supersedes the profession's espoused values of subjective engagement, humanly involved relations, and embodied practices (Hartrick, 1997, 2002a, 2002b; Hartrick Doane, 2002a, 2002b). Subsequently, neither practice nor education settings are structured in ways that support nurses to move into practice and/or education in a humanly involved way that is consistent with those values. The overriding desire for knowledge (as a thing to be obtained or deposited) and methods that will solve any problems arising in practice/teaching dominates. And just as giving authority to methods can hinder responsive and competent nursing practice, (Hartrick, 2002a, 2002b; Hartrick Doane, 2002a; Hartrick Doane & Varcoe, 2005) the authority of educative method can hinder the living process of learning/teaching. We concur with Ironside (2003) who contends that nursing requires " . . . discipline-specific pedagogies that are responsive to the pressure and contingencies of nursing practice" (p. 510). She calls for shifting students' and teachers' attention away from an emphasis on issues of knowledge acquisition (i.e., cognitive gain) and application to thinking and learning as practices to be fostered.

Learning and Teaching as More Than Method

As a result of the banking approach to education and an objective, fact-oriented, pedagogical language that has had firm roots in nursing since the early 20th century (Hodges, 1997), nurse educators have sought curriculum development and teaching strategies that appear as precise and scientific as possible. For example, whether it be to undertake the development of a formal nursing curriculum or to create a professional development workshop, nurse educators often rely on the knowledge and methods developed in the field of adult education (such as formal instructional design methods) to ensure they know how to do and are doing sound curriculum development and teaching practice. This reliance on external methods rests on the assumption that the methods developed in the field of education give credibility to their work and that those methods can serve as the foundation for nursing education.

While there is no doubt that knowledge from the field of adult education can serve as a resource to nurse educators, the problem lies with where authority is placed. The reliance on educational theory and method often results in nursing and nurses losing the authority for the enterprise of nursing education. Moreover, developments in the field of education that have potential relevance and benefit for a more humanly-involved process of teaching and learning have not been well integrated (Schön, 1987; hooks, 1994, 2003;

Friere, 1988; Giroux, 1991). As authority is bequeathed to educational methods, the people involved in the educational endeavor—namely nursing students and teachers—lose sight of their own knowledge and expertise (Hartrick, 2002a, 2002b). The result is what Berman (1981, 2000) describes as a nonparticipatory way of being.

Educational methods, including instructional design techniques and strategies, gain authority over how students are introduced to nursing, how nursing knowledge is presented and so forth. Following the method, covering the deliverables (e.g., content) and meeting the benchmarks (e.g., learning objectives) becomes the center of the educational enterprise. As the teaching of content overrides meaningful participation (of both students and teachers) in the spontaneous, uncertain, and relational process of learning and practicing nursing, objective knowledge relegates subjective, experiential meaning making and practical knowledge to the margins of knowing. Subsequently, in many ways nurses learn to not only give authority to objectively derived knowledge but to overlook their own knowing in the moment of the practice encounter. As their subjective/experiential knowledge is sanctioned and overridden by rational and objective knowledge and method in both clinical and educational settings, they miss the opportunity to become acquainted with themselves as knowers, to figure out how their approach to knowing and knowledge is shaping their everyday nursing practice (Diekelmann, 2002; Diekelmann, Swenson, & Sims, 2003; Doane, Pauly, Brown, & McPherson, 2004).

An example of this overriding of authority is offered by Diekelmann, et al. (2003) in their critique of contemporary nursing education by specifically questioning the authority ascribed to the method of problem-based learning. These authors' present their view on problem-based learning and claim it is focused on content (i.e., cognitive gain) through the ". . . application and synthesis of content and the acquisition of skill toward solving teacher-specified problems" (Diekelmann et al., 2003, p. 104). Diekelmann et al., (2003) based on this view, subsequently call for reform in nursing pedagogy toward learning that ". . . shifts from lecturing and providing content . . . to a new conversation with students who pool their resources and knowledge to learn what they each needed to know . . . to fit their lives as clinicians" (p. 104). This drawing forth and building upon learners' existing knowledge and experience—that is, enlisting what students already know as the requisite knowledge for entering into meaningful learning, enables the teacher to highlight and build upon learners' capacities. Any new content (e.g., theory, experiences) is then critically examined, linked, and integrated into the existing knowledge and capacity of the learner rather than overriding it.

BEING IN-RELATION WITH KNOWLEDGE

All learning and all nursing practice involves an engagement with knowledge. This engagement requires the formation of a relationship to knowledge. As described above, depending on how learning/teaching is structured students engage and relate to knowledge differently. For example, if learning/teaching is grounded in the assumption that knowledge offers us facts or truths that are to be deposited, students (and teachers) will engage with knowledge differently than if learning/teaching rests on the pragmatic assumption that there is no such thing as truth—that all so-called knowledge requires scrutiny. As we highlighted above, the way students are in-relation with knowledge is not only a result of how they think of knowledge, but also how learning processes are structured. And, depending on how the educational endeavor is structured and how students are subsequently invited to relate to knowledge, what it is that is learned, and how that learning is used in the world will differ. For example, the approach to knowledge and learning and the particular way of relationally engaging with knowledge that is fostered in nursing education ultimately shapes the authority that nurses give knowledge in their practice, which knowledge they give authority to, the way in which they use and rely on knowledge, the way they continue to develop knowledge when in practice and so forth. Given that how nurses are guided to learn to know and think about knowledge profoundly shapes everyday nursing practice, our approach to learning/teaching must be in satisfactory relation with the way we want nurses to relate to knowledge in practice settings. That is, any learning situation must support a way of living and relating to knowledge that helps them to see how knowledge itself is useful in everyday moments of practice. For example, by beginning with what students already know and engaging them in a critical examination of new ideas and experiences, the opportunity to raise larger questions about how they live and relate to knowledge is created. That is, in exploring what they already know and linking any new content to that existing knowledge the opportunity is created to raise questions such as, How do you know what you know? What knowledge are you giving authority to? What leads you to give authority to that particular knowledge? How might your knowledge be expanded? What questions does your knowing not address? Through this process students not only develop more knowledge but simultaneously develop the skills and capacities that support critically reflective practice.

Aligning Education with Our Practice Vision

I remember how I spent the rest of my day after that nurse educator made her request. In inviting me to be a preceptor, it was almost as if she had made the space for me to unpack my assumption that seniority and expertise were the unquestioned criteria for being a good nurse and a good teacher. I wonder now what specifically the educator noticed about how I practiced nursing, both when I had the necessary knowledge to provide care and when I proceeded to know more. When caring for families of dying infants I knew that I moved back and forth between what I knew and had learned from other parents, but also tried to approach each family in a way that opened space for them to figure out and tell me what they needed. Could this moving back and forth between my knowing and being responsive to their needs be helpful when working with another nurse learning to work in the NICU? Could it be that similar to how I worked with families, the educator wanted me to engage with the new nurse in such a way as to invite her to inquire into her own knowledge—to learn about what she already knew and what she needed to know to provide effective care to critically ill infants and families? As I thought about this it occurred to me that this way of teaching—this inviting inquiry into knowledge—was at odds with my own experience of learning nursing. As a student I had never really been invited to explore my own knowledge in that way. As I continued to grapple with how I might be as a preceptor, I felt a bit lost—how might I teach based on these insights about knowledge and neonatal nursing care? Did it mean that "good teaching" could reflect "good nursing practice"?

This questioning is reflective of a pragmatic view of knowledge and the recognition that nurses' own relationship to knowledge shapes their everyday practice. As teachers we have found ourselves in a constant process of rethinking our teaching practice. We continually question how we might structure the learning/teaching of nursing in ways that will foster what it is we hope to see in practicing nurses. Since our ultimate goal as nurse educators is to support the development of nurses who consciously and intentionally develop, revise, adapt, expand, and alter nursing knowledge and practice to be responsive to particular people in particular relationships and contexts (Hartrick Doane & Varcoe, 2005), at the heart of any educational endeavor is our desire to foster students' capacities to intentionally and consciously choose how they live knowledge. To become more responsive to the relationships and contexts in which they practice, nurses need to have the opportunity to explore their own way of knowing and how they relationally engage with knowledge.

Subsequently, one of our pedagogical intents is to create the opportunity for students to see that what makes them successful learners. The attributes of curiosity, critical questioning, intentional scrutiny, ability to tolerate uncertainty, the desire to know more, openness to new perspectives, and so forth, are significant components of becoming safe and competent practitioners. Developing learning/teaching practices that support nurses to become inquirers, and also to be conscious and intentional agents of their living knowledge in practice, is a vital aspect of this process. Through such a process students are able to experience the parallels between the practice of nursing and the practice of learning/teaching and to recognize how both forms of practice involve active inquiry (Hartrick Doane & Varcoe, 2005).

INQUIRING INTO KNOWLEDGE AND MOVING BEYOND METHOD: SOME WORKING ASSUMPTIONS

What happened when I began the preceptorship? How did recognizing my own knowing about neonatal nursing practice and what good teaching might be about inform how I took up the responsibility of being a preceptor? What knowledge of neonatal pathophysiology was important? What did this mean for how I went about working with the nurse I was preceptoring—for the method I used as a teacher? I recall feeling a sense of relief after realizing that a full bucket of knowledge was not the prerequisite for being a good teacher. It was almost as if being released from the responsibility of being an expert actually allowed me to tap into what I actually did know. And I began to see that I had something to offer the new nurse. As the preceptorship unfolded and we inquired into her knowing, it was clear that there was particular knowledge that was new to her, like the methodology of newborn assessment. But there were many times that we shared questions and set about codeveloping the knowledge we needed to provide care. Part of why we were able to do this was that we both seemed to share a curiosity about learning and teaching. This seemed to help her believe she had the capacity to enter into her own knowledge development with some inquiring abilities for this new practice area.

On what basis, then, might the nurse proceed to teach the new nurse in the above example? Understanding the significance of how one relates to knowledge for nursing practice and the synergy between good learning/teaching and good nursing practice calls for an alignment of learning/teaching with nursing practice. And first and foremost is the importance of a learning/teaching relationship that respectfully supports differences and that nurtures curiosity. Such a relationship does not require that students and teacher be similarly matched, but rather that there is as Rogers (1969) describes unconditional positive regard, especially during experiences where differences between students and teachers arise.

Recalling the words of William Yeats, who suggests that education is not filling a bucket but lighting a fire, we believe that teaching ought to be structured not according to substantive content and/or educational methods but in accordance with the ever-changing process of nursing practice. As stated previously, focusing our teaching on lighting fires is quite different than undertaking the job of filling buckets. For example, if we want to light fires that inspire students to delve deeply into questions of practice and actively inquire into the knowledge they have and are living through their actions, we need an approach to learning/teaching that brings us (students and teachers) into satisfactory relation with knowing and knowledge development in nursing practice.

Interestingly, four decades ago Hassenplug (1964) challenged nurse educators to pay close attention to how nursing practice ought to shape nursing education:

> *The future of nursing education and nursing itself probably depends on good teaching. It is difficult to say just what the good teacher of nursing does, but it is obvious that she [sic] does more than impart knowledge and teach skills. Somehow she [sic] introduces the student to the subject of nursing in such a way that the student desires more knowledge and the understanding of how to acquire it. Thus, the student is inoculated with the spirit of inquiry and the excitement of discovery. (p. 3)*

It is this spirit of inquiry that lights the fires of learning. Therefore, in this final section, we offer some working assumptions that we have found helpful in guiding our teaching in this way. In presenting these assumptions, we want to emphasize that we are not "throwing the baby out with the bath water." That is, we are not suggesting that substantive content, educative methods, and teaching strategies are not useful extrinsic tools that we can enlist to enhance learning/teaching effectiveness, and we fully expect that as teachers we will continue to tap each of these. Rather, what we are challenging is the idea of giving content and methods overriding authority in the educative endeavor, bequeathing more authority to content and method than to students as learning people and to ourselves as teachers. And we are suggesting that it is important to reconsider the sense and purpose of method in nursing education (Hartrick, 2002a, 2002b). In particular, we are arguing that what is needed is a more **critical relationship** with teaching methods. In order to ensure that nursing and the people involved in learning "take center stage", content and methods need to become useful tools and resources as opposed to the substance of nursing education.

The following assumptions help us maintain that authoritative balance (Box 5.1):

- Nursing is responsive knowing-in-action.
- Objective/theoretical knowledge is a pragmatic tool.
- Nursing practice and education require creative capacity.

BOX 5.1 WORKING ASSUMPTIONS—KEY POINTS

ASSUMPTION 1: NURSING IS RESPONSIVE KNOWING-IN-ACTION.

- Knowledge is understood and enacted in particular relationships and contexts.
- Teachers and students need to constantly inform and reform their thinking about effective knowledge and methods for practice in particular situations.
- Knowledge and knowing are shaped by who we are and who we are becoming.

ASSUMPTION 2: OBJECTIVE/THEORETICAL KNOWLEDGE IS A PRAGMATIC TOOL.

- Knowledge helps us to be more responsive practitioners.
- What counts as knowledge is a question of relevance and responsiveness.

ASSUMPTION 3: NURSING PRACTICE AND EDUCATION REQUIRE CREATIVE CAPACITY.

- Reflecting on living experience can spark creative capacity.
- Teachers need to support the development and expression of students' imaginations.
- Creativity requires paying attention to your own and students' knowing in the moment.

Working Assumption 1: Nursing Is Responsive Knowing-In-Action

As we described above, we believe the goal of nursing education is the development of nurses who consciously and intentionally develop, revise, adapt, expand, and alter nursing knowledge and practice to be responsive in particular relationships and clinical practice contexts. We propose one way to foster students' capacities in this regard is to think of nursing practice as responsive knowing-in-action (Hartrick Doane & Varcoe, 2005). Nursing as knowing-in-action means that any nursing response is understood to be enacted by particular people within particular relationships and contexts. This educative assumption leads us to intentionally encourage students to identify and pay attention to their own particular knowing-in-action; that is, to listen to personally and professional significant meanings as they arise, to question how they as individuals are constituting those meanings, and to consciously and intentionally question the multiple social, organizational, and cultural forces pressing in upon them s they do so (Hartrick Doane & Varcoe, 2005a). For example, working with a family experiencing newborn death as teachers we would ask a student to critically consider how his or her theoretical understanding of grief, his or her own personal experiences of loss, the culture in the neonatal unit around infant death, the response of a particular family and so forth shape their knowing-in-action; that is, his or her response to that particular family. Seeing students as knowers-in-action reminds us to move beyond the dichotomies of objective and subjective knowledge and help students pay attention to how different forms of knowledge are coming together at any particular moment. For example, helping students tune into their bodily experiences and emotions arising from caring for critically ill infants is an important source of knowing about how to provide responsive care to both the infant and his or her family. The assumption highlights our educative responsibility to facilitate the development of mindful critical awareness and attunement to subjective experience and knowing, as well as the development of critical analytic skills to examine contextual and relational forms of knowledge. This assumption calls us to see the active nature of knowing, and to encourage students to explore, articulate, and enlist their subjective experiences as they critically reflect on and analyze their knowing-in-action. The assumption also highlights how theoretical knowledge is affected by context and how a significant amount of learning takes place in its context of use—or in action (Eraut, 1994). It directs us to create opportunities for students to access and perhaps alter what they already know and do intuitively without conscious awareness. And similar to how nurses approach their work in clinical practice settings, it spurs us as teachers to constantly inform and reform our thinking about what constitutes effective methods of practice in particular (learning) situations. This means that students and teachers may together try out certain types of theories about, for example, promoting the health of immigrant women. Together they could examine how certain theories or knowledge guides them to a greater or lesser degree to question taken for granted assumptions about the meaning of being an immigrant. This may be particularly relevant for a substantive curricular focus on diversity in women's experience of health. Teachers can then ask themselves how they might continually inform and reform their teaching practices in ways that are more adequate for curricular content and for creating meaningful learning experiences for students.

Overall, the above assumption highlights how nursing practice involves nurses' personal identity and involvement in their practice and obligations to act in professional and ethical ways. Thus, it reminds us to invite nurses to tune into the ways they are being as practitioners as well as what they are doing. For example, how nurses are presenting themselves during particular treatments (body posture, nonverbal cues) provides the context within which particular treatments are administered. Neonatal nurses, for instance, will often calm and soothe infants by holding their limbs in flexion while performing certain procedures. Parents often see this mindful, calming approach as equally important to their infants care as the therapeutic treatments alone. By creating opportunities for students to grapple with questions of "Who am I?" and "How am I compelled to act?" there is the potential to develop the ability to live these questions out within the relational and contextual complexities of everyday practice (Hartrick Doane, 2002a). These seemingly abstract questions offer a pragmatic compass for ethical nursing practice (Hartrick Doane, 2002b). Specifically this grappling with who am I as a nurse/person enables them to navigate through challenging practice contexts and situations, to see how they shape and are being shaped by particular forces in organizations and to determine their own bottom lines. For example, when they see end-of-life decisions being made that are ethically questionable this self-knowledge enables them to critically sort through the complexities of the situation and decide how they might effectively address ethical issues arising.

Creating the space to help students learn about themselves as persons situated in particular contexts and relationships means they may be more apt to understand how their knowing and knowledge is shaped by who they are as people. It directs us as teachers to move learning to a deeply personal level—to move questions beyond "how do I make decisions" to "what does how I make decisions tell me about who I am and how I practice?" (Hartrick Doane, 2002a). In so doing, we invite students—and ourselves—into critical relation with knowing and with developing knowledge. Thus, together we can begin to question the taken-for-granted truths about what constitutes right and good actions in nursing practice.

Working from the assumption of nursing as responsive knowing-in-action also directs us as teachers to move closer to ourselves. Through this assumption, we are reminded to question our own knowing and action (i.e., such as the methods we employ) to consider how our own identity, our relationships, location, and context shape our practice as educators.

Working Assumption 2: Objective/Theoretical Knowledge Is a Pragmatic Tool

Nurse educators have always been faced with a myriad of theoretical possibilities for fostering the learning of nursing. We suggest that when rethinking knowledge from a pragmatic perspective the questions of "which theories do I teach?" and "which theory will provide the best foundation for nursing practice?" is answered differently.[3] As James (1907) contends, theories are "instruments, not answers to enigmas, in which we can rest" (p. 147). From this perspective, theoretical knowledge is something that can help us move forward and aid us in being more responsive in practice, rather than as something in which we ground ourselves. This means that rather than beginning with content we enlist theoretical knowledge to help us to get into satisfactory relation with our experiences (James, 1907) and be more responsive to the people we are working with (Hartrick Doane & Varcoe, 2005a; 2005b).

From this pragmatic perspective, then, the question of which theory to teach does not call for us to merely make a choice between theories. Rather the question of which theories is actually more a question of relevance and responsiveness. And this question is one that we continually ask in each moment of our teaching. Specifically, the questions we live as educators are: Which theories can most enhance the student's sensitivity and ability to be responsive in particular moments of practice? Which theories will promote critical analysis of the complexities within situations and ultimately help students imagine and act in ways that are tailored to fit particular situations?

For example, rather than trying to decide whether or not family systems theory or some other theoretical approach to family nursing is the best basis for teaching and learning about facilitating the health of families, the educative assumption theory is a pragmatic tool which leads us to draw upon a range of theoretical ideas that are responsive to the particularities of families' health care needs, life situations, and the various contexts in which families and nurses interact (Hartrick Doane & Varcoe, 2005b). Therefore, this assumption leads us to not only choose the content of our

---

[3] Taking a stance on objective/theoretical knowledge as a pragmatic tool does not imply that we are assuming a relativist or anything-goes position. Claiming that there are many right theories for nursing, and that such rightness is determined by the theories' ability to solve real problems in the real world (Rorty, 1999) does not imply that there are no preferred realities and truths. However, preferred truths or theories are determined by their contribution to responsive nursing practice. For example, with regard to the issue of dehumanizing practices, the question becomes, Which theories best support us to fully address the complexities of the situation, and analyze and articulate responsive actions consistent with the shared human-caring values underlying the practice of nursing?

courses based on that question, but also spontaneously tap into other relevant theories in particular teaching moments. For example, hearing a student label and/or stereotype someone by referring to them as a drug addict, we might draw upon cultural theory or poststructural theory to engage students in a critical consideration of how labeling and stereotyping shapes and constrains nursing practice.

Working Assumption 3: Nursing Practice and Education Require Creative Capacity

As educators, we have come to believe that nursing practice is a creative process and that a pedagogy that supports the development of creativity offers a powerful foundation for learning and teaching nursing (Hartrick, 2002a; Hartrick Doane, 2002a). Subsequently, as teachers we strive to cultivate **creative capacity** in students. We invite them to creatively engage in their living experiences and creatively be in relation to their learning so as to support their knowledge development. In such creative processes, the spark of hidden internal forces, including emotion, care, and commitment, works in tandem with reason, the work of honing, limiting, and clarifying to give form (Vogt, 1987). Working from this assumption of creativity, our intent as educators is to not only promote conscious awareness of practice, but also to support students to recreate their knowledgeable practice in particular situations.

Attention to creativity directs nurse educators to support the development and expression of students' imaginations—to help them develop the capacity to understand and reimagine their own responsibility of participating in a community such as nursing. Facilitating learners' development involves cultivating both cognitive maturity and a conscious, intentional awareness that becomes the basis for creative and responsive knowing-in-action. This is different from teaching students about knowledge for nursing practice where learners are actually taught to apply particular ideas in practice. Rather, guided by this educative assumption, students are encouraged to examine their location and power while thoughtfully and critically attending to seemingly established truths in nursing. This assumption compels us to bring theories and concepts as raw material for students' creative processes. It leads us to continually inspire students to revise, adapt, expand, and reimagine possibilities for nursing practice within particular relationships and situations. In this way it shifts away from thinking of truth as a thing to understanding truth as an active process of interpreting. At a pragmatic level this living approach to truth spurs us to ask students how they might enhance their practical, affective, relational, and reasoning skills so that they become more able to meet the needs of their patients and colleagues in practice.

This educative assumption also reminds us to listen carefully to how students are creating their knowing in the moment. For example, we listen to how they are creatively using theories to name and understand their nursing practice. In learning to practice in the neonatal unit, students might potentially draw on theories about infant vulnerability following preterm birth since these theories are relevant in highlighting aspects that a neonatal nurse needs to notice, assess, question, and evaluate within the context of care giving. However, theory in this situation is not enough since nurses require the creative ability to determine the relevance of this knowledge to particular families in particular situations (Hartrick, 2002a; Hartrick Doane, 2002a). Thus, this working assumption of creativity reminds us of the shifting nature of all theory and knowledge (all knowledge has limitations and a shelf-life)—and that a students' knowing in any moment of practice is a synergy of their relational knowing of a particular baby/family, their past and present knowing as well as their desire for more knowledge (future knowing). Guided by our creative intent as teachers, we are directed to listen carefully to how students are presenting themselves in knowledge (for example family knowledge, theoretical knowledge, physical assessment knowledge, and so forth), what knowledge they are drawing and not drawing on, what efforts they are making and might need to make to know more, and how we might support their creative ability to bring their knowledge to form in order to inform and/or reform their practice.

The reader might question at this point if there is no truth, how can one reason, because surely reason must be founded on something.

Caputo (1987) describes (and we agree) how the view of reason is merely a socially constructed view of reason that has been used to exclude voices that have been criticized as primitive, passionate, or emotional in the march of enlightenment and progress. Caputo (1987) argues for our ability to emancipate ourselves and others from this limited view of reason. He reminds us that reason has to do with action and responsiveness—and in this way his perspective of reason is in line with the pragmatic view of knowing that we are proposing.

> *If things are in flux, in undecidable drift and slippage, and if reason is to respond to things, to keep up a correspondence with them (according even to the most classical demand of metaphysics of truth), reason must play it loose, be capable of unexpected moves, of paradigm switches, of following up unorthodox suggestions. The most reasonable view of reason denies that you can write a handbook about the way reason works. (Caputo, 1987, p. 228)*

Rather than making humanness subservient to reason and method, redescribing reason makes reason and method subservient to humanness. Drawing from Heidegger, Caputo (1987) suggests replacing method with a deeper appreciation of *methodos,* which is "the way in which we pursue a matter" (p. 213).

FROM ASSUMPTIONS TO PRACTICES: MAKING IT HAPPEN

Based on the three assumptions presented in the previous section, we will explore strategies or processes that we as nurse educators employ in our practice. Our intent in providing these processes is not to offer methods but rather examples of possibilities arising from the working assumptions. Many educators may find that the guiding assumptions are sufficient in sparking their own creative teaching ideas. Others may choose to try out some of the processes suggested here as a means to developing their own approaches. It is important to emphasize that our hesitancy in offering this suggestion is fueled by our desire to resist perpetuating the thing we are challenging. That is, we do not wish to promote the turning of strategies and processes into prescriptive method that will, in our view, stifle educators' own creative capacity to develop practices based on their own conscious, intentional, living knowledge of nursing education and nursing practice.

The practices that flow from the working assumptions will be explored next. They are:

- Rethinking knowledge.
- Bringing learners closer to themselves.
- Learning moments.
- Attending to particulars.
- Teachers in-relation with knowledge.

Rethinking Knowledge

The working assumptions outlined above offer some direction for how to create space for students to intentionally and consciously engage with knowledge. First, since nursing practice involves responsive knowing-in-action, any learning of theory must speak to the subjective and objective experiences and ways of knowing in nursing practice (Hartrick Doane & Varcoe, 2005b). Thus, new knowledge must be taken up, tried on/out, and lived. Second, since students' personal identity is deeply implicated in how they learn and develop knowledge, they require opportunities to see how existing theory *is* or is *not* relevant to their own process of becoming a nurse. Third, if we suggest that objective/theoretical knowledge is a pragmatic tool, any theory needs to be explored for its usefulness in particular situations.

With these assumptions and directions in mind, one strategy we have used with students is to have them choose and live different theories in practice. For example, when teaching nursing ethics, we might ask students to take the ethic of justice and try to live that theory during one clinical day and on the next day try out and live feminist ethical theory. Students are directed to employ the theories to help them create their moment to moment practice throughout the day. The theory is to be used to direct their attention, to make decisions, and to determine action. As they live out the theories, students are asked to pay close attention to:

- Their personal experience (e.g., how comfortable/uncomfortable it felt, what specifically felt good/did not feel good, etc.).
- Their conscious thinking processes (e.g., what each theory directed their attention to, what factors and values became part of their reasoning process).
- What decisions they ultimately made and how right (using personal and professional ethical values) those decisions felt.
- What actions they engaged in.
- What seemed to not be addressed by each particular theoretical stance.

In seminar we then debrief their experiences. In this debriefing, we seek to inquire deeply into the students' experiences going beyond questions of What do I think about the theories? Which was the best one? to questions of experience and their own processes of knowing. Questions we might ask include: How did the theory help you name and clarify what mattered? How did what matters or what you value change as you moved between the theories? What assumptions and limitations can you see underlying the theories? What did good nursing practice look like with each? How did your view of good practice fit with your own sense of how you ought to be? How did your approach to practice fit with the people you were nursing that day? In what ways did the theory support and/or constrain your responsiveness to relationships and context? How did the theory help you sort through the complexities of your everyday work and the many forces that shaped your work and day? How did each theory help you create your own responsive practice in the particular situations of the day? How is your own responsiveness reflective of the shared values about nursing practice? What other knowledge(s) did you need to bring to your practice?

As students try out theoretical ideas and we explore these questions together, the opportunity is created for them to practice attuning to their subjective experience and accessing that knowledge in the moment. They have the opportunity to critically examine theoretical knowledge in light of the professional practice of nursing and examine the particular knowledge(s) and the sociopolitical stance the theories perpetuate. In addition, students have the opportunity to learn about themselves including the taken-for-granted knowing that they currently bring to their practice, to learn from families, and to question how all of that knowing might enhance what they see, what they attend to, what they give value to, and how they respond. Through this process, students have the opportunity to grapple with: How does theory and experience inform me and how might I recreate my own living knowledge to enhance my ability to meet the needs of patients/families.

Bringing Learners Closer to Themselves

The working assumptions outlined earlier also direct us to create ways of bringing learners closer to themselves. The understanding that nursing is a responsive practice that is shaped by nurses' personal identity means teachers need to find ways to help students to be in-relation with themselves and with their own knowing and developing knowledge. Thus, it is important to create learning spaces where students' drop into themselves, to listen, hear, and come to know themselves as nurses (Hartrick Doane, 2002a). We use their living experience as the medium for learning. We might ask them to name a seemingly simple decision they made that week in their practice setting such as how they decided which patient call bell to answer first. Working together, student and teacher examine their decision-making process through questions such as: What are you aware of as you contemplate which bell to answer? What are you thinking? How do you actually set priorities? What is informing your practice and decision making? What contextual elements are shaping you in that moment? Do you see an alliance with any particular theoretical perspective or principle? What personal, professional, and societal values and assumptions are you basing your decisions on? And so forth. One way we have purposefully attempted to do this is through expanding our approach to learning moments.

Learning Moments as Strategy

If we take a view of nursing as responsive knowing-in-action this tells us that any moment is potentially a learning moment. Since knowing and nursing practice are not solely rational processes that unfold in a linear fashion, there are many moments in students' lives, beyond the classroom or clinical setting, that foster their capacities to practice nursing. For example, the illness or death of a family member holds a good deal of learning for students developing knowledge for nursing practice.

Based on the assumption that the learning of nursing can occur anywhere and anytime, we intentionally strive to use the time we have with students to potentiate learning outside of the classroom and/or clinical time. That is, we see the time we are with students as a small portion of the actual learning moments they have in a day, so we purposefully attempt to capitalize on learning that occurs beyond formal settings. For example, as students begin developing the skills of conscious attunement and discernment we encourage them to start employing those skills as they go about their everyday lives. Often they return to class with more raw material from which to recreate their living knowledge. Perhaps one of the greatest challenges in fostering learning moments is knowing when to bring in our own knowledge (Hartrick, 2002b). That is, there are times when offering our own knowledge can help students name and clarify their own. However, there is also the potential for our knowledge to be offered in such a way that it shuts down the student's own relation to their knowing and creative process of knowledge development. We find this tension to be particularly present when a student is struggling and experiencing great anxiety about what to do in a particular situation. Overall we attempt to not try and make the anxiety better or alleviate it, but rather enlist the students' experience and support them as they work through their anxiety, enhance their understanding, and continue to create their own living knowledge of themselves and of nursing. For example, some students bring a particular experience of patient care into the classroom and describe how something was not right. They are drawing on a gut feeling or bodily sense that something may have been unattended to or done poorly. In our experience this is not uncommon when students are involved in caregiving for patients at the end of life. Our view is that enlisting this bodily sense, tuning into and (not away from) the gut feeling, and exploring how students' own experience and values about care at the end of life are influencing them, opens a place where they can see how they are creating their own living knowledge of themselves and nursing.

Attending to the Particulars as Strategy

A particularly powerful way to cultivate creative capacity is to help students learn to pay attention to the particular (Hartrick Doane & Varcoe, 2005a). The particulars of situations create discerning insights that indicate the presence of relevant dimensions of practice (Jaeger, 2001). Sensitivity to particularity enables nurses to be both intellectually and emotionally attuned to perceive, interpret, and respond to what may be relevant in a given situation.

To assist students to learn this skill of attuning to the particular, we attempt to cultivate the skills of observation and critical questioning. We ask them to scrutinize situations, theories, and experiences in order to notice the particularities within them. This may involve directing their attention to the particularities of the sociopolitical context (e.g., what particular values seem to be shaping the situation?), to relational particularities (e.g., how is power playing out between the nurse and the physician?), and to particularities of people in the situation (e.g., what is this particular patient asking or experiencing?). Other scrutinizing questions include: What is happening in this situation? What seems to be significant in this situation? What makes it significant? What informs what you see as significant? What subtle aspects have significance to the situation? What particular aspects are different people highlighting as significant? And how does your particular way of looking shape and perhaps constrain what you see?

In our desire to cultivate creative capacity, we also attempt to involve students in varying approaches to deliberation including both rationalistic concepts and methods of analysis and others such as intuition, emotions, subjective experience, values, and sensitivity. In addition, we attempt to highlight the connections between what students already know and are familiar with (e.g., the clinical assessment skills of observing, interpreting, clarifying their understanding of the importance of looking for subtle clinical signs) and responsive nursing practice. In this way, students spontaneously become more attuned to the complexities of nursing practice and the conscious, responsive, intentional way of being that knowing in action calls forth.

Teachers In-Relation With Knowledge as Process

As teachers we begin with the assumption that students bring self-knowledge and capacities to learn nursing. We invite students to be who they are, both in the way we offer knowledge and in the way we live in-relation with them. We purposefully attempt to be ourselves and to explicitly name how it is we have chosen to live and practice nursing. At the same time we bring in guests who are different from ourselves and yet exemplify how responsive knowing in action is visible in nursing practice.

Teachers working from the pedagogical processes we have proposed may find their greatest challenge to be living the thing they are teaching. Making space to stay attuned to how we are in-relation to knowing and knowledge is both a classroom practice, a way of being as a teacher and the humanly-involved nature of nursing practice. One way we attempt to stay attuned as teachers is to continually ask ourselves the following question: Am I living my knowledge in a way that is responsive and will cultivate students' learning and becoming as nurses?

SUMMARY

In closing, we echo Palmer's (1998) thoughts on being good teachers and invite you to think about how rethinking knowledge and moving beyond method may foster students' abilities to be in-relation with, or connected to, their knowing and knowledge development.

> *. . . good teachers possess a capacity for connectedness. They are able to weave a complex web of connections among themselves, their subjects, and their students so that students can learn to weave a world for themselves. . . . The connections made by good teachers are held not in their methods but in their hearts—meaning* heart *in the ancient sense, as the place where intellect and emotion and spirit and will converge in the human self. (p. 11)*

It has been our intent to imagine possibilities for nursing education by examining how it could be more closely aligned with, and flow out of, the practice of nursing. We offer the working assumptions and practices as creative resources and tools to assist you in your learning/teaching work and hope that they spark further conversation about how we may go about achieving our ultimate goal as nurse educators; that is, to support the development of nurses who consciously and intentionally develop, revise, adapt, expand, and alter nursing knowledge and practice to be responsive to particular people in particular relationships and contexts. Rather than assuming that it is substantive knowledge and/or educative methods and strategies that lead to high-quality learning/teaching we invite you to consider how, similar to nursing practice, exemplary teaching lies in the way that educators engage with the people they are teaching and how they approach and live nursing knowledge.

LEARNING ACTIVITY

The focus of this learning activity is to have students engage in a critical analysis of how particular knowledge(s) either enhances or constrains their ability to effectively respond to a particular patient or family for whom he or she has provided care.

1. Ask the student to list the kind of knowledge they may require to care for a particular patient, like a preterm infant. Likely they will list knowledge of neonatal pathophysiology, intrauterine growth and development, and knowledge of nursing care for vulnerable and fragile preterm infants.
2. Ask them to think about what knowledge of the family may help them provide responsive and effective care.
3. Ask the students to consider what being-in-relation with these multiple sources of knowledge looks like. When will particular knowledge(s) become important, in the foreground, and when will particular ways of knowing enter the background? Ask the students to describe how they go about deciding foreground/background knowledge or ways of knowing in particular relationships.
4. Summarize by having the students critically examine how particular knowledge can either enhance or constrain the possibilities for good nursing care during particular moments of practice. Ask students to think about how they are developing creative capacities that help them identify how particular knowledge in particular moments of practice makes possible responsive, effective nursing care for specific patients/families.

RESOURCES FOR EDUCATORS

PLANNING THE TEACHING/LEARNING EXPERIENCE

Questions to Support a Thoughtful Reading

1. What might be similar elements or characteristics between good nursing and good teaching?
2. Think about your favorite nursing instructor or recall a teacher who inspired you to learn. How did he or she nurture you as both a learner and becoming a nurse?
3. Can you recall being a patient or when a family member was a patient? Can you describe what good nursing care looked like during that time? Do you see similarities with how as a learner you might describe good teaching?

Tips for Developing a Student-Centered Learning Environment

- Encourage students to foster the integral relationship between their personal and professional selves.
- Create the space for learners to see how who they are as a person shapes who they are as a nurse.
- Encourage examination of particularities (i.e., what is unique, significant, similar, different).
- Pay attention to how you are taking up and expressing knowledge and how that is shaping you in particular moments of your teaching practice.

EVALUATING THE TEACHING/LEARNING EXPERIENCE

Questions to Elicit Feedback from Students on Their Learning

1. Am I valued for who I am as a teacher/learner?
2. Do I create and engage in opportunities to explore how who I am as a person affects how I teach/learn?
3. How might I articulate my relationship to knowing and knowledge development? What makes it critical or uncritical? To whom do I give authority in teaching/learning nursing?

Sample Evaluation Strategies

Guided by the question, have I and my teaching made a difference?, think about what making a difference to students' learning means within the context of the course you are teaching. List the elements of what making a difference looks like. Then, ask yourself, what are the signposts of learning that I believe make this difference visible? For example, we believe signposts from our teaching practice are tuning into the following kinds of questions:

1. Are students drawing on bodily sensing and responses in situations of nursing practice?
2. Are students drawing on various ways of knowing in order to continually scrutinize how particular knowledge enables them to be effective and responsive in nursing practice?
3. How do students describe the integral relationship between their personal and professional selves?
4. How do students link who they are with what they do?
5. How do students live truth critically and intentionally?
6. How do students pay attention to the particulars of nursing practice?

References

Berman, M. (1981). *The reenchantment of the world.* Ithaca, NY: Cornell University Press.

Berman, M. (2000). *The wandering god. A study in nomadic spirituality.* New York: State of New York Press.

Bevis, E. & Watson, J. (1989). *Toward a caring curriculum: A new pedagogy for nursing.* New York: National League for Nursing.

Caputo, J. D. (1987). *Radical hermeneutics: Repetition, deconstruction, and the hermeneutic project.* Bloomington and Indianapolis: University Press.

Diekelmann, N. (2002). "Pitching a lecture" and "reading the faces of students": Learning lecturing and the embodied practices of teaching. *Journal of Nursing Education, 41(7)*, 97–99.

Diekelmann, N., Swenson, M. M, & Sims, S. L. (2003). Reforming the lecture: Avoiding what students already know. *Journal of Nursing Education, 42*(3), 103–105.

Doane, G., Pauly, B., Brown, H., et al. (2004). Exploring the heart of ethical nursing practice: Implications for nursing education. *Nursing Ethics, 11*(3), 240–253.

Eraut, M. (1994). *Developing professional knowledge and competence.* London: Falmer Press.

Eraut, M. (2000). The intuitive practitioner: A critical overview. In T. Atkinson & G. Claxton, (Eds.), *The intuitive practitioner: On the value of not always knowing what one is doing.* Buckingham: Open University Press.

Freire, P. (1988). *Pedagogy of the oppressed.* New York: Continuum.

Giroux, H. (1991). Beyond the ethics of flag waving: Schooling and citizenship for a critical democracy. *Clearing House, 64*(5), 305.

Habermas, J. (1987). *Knowledge and human interest* (Translated by J. Shapiro). Cambridge: Polity Press.

Hadot, P. (1995). *Philosophy as a way of life: Spiritual experience from Socrates to Foucault.* New York: Blackwell.

Hartrick, G. A. (1997). Relational capacity: The foundation for interpersonal nursing practice. *Journal of Advanced Nursing, 26*(3), 523–528.

Hartrick, G. (2002a). Transcending the limits of method: Cultivating creativity in nursing. *Research and Theory for Nursing Practice. An International Journal, 16*(1), 53–62.

Hartrick, G. (2002b). Beyond behavioural skills to human-involved processes: Relational nursing practice and interpretive pedagogy. *Journal of Nursing Education, 41*(9), 400–404.

Hartrick Doane, G. (2002a). In the spirit of creativity: the learning and teaching of ethics in nursing. *Journal of Advanced Nursing, 39*(6), 1–8.

Hartrick Doane, G. (2002b). Am I still ethical? The socially-mediated process of nurses' moral identity. *Nursing Ethics, 9*(6), 623–635.

Hartrick Doane, G. (2003). Through pragmatic eyes: Philosophy and the re-sourcing of family nursing. *Nursing Philosophy, 4*(1), 25–33.

Hartrick Doane, G. & Varcoe, C. (2005a). *Family nursing as relational inquiry.* Philadelphia: Lippincott Williams & Wilkins.

Hartrick Doane, G. & Varcoe, C. (2005b). Toward compassionate action: Pragmatism and the inseparability of theory/practice. *Advances in Nursing Science, 28*(1), 81–90.

Hassenplug, L. W. (1964, August). Editorial. *Journal of Nursing Education, 3.*

Hodges, H. F. (1997). Seeking balance to dialectic tensions in teaching through philosophic inquiry. *Image: Journal of Nursing Scholarship, 29*(4), 349–354.

hooks, b. (1994). *Teaching to transgress: Education as the practice of freedom.* New York: Routledge.

hooks, b. (2003). *Teaching community: Pedagogy of hope.* London: Routledge.

Ironside, P. M, (2003). New pedagogies for teaching thinking: The lived experiences of students and teachers enacting narrative pedagogy. *Journal of Nursing Education, 42*(11), 509–516.

Jaeger, S. (2001). Teaching health care ethics: the importance of moral sensitivity for moral reasoning. *Nursing Philosophy, 1,* (2) 131–142.

James, W. (1907). *Pragmatism: A new name for some old ways of thinking.* New York: Longmans, Green and Company.

Moccia, P. (1988). Curriculum revolution: An agenda for change. In *Curriculum revolution: Mandate for change.* (pp. 53–64). New York: National League for Nursing.

Palmer, P. J. (1998). *The courage to teach: Exploring the inner landscape of a teacher's life.* New York: Jossey-Bass.

Rogers, C. (1969). *Freedom to learn.* London: Charles E. Merrill.

Rorty, R. (1999). *Philosophy and social hope.* London: Penguin.

Schön, D. (1987). *Educating the reflective practitioner.* New York: Jossey Bass.

Thayer-Bacon, B. J. (2003). *Relational epistemologies.* New York: Peter Lang.

Vogt, K. D. (1987). *Vision and revision: The concept of inspiration in Thomas' Mann's fiction.* New York: Peter Lang.

Theories and Concepts to Guide Distance Education Using Student-Centered Approaches

Chapter 6

Victoria S. Murrell
Cynthia K. Russell
Margaret T. Hartig
W. Dean Care

An advanced nurse practitioner and educator of many years, Michael knew that nursing education had a long history of innovation. It was now time to better utilize the Internet, fast becoming one of the most common resources for information exchange, for educating nurses. At issue was how best to go about changing a traditional teaching institution—one that offered solid instruction, broad learning, and good clinical experiences in a face-to-face environment—to an institution with the same high standards and experiences presented at a distance. Was it possible to educate and train people via the Internet in such a hands-on profession? Could the Internet be harnessed to bring education to people who otherwise might not be able to get that education? Was it possible to teach and learn the skills of practice in such a remote (nonhands-on) way?

Michael began his research into what other educational institutions were doing, only to find a deficiency of solid research about best practices in distance education. Might there be some basic learning theory that would lead the way and provide some ideas for ensuring that the educational experience would take into account the needs of the students?

INTENT This chapter provides an overview of the educational theories that build a framework for philosophies of teaching and learning. It will focus on theories of student-centered learning and adult education, specifically within the context of teaching and learning at a distance. We will also consider the implementation of student-centered educational theories and their impact on teaching and learning at a distance. The chapter concludes with a brief look at issues vital to distance education: the nature of nursing education, the impact of technology, the cost and time associated with student-centered learning, and the common problem of information management.

OVERVIEW

WHAT *IS* DISTANCE EDUCATION?

Distance education is a descriptor for teaching and learning that takes place outside of what we know as the traditional, face-to-face classroom. The concept of distance education has enjoyed a surprisingly long history in western education. Distance learning dates back to Plato when he published Socrates' Dialogues (circa 360 B.C.) (Klass, 2000). By committing his teachings to the written word, Plato introduced a new technology to education that enabled his students to experience and interpret the words and thoughts of their teacher without being face-to-face with him. Throughout the Middle Ages, the Renaissance, and the Industrial Revolution, the increasing availability of the written word meant teaching and learning could take place outside of a classroom.

Learning modalities continued to be influenced as education became more available and new resources and technologies developed as a result of the Industrial Revolution.

The expansion of postal services increased the accessibility of education at a distance via the correspondence course. As early as 1892, Pennsylvania State University offered for-credit distance education courses in the United States (Banas & Emory, 1998). With the evolution of more ubiquitous and less expensive audio and video technologies during the 1950s and 1960s, correspondence courses expanded from primarily text-based materials into multimedia presentations combining text, sound, and visual materials. Students who could not attend in-person classes gained access to the content in **independent studies**, although often as passive and impersonal learning experiences. The widespread presence of televisions, and then of videocassette players, encouraged development of video-based materials. Video materials provided a wider array of content and addressed visual learning needs, though the teaching mode usually remained a one-way experience.

Development of the **World Wide Web**, as well as other resources offered by the **Internet**, has dramatically increased the modes and methods of educating in a noncontiguous space. Communication via the Internet has introduced a new world of potential to distance education. Ways of delivering, receiving, and responding to course content are now available to learners on both sides of the lectern. In addition to new methods of interaction between faculty and students, these technologies have the capacity to change isolation to interactivity. The advent of the World Wide Web following the development and widespread dispersal of the graphical user interface (GUI) browsers in the late 1980s and early 1990s, as well as the subsequent development of interactive and user-friendly technologies, presents the potential for new teaching and learning methodologies.

In many cases, however, the same traditional teaching processes are still at work in current educational programs. Faculty who teach in distance course offerings send instructive information, perhaps with some follow-up questions and answers, and an assessment to the student who then sends back answers. The use of electronic mail (e-mail) to exchange information between faculty and students has provided a much more immediate rate of communication between teacher and learner, but speed alone does not improve learning. Possibilities associated with the wealth of a constantly increasing flow of knowledge and interactive formats also reinforce the need to examine teaching styles. Educators must consider **student-centered teaching** approaches that acknowledge both lifelong learning, necessitated by the information explosion, and the versatility of the delivery technology that makes multiple ways of learning and understanding possible.

The Web fueled an explosion of available information and communication that moved Western society deep into the Information Age. By 1996, freshmen in college had access to more information in one year than their grandparents received in an entire lifetime (Oblinger & Rush, 1997). This sudden increase in information, the ubiquity of technology in the workplace, the importance of dynamic knowledge use and acquisition, the need for lifelong learning, and competition for work among talented people across the world undeniably changed the face of education for both the teacher and the learner. Implicit in that changing paradigm is the understanding that as the flow and management of information changes, so must those of us in the classroom—on both sides of the lectern.

PHILOSOPHICAL PERSPECTIVES: FRAMING A STUDENT-CENTERED APPROACH TO DISTANCE EDUCATION

An understanding of the theories that support student-centered learning provides a scaffold for the development of teaching modalities. Educational theory is in constant development as techniques are discovered and rediscovered, implemented, and evaluated both by those in the field and in the field of educational research and psychology.

Educational Theories

The theories on which methodologies are developed can provide educators with a clear indication of what others have constructed as sound educational practice. (See Chapter 1 for a full discussion of the philosophical and theoretical grounding of student-centered learning. Box 6.1 provides a quick comparison of the different viewpoints.) The concept of **active learning**—increased engagement of students with the learning process with the ultimate goal of integrating and applying new knowledge—evolved from the development of **cognitive theory**, which espouses that learning takes place when information is perceived, attended to, and stored into long-term memory. **Cognitivists** generally believe that knowledge is generated when information is integrated or assimilated into a framework of existing knowledge (Bruner, 1966; Piaget, 1970). This process occurs differently in different people, thus the need for a variety of teaching methodologies. The important concept for cognitivists is the attendance to what needs to be learned. Students need to desire or value the content to be gained; otherwise the information moves into short-term memory and is quickly discarded.

BOX 6.1 EDUCATIONAL THEORIES

THEORY	KEY POINTS	NOTED RESEARCHERS
Cognition	• Learning is a biologically-based process and is somewhat dependent on maturation. • Knowledge is generated when new information is assimilated with existing knowledge. • Interaction with the environment is key to acquiring new knowledge.	Jean Piaget, Jerome Bruner
Behaviorism	• Learning occurs when the individual is motivated by the potential reward or the avoidance of punishment, by reinforcement provided by teachers.	B.F. Skinner
Social behaviorism	• Interaction with others is key to the learning process.	Albert Bandura, Lev Vygotsky

Behaviorists (e.g., Skinner, 1968) theorized that learning resulted from rewards gained from a specific action (e.g., a good grade from a well-written paper). **Social behaviorists** (e.g., Bandura, 1977; Vygotsky, 1978) believed that learning resulted from the synergies developed from interaction with others. Like Piaget, the behaviorists believed that students constructed knowledge from their experience, but the social behaviorists proposed that knowledge construction occurs within a framework of learning with and from other people, not just from the environment.

While the teaching and evaluation methodologies that developed from these learning theories have ranged from practical (students must have "hooks" on which they can hang new information) to one-dimensional (learners are motivated solely by grades), student-centered learning has evolved primarily from the cognitivist point of view. This teaching approach focuses on the students, not the teachers, during the teaching and learning experience; that is, the learning experience should encompass more learner involvement. The learner must be more active than passive. While the component of sharing expertise must not be lost, student-centered learning requires a shift toward greater engagement on the part of the student than is possible in the traditional lecture or classroom scenario.

Teaching and Learning With Adults

The term **androgogy** was coined in the 19th century to describe the art and science of teaching adults. As the development of educational theories focused on **pedagogy** (the teaching of children), both John Dewey (1938) and Malcolm Knowles (1970, 1975, 1984) proposed that adult learners particularly benefit from collaborative, participatory educational practices. Encouraged to learn by both extrinsic and intrinsic motivation, adults become ready to learn when they experience a life situation where they need or want to know and thereby value acquiring the new skill, knowledge, or attitude. This pragmatic attitude also extends into the adult need to know why they should learn something.

Knowles (1970) referred to as the father of adult learning, saw the education of adults more as a process of self-directed inquiry. According to Knowles, adults prefer to decide for themselves what they want to learn and enter into the learning process with a task-centered orientation. Compared to children and teenagers, adults bring a far different volume and quality of experiences to learning that help them connect learning experiences to past experiences. These life experiences enhance learners' abilities to guide their education and fuel their expectations to participate in the educational process. Learning experiences are often more meaningful and more likely to result in integrating new knowledge when learner expectations are met.

Teacher-Centered Education

Models of distance education in many ways mirror models of teaching and learning in the traditional classroom. The continuum of models is anchored by two theoretically opposed approaches to educating: teacher-centered and student-centered. In the **teacher-centered teaching** paradigm, the focus is on the instructor, who provides mostly unidirectional information to a group of students. In many cases, this approach provides a passive educational experience for the students.

One of the most typical teacher-centered models is that of **lecture**, whereby the instructor provides information, usually verbally but sometimes with written or graphical documentation. Whether it takes place in a large or small group, lecture normally involves little student involvement, other than the activity of note taking and perhaps one-on-one questioning of the instructor. According to the 2001 report on the Condition of Education, published by the U.S. National Center for Education Statistics, 83% of reporting higher education faculty used the lecture format as their primary instructional method in at least one class taught for credit in fall 1998 (NCES, 2001).

Developing and presenting a well-delivered lecture requires valuable active learning on the part of the instructor. Students attending a lecture, on the other hand, are involved in little more than ingesting (not *digesting*) information and writing notes. This does not provide the learner with effective or efficient learning opportunities and, for many students in a lecture hall, the educational experience is a passive one with little processing. Furthermore, research has shown that the efficiency of learning via lecture is poor. In one often-cited study (McLeish, 1968), researchers found that students' notes and their performance on an immediate assessment of the lecture material produced a maximum of 42% of the material provided during lecture. A week later, students could only recall 17% of the lecture material without use of notes.

Some distance learning emulates a lecture hall. Instructors put their lectures (text-based or **multimedia**) **online**, and students are tasked with comprehending and processing information as best they can. This distributed classroom model differs from the live lecture in that students have the option to reread or replay parts of the lecture that are unclear, allowing them to review the information at times of their choosing. However, there is little or no interaction with other students and limited interaction with the instructor. Students are left to read, research, and integrate material on their own without the benefit of the instructor's expertise and guidance. While active, student-centered learning is far more productive and efficient for the student, it is surprisingly underutilized in postsecondary education. Research has consistently shown that learning is more permanent and meaningful when learners take an active role in the process (Jones, 2003).

Student-Centered Education

In student-centered learning, the instructor takes on a role more like that of an information facilitator. Faculty move from the central focus, or sage-on-the-stage, to the supporting function of guide-on-the-side. Students' involvement and participation become the focus of the teaching and learning process, and their engagement prompts them to be more involved interactively with the learning material. Piaget (1952) theorized that learners cannot be taught but must be forced into a state of disequilibrium that resulted from the learner's attempt to reconcile new environmental stimuli with that which was already known. The need to alleviate this imbalance provides the impetus for cognitive reconciliation, and the learner's accommodation of the environmental input into the cognitive structure, provides equilibrium; a state of balance between the cognitive and the environment. Such an adaptive, dialectic model of learning describes the interaction of the individual learner with the environment, which results in the progressive development of knowledge. The central challenge for educators is to maximize engagement for learners, thus providing them with the stimuli to grow.

IMPLEMENTING A STUDENT-CENTERED APPROACH IN DISTANCE EDUCATION

Educating well challenges the most experienced teacher. Doing so at a distance adds another layer to a complex process. While some think that distance learning means making text-based lectures and associated questions available for students to access via the Web, others know that doing a good job of teaching at a distance requires much more than dispensing information for self-teaching. Providing student-centered learning possibilities poses an exciting yet reachable challenge.

Student-centered instruction is about the active, two-way communication of information and understanding. Models for distance education are restricted only by the instructors' imagination, institutional infrastructure, and students' technological capacity. The distance educator's challenge is to design and provide curricular content that is androgogically sound and available to the learner without requiring face-to-face delivery of that content by the teacher. In a distance setting, this may involve the use of multimedia technology, such as audio, video, and interactive programs or Web sites. However, technological capacity is only one framework for structuring learner-centered distance education opportunities. The more important challenge in student-centered education is creating the environment for learning. Learning theories support that such an environment must involve consistent, focused, two-way communication between the student and the teacher as well as communication among all members of the learning community.

There are many options for the communication of information in a distance education scenario. Along with the traditional venues (books, articles, video, or audio), there are electronic mail (e-mail); Web-enhanced or Web-enabled materials; Web-based resources; videoconferencing (desktop or H.323); interactive television; and telephone conferencing, to name a few. Many of these venues promote an active learning process, with the capability of engaging the kinesthetic, visual, and auditory modes of the learner. Many of these methods can be implemented **synchronously** or **asynchronously**, depending upon the intent of the instructor, the content of the teaching, and the best use of available resources.

Synchronous Approaches

Synchronous options require that the participants be in the same space (whether copresent in a classroom setting or in cyberspace) at the same time in order to attend to the material. Some describe synchronous approaches in distance education as more closely matching the traditional classroom lecture model in its flexibility and immediacy, both of which effectively accommodate learning (Ellis, 1997). At a distance, synchronous activities are designed for one-way or two-way communication that may be based in text, audio, visual, or any combination of the three (Table 6.1).

Advocates of synchronous approaches highlight several advantages of same-time, same-space activities. Synchronous options facilitate group building, brainstorming,

TABLE 6.1 TECHNOLOGY-ENHANCED LEARNING OPTIONS

While most of these can be categorized based on implementation, these options for exchanging information are grouped according to their more common uses.

	TEXT/VISUAL	AUDIO	AUDIOVISUAL
One-way	Lecture notes PowerPoint presentations Journal articles (scanned or via library database) Weblogs	Streaming audio Cassette tapes CD-ROM	Streaming lecture via • Cable • Web • Satellite • Videotape • CD-ROM
Two-way	Web-based chat Discussion boards Weblogs (with comments) E-mail	Telephone Web-based chat with audio enhancement using telephone or Voice over IP (VoIP)	Classroom videoconferencing: • Learn Linc • I-Net • Interactive TV Desktop videoconferencing: • NetMeeting • H.323 • PolyCom • CuSeeMe Application sharing

decision making, and cooperative learning (Collison, Elbaum, Haavind, & Tinker, 2000; Duffy & Kirkley, 2004). These social learning activities may be undertaken using asynchronous mechanisms such as e-mail and discussion boards, but synchronous modalities offer opportunities for more immediate and fulfilling interactions. Cooperative learning, among classmates and between students and faculty (whether regular faculty or experts in a field), is enhanced with synchronous connections that extend worldwide (Van Dusen, 1997). Synchronous environments offer students the opportunity to gain skills in delivering formal presentations under similar conditions as offline settings (Collison, et al.). Finally, although conventional wisdom says that in online courses, asynchronous communication should be the dominant mode of interaction because of its purported reflective and time-flexibility benefits (Schlager, 2004), researchers have found that students in synchronous online environments prefer having more rather than less synchronous interactions (Ruhleder, 2004) and have a sense of familiarity within their group that is in contrast to the more formal tone of student groups who use asynchronous modalities (Duffy & Kirkley).

Synchronous approaches to distance education offer several challenges to those who wish to incorporate these activities. One easily forgotten challenge to incorporating synchronous approaches is the complexity of scheduling a same time session with multiple participants who may reside across several time zones and have complicated personal schedules (Collison, et al., 2000). Considerable financial and personnel resources are required to implement many of the more sophisticated aspects of synchronous environments, including: interfacing with various technology capabilities at distant sites (whether classroom or home/office); the bandwidth required to deliver high quality audio and video (if detail is important), the costs of setting up special rooms at centralized locations or of purchasing the necessary hardware/software and, possibly upgrading personal computers; and, the technical support that is required for the setup, use, and maintenance of synchronous activities (Collison, et al., 2000; McGreal & Elliott, 2004).

Online learning is often touted as a leveling mechanism, wherein all students, whether shy or outgoing, will be able to fully engage with the content, faculty, and fellow learners. Synchronous text-based chats are often used, yet in this learning environment students' typing abilities become pre-eminent, resulting in dominance in the chat session going to the fastest typists (McVay Lynch, 2004; Palloff & Pratt, 2001). The requirement of synchronous modalities for students to engage in quick thinking in real time means that students who are not quick typists or thinkers may do no better—or even worse—in the synchronous chat environment (Duffy & Kirkley, 2004).

Synchronous chats are often touted for their contributions to learning, yet some faculty eschew chats because of what the learning literature has to say about such environments. In reviewing some of the literature on chats, Polin (2004) describes chats as a "resource-poor environment for conversation, especially intellectual conversation" (p. 32). Text-based chats poorly support some of the communication devices that humans use to infer meaning to communication, such as intonation, variations in vowel length, and stress, and are subject to misinterpretation (Polin, 2004). Text-based chats are also typically unable to explore material in-depth because of turn-taking constraints and the multiple threads of social, logistical, and content-focused conversation (Duffy & Kirkley, 2004).

Asynchronous Approaches

Asynchronous learning does not require that participants share the same time or space to contribute to or benefit from the content of the interactions. Although the term asynchronous has acquired increased use in the discussion of distance education, the concept is not new. It often requires individual work to be done outside of the structured or supervised environment of the classroom. For example, homework can provide students with asynchronous learning opportunities. The main tenet in asynchronous activity is that it does not have to occur in the same time or place with another person. Examples of asynchronous methods include individual research (reading, literary searches, Web quests), e-mail, watching and/or listening to video and/or audio, and online discussion boards.

Online discussion boards are one of the more dynamic and multidirectional methods of communicating at a distance. Discussion boards are designated Internet sites that provide space to display comments and/or answers to course questions. Responses to this content are collected in a listing below the original content so a reader can follow the flow of thought. Additional responses can be added as readers desire to extend the conversation.

Discussion boards allow for the kind of discursive activity that enables learners to become more engaged with the course content as well as with each other and their faculty.

Much less spontaneous than a synchronous chat (which would be like a face-to-face conversation), discussion boards provide the opportunity for a written exchange, based on readings or research, which can challenge the learners' ideas in order to generate a more robust understanding of the course content and its implications.

Several studies have shown that use of discussion boards increased and enhanced communication among and between class participants regarding course content, thereby fostering the practical application of knowledge and allowing learners to be more actively engaged in their educational process as a result of participation in online discussions (Bennett, 2000; Irvine, 2000; Pena-Shaff, Martin, & Gay, 2001; Polhemus & Swan, 2002; Teikmanis & Armstrong, 2001). It is becoming more commonplace for discussion boards to be used as a complement to, or replacement of, face-to-face instruction, both incorporated into course management systems or used as a stand-alone application. When utilized constructively, online discussions can promote student involvement—the major component of active learning. Participation in Internet-based communication encourages student interactions and engagement both with each other and the course material. Box 6.2 provides a quick list of the advantages of utilizing discussion boards.

Increased attention is being given to researching nontraditional teaching strategies that promote active learning. In one study, comparisons between the two groups using several performance instruments over four semesters indicated that the active learning approach had no adverse effects on student performance. In fact, students in an active learning classroom showed significant improvement in performance relative to students in a lecture-based course during the first semester of the study (O'Sullivan & Copper, 2003).

Irvine (2000) reviewed student communications in an undergraduate educational technology course. Her research analyzed the types of discussion that took place in e-mail, Web-based, and chat communication settings; the amount of discussion that took place in each setting; and the quality of the discussions in each setting. During a one-semester course, 42 students were asked to participate voluntarily in e-mail, discussion board, and/or chat. At the end of the term, there were a total of 279 postings from e-mails, discussion boards, and chat rooms that were analyzed by separating comments into those that concerned procedural statements and those that were content-related. Irvine found that far more postings were content-driven rather than procedural,

BOX 6.2 ADVANTAGES OF ONLINE DISCUSSION BOARDS

- Internet-based bulletin boards can provide a space in which learners can both assimilate and synthesize the subject content.
- Discussion board technology is an asynchronous one—that is, users can go to the specific Internet site at any time to read or create postings. Communication can occur with others through postings made within the individual's timeframe.
- Users of a discussion board do not have to be at the site at the same time to communicate, unlike those using chat rooms, which require synchronous attendance.

indicating that the students used the online venues to communicate about the substance of the course rather than the mechanics. More references were cited and longer statements were made in e-mails and discussion board postings than in chat rooms.

Of the students who participated in the Internet-based communications, 85% indicated that the discussions changed or influenced their opinions and 100% indicated their knowledge of content improved. All students participated in the discussion board communications, and nearly 100% participated in chat, a much larger percentage than would typically participate in a face-to-face classroom setting of 42 students. Irvine's findings show that providing the opportunity for students to engage in thoughtful, content-based conversations about the topic under study may result in deeper understanding and greater learning gains.

Pena-Shaff, Martin, and Gay (2001) found that with the appropriate course design, online discussion may not only encourage collaborative learning, but also may help to engage students in a process of self-reflection. Discussions provide students with the opportunity to analyze and reflect on their own as well as other students' points of view when presented in a format that allowed time to organize the thoughts and ideas to be communicated. Using a theoretical framework based on the work of Henri and Zhu (Henri, 1991; Henri & Rigault, 1996; Zhu, 1996), Pena-Shaff et al., (2001) focused on the students' epistemological growth and knowledge construction using different electronic communications media. Twenty-four graduate students participating in a 14-week course at Cornell University used different tools for class discussions, brainstorming, and group activities, either out of class or during class time. These tools were accessed through the class Web site, which served the central resource for students. Analysis of the data showed that

> *. . . asynchronous discussion environments increased the opportunity for participants to develop sophisticated cognitive skills such as self-reflection, critical thinking and in-depth analysis of the course content, supporting the purposeful construction of meaning. The need to articulate one's own argument in this type of text-based environment encourages students to engage in analytical and reflective action. This process helps students construct purposeful arguments and transmit them to an audience. (Pena-Shaff et al., 2001, p. 65)*

Several other published studies uphold the thesis that Internet-based communication encourages student-student exchanges and interactions with the course material. Polhemus and Swan (2002) conducted a qualitative study of postings made by graduate-level students in various education courses and concluded that the integration of multiple perspectives facilitated the construction of knowledge both individually and communally. Participants in the study were volunteers from different courses during two semesters. They were asked to respond to questions regarding discussion board participation and their particular online community and to think aloud on videotape while reading and responding to required discussions for that particular module or week. Additionally, they were asked to answer follow-up questions regarding their interactions with the discussion messages, why they interacted in specific ways, and what they thought about the online community. The researchers analyzed not only the content of posted messages, but also students' reactions to and interpretations of the messages of others. Students reported that learning took place as they compared alternative perspectives and that they used the discussion board to prime their thought processes when composing messages to others. The discussion board provided resources for students to process their thoughts in a different manner from what could be expected in a lecture setting.

The construction of knowledge promoted by participation in online communication was supported in other research. Wang, Newlin, and Tucker (2001) conducted a discourse analysis of over 8,500 lines of text logged from a course-based chat room. Statistical analysis showed substantive correlations between the number and types of communications and final course grades. Additionally, Teikmanis and Armstrong's (2001) analysis of their course-based discussion boards led them to conclude that despite the potential isolation of Internet and e-mail-based communications, discussion boards may facilitate an important shift from teacher-orchestrated to student-centered learning.

Online discussion boards, implemented appropriately and thoughtfully, can provide important venues for active learning. Internet-mediated communication can also invite different levels of participation that may not be as prevalent in the face-to-face classroom.

Gender and Learning Styles

Research on communication structures shows women prefer conversational environments where opportunities for interrelation of thoughts and actions are provided. Men, on the other hand, are socialized early on to be argumentative and competitive and to appreciate individualized learning (Schwartz & Hanson, 1992). This sometimes provides an environment of intimidation for women, some of whom do not wish to become engaged in antagonistic dialog. In their study of gender and adult learning styles, Philbin, Meier, Huffman, & Boverie (1995) found that "traditional education is directed towards and appeals more to men since it is primarily abstract and reflective. Women learn better in hands-on and practical settings, emphasizing the realm of the affective and doing" (p. 491). The results of this study indicated that women learn best when watching and feeling or doing and thinking, and men learn best when thinking and watching.

Some students at a distance experience social isolation, which can have a significant impact on the level of participation in course communication (Furst-Bowe & Dittmann, 2001). Reduced face-to-face contact can impair communication due to lack of verbal and visual cues, although ironically the sense of anonymity can also encourage more openness in conversation. The effects of isolation seem to be more pronounced in female students who yearn for more intimacy in communication venues. Appropriate use of computer-mediated methodologies, such as well-moderated discussion boards, along with awareness and sensitivity to the need for communication cues can help dilute this real or perceived isolation (Johnson & Huff, 2000).

Such gender differences can pose a challenge to instructors who need to engage distance education students. In the face-to-face classroom, body language, facial expressions, and verbal cues provide the facilitator with information needed to adjust pace, to review or skip over content, and to insert different activities when one does not provide the expected result. At a distance, these considerations must be made prior to class so that any potential barriers to learning can be removed.

Depending on the methodologies used by the instructor, learning at a distance can actually give female students an advantage. Learning materials that incorporate active learning using constructivist principles (initiating the learner's production of his or her knowledge by encouraging the synthesis of new information with learner experiences) would not only meet the learning needs of women but would cultivate those abilities in men. This approach would also answer the needs of students with different characteristic learning preferences. Providing differences in the way information is to be taken in (using sight, sound, touch, smell, taste or approaching a topic in a concrete or abstract way) as well as the way information is processed (reflective thinking, practice, experimentation, research, etc.) can give a wide berth to the variety of learning preferences that manifest themselves in the "classroom."

Interactivity

Interactivity is an important component of the learning process (Bork, 2001). The dialectical nature of learning via distributed communication has the potential to push learners toward meaning-making, engendering a greater sense of learner control of their learning experiences as well as enhancing their self-efficacy (Miller, 2001). These are essential variables in the learning process. For postsecondary and adult learners, it is especially important that they know why they are being asked to acquire new knowledge, skills, or attitudes so that they will become engaged with the content and own their learning. They will be better able to strategize, to participate in the formation of purpose (Dewey, 1938), to transfer knowledge, and to solve problems with creativity. They will also be able to apply and integrate more appropriately what they have learned, increasing their generativity (Knowles, 1970). The ultimate goal is for adult learners to become facile, lifelong learners.

KEY ISSUES FOR STUDENT-CENTERED DISTANCE EDUCATION IN NURSING

Education of Nurses

Distance education of nurses poses a particular challenge. In addition to the theoretical knowledge base required for practice, as members of a practice discipline, nurses at undergraduate and graduate levels must acquire technical, or clinical, skills. Such skills have traditionally been taught during on-campus clinical laboratory sessions or during clinical rotations with faculty. Challenges exist in how to convey these skills, as well as how to evaluate students' acquisition of these skills, via distance. Some institutions address the issue by requiring some on-campus visits so that faculty can work with and evaluate students' clinical skills. Another mechanism for addressing the issue is for faculty to ensure that distant preceptors are familiar with the clinical skills students at specific levels need to acquire. Preceptors can then provide opportunities for students to practice these skills and demonstrate their competency. To date, literature on distance education in nursing has been noticeably quiet about this important issue.

Impact of Technology

Technologies are neutral and influence the environment by creating the potential for ongoing change. The mere existence of electronically mediated technology does not change learning unless we consciously change the teaching environment. If educators do not take the lead in this change, other societal forces will. This will leave educators as the followers, struggling to keep up, rather than being the ones who define creative and meaningful educational experiences based on sound educational theory.

There are many issues related to the use of electronically-mediated technology in the teaching and learning process. While the availability of technology is of less importance as technologies become more ubiquitous, availability can engender a have/have not scenario. Less and less the issue is whether or not the technology is available. More important is the quality of the available technologies and the ability to afford them. The ever shifting digital divide most severely affects those who are without these resources, and, as the cutting edge bleeds, so do the users. A recent study of broadband availability in the United States indicates that there is:

- Little evidence of unequal availability based on income or on Black or Hispanic concentration.
- Mixed evidence concerning availability based on Native American or Asian concentration.
- Decreased availability in rural locations.
- Increased availability in areas of large market size, higher educational levels education, Spanish language use, and telephone company presence (Prieger, 2003).

While this study did not consider the resources individuals must have to obtain available services, it presents important information to be considered in the implementation of required technology in any curriculum.

Cost

The monies involved in the investment of technologies can be significant, both for the educational institution and for the individual. Historically, an infusion of monies placed educational institutions on the cutting edge, whereas that kind of investment now is required to merely maintain pace with peer institutions (Brynjolfsson, Hitt, & Yang, 2002). The value added by the purchase of technologies is not intrinsic and depends on how and why the technology is utilized (Ginsburg, 1999). However, for the individual without appropriate technology, disadvantages increase in relation to access to information, economic opportunities, and educational options (Lu, 2001; Prieger, 2003).

Time

Time is a component that is equally distributed. For those who have traditionally used lecture styles, moving to distance education can require an incredible investment of time. If an educator only types up lectures to place online, it requires some investment of time. Moving beyond merely placing lectures online requires a more significant investment of time, as educators conceptualize how to engage students in meaningful ways and then work with instructional designers or develop a new skill set for themselves. However, it is imperative that educators rethink the way that we teach so that we can better respond to students' needs and to the limitations and benefits of various methodologies.

Information Management and Lifelong Learning

More and more, **knowledge workers** must remain cognitively nimble, constantly honing the ability to filter information appropriately for their needs. As previously noted, the amount of available information compounds exponentially, making it more important to be able to utilize critical thinking skills in determining what is valid, significant, and timely. No longer can anyone know it all; we must each discover and maintain our own epistemological compass.

As educators, the need to understand learning processes becomes more important as the amount of available information and knowledge continues its exponential growth. Learning situations that focus on didactic, fact-based objectives rather than development of critical thinking skills require proactive efforts to change the educational focus from acquisition of time-limited, discrete knowledge to an emphasis on lifelong learning. It is imperative, therefore, given what we know about adult learners, to enable people to learn in the way they know best. This encourages successful negotiation of the complexities of contemporary life, effective and efficient working, and the maintenance of status quo skills that have an increasingly shortened shelf life.

SUMMARY

The advent of a ubiquitous Internet has led to studies considering the impact of information technology on human learning and how it might be used to enhance the generation of knowledge. Given the importance of an engaged learner, it is essential that the content be presented in ways that challenge the learner to comprehend and actively process the information so that it results in useable knowledge. This may call for reevaluation of teaching strategies to determine what may work best in different venues. What may work in the face-to-face classroom may not be effective in the distance education setting and, indeed, could be detrimental. Shared information about best practices in distance education should facilitate continued learning among nurse educators and their students.

LEARNING ACTIVITY

Implementing a student-centered approach to online education requires the teacher to consciously engage students as involved and active participants in the learning process, both synchronously and asynchronously. Consequently, it is important for instructors to assess their experiences with enhancing student involvement and, particularly, the implications of this for synchronous and asynchronous online environments.

Consider one or two recent courses with which you've been involved, whether as solo faculty, coteacher, or learner. Using the chart below, provide specific examples from your course(s) that reflect how you implemented each aspect. Use the two columns on the far right-hand side to identify ways that an educator could incorporate more of a student-centered approach for each item.

	MY SPECIFIC COURSE EXAMPLES		HOW CAN I INCORPORATE A MORE STUDENT-CENTERED APPROACH?	
ASPECT	Asynchronous approaches	Synchronous approaches	Asynchronous approaches	Synchronous approaches
Interaction with faculty				
Interaction with peers				
Active learning				
Teacher-centered aspects				
Student-centered aspects				
Respect for different learning styles				
Preparation for lifelong learning				

RESOURCES FOR EDUCATORS

PLANNING THE TEACHING/LEARNING EXPERIENCE

Questions to Support a Thoughtful Reading

1. How does use of technology allow/support a different allocation of responsibility for learning?
2. Discuss examples of different uses of time and space in distance education.
3. Is there content that might be taught more effectively in a distance mode rather than a traditional classroom?
4. What societal factors have influenced the evolution of distance education?
5. What changes would you make to your teaching style to become more adult focused? And why?
6. How might a learning experience be structured to promote development of active learning?
7. What teaching strategies do you need to develop in order to adopt a student-centered approach to distance education?

Tips for Developing a Student-Centered Environment

- Utilize Web resources as a source of comparison between your course's goals and objectives and those of others. Can you glean ideas from how other people are teaching the content?
- Maintain all of your course documents in separate folders on your hard drive and in your course management system/Web site. This will make it easier for you and for the students to find the information.
- Organize your course materials in logical format and stick with that format throughout the course. Post information alphabetically or chronologically, but consistently.
- Use e-mail to let your students know when materials have been added or deleted from your course site.
- Identify information as either necessary for the course or for enrichment purposes.

EVALUATING THE TEACHING/LEARNING EXPERIENCE

Questions to Elicit Feedback from Students on Their Learning

1. Describe the benefits and disadvantages of discussion board postings compared to the typical responses of students in a traditional classroom.
2. Differentiate between the benefits of synchronous and asynchronous learning environments.

Sample Evaluation Strategies or Tools

FACTORS TO CONSIDER WHEN CHOOSING SYNCHRONOUS OR ASYNCHRONOUS MEANS

FACTOR	SYNCHRONOUS	ASYNCHRONOUS
Learners' level of autonomy	Learners are not autonomous and require a scheduled program to keep them engaged	Learners are autonomous
Learners' typing ability	Learners type well	Learners do not type well
Learners' need to learn	Learners have the same or similar needs	Learners have diverse needs
Learners are available	At the same time	At various times
Where are the learners located?	Located in close or same time zones	Located in diverse time zones
Learners prefer to learn or instructors prefer to instruct	Experts online or in discussion with fellow students in chat sessions	Discovering new information and progressing at their own pace
Number of learners	Small number using chat	Larger numbers

Reflective Questions for Educators

1. Think about a time when your teaching was most effective. What made it so effective? What teaching methods did you employ? What outcomes did students demonstrate?

2. Analyze your teaching style (or trade off and have a peer critique yours while you critique your peer's). Consider if your teaching style takes learning style differences into account.

3. Most faculty members have strong role models and experience in teacher-centered learning. Reflect on your personal attitudes toward student-centered learning. Is this a philosophy you can embrace? What changes will you have to make to become student-centered? What resources and feedback will help you know if you have achieved a student-centered approach?

References

Banas, E. J., & Emory, W. F. (1998). History and issues of distance learning. *Public Administration Quarterly, 22*(3), 365–383.

Bandura, A. (1977). *Social learning theory*. New York: General Learning Press.

Bennett, J. P. (2000). Assessing the potential of electronic discussion groups to enhance learning in a classroom-based course. Paper presented at the ED-MEDIA 2000, Montreal.

Bork, A. (2001). *What is needed for effective learning on the Internet?* Retrieved October 17, 2005, from http://ifets.ieee.org/periodical/vol_3_2001/bork.html.

Britannica.com. (2004). Retrieved May 17, 2004, from http://www.britannica.com

Bruner, J. (1966). *Toward a theory of instruction*. Cambridge, MA: Harvard University Press.

Brynjolfsson, E., Hitt, L. M., & Yang, S. (2002). *Intangible assets: Computers and organizational capital*. Washington, DC Brookings Institution.

Collison, G., Elbaum, B., Haavind, S., et al. (2000). *Facilitating online learning: Effective strategies for moderators*. Madison, WI: Atwood Publishing.

Dewey, J. (1938). *Experience and education*. New York: Collier Books.

Drucker, P. F. (1959). *Landmarks for Tomorrow*. New York: Harper & Row.

Duffy, T. M., & Kirkley, J. R. (Eds.). (2004). *Learner-centered theory and practice in distance education: Cases from higher education*. Mahwah, NJ: Lawrence Erlbaum Associates.

Ellis, B. (1997). *Virtual classroom technologies for distance education: The case for on-line synchronous delivery*. Retrieved October 17, 2005, from http://www.detac.com/solution/naweb97.htm.

Furst-Bowe, J., & Dittmann, W. (2001). Identifying the needs of adult women in distance learning programs. *International Journal of Instructional Media, 28*(4), 405–414.

Ginsburg, L. (1999). Educational technology: Searching for the value added. *Adult Learning, 10*(4), 12–15.

Henri, F. (1991). Computer conferencing and content analysis. In A. Kaye (Ed.), *Collaborative learning through computer conferencing* (Vol. 90, pp. 117–136). Berlin: Springer-Verlag.

Henri, F., & Rigault, C. (1996). Collaborative distance learning and computer conferencing. In T. Liao, (Ed.), *Advanced educational technology: Research issues and future potential* (Vol. 145, pp. 45–76). New York: Springer.

Irvine, S. E. (2000). *What are we talking about? The impact of computer-mediated communication on student learning*. Paper presented at the SITE 2000.

Johnson, M. M., & Huff, M. T. (2000). Students' use of computer-mediated communication in a distance education course. *Research on Social Work Practice, 10*(4), 519–532.

Jones, L. L. C. (2003). Are lectures a thing of the past? *Journal of College Science Teaching, 32*(7), 453–457.

Klass, G. (July 2000). *Plato as distance education pioneer: Status and quality threats of internet education*. Retrieved October 17, 2005, from http://firstmonday.org/issues/issue5_7/klass/.

Knowles, M. S. (1970). *The modern practise of adult education: Andragogy versus pedagogy*. New York: New York Association Press.

Knowles, M. S. (1975). *Self-directed learning: A guide for learners and teachers*. Chicago: Follett Publishing Company.

Knowles, M. S. (1984). *The adult learner: A neglected species* (3rd ed.). Houston, TX: Gulf Publishing Co.

Lu, M.-T. (2001). Digital divide in developing countries. *Journal of Global Information Technology Management, 4*(3), 1–4.

McGreal, R., & Elliott, M. (2004). *Technologies of online learning (E-learning)*. Retrieved May 4, 2004, from http://cde.athabascau.ca/online_book/pdf/tpol_chp05.pdf.

McLeish, J. (1968). *Lecture method in teaching.*Unpublished manuscript, Cambridge.

McVay Lynch, M. (2004). *Learning online: A guide to success in the virtual classroom.* New York: Routledge-Falmer.

Miller, B. L. (2001). Technology and learning in the undergraduate classroom. *DAI, 62*(04A), 197.

National Center for Education Statistics (NCES). (2001). *The Condition of Education 2001 (NCES 2001–072)*. Washington, DC: U.S. Government Printing Office.

Oblinger, D., & Rush, S. (1997). *The Learning Revolution*. Boston: Anker.

O'Sullivan, D. W., & Copper, C. L. (2003). Evaluating active learning. *Journal of College Science Teaching, 32*(7), 448–452.

Palloff, R. M., & Pratt, K. (2001). *Lessons from the cyberspace classroom: The realities of online teaching.* San Francisco: Jossey-Bass.

Pena-Shaff, J., Martin, W., & Gay, G. (2001). An epistemological framework for analyzing student interactions in computer-mediated communication environments. *Journal of Interactive Learning Research, 12*(1), 41–68.

Philbin, M., Meier, E., Huffman, S., et al. (1995). A survey of gender and learning styles. *Sex Roles: A Journal of Research, 32*(7–8), 485–494.

Piaget, J. (1952). *The origins of intelligence in children* (M. Cook, Trans.). New York: International Universities Press, Inc.

Piaget, J. (1970). *The science of education and the psychology of the child.* New York: Grossman.

Polhemus, L., & Swan, K. (2002). *Student roles in online learning communities: Navigating threaded discussions.* Paper presented at the World Conference on E-Learning in Corporations, Government, Health, & Higher Education.

Polin, L. (2004). Learning in dialogue with a practicing community. In T. M. Duffy & J. R. Kirkley (Eds.), *Learner-centered theory and practice in distance education: Cases from higher education* (pp. 17–48). Mahwah, NJ: Lawrence Erlbaum Associates.

Prieger, J. E. (2003). The supply side of the digital divide: Is there equal availability in the broadband Internet access market? *Economic Inquiry, 41*(2), 346.

Reinert, B., & Fryback, P. (1997). Distance learning and nursing education. *Journal of Nursing Education, 36*(9), 421.

Ruhleder, K. (2004). Interaction and engagement in LEEP: Undistancing "distance" education at the graduate level. In T. M. Duffy & J. R. Kirkley, (Eds.), *Learner-centered theory and practice in distance education: Cases from higher education* (pp. 71–90). Mahwah, NJ: Lawrence Erlbaum Associates.

Schlager, M. (2004). Enabling new forms of online engagement: Challenges for e-learning design and research. In T. M. Duffy & J. R. Kirkley, (Eds.), *Learner-centered theory and practice in distance education: Cases from higher education* (pp. 71–90). Mahwah, NJ: Lawrence Erlbaum Associates.

Schwartz, W., & Hanson, K. (1992). *Equal mathematics education for female students*: ERIC Clearinghouse on Urban Education; New York.

Skinner, B. F. (1968). *The technology of teaching.* New York: Appleton-Century-Crofts.

Sorrells-Jones, J., & Weaver, D. (1999a). Knowledge workers and knowledge-intense organizations, part 1: A promising framework for nursing and healthcare. *Journal of Nursing Administration, 29*(7/8), 12–18.

Sorrells-Jones, J., & Weaver, D. (1999b). Knowledge workers and knowledge-intense organizations, part 3: Implications for preparing healthcare professionals. *Journal of Nursing Administration, 29*(10), 14–21.

Teikmanis, M., & Armstrong, J. (2001). Teaching pathophysiology to diverse students using an online discussion board. *Computers in Nursing, 19*(2), 75–81.

Van Dusen, G. C. (1997). *The virtual campus: Technology and reform in higher education. ASHE-ERIC Higher Education Report Volume 25, No. 5.* Washington, DC: George Washington University Graduate School of Education and Human Development.

Vygotsky, L. S. (1978). *Mind in society.* Cambridge, MA: Harvard University Press.

Wang, A. Y., Newlin, M. H., & Tucker, T. L. (2001). Computers in teaching. A discourse analysis of online classroom chats: Predictors of cyber-student performance. *Teaching of Psychology, 28*(3), 222–226.

Weaver, D., & Sorrells-Jones, J. (1999). Knowledge workers and knowledge-intense organizations, part 2: Designing and managing for productivity. *Journal of Nursing Administration, 29*(9), 19–25.

Webopedia.com. (2004). Retrieved May, 2004, from http://www.webopedia.com/

Zhu, E. (1996). Meaning negotiation, knowledge construction, and mentoring in a distance learning course. Paper presented at the National Convention of the Association for Educational Communications and Technology, Indianapolis, IN.

Additional Resources

Anderson, T. & Elloumi, F. (Eds.). *Theory and practice of online learning.* Athabasca, Alberta, CA: Athabasca University. Retrieved October 17, 2005, at http://cde.athabascau.ca/online_book/.

Baker, A. C., Jensen, P. J., & Kolb, D. A. (2002). *Conversational learning: An experiential approach to knowledge creation.* Unpublished manuscript.

Duffy, T. M. & Kirkley, J. R. (Eds.) (2004). *Learner-centered theory and practice in distance education: Cases from higher education.* Mahwah, NJ: Lawrence Erlbaum Associates.

Kearsley, G. *Explorations in learning and instruction: The theory into practice database.* Retrieved October 17, 2005, at http://tip.psychology.org/.

Miller, B. L. (2001). *Technology and learning in the undergraduate classroom.* DAI, 62 (04A), 197.

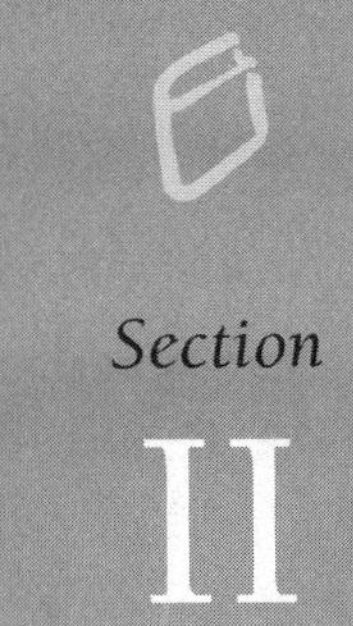

Section

II

METHODS AND APPROACHES TO STUDENT-CENTERED LEARNING IN NURSING

Chapter 7

Beyond Case Studies in Practice Education: Creating Capacities for Ethical Knowledge Through Story and Narrative

Helen Brown
Patricia Rodney

As a clinical teacher in neonatal nursing, I have noticed how clinical post-conferences are an important place for teaching and learning about the ethical dimensions of nursing practice.[1] When students and teachers come together at the end of a clinical shift, it seems there is a certain kind of openness and curiosity that emerges as they work together to make sense of and learn from clinical practice. Students reflect on their day and try to determine if they missed anything or if they effectively met the needs of the infants and families in their care.

During case study presentations, students spend a great deal of time speaking about their objective evaluations of the care they have provided, drawing primarily on the facts about a woman's labor and birthing events, an infant's birth experience, his or her trajectory following admission to the neonatal intensive care unit and pertinent diagnostic findings and treatments. Novice neonatal nurses tend to focus primarily on their ability to meet the physiological needs of the infant through making sense of x-ray reports, lab results, medication infusions, ventilator settings, and so on. They are also asked to comment on any ethical issues that arise when caring for their selected patient. Yet, when students try to speak about what is ethically relevant about caring for an infant and family, and what kind of knowledge they need to practice ethically in relation to the infant and family, they often appear unable to do so. This has led me to wonder how certain teaching methods either facilitate or constrain students' knowledge-generating capacities for being moral agents in practice. Why and how do some methods more effectively tap students' capacity for creating knowledge about becoming ethical practitioners than others?

[1] The first-person "I" is that of author Helen Brown.

INTENT

In this chapter our intent is to explore the promise of stories—specifically as relayed through narratives—in teaching nursing ethics. We begin by contrasting this approach with the traditional use of case studies in teaching and learning nursing ethics and propose that the rich inductive opportunities created by narrative better support the relational and contextual nature of nurses' ethical practice. While our focus is on narratives and stories for teaching nursing ethics, we believe that what we have to say resonates with much of what is being called for in nursing education; that is, to find ways to see how the practice of nursing could more intentionally inform the education of nurses.

Many narrative theorists say that human beings live a storied existence (Frank, 1991, 1995; Kohler Riessman, 1993). This means that most of what we experience can be relayed in narrative form and that we have a natural tendency to make sense of experience through telling stories about it. When turning toward nursing practice, much of what nurses learn about patients' health, healing, and illness experiences come to us in stories and narratives. In particular, stories can effectively reveal the moral and ethical nature of health care practice (Carson, 2001; Nisker, 2004). In this chapter we will show how narratives and stories hold possibilities for creating the capacity for developing ethical knowledge in nursing and acting as moral agents in practice.

We begin by briefly presenting our views on nursing ethics particularly for how these views inform our thinking on teaching ethics in nursing. Next we explore how the traditional methods of case study widely used in health care ethics may limit or constrain the development of ethical knowledge, especially if such teaching methods fail to acknowledge the relational nature of nurses' **moral agency** and **ethical practice**. Our critique of case methods in ethics education arise from our view that knowledge about being ethical in nursing practice is inseparable from everyday experience and thus cannot be taken out of the context in which it originates. Since we know that every moment in nursing practice is imbued with ethical questions and challenges (Rodney, Brown, & Liaschenko, 2004), and that moral agency is enacted within particular relationships and contexts (Mackenzie & Stoljar, 2000; Sherwin, 1998), it seems timely to explore how narratives and stories bring learners closer to the everyday ethical moments in practice as a way to develop ethical knowledge in nursing.

OVERVIEW

INTRODUCTION

The opening scenario turns our attention to how teaching practices and methods work together to actively engage students in their own learning. As teachers we know that students are more likely to become engaged in their own learning when they are involved in creating their educational experiences. For example, when students are asked to participate in refining the evaluation strategies for a course they often shift from focusing entirely on what the teachers want toward asking what might help them learn the course content. When students are actively engaged in inquiring into what may help them learn the course content, they are more likely to tap their own capacities as a learner, rather than just jumping through hoops to complete a course.

In this chapter we join other authors in suggesting that there has been scant attention paid toward developing pedagogical methods and strategies in nursing that recognize the necessity for learners to develop their own voice in order to participate in and contribute to the knowing process (see Diekelmann, 2002; MacDonald, 2002; Munhall, 1988; Romyn, 2000). Many of the ideas and strategies in this book, particularly the influence of social constructionism and reflective learning processes, are fundamental to what we propose here. We echo ideas of other authors in this book by proposing ways to bring learners into their educative experiences. More specifically, in this chapter we propose that **narratives and stories** hold potential to bring learners into the everyday moments of ethical practice as an effective way to teach and learn ethical practice in nursing.

Before we move further let us describe what we mean by narrative and stories. While the terms story and narrative are often used interchangeably (Nisker, 2004), we consider story to be the broader category, a vehicle that implies a plot with a beginning, middle, and end. Stories may take many forms, where narrative is one means of expressing stories. The various forms of narrative include not only written or spoken accounts but poems, short stories, plays, and films (Nisker, 2004, p. 289). For the purposes of this chapter, then, we will be thinking of written or spoken narratives that convey part of a story. They may be brief or long, but what they share is attention to personal experience and context, not just a (supposedly) objective reporting of facts.

We will use a narrative entitled "About Mr. Johansen" (which is itself one glimpse into a broader story) to help us explain some of the limitations of traditional approaches to case studies in teaching and learning nursing ethics. Parts of the narrative are woven throughout the chapter to illuminate strategies for teaching and learning nursing ethics.

TEACHING AND LEARNING ETHICS IN NURSING

Understanding Nurses' Ethical Practice

The area of study and research about nurses' ethical practice is known as the field of nursing ethics. This area of interest in nursing is rapidly expanding and is now seen as a distinct area of inquiry. As a result, a great deal of information has been generated about how ethical practice in nursing can be taught and learned. This means that nurse educators are asking questions such as "how do nurses learn to be ethical?" and "what theories and knowledge do nurses need to practice ethically?" The response to questions such as these can help educators design curricula and learning experiences to prepare nurses for the realities of nursing practice. Theorists and educators have learned that attention to everyday practice realities and the moral nature of nursing work is critical for developing knowledge about being and becoming ethical practitioners (Benner, 1991; 2000; Brown, Rodney, Pauly, Varcoe, & Smye, 2004; Rodney, Brown, et al., 2004; Tschudin, 2003). One of our colleagues in a program of nursing ethics research proposes that nursing ethics is "a deeply personal, embodied process . . . where being and becoming a moral agent requires the cultivation of mindful, critical awareness and attunement to emotion and bodily experience" (Doane, 2004, p. 433). Taking this view about nursing ethics raises the question of how to help students learn about ethical practice as both a subjective, embodied experience, and a reasoned method of decision making and analysis. For example, drawing on formal ethical theories may help students participate in reasoned decisions about the allocation of resources based on principles of fairness and justice. But they also need to be able to see how their own responses to particular patients and their values about what fairness means in certain situations is shaping how and what they advocate for when attending to patients' needs. Student nurses in our research spoke of the profound emotional turmoil that persisted when they felt as though they were not able to uphold their standards for ethical patient care. For instance, one nurse spoke about the need to carry her heavy heart with her as she went about her daily work—a heavy heart that resulted from an unresolved ethical issue where she received little collegial or organizational support. She described her experience of being ethical, or unethical, as related to the embodied feelings of a heavy heart—it became a trigger for her to ask more questions about what she was participating in and on what basis she was advocating for her patient's wishes and needs. Having the chance to discuss such feelings and responses is important when exploring how nurses identify themselves as moral agents and ethical practitioners.

Being ethical in nursing requires turning toward, and not away from (as some traditional ethical theories espouse), the interrelationship between objective and subjective experience, and reasoned and emotive decision making. It is important to note that some contemporary theorists see health care ethics as "fundamentally to do with the quality of relationships that we live in the moral communities we inhabit" (Doane, 2004, p. 34). Such views raise questions about the adequacy of traditional approaches for teaching and learning ethics. Teaching and learning ethics in nursing could more effectively flow from seeing nurses' ethical practice as both **relational** and **contextual**. Seeing ethical practice as relational and contextual implies that how nurses construct knowledge about being ethical is always in and through their relations with others in particular contexts. In other words, what nurses come to see as ethically relevant often arises from working closely with each other, their interdisciplinary colleagues, by accounting for the lived experiences and perspectives of their patients, and by revealing how their practice environment influences what they might see and know in any moment of practice.

Next we explore how case studies have been used in ethics education and why this has been problematic in nursing education. We then explore how narratives and stories can help students tap their own capacities for developing ethical knowledge.

The Use of Case Studies in Ethics Education

Let us start by reflecting briefly on the uses of cases in ethics education in general and then speak about why they may be limiting for teaching and learning nursing ethics.

The reason that case studies are frequently employed in ethics education—and education more broadly—is because they can foster in-depth analysis, application of concepts and theory, insight development, and creativity (O'Connor, 2001; Pattison, Dickenson, Parker, & Heller, 1999; Reilly & Oermann, 1992; Veatch & Fry, 1987) (Box 7.1).

Case studies can also be used for evaluative purposes as they can generate evidence of students' application of their cognitive skills (O'Connor, 2001). Overall, case studies, particularly in health care and nursing ethics education, can provide opportunities for students to better appreciate the interrelationship between theory and practice.

In health care ethics education, case studies have traditionally been presented in a brief narrative form, but what distinguishes them from narrative (as we are using the term) is that cases are generally presented as a closed set of information. This means that students most often are asked to work with the information that is presented in the case, and are not necessarily encouraged to pursue other points of view, contextual information, and so on. Students are frequently also asked to apply an ethical decision-making framework to a particular case study and, when guided in this way, students may or may

BOX 7.1 PURPOSES OF CASE STUDIES IN NURSING EDUCATION

- Examine the relationship of multiple phenomena in the clinical situation.
- Enlarge students' knowledge base.
- Develop skills in problem solving in critical thinking.
- Examine multiple approaches to problems, compare them, and decide upon approaches to be used in particular situations.
- Provide a supporting rationale for decisions made.
- Organize ideas logically in written form.

Adapted from Reilly, D. E. & Oermann, M. H. (1992). *Clinical teaching in nursing education* (2nd ed., p. 169). New York: National League for Nursing.

not seek out the full scope of additional information required to determine an appropriate course of action. The traditional use of case studies in ethics education helps students to apply their knowledge and try out decision-making models, but such use does not necessarily help them to explore the richness of human experience and the complexities of the sociopolitical contexts in which such experience takes place.

It is important to note that there are ways of using case studies that do draw forth the relational and contextual aspects of knowledge and experience and that are more consistent with the narrative approaches we suggest here. However, in the field of health care ethics education there has been a traditional tendency to use cases in ways that reflect rational, objectified accounts of human experience and health care practice (Carson, 2001; Kaufman, 2001; Nisker, 2004). How the case is used can also constrain or enhance students' efforts to see relevant contextual meanings and experience beyond the objective facts. In the hands of one educator, a case discussion may be reduced to a (purportedly) logical discussion of facts and alternatives, while the same case in the hands of another educator may encourage a richer exploration on the part of the students and the educator.

Even though we agree that case studies can provide significant advantages for educators and learners, we feel strongly that when teaching and learning about the nature of being a moral agent in nursing practice, certain limitations exist. These limitations are most often evident in a lack of attention to context, values, and power dynamics in nursing practice. We support the suggestion by Pattison et al. (1999) that a critical question must be raised about how case studies are constructed and used for teaching ethics so that we enlist these methods with greater discrimination and awareness. When teachers use cases in a purportedly objective, context-free manner, stripped of what are seen as extraneous variables, it becomes next to impossible for students to appreciate the effects of values, relationships, and context on their efforts to be moral agents in practice (Rodney & Street, 2004). The following narrative will help us to illustrate the limitation of case studies for learning ethics, particularly within the context of unraveling the effects of values, relationships, and contexts. The narrative has three dimensions we will work with: the use of a clinical case study, an ethical analysis of the case, and a reflection on the position of the clinical instructor.

ABOUT MR. JOHANSEN

My name is Han Chui, and I am a clinical nurse educator conducting a postconference with fourth-year undergraduate nursing students in the last week of their final practicum.[2] *I have nine students with me in the postconference, which is taking place in a conference room in a large teaching hospital. The students are assigned to preceptors in a variety of units in the hospital and have come together for a final two-hour postconference to share their experiences and reflect on what they will be taking forward into their practice as registered nurses. One of the students, Sarah Miller, has her preceptorship on an acute medical unit. Before the postconference, she told me that she wanted to talk about a patient she had been caring for, Mr. Johansen, especially the ethics involved in decision making about his care.*

[2] This story is adapted from Rodney (1997) and McPherson, et al. (2004).

When Sarah speaks in the postconference, she tells the other students and myself that Mr. Johansen is an elderly man who had been living with his daughter until he had had a stroke, and he has been in the hospital on the general medical unit for approximately two weeks. Following admission, he suffered acute delirium which seemed to resolve somewhat but, worsening now—he is increasingly confused. Sarah explains that Mr. Johansen's daughter, Ingrid, is in to visit him every day. Ingrid appears knowledgeable, having read up on stroke, dementia, and delirium. Sarah tells us that by asking many questions, Ingrid seems to have driven the physicians away. Furthermore, Sarah says that when she and her preceptor tried to draw Mr. Johansen's increasing confusion and delirium to the attention of the charge nurse, they received an abrupt and sarcastic response. The charge nurse said that Mr. Johansen "is not going to make it out of here anyway" and "we are too busy with more critical stuff to worry about every old person's confusion."

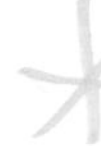

Sarah goes on to tell us that she and her preceptor believe that Mr. Johansen's worsening confusion is related to a probable urinary tract infection (UTI). However, they have not yet been able to get the attending physician in to assess the patient, and Sarah says that she knows that her preceptor's workload is heavy. So that once Sarah is gone, she will not have extra time to track down a physician. In the meanwhile, Sarah says that when she reported off to come to the postconference, Mr. Johansen was lying in bed with his legs over the side rails, picking things out of the air. His daughter was at his bedside, clearly distressed. Sarah says she did the best she could before she left, but she knew it was not enough.

As she finishes her story, I can sense how distressed Sarah still is. And I can see her distress mirrored in the faces of the other students. I wonder how I should proceed. . . .

Han's narrative raises a broad scope of issues about ethical practice for all the members of the health care team, and about the interface of nursing ethics and nursing education. While we will not be able to address all the issues in this chapter, we can raise some important points about the substance of how decisions ought to be approached in Mr. Johansen's situation, what we need to know about him and his family, and what we need to know about the context within which his treatment and care are being delivered. We can also raise some important points about how Mr. Johansen's story might be told, and what this means for attending to his situation and for the teaching and learning of ethics. Finally, we can reflect on Han's situatedness as a clinical instructor, and the nature of the support he, the students, and the preceptors need. In other words, we also ought to pay attention to Han's experiences as an instructor who may find himself in conflict with staff and/or management on the unit at the same time as he is trying to help everyone involved.

A Decontextualized View

Using a traditional ethics case study approach, we would likely summarize Mr. Johansen's story as follows:

Mr. Johansen, an elderly man who suffered a stroke, is experiencing increasing confusion. His daughter and the nurses involved in his care believe that he should be assessed and treated. His attending physician and the charge nurse feel this is a waste of scarce resources. Should he be assessed and treated or not? [3]

[3]Adapted from McPherson, et al. (2004), p. 110.

In this kind of traditional approach, we might look for more information and flesh out more details of the case, but the tendency would be to treat the decision as a binary or yes or no question when examining how health care providers ought to act toward Mr. Johansen and his family. We would not be likely to fully explore questions about his family context, support for his daughter, the knowledge of the staff about gerontology, the impact of the workload on the rest of the unit on the treatment and care Mr. Johansen is receiving, and so on. Importantly, we would also not be likely to explore the nature and history of the interdisciplinary team relationships on the acute medical unit, or the experiences and feelings of Sarah and her preceptor.

In the practice and the teaching of health care ethics, it used to be common to focus on cases stripped of context. As we have already stated, the use of cases is not in and of itself problematic—indeed, cases "function as the salvation of ethics teaching and discourse" as people become "interested and engaged" (Pattison, et al., 1999, p. 42). The problem lies in how cases have tended to be uncritically used, as they are too often written in an authoritative voice as if they are fact, thereby obscuring alternate voices, significant contextual features, enactments of power, and hidden value judgments (Carson, 2001; Nisker, 2004; Pattison, et al., 1999). Such problems are evident in the summary above of Mr. Johansen's situation; for example, his daughter's perspective is missing, the context of a treatable UTI is overlooked, and he is seen as wasting resources. The uncritical use of cases in health care ethics to some extent mirrors the history of the use of ethical principles (autonomy, beneficence, nonmaleficence, and justice).

Although the principle-oriented approach to health care ethics has been widely accepted, over the past two decades or so there have been serious concerns raised about its adequacy. Principle-oriented ethics has been criticized for relying on ethical principles to the exclusion of other variables known to influence ethical practice, for not reflecting the breadth and diversity of concepts available in the general ethics literature, and for fostering a prescriptive, formal approach by which principles are applied in a process-dominated manner (Penticuff, 1991, pp. 236–240). As with case method, this does not mean that ethical principles are not useful—they provide significant moral guidance, but need to be used in a more thoughtful manner and supplemented with other ethical theory, such as cross-cultural and feminist theory (Rodney, Pauly, & Burgess, 2004). Reflecting back on Mr. Johansen's situation, this means that we would certainly be interested in his uniqueness and self-determination (autonomy), want to promote comfort (beneficence and nonmaleficence), and we would want to provide fair access to resources based on his needs (justice). However, as stated earlier, we would want to be interested in context, values, and relationships as well, especially the power in those relationships. The traditional approach to cases and ethical principles will not easily get us there.

We are compelled to question why case studies tend to be used to draw learners into the lives of others without an explicit intent to draw them into such lives through knowing about themselves. And because we believe that in nursing arises from seeing ethics as a personal and embodied experience (Doane, 2004), it seems worthy to ask about how we might invite learners into their knowing about ethics and ethical practice as the place from which they developed knowledge about being in ethical relation to colleagues, patients, and broader contexts in which they practice. Thus, if Han engages Sarah and the other students in the postconference in a decontextualized approach to Mr. Johansen's situation, he may miss the opportunity to tap his own capacity for teaching ethics, and possibly students' capacities for learning about the ethical challenges and moral dimension of nursing care of this patient and family. For instance, he would not be able to help the students to reflect on the difficult situation Mr. Johansen's daughter, Ingrid, is in, including how she might be supported. And it would be difficult to help Sarah and the other students think about the power dynamics in the interdisciplinary team, and to think about how they might move forward constructively as students and pending graduates in the face of such power dynamics. Indeed, Han himself would not be encouraged to reflect on his own role on the medical unit, and how he might support Sarah and her preceptor to have their concerns heard.

Nurses as Isolated Agents

Thus far, our main concern about a traditional decontextualized view of cases is that such a view may limit the **moral sensitivity** and agency of nurses and other health care providers, and ultimately, not help patients and families such as Mr. Johansen and his daughter. In nursing, we are coming to understand that nurses' moral agency arises from their ability to tune into their emotional and embodied experience and from their ability to see the influence of contextual factors and interdisciplinary relationships, including how these influences affect their ability to act ethically (Brown, et al., 2004; Rodney, 1997; Rodney et al., 2002; Benner, 1991, 2000; Nortvedt, 2004; Scott, 2000). Being morally sensitive requires being tuned into seeing how relationships and context shape any moral action undertaken. Sarah and her preceptor, for example, are noticing what is ethically relevant by trying to tune into their own responses, those of Mr. Johansen, Ingrid, and the interdisciplinary team. Their ability to remain sensitive in ways that are ethically relevant requires that they see the interrelationships between their practice, their own emotional and embodied responses to the situation, and the contextual and experiential aspect of Mr. Johansen's life. Cultivating such sensitivity requires a different approach to ethics education than we have employed thus far. We need to get away from the predominant view of nurses (and others) as isolated moral agents who operate in a rational manner regardless of context or emotion (Doane, 2004; Nortvedt, 2004; Scott, 2000).

Through the research we, and other colleagues at the University of Victoria School of Nursing, have engaged in with practicing nurses, we have learned that in order to provide what they see as ethical care, nurses confront multiple challenges. For example, nurses are often being asked to do more with less, particularly in terms of resources and support, as they face excessive workloads, fewer accessible and visible nursing leaders, and increasingly complex patient care situations. Within this context of excessive workload and patients with complex needs, conflict with other health care team members arise as each team member struggles to provide safe, competent, and ethical care. Related to these challenges in the practice environment is an erosion of nurses' moral identity (how they see themselves as moral agents), since nurses are finding it harder and harder to practice in ways they believe to be ethical (Hartrick Doane, 2002; Rodney, et al., 2002; Storch, Rodney, Pauly, Brown, & Starzomski, 2003; Varcoe, et al., 2004). Such barriers were operating in Sarah's account of Mr. Johansen's situation. As we have indicated, many in the field of ethics, and particularly within feminist ethics, have critiqued a rationality approach to the search for moral truth. Consequently, many have seen ethical conduct as being about much more than theories and codes of moral rules and codes that nurses could be taught and could apply in practice (Bauman, 1993; Doane, 2004; Gadow, 1999; Heckman, 1995; Nortvedt, 2004; Scott, 2000; Sherwin, 1992, 1998). Nussbaum (2001), among others, claims that although rationalist approaches to ethics help us to see our moral choices, each and every moral situation is complex and highly nuanced. Doane (2004), citing Walker (1999), suggests that the "danger of an overemphasis on rational principles is that they divorce people from their own identities and thereby risk destroying people's motivation to be moral" (p. 434). Thinking back to Han's narrative "About Mr. Johansen," this means that Han ought to engage Sarah and the other students in the postconference in a way that helps to uncover more about the complexity of Mr. Johansen's and Mr. Johansen's family's situation. As we have said earlier, he also ought to make it more possible for the students to engage in reflecting on the difficult situation Mr. Johansen's daughter is in, including how she might be supported. And he ought to help Sarah and the other students think about the power dynamics in the interdisciplinary team, and to think about how they might move forward constructively as students and pending graduates in the face of such power dynamics. This should include Han's own reflections on his role on the medical unit, and how he might support Sarah and her preceptor to have their concerns heard. Creating a climate where it is safe for the students to raise diverse viewpoints is imperative toward the goal of revealing power dynamics at play (Chinn, 2001), those that unfold in the classroom, and in nursing practice itself.

Creating a safe environment for students to raise diverse viewpoints begins with having students examine their own enactment of power is ways that positively or negatively affect their learning and those of their classmates. For example, students need to be encouraged to listen attentively to each other's concerns and feelings arising in clinical situations. This means not evaluating one another's responses and questions as good or bad but creating a place where each student can develop insight into how and why they are having the response they are. In the case of health care team power dynamics, it is important to have students explore how various team members are enacting power and ask them to think about why this is happening. Is there a history of certain voices being silenced in this clinical care area? Are family members seen as active participants in all decisions about their members care? Do nurses' and physicians' knowledge about the situation complement one another or compete? Trying to peel back the layers of what is going on in ways that are nonevaluative and nonjudgmental can create a learning situation where students feel free to take risks, pose difficult questions, and learn more about themselves as nurses. It is our contention that shifting from a case study approach toward a narrative and storytelling approach will be of great assistance to Han and the students as they seek to become responsive to Mr. Johansen and his family's needs. Such a shift will also help relationships among the interdisciplinary team members. We turn now to a relational view of ethical knowledge in general, and narrative approaches more specifically.

A CAPACITY FOR ETHICAL KNOWLEDGE

As many chapters in this book attest, learning requires a relationship to knowledge. Here we extend this claim to suggest that how we see ethical practice in nursing and the contextual and relational nature of nurses' moral agency is important for how we go about developing **ethical knowledge**. Taken together, these two ideas underpin our belief that the capacity to develop ethical knowledge arises from seeing nurses as always in relation to themselves, others, and the contexts in which they work. Therefore, there is no such thing as asking learners to stand outside of their experiences of themselves, patients, colleagues, and the context of nursing practice so as to develop knowledge about being ethical practitioners. Or, as Dewey (1922) proposes, knowledge is not some kind of *fixed state of knowing something, but is more about an ever-increasing and evolving relationship to experience*. Everyday experience is always a site where knowledge is being developed and as a result it becomes ". . . an active, working aspect of life" (Dewey, 1922, p. 59). We aim toward a similar notion of ethical knowledge in nursing, where it is a dynamic, living knowing that relies on learners being implicated in all aspects of learning.

Reason and Bradbury (2001) claim that one of the greatest challenges we face in the Western world is how particular educational methods have tended to subvert our own capacities to create knowledge. These authors suggest that in order to create knowledge that is worthwhile and practical we might consider ". . . taking back the capacity to create one's own knowledge particularly in light of the repressive and damaging educational experiences many of us have endured" (Reason & Bradbury, 2001, p. 56). We do not mean to imply that case studies are necessarily the source of repressive or damaging experiences for nurses, yet we do believe that for nurses to learn about becoming ethical practitioners they ought to engage with, or develop a relationship with, their own knowledge-generating capacities. We believe that this will help them to be morally sensitive to the needs of patients, families, communities, and nurses' interdisciplinary colleagues.

Through work in feminist ethics and feminist pedagogy there have been varying criticisms of moral and ethical knowledge when viewed as disembodied from persons (Heckman, 1995; Nussbaum, 2001; Sherwin, 1992, 1998; Walker 1999). This work has attempted to replace the disembodied moral knower with the relational self. The knowledge constituted by a relational self is a different kind of knowing than that arising from seeing knowledge as residing outside of persons.

> *The relational self produces knowledge that is connected, a product of discourse that constitutes forms of life; it is plural rather than singular. [The feminist theorist] Gilligan hears moral voices speaking from the lives of connected, situated selves, not the single truth of disembodied moral principles. She hears these voices because she defines morality as plural and heterogeneous. (Heckman, 1995, p. 30)*

Through our research into ethical practice, nurses have shared stories of how they see ethical practice as something that they are and not something that is *applied* to nursing practice. Such a view challenges existing ways of thinking about ethics and moral conduct in professional disciplines, including nursing. Coming to see nursing practice and nurses' moral agency through a relational view means that the teaching and learning of nursing ethics ought to flow similarly. We ought to see learners as knowers in relation to themselves and others in the process of learning ethics and when becoming moral agents in practice. One of the ways to tap this capacity to create ethical knowledge is to bring learners into relation with their experience of ethics in practice. Given that it has been proposed that we, as human beings, have an "impulse to narrate" (White, 1980, p. 5), it may be that this impulse is a capacity for developing ethical knowledge in nursing practice.

A Narrative Approach to Ethics Education

Narrative-based approaches to health care and ethics education are gaining increasing attention in the literature (Brody, 2003; Clarke, 2000; Frank, 1991, 1995; Gadow 1999; Nisker, 2004; Tschudin, 2003). Arising from a critique of traditional bioethics as based on the tenets of Western rationalist approaches to moral theory, it is not surprising that narrative and story are helping to broaden the boundaries of ethical inquiry. Narrative and story foster interest in context, as well as analyses of moral problems in relation to structural, cultural, and political sources and the complexity of patient and practitioners' moral experience and problems. Kaufman (2001) suggests that clinical narratives open the content of ethics to a range of underdiscussed topics that are deeply troubling to practitioners and patients and their families. She also claims that narrative helps to expand the scope of ethical discussion to show how ethical deliberation and actual problem solving are "dynamic activities situated in local worlds where explicit institutional demands and expectations shape practice" (Kaufman, 2001, p. 13). Therefore, narrative and stories bring learners into relation with relevant aspects of practice for being moral agents (Box 7.2). As noted previously, values, relationships, and power have been found to be highly relevant and relatively unrecognized aspects of ethical practice in nursing.

Nisker (2004) claims that it may be the difference in the "thickness" or "thinness" of cases in ethics that contribute to their success in helping to bring us closer to the "insights into the moral problems of humanness" (p. 286). He claims that learning ethics requires bringing students closer to the person at the center of the ethical issue being explored. We suggest that it is about bringing learners closer to the people they are caring for as the basis for developing ethical knowledge, and that this closeness can be more fully facilitated by helping learners see how they are implicated in, and related to, their own knowing about being ethical. In other words, our view of shifting toward narrative and stories for helping students developing capacities for ethical knowledge arises from

BOX 7.2 PURPOSES OF NARRATIVES IN HEALTH CARE ETHICS

- Bringing the learner to the position of the person requiring health care.
- Approximating empathy for the person at the center of decision making.
- Engaging learners in different ways of perceiving the world.
- Providing more depth in ethical analyses and more possibilities for empowerment.
- Promoting public discussions of ethical issues and related policy.

Adapted from Nisker, J. (2004). Narrative ethics in health care. In J. Storch, P. Rodney, & R. Starzomski (Eds.), *Toward a moral horizon: Nursing ethics for leadership and practice* (pp. 291–294). Toronto: Pearson-Prentice Hall.

seeing both themselves and patients at the center of the knowing and learning process. As Carson (2001) explains:

> *Stories allow students to evaluate themselves as practicing nurses, to see their practice as a mix of professional duties and personal choices. Sometimes they do not like the nurse they see, but they come to realize that nursing practice may be a conflict between the personal and the professional. This more reflective researching of their own story/practice can help the student see or become more conscious of themselves as practitioners. (p. 20)*

Tirrell (1990) posits that telling stories creates the possibility for developing the capacity to be a moral agent since it can help us develop a sense of self, a sense of self in relation to others, and the capacity to justify our decisions. The capacity to be ethical also involves understanding, or attempting to understand, others. Since a story is a special kind of account, it recognizes and relies on the idea that nurses and patients are particular people living at a time within a particular context. It helps us articulate our own lives, and those of others, to learn nursing. When telling their own stories, students may see what kind of stories they can tell; in this way telling a story can be a sort of self-inquiry. As teachers and students we find out what we think by listening to what we say and write. In this way telling or writing stories helps us to find out who we are (Nussbaum, 2001). Yet, stories do not just tell us who we are, who we have been, they tell us what we are capable of and they tell us whom we might be. Stories provide us ". . . with a way of exploring, logically and emotionally, actions occurring in context, actions performed by agents with particular beliefs, motives, and desires" (Tirrell, 1990, p. 117).

Skott (2001) proposes ". . . in the framework of nursing as a human science with a focus on personal lived experience, theoretical nursing literature contains narrative as a rediscovered form of knowledge" (p. 249). It has been proposed that narrative and story hold moral force, healing power, and contain an emancipatory thrust that has been missing from patients' stories of illness and for making visible aspects of nurses' work. Vezeau (1994) cites the value of narrative as not revealed through answering questions, but rather with discovering questions that were invisible before the narration. She argues that "narratives should provide mirrors and lamps to illuminate issues usually concealed" (p. 54). In the teaching and learning of ethics, we propose that the issues to be revealed are the contextual and relational aspects of nurses' moral agency and their capacity to be in relation with their own knowledge development about being ethical practitioners. By suggesting that narrative and stories are valuable for learning about nursing ethics, we do not intend to advocate an uncritical reliance on stories implying that they contain all the answers to what nurses need to practice ethically. We acknowledge that narratives can be constructed and stories told in ways that advance the power and position of some groups while disadvantaging others. We also recognize that the limits of our knowing that are expressed in narrative and story are based on our different subject positions. How the physician caring for Mr. Johansen tells his or her story may serve a particular purpose, one that eclipses the concerns and interests of Mr. Johansen's daughter. And someone charged with bed utilization based on patient need may construct the story quite differently. What we want to point to here is the idea that narratives and stories are constructed in certain ways and reflect the complex interplay between the subject positions of the tellers and listeners. It is equally important to examine how we, as teachers, construct and relate to our own stories and those of students. Doing this requires particular skills of tracing how we are in relation to ourselves and others—both in what we know and narrate and how we know and tell. We will now explore ways of using narrative and story to bring learners closer to their knowledge-generating capacities.

ENLISTING NARRATIVE AND STORY AS ETHICS TEACHING STRATEGIES

Before describing how narrative and story can be used as ethics teaching strategies, we want to pick up on an idea proposed in Chapter 5 that suggested that teaching methods ought to serve rather than constrain our teaching intent. If we intend to bring students into relation with their own knowledge-generating capacity, then it is necessary to question how our methods actually help us do this. For instance, given that Nisker (2004) claims that one of the purposes of narrative in health care ethics may be to have "long term effects on the structure of the self by extending a reader's psychic map to . . . unfamiliar territory, taking in new values and knowledge and knowledge of other ways of seeing the world" (pp. 188–190), it is critical that his methods serve this purpose. Nisker (2004) does not ask students to step back from their stories and experiences or to bracket their values and beliefs about the experience being narrated. In fact, Nisker (2004) speaks of how he uses drama to bring students into feeling, experiencing, and imagining the lives of others. The method serves learners' efforts to develop knowledge rather than asking them to step back so as to learn. Finally, it is being questioned if case methods may effectively help practitioners learn ethics since cases are generally social constructions that may reflect ". . . the author's values and assumptions" (Carson, 2001, p. 198). It seems worthy and timely to ask how we could create learning opportunities where students become authors and editors in their knowledge development.

We will now describe how narrative and stories can be integrated in ethics teaching strategies by outlining how and what possibilities narrative and stories hold for learning about ethical practice. Our aim here is to provide ways that teachers can connect students to their own stories and those of patients, families, and colleagues in meaningful ways.

Finding Narratives and Stories

Integrating narratives and stories as ethics teaching tools begins by creating a culture or spirit in the class that encourage what McDrury and Alterio (2002) describe as a "storytelling culture" (p. 156)—a place where experience and speaking and writing in the first person is valued, and where teaching and learning expertise is embodied within people, not only within course textbooks and expert authorities. This means that Sarah, in Mr. Johansen's case, finds a place where her feelings and insights about his care are seen as valued and important for learning. This also means speaking from our experience as teachers and encouraging students to speak about their experience with ethical issues in practice for how they live on in present modes of understanding. Han might share his own feelings of sadness and frustration in confronting negative attitudes toward the elderly, for example.

Narratives and stories are always about something. This something may only be known to the teller and may become known to the listener through its telling. Narrative and stories often become something more and different based on how the listener engages with the story. For instance, Han may pose questions to Sarah that help her to see additional aspects of the situation, such as how her preceptor may approach her colleagues and present her concerns about this patient's confusion and the team's lack of response to their concerns.

One of their most salient features of narratives and stories is their ability to attend to the emotional dimensions of moral situations, which many scholars have come to see as prerequisite to moral sensitivity (Nortvedt, 2004; Scott, 2000; Thayer-Bacon, 2003). Thayer-Bacon (2003) explains:

> *It is not the case that reason is in opposition to emotions. Such a view of reason is impoverished, for reason and emotions are really very closely intertwined. Our emotions stir us and move us to act; they are expressions of doubt, love, concerns, hate, fear, and surprise, for example.* (p. 120)

This implies that stories and narratives arise from places that may have previously been deemed as irrelevant for learning about ethical practice. Traditionally, emotions have been viewed as contaminants of moral deliberation and not relevant for discerning ethically relevant issues in professional practice. We believe that ethical issues, more often than not, show themselves through our emotional and bodily responses, such as gut feelings and questions from the heart. Asking students about their emotive and embodied responses to particular situations expressed narratively (in either written or spoken form) helps them to tap into this discerning source of ethical knowledge.

In the postconference where Mr. Johansen's story is being recounted, for instance, by continuing the dialogue with the students, Han could encourage them to think about how their feelings of outrage and sadness sensitize them to end-of-life care and resource allocation. And he could encourage the students to talk about how they, and the rest of the nursing staff, could work with their feelings of powerlessness. Narrating is also a practice, as it gives us a way to imagine, try out, and see something in a new way through a reflexive awareness. Each telling constructs a new reality, helping learners to learn about themselves and others and their actions. The story itself may be less important than what may happen in the telling. To illustrate, by making it safe for Sarah to tell more of Mr. Johansen's story, Han may be helping her, and her fellow students, feel more confident in having their voices heard. The story becomes about Mr. Johansen's care and about how nurses' moral agency may be constrained by the organizational structures and interdisciplinary relationships that create the context in which these particular nurses are practicing.

Another important way in which stories and narratives can be found[4] is by thinking about how narratives reflect cultural practices of health and health care (Gadow, 1994;

[4]We are not implying that stories and narratives are out there waiting for teachers to find them. Stories and narratives are always situated and local and only come into being through a person's engagement in some sense-making experience. Tuning into where and how stories are told and narratives constructed helps us to see the myriad ways in which experience and events come into a spoken form.

BOX 7.3 SEEKING STUDENTS' NARRATIVES

Ask students to think about stories that are told repeatedly in practice. For example, are there stories about noncompliant patients being told over and over? Are there stories about interfering family members, about doctors trying to play "God", or about some patients as less deserving of care than others? What do you see reoccurring in your practice that you think has an ethical dimension? Are they able to see how these stories either hold up or are challenged? Are there stories about family members who interfere in their family member's care in ways that create a certain narrative about what good and bad interfering looks like? Asking students to find and construct their own stories while at the same time noticing those being told around them will help them to see how their own stories can never stand completely outside the broader cultural narratives of health care. That is, they come to recognize the influence of the context on themselves as well as on patients, families, and other health care providers.

Stivers, 1993). In other words, when particular stories are told over and over again sometimes they become viewed as a truth or something that defies critical scrutiny. It is almost as if the narrative gains momentum in ways that function to pull the wool over our eyes. Such is the case in health care when particular ways in which medical narratives of disease and illness separate the person from their illness, the body from the person's experience of being ill. For instance, a narrative about the body as an object, and about how our thoughts, feelings, and experiences can be seen separately from disease and illness processes, gains momentum and assumes a status of truth (Brody, 2003; Frank, 1991, 1995; Nisker, 2004). This objectified view of bodies as objects has become a cultural narrative in health care. Looking for ways in which certain stories and narrative become uncontested truths can also help students to see how what they tell and narrate is always in relation to, and inseparable from, what gets told and narrated in health care generally. For example, Han could ask the students in the postconference to reflect on the possible meanings behind the charge nurse's statement that Mr. Johansen is someone who is "not going to make it out of here anyway." Asking students to think about what they construct as stories can then be contrasted with the broader narratives shaping health care (Box 7.3).

Constructing Narratives and Telling Stories

Narratives and stories are constructions and meaning-making mechanisms that we employ to understand and make sense of our experiences and the world generally. Stories and narrative are therefore constructed for particular reasons. This means that stories and narrative can be constructed differently depending on the context in which they are shared. Stories and narrative are not about getting it right, they are more about construction and articulation. This means that students and teachers require critical awareness when inquiring into how stories and narratives are shared, and for what purpose. Teachers can ask students to think of an experience and then share it in more than one context, paying attention to how it is told, and if it varies at all. They can then ask themselves why this might be. How stories are told and how we hear them is dependent on our particular moral values by which we live. Was the narrative constructed and told to elicit a particular response, to show something of the teller, or to ask a question?

Returning to Mr. Johansen's story, by shifting from a case study approach toward narrative and story telling in the clinical postconference, Han could help the students, himself, and ultimately the members of the health care team, to have a richer and more nuanced appreciation of the experiences of Mr. Johansen, his family, and all those involved in his care. The narrative summary that Han and his students could cocreate would furnish a much stronger platform for ethical action than a traditional ethical case study summary. Han's own narrative already furnishes a strong start. If continued by Sarah, part of the narrative might read as follows:

I came into this postconference feeling so frustrated. My preceptor and I just seemed to have failed our sickest patient and his daughter today. My patient today is Mr. Johansen. He is a 76-year-old man who recently had a pretty serious stroke, and he's experiencing worsening confusion, including periods of some pretty scary delirium. His daughter, whose name is Ingrid, and my preceptor, as well as the other nurses who have been caring for him for the past few days, have noticed this change and think that it may be the result of a treatable problem, maybe a urinary tract infection, But when my preceptor spoke to Mr. Johansen's doctor, he brushed her off. And the charge nurse seems to think we should quit wasting our time worrying about an old person who is dying. I felt sick when I heard her say that. My preceptor and I don't know what to do. We can't get anyone to listen to us.

I felt terrible when I left his room. His legs were hanging out over the side rails and my preceptor was trying to help. The room seemed so crowded and cluttered—it's a noisy four-bed room—and his daughter was sitting crying in the corner.

So I have come to this postconference wanting some help. This isn't right, and I want to help. What can I do?

Writing the story in this way brings the teller and listener into seeing ethical dimensions that may have been previously unseen. It provides an open set that students and practitioners are encouraged to continue to explore. The ethical dimensions of Mr. Johansen's story could then be written as questions:

1. *What authority should the voices of the daughter and the nurses have in this decision-making process? How are they reflecting Mr. Johansen's interests?*
2. *Should Mr. Johansen be offered medical assessment and treatment that may well improve the quality of his life even though it will not likely change its duration? What symptom management can be achieved?*
3. *How can the well-being of Mr. Johansen's family be attended to as they face his uncertain prognosis and possible death?*
4. *How can the staff, students, and Han deal with the interdisciplinary team conflict that has exacerbated this situation?*
5. *How can Han and the students support the nursing staff to work toward interdisciplinary team and family meetings to discuss all of the above?*
6. *How can Sarah make sense of her emotional and bodily response to the suggestion that Mr. Johansen is wasting resources?*

7. *How can Sarah and her preceptor—as well as the other students—be supported to see possibilities for their own agency in conflicted situations such as this?*
8. *What support will Han himself need as he works to support others in this situation?*[5]

Expanding Narratives and Stories

How might aspects of students' experiences become more visible through narrative and stories? In Han's narrative about Mr. Johansen, he helps us to tune into additional questions that allowed both the teller and listener to see more nuanced aspects of the situation. Asking students to tune into how a listener's question moves them to a new place may help them see how diverse perspectives can expand a field of view. This skill is fundamental to being able to act ethically toward others, through cultivating the capacity to try to understand and acknowledge the lives and experience of patients and families.

It has been proposed that stories shift the ground under people and in that way change the world (Clarke, 2000). This may sound ambitious and even idealistic, yet we can likely each recall a time that a story and experience told to us dramatically altered the way we see and think about things now. This tells us something about how students' and teachers' stories alike have the potential to draw us in, helping us to see aspects of ourselves and our responses in a new way. This skill of being able to tune into emotional and embodied aspects of moral experience has also been proposed as necessary to moral sensitivity and ethical action (Bowman, 1995; Nortvedt, 2004; Nussbaum, 2001).When students tell stories in which they see ethical difficulty, such as those expressed by Sarah, the story itself can draw other students in as they imagine being in Sarah's position now or in the future. Through the integration of other students' perspectives, Sarah herself may see her own narrative expanding through the critical reflections of others. As an in-class activity this process could be structured by asking each student to speak about what they noticed in the story and their response to hearing about Mr. Johansen. Students could then be invited to share what they each hear in Sarah's story through what they notice and their response. Each student could then tell their story of Mr. Johansen through what it was like to hear Sarah's. The story Sarah brought expands through multiple perspective and understandings, while still acknowledging and honoring the story as it came through Sarah into the group. Thus, there is no complete or more truthful account to be generated, but additional threads woven into the tapestry of students' learning.

Reconstructing Narratives and Stories

Narratives and stories provide us with a particular perspective on situations. We each tell stories based on an often unconscious selection of people and events to understand, make sense, and/or make specific points. In this chapter we have proposed that context (the environment within which nurses' work) also significantly impacts events, how they are narrated, and our relationships with others. In learning about ethical practice in nursing we see it as imperative that narrative and stories are learned from in ways that reveal how context and relationships influence what is told and how we make sense of

[5]Adapted from McPherson, et al. (2004), p. 110.

everyday practice realities. Since teaching and learning ethics mostly occurs in a group setting, the final strategy to be discussed is how stories and narratives can be used to facilitate dialogue and exploration of multiple perspectives in groups.

Facilitating students' abilities to engage in dialogue with others about their clinical experiences through narrative and stories can help them to see both differing realities and new realities (McDrury & Alterio, 2002). For example, as Han shares his narrative describing Mr. Johansen's situation, students can begin to see how the cultural framework of professional nursing shapes what and how Han does this. This not only challenges the teller to develop new insights or understandings (such as how to use the language of resource allocation to advance his position on Mr. Johansen as deserving of care and attention), it also invites the listener (the students) into another layer of understanding. As Han and the students move toward new and deeper understandings, new possibilities or realities become imagined. Sarah and her preceptor may find a new way to act as moral agents on behalf of Mr. Johansen and his daughter.

Telling stories in groups so as to learn about ethical practice in nursing enables tellers and listeners to see the emotional and affective dimension of stories, comprehend the complexity revealed through multiple perspectives, and acknowledge various ideas for moral action that account for the relational and contextual realities of practice. One way is to ask students to select a story offered by a classmate. Listeners are encouraged to carefully attend to the teller and not become focused on creating a response story from their own experience. Ask students to imagine how they might feel in a similar situation. Listeners can be encouraged to keep track of their responses to the story and its telling and can be given a chance to clarify any perceptions when the story has been told. Together the teller and the listeners identify key people involved, insights, feelings, facts, and questions. As we indicated earlier, the story can then be reconstructed based on collective insights and questions, while still honoring the original version. This can occur in a written or verbal format, or ideas and insights can be represented in images, drawings, or other vehicles or modes of expression. The final part of this activity could engage students in a discussion of what they came to see through their diverse perspectives and the insights they have gained.

The aim is not to reach a consensus story where all differences in perspectives is collapsed. Rather, the aim is to create opportunities for learners to notice, make sense, and create meaning through the various perspectives and insights that emerge. Returning to the reflection on the clinical postconference that began this chapter, it may be that bringing students into an exploration of one infant's care together creates a possibility for seeing ethically relevant aspects of his or her care through such a process. One student could be responsible for telling the infant's story and through the various insights and questions raised, a new story could emerge that reveals how novice neonatal nurses may learn about being a moral agent in practice.

SUMMARY

In this chapter, we have explored the promise of stories as relayed through narratives in teaching nursing ethics. We have contrasted this approach with the traditional use of case studies, arguing that the rich inductive opportunities furnished by narrative better support the relational and contextual nature of nurses' moral agency.

In closing, we would like to echo the philosopher of education, John Dewey's (1922), idea that inquiry stems from a felt need and that interest is an expression of felt desires. Our work focusing on ethical practice in nursing has stemmed from a felt need and expressed desire to more accurately account for the nature of nurses' moral work, particularly for how this shapes what it means to be a moral agent and act ethically in everyday practice. Dewey also views the personal experiences of learners as the vehicle through which inquiry skills for lifelong learning are developed. Bringing both of Dewey's insights to bear on this discussion has helped us to see how nurses' everyday practice experience of caring for patients could be more effectively tapped as a capacity for developing ethical knowledge. Narrative and story hold much possibility for helping nurses to discern their own values in relation to what is good for patients and to investigate conflicting values and power relations. Narrative and story can also help us to value the life experiences and cultural identities of nurses as moral agents whose unique, contextualized perspective and position have been less than visible through the traditional use of case studies. We would like to offer the challenge to ourselves as educators to tap our own storytelling and narrative capacities so that we may facilitate those of students to become critical autobiographers of our own lives as nurses.

LEARNING ACTIVITY

The purpose of this activity is to facilitate students' capacity to see how they live in and through the stories they tell. It also helps learners to see how being in relation with others, such as classmates, can reveal additional understandings to an experience when narratives are shared with others. It also helps students to think about how stories may give them a place to try out various courses of action in practice.

1. Ask students to think of an experience from practice that is currently intriguing them. Or ask them to recreate a clinical experience in a role play.
2. Ask them if they were to tell a story about this experience or clinical scenario what would the story be about and how would they tell it. How is their particular story being shaped by fellow students or other care providers in their practice area?
3. Write the story down.
4. Share the story in pairs.
5. Have the students ask each other why each of them chose the particular situation and why they constructed the story in the way they have. Ask them to compare how their stories are similar and/or different.
6. Ask the students to identify possible implications for their own practice and how they see themselves as nurses if they were to reflect on the story in more depth.
7. What possibilities for making sense of the ethical dimensions of the story arise?
8. What are they able to see and/or not see that may be ethically relevant?
9. Can they see themselves acting as a moral agent in the story?
10. What possibilities for future moral action and ethical deliberation arise?
11. What did you learn about yourself and from your partner as a result of sharing the story?

RESOURCES FOR EDUCATORS

PLANNING THE TEACHING/LEARNING EXPERIENCE

Instructions for Educators

One of the most challenging aspects of teaching ethics in nursing is to help students to see what they are concerned about as ethically relevant. This is likely due to the influence of biomedical principlism and the way in which ethics has been taught. When nurses see ethics as something out here and not in here (in themselves), they tend to only speak about ethical issues in those terms. Thus, asking students to bring stories of ethical issues to the classroom can be met with blank stares. In order to create a culture for storytelling, we also need to create a culture for ethics as embodied and personal so that students see their how both their emotional and intellectual experiences are the basis for the narrative and stories they share in class.

To do this ask students to tell you about a patient care experience that did not sit well for them, one where they had a gut feeling that something was wrong or that something bad was going to happen. Acknowledging that emotions and gut feelings are moral cues can be a powerful invitation for learners to share their stories of practice. And it is our responsibility as teachers to be clear about ethics as it lives in each of us so we can speak about tuning into those experiences as the basis for becoming morally sensitive practitioners. Ask students to see if the story they shared is also being shaped by a broader narrative in health care. For example, is a student's concern about not providing adequate care to a patient being shaped by the narratives of efficiency and scarce resources? Is the student's feeling of not meeting a patient's needs also being influenced by organizational downsizing and a "do more with less" narrative that is living within his or her particular practice area?

EVALUATING THE TEACHING/LEARNING EXPERIENCE

Sample Evaluation Strategy

Seeing ethical practice as something nurses are and not just something they do requires that evaluation strategies reflect the degree to which learners are aware of and in tune with how their own ethical values are shaping their views on a particular situation. For example, when students undertake an ethical analysis of an issue in practice, such as when some patients are seen as more deserving of care than others do, students are required to critically reflect on how their views of deservedness may potentially play out in the way they go about making decisions about prioritizing patient care. This means the student could respond to the question, "How are my own ethical values shaping my practice?" The degree to which students willingly inquire into and critically reflect upon this interface, between ethical values and practice, could be a criterion upon which assignments or presentations are evaluated.

References

Bauman, Z. (1993). *Postmodern ethics*. Oxford, UK: Blackwell.

Benner, P. (1991). The role of experience, narrative and community in skilled ethical comportment. *Advances in Nursing Science, 14*(2), 1–21.

Benner, P. (2000). The roles of embodiment, emotion and lifeworld for rationality and agency in nursing practice. *Nursing Philosophy,* 1, 1–14.

Bowman, A. (1995). Teaching ethics: Telling stories. *Nurse Educator Today,* 15(1), 33–38.

Brody, H. (2003). Stories of sickness (2nd ed.). Oxford, England: Oxford University Press.

Brown, H., Rodney, P., Pauly, B., et al. (2004). Working within the landscape: Nursing ethics. In J. Storch, P. Rodney, & R. Starzomski (Eds.), *Toward a moral horizon: Nursing ethics for leadership and practice* (pp. 126–153). Toronto: Pearson-Prentice Hall.

Carson, A. M. (2001). That's another story: Narrative methods and ethical practice. *Journal of Medical Ethics 27*, 198–202.

Chinn, P. L. (2001). *Peace and power: Building communities for the future* (5th ed.). Boston: Jones & Bartlett.

Clarke, L. E. (2000). *Making meaning in medicine: The role of narrative and storytelling in clinical ethics.* Unpublished master's thesis, Department of Adult Education, Community Development, and Counseling Psychology, University of Toronto.

Dewey, J. (1922). *Human nature and conduct*. New York: Henry Holt.

Diekelmann, N. (2002). "Pitching a lecture" and "reading the faces of students": Learning lecturing and the embodied practices of teaching. *Journal of Nursing Education, 41(3)*, 97–99.

Doane, G. (2004). Being an ethical practitioner: The embodiment of mind, emotion and action In J. Storch, P. Rodney, & R. Starzomski (Eds.), *Toward a moral horizon: Nursing ethics for leadership and practice* (pp. 433–446). Toronto: Pearson-Prentice Hall.

Frank, A. (1991). *At the will of the body*. Boston: Houghton Mifflin.

Frank, A. (1995). *The wounded storyteller: Body, illness, and ethics.* Chicago: University of Chicago Press.

Gadow, S. (1994). Whose body? Whose story? The question about narrative in women's health care. *Soundings, 77*(3–4), 295–307.

Gadow, S. (1999). Relational narrative: The postmodern turn in nursing ethics. *Scholarly Inquiry for Nursing Practice, 13*(1), 57–69.

Hartrick Doane, G. (2002). Am I still ethical? The socially mediated process of nurses' moral identity. *Nursing Ethics, 9*(6). 623–635.

Heckman, S. J. (1995). *Moral voices, moral selves.* University Park, PA: Pennsylvania State University Press.

Kaufman, S. R. (2001). Clinical narratives and ethical dilemmas in geriatrics. In B. Hoffmaster (Ed.), *Bioethics in social context* (pp. 12–38). Philadelphia: Temple University Press.

Kohler Riessman, C. (1993). *Narrative analysis*. London: Sage.

MacDonald, G. (2002). Transformative unlearning: Safety, discernment and communities of learning. *Nursing Inquiry 9*(3), 170–178.

Mackenzie, C., & Stoljar, N. (2000). *Relational autonomy: Feminist perspectives on autonomy, agency and the social self.* New York: Oxford University Press.

McDrury, J. & Alterio, M. (2002). *Learning through storytelling.* Palmerston North, New Zealand: Dunmore Press Limited.

McPherson, G., Rodney, P., Storch, J., et al. (2004). Working within the landscape: Applications in health care ethics. In J. Storch, P. Rodney, & R. Starzomski (Eds.), *Toward a moral horizon: Nursing ethics for leadership and practice* (pp. 98–125). Toronto: Pearson-Prentice Hall.

Munhall, P. L. (1988). Curriculum revolution: A social mandate for change. In National League for Nursing, (Eds.), *Curriculum revolution: Mandate for change* (pp. 217–230). New York: National League for Nursing.

Nisker, J. (2004). Narrative ethics in health care. In J. Storch, P. Rodney, & R. Starzomski (Eds.), *Toward a moral horizon: Nursing ethics for leadership and practice* (pp. 285–309). Toronto: Pearson-Prentice Hall.

Nortvedt, P. (2004). Emotions and ethics. In J. Storch, P. Rodney, & R. Starzomski, (Eds.), *Toward a moral horizon: Nursing ethics for leadership and practice* (pp. 447–464). Toronto: Pearson-Prentice Hall.

Nussbaum, M. C. (2001). *Upheavals of thought. The intelligence of emotions.* Cambridge, UK: Cambridge University Press.

O'Connor, A. B. (2001). *Clinical instruction and evaluation: A teaching resource.* Sudbury, MA: Jones & Bartlett.

Pattison, S., Dickenson, D., Parker, M., et al. (1999). Do case studies mislead about the nature of reality? *Journal of Medical Ethics* 25(1), 42–46.

Penticuff, J. H. (1991). Conceptual issues in nursing ethics research. *Journal of Medicine and Philosophy, 26*(3), 235–258.

Reason, P. & Bradbury, H. (2001). *Handbook of action research: Participative inquiry and practice.* Beverly Hills, CA: Sage.

Reilly, D. E., & Oermann, M. H. (1992). *Clinical teaching in nursing education* (2nd ed.). New York: National League for Nursing.

Rodney, P. A. (1997). *Towards connectedness and trust: Nurses' enactment of their moral agency within an organizational context.* Unpublished doctoral dissertation, University of British Columbia, Vancouver, BC.

Rodney, P., Brown, H., & Liaschenko, J. (2004). Moral agency: Relational connections and trust. In J. Storch, P. Rodney, & R. Starzomski (Eds.), *Toward a moral horizon: Nursing ethics for leadership and practice* (pp. 154–177). Toronto: Pearson-Prentice Hall.

Rodney, P., Pauly, B., & Burgess, M. (2004). Our theoretical landscape: Complementary approaches to health care ethics. In J. Storch, P. Rodney, & R. Starzomski (Eds.), *Toward a moral horizon: Nursing ethics for leadership and practice* (pp. 77–97). Toronto: Pearson-Prentice Hall.

Rodney, P., & Street, A. (2004). The moral climate of nursing practice: Inquiry and action. In J. Storch, P. Rodney, & R. Starzomski (Eds.), *Toward a moral horizon: Nursing ethics for leadership and practice* (pp. 209–231). Toronto: Pearson-Prentice Hall.

Rodney, P., Varcoe, C., Storch, J. L., et al. (2002). Navigating toward a moral horizon: A multi-site qualitative study of nurses' enactment of ethical practice. *Canadian Journal of Nursing Research 34*(3), 75–102.

Romyn, D. (2000). Emancipatory pedagogy in nursing education: A dialectical analysis. *Canadian Journal of Nursing Research, 32*(92), 119–138.

Scott, P. A. (2000). Emotion, moral perception, and nursing practice. *Nursing Philosophy, 1*, 123–133.

Sherwin, S. (1992). *No longer patient: Feminist ethics and health care.* Philadelphia: Temple University Press.

Sherwin, S. (1998). A relational approach to autonomy in health care. In S. Sherwin (Coordinator), *The politics of women's health: Exploring agency and autonomy* (pp. 19–47). Philadelphia: Temple University Press.

Skott, C. (2001). Caring narratives and the strategy of presence: Narrative communication in nursing practice and research. *Nursing Science Quarterly, 14*(3), 249–254.

Storch, J., Rodney, P., Pauly, B., et al. (2003). Listening to nurses' moral voices: Building a quality health care environment. *Canadian Journal of Nursing Leadership, 15*(4), 7–16.

Stivers, C. (1993). Reflections on the role of personal narrative in social science. *Signs: Journal of Women in Culture and Society, 18*(2), 408–425.

Thayer-Bacon, B. J. (2003). *Relational (e)pistemologies.* New York: Peter Lang Publishing.

Tirrell, L. (1990). Storytelling and moral agency. *The Journal of Aesthetics and Art Criticism, 48*(2), 115–126.

Tschudin, V. (2003). Narrative ethics. In V. Tschudin, (Ed.). *Approaches to ethics: Nursing beyond boundaries* (pp. 61–72). Edinburgh: Butterworth Heinemann.

Varcoe, C., Doane, G., Pauly, B., et al. (2004). Ethical practice in nursing: working the in-betweens. *Journal of Advanced Nursing* 45(3), 316–325.

Veatch, R. M., & Fry, S. T. (1987). *Case studies in nursing ethics.* London: Lippincott.

Vezeau, T. M. (1994). Narrative inquiry in nursing. In P. Chinn, & J. Watson, (Eds.), *Art and aesthetic of nursing* (pp. 41–66). New York: National League for Nursing.

Walker, L. J. (1999). The perceived personality of moral exemplars. *Journal of Moral Education, 28*(2), 145–163.

White, H. (1980). The value of narrativity in the representation of reality. *Critical Inquiry, 7*, 5–27.

Additional Resources

Benner, P. (1984). *From novice to expert: Excellence and power in clinical nursing practice.* Menlo Park, CA: Addison-Wesley.

Diekelmann, N. (1991). The emancipatory power of the narrative. In *Curriculum revolution: Community building and activism* (pp. 41–62). New York: The National League for Nursing Press.

Diekelmann, N., & Diekelmann, J. (2000). Learning ethics in nursing and genetics: Narrative pedagogy and the grounding of values. *Journal of Pediatric Nursing, 15,* 226–231.

Chapter

8

Story-Based Learning: Blending Content and Process to Learn Nursing

Lynne E. Young

Teaching is even more difficult than learning because what teaching calls for is this: to let learn. The real teacher, in fact, lets nothing else be learned than learning. . . . the teacher is ahead of [her] apprentices in this alone, that she has still more to learn than they—[he or she] has to learn to let them learn. (Heidegger, 1968, p. 15)

INTENT The intent of this chapter is to introduce readers to story-based learning, a student-centered pedagogical model that is designed to guide teaching clinical decision making in nursing in the spirit of letting learn. Following a discussion of its origins in case method teaching and problem-based learning, the story-based learning model, a student-centered approach to teaching nursing, is introduced and discussed. An overview of its development is presented featuring a discussion of challenges and possible solutions. The chapter concludes with reflections on the paradox of student-centered teaching and a summary of the benefits of using such a model to teach nursing practice.

OVERVIEW

BACKGROUND TO THE MODEL

Letting learn is a radical departure from traditional nursing education practices in which the teacher is the expert and the student the passive recipient, clean slate, or empty vessel. Such a radical departure is a most unsettling notion for teachers and students alike (Grkovic, 2005; Hiemstra & Brockett, 1994; Slusarski, 1994; Taylor, 1986, 1991; Woods, 1994). Letting learn shifts the focus from what the teacher sets out in behavioral objectives for the student to follow, to the student finding her or his way through assigned materials to identify what he or she needs to know (Taylor, 1991). Memorizing facts is replaced by acquiring knowledge for some purpose. Regurgitating facts is replaced by discovering what it is like to find personal meaning in learning, and vicariously to own knowledge. Yet, how does a teacher teach toward such learning? How is such learning evaluated? How is a student motivated to learn for herself? How does a nurse educator let students learn clinical decision making toward enhanced professionalism? The story-based learning model (SBL) is a guide for letting nursing students learn about clinical decision making.

Case method teaching (CMT) (Christensen & Hansen, 1987) and problem-based learning (PBL) (Barrows & Tamblyn, 1980), approaches to teaching that encourage self-directed learning, informed the development of SBL. As a pedagogical tool, SBL guides students through a decision-making process that simulates everyday nursing practice. Consistent with the tenets of constructivism and social constructivism, SBL calls for students to build on existing clinical knowledge and learn through interaction with others. SBL rests on principles of education specific to preparing professionals for practice:

- Active learning develops responsible engaged learners.
- Personalizing learning renders learning relevant and meaningful.
- Introducing concepts and content in context expands awareness.
- Sequencing the presentation of material supports knowledge acquisition.
- Strategies that require students to learn how to learn, to think critically, and to attend to emotions goes some way to preparing mature, flexible, thoughtful professionals.
- Learning in groups prepares a professional for team work.
- Developing information literacy is a skill that can be used to manage the current information explosion (Bruner, 1966, 1996; Callister, Matsumura, Lookinland, Mangum, Loucks, 2005; Cunliffe, 2002; Knowles, 1975; Lindemann, 2000; Rideout, 2001; Weaver, 1993).

Using the model as a guide for learning integrates and builds on what students have learned through their studies in a **caring curriculum**. Its application reinforces and further develops **habits of mind** cultivated throughout the curriculum that will eventually evolve into tacit knowledge for professional practice. SBL thus serves as a metacognitive strategy bridging between explicit and tacit knowing. With SBL, the educator has a tool to not only let students learn, but also an approach to teaching that provides students with opportunities to begin transforming explicit knowledge into tacit knowledge.

Story-Based Learning Model: Its Raison d'Etre

SBL is a product of necessity. I was charged with delivering a final theory course in a caring curriculum where students were asked to bridge nursing worlds located with different **paradigms**. With its philosophical foundations of **phenomenology**, **feminism**, **critical social theory**, **humanism**, and the curriculum meta concepts **caring** and **health promotion**, the curriculum is located within a paradigm referred to as the humanistic, naturalistic, or holistic (Bensing, 2000; Morse, 1995; Thompson, 2003; Vinicor, 1995). Here, health is understood to be constructed by the social, and health experience is understood to be shaped by dominant values and interests, including those that are gender based. Meanings of illness and health are constructed by the person living the experience, meanings that are unconsciously shaped by dominant ideologies. Caring is a partnership in which the person is the focus of care. Decisions are coconstructed and intentionally aligned with the interpretations of the one(s) in care. Decisions are carefully thought through so that it is the interests of the individual, family, community, and/or populations that are served. Such clinical decision making is a collaborative, relational, interpretive process. In contrast, acute care nursing commonly occurs in a highly medicalized context, one in which health is envisioned as the absence of disease, the health professional as the expert, empirical truths reign supreme, and patients are objectified and decontextualized individuals (Malterud, 2001;Young & Wharf-Higgins, 2004). In contrast to the holistic paradigm, treatment goals are often established with little or no meaningful input from the patient (Dordrecht, 2002). These two perspectives are in stark contrast and dominate the conceptual worlds of student nurses studying in a caring curriculum who are thinking through the care of a person with an acute illness. Thus, I was faced with guiding students to apply new paradigm ideas in old paradigm contexts. This was the challenge. Where to begin? (See Chapter 16 for a discussion of the caring curriculum as revolution.)

Reflecting on being a student in a critical care nursing course, I recalled spending endless hours sitting in a classroom listening to lectures about the intricacies of the workings of body parts, a quintessentially biomedical approach to teaching. This, I thought, was not the way to bridge between the holistic and biomedical paradigms. Are there not ways to teach nursing that resonate with the tenets of the holistic paradigm? I began to read and talk with people and found two promising strategies—case method teaching and problem-based learning. I learned that case method teaching (CMT), and its offspring, problem-based learning (PBL) were developed to bridge between classroom learning and professional practice in such professions as nursing, education, law, medicine, accounting, and business. Both strategies are student-centered, similar to the caring philosophy of nursing that considers the client to be the center of care. This seemed a promising place to start.

CMT precedes PBL as a pedagogical strategy. The origins of CMT can be traced back to the Medical Society of New Haven in 1788 (Tomey, 2003). But it was Harvard professors in Law and Business who invested a good deal of time and energy to develop the use of cases in teaching into a pedagogical strategy, a strategy that is now considered an educational innovation in many countries (Garvin, 2003). CMT requires students to raise questions, and explore in **dialogue** with the instructor and each other, the relative benefits of potential decisions from a list of alternatives toward an evolving and ever deepening understanding of the field (Wassermann, 1994). CMT places students in learning situations in which making thoughtful decisions becomes a habit (Garvin, 2003).

Medical education reformers began to use CMT as a way to combine science with clinical medicine. PBL emerged as a bona fide teaching strategy for medicine in the 1970s at McMaster University Medical School (Neufeld & Barrows, 1974). PBL has revolutionized medical education around the world, and has been adopted by numerous other health sciences disciplines, including nursing. PBL serves as the basis of curricula, courses, or merely one, of learning activities. Problem-based learning requires learners to discover what they need to know to competently address a practice-related problem (Woods, 1994). The idea of addressing a problem is grounded in the work of Dewey (1963/1938) who recognized that learning occurs when the learner is confronted by a cognitive challenge such as a problem that needs to be thought through. In PBL, the problem is posed as a clinical case. Learners read the case and begin by articulating what they need to know to competently address the situation. These are called their learning issues. Students list their learning issues, then address these issues drawing on a range of resources. The expectation is that in the process of accessing resources, the students will develop skills with information literacy. Following individual work, students are convened in small groups to discuss what they have learned to solve the problem. Thus, PBL is a problem-oriented, student-directed strategy designed to provide learners with opportunities to build on existing knowledge, acquire information literacy skills, learn from each other, practice clinical decision making, and acquire cognitive cues to guide future clinical decision making in real world situations (Rideout, 2001; Schmidt, 1993; Woods, 1994). CMT and PBL are student-centered pedagogies that let the students learn while they acquire skills for real world application. (See Chapters 10 and 11.)

As student-centered pedagogies, CMT and PBL resonate with the idea of client-centeredness central to the caring curriculum. Common to these pedagogies and to client-centered nursing (Young, 2002) are the notions of shared responsibility, collaboration, and learning through dialogue. Thus, using these strategies in the nursing classroom, I reasoned, would allow for congruence between how I was teaching and what I was teaching. Recalling that social cognitive learning theory (Bandura, 1986), and related empirical research, suggest that learning occurs through modeling, modeling what I was teaching would be a way to reinforce learning. As I was pondering these matters, medical faculty in my community were preparing to assume tutor roles in a PBL curriculum. I was fortunate to join them for a few introductory sessions, including a mock PBL session. The sessions convinced me that PBL had the potential to bridge between classroom and clinical learning, and to provide opportunities for students to integrate all that they had been required to learn in the curriculum. Paradoxically, in learning about PBL, I learned about new developments in medical education; new paradigm thinking is not only evident in nursing, but also in medicine (Malterud, 2000; Pauli, White, & McWhinney, 2000). Perhaps this bodes well for changing practice patterns in settings such as acute care nursing.

To better understand the issues related to using PBL, I turned to the literature. Three recent evaluation studies of PBL report the main themes that appear in the empirical literature on PBL since 1974. Rideout, et al. (2002) conducted a robust evaluation in which nursing students in a conventional program were compared to those in a problem-based curriculum. Students' performance on RN exams did not differ significantly, however the students in the PBL group were more satisfied with their learning experience and their relationships with instructors. Results of a recent qualitative study in which PBL was evaluated for its effectiveness in nursing education in Hong Kong demonstrated that PBL was effective in terms of facilitating critical reflection and debate, self-directed learning, and cooperative learning (Lee, Wong, & Mok, 2004). An insightful evaluation study was conducted by Azila, Sim, and Atiya (2001) who concluded that PBL requires an investment of time and a paradigm shift with regard to the roles of students and teachers. PBL holds promise as a student-centered teaching strategy but is not without its own challenges and controversies.

Case method teaching is more a philosophy and a related set of principles than a distinct strategy like PBL. Evaluations of teaching with cases generally appear in the literature in relation to PBL-style applications, for example. Since PBL afforded theoretical congruence with some aspects of the caring curriculum, and its empirical evaluations were favorable, PBL seemed like a reasonable model to adopt. My concern was that PBL generally required a student to teacher ratio of 6:1 in small group work, yet I would be faced with a 25:1 student to teacher ratio. Since our students had completed formal preparation in group work, I decided to risk using PBL despite this skewed ratio.

During the introduction of PBL to students in our program, I conducted formative and summative evaluation to inform its adaptation. Data was gathered in focus groups with students, individual interviews with faculty, and appeared as memos of my reflections. Consequently, the PBL model was adapted and became story-based learning. This adapted version of PBL differed from PBL in three ways:

1. It used stories or narratives rather than the more conventional objectified cases.
2. It drew specific attention to socioeconomic and political factors.
3. It was presented as a circular, iterative rather than linear process.

Regarding changing the title, removing "problem" from the title was political. Although the idea of using problem in the title was reasoned from an educational scholar's perspective, when used in the nursing context, the use of the term problem in the title struck a sensitive chord. Held wisdom is that nurses focus on strengths not problems. Hence problem was removed from the title of the model. Stories written for SBL are stories of nurses' or their clients' tensions, issues, dilemmas, enigmas, and challenges. Regarding the shift from cases to stories, students and faculty noted that cases written in a

BOX 8.1 A CONVENTIONAL CASE—DOROTHY MCGUIRE

You have been asked to care for Mrs. McGuire, an 83-year-old widow from New Westminister. She was admitted yesterday for a cystoscopy for a possible diagnosis of bladder cancer, an intervention she had today. Mrs. McGuire returned from the operating room (OR) at 10:00 A.M. and it is now 8:00 P.M. You notice a moderate amount of blood in her urine despite the continuous bladder irrigation that she is on. Your assessment indicates that she is a tiny woman (her chart notes that she is 4′11″ and 102 lbs and that she has recently lost 6 pounds), her blood pressure is 150/90, pulse 80 and regular. Mrs. McGuire is a pleasant lady, but you have growing concerns about her mental status. On assessment, she is disoriented to time and date even though you have oriented her on several occasions since the beginning of your shift.

conventional manner objectified and decontextualized the patient, and this was incongruent with the notion of understanding lived experience in context, a notion central to the curriculum. Thus, the cases evolved into stories in which actors were richly contextualized to emphasize the effects of sociopolitical and economic factors on illness experiences. Further, the stories were written as narratives to elicit emotion to better emulate the full scope of the lived experience. Similarly, Yamada and Maskarinec (2004) note these same weaknesses in conventional PBL cases, and propose that PBL cases should be written as narratives that draw in the effects of sociopolitical and economic factors on illness experiences. To exemplify the difference between a case written in a conventional manner and a case story, refer to Boxes 8.1 and 8.2. The case in Box 8.1 is written in the conventional way where the patient is objectified. In Box 8.2, the case is

BOX 8.2 A CASE STORY—MRS. RANJIT SANKRIT, ROOM 356

Voices, male and female. So many words I don't understand . . . sodium, potassium, I know those words. Now, cold pressure on my chest. Please cover my breasts. . . . why can't I say it, my mouth won't work my eyes won't open. Drugged, I am drugged. . . .

My patient this morning, Ranjit Sankrit, is a diagnostic and nursing challenge for sure. When she was dialyzed yesterday, her blood pressure plummeted and dialysis had to be discontinued. That must have been so distressing for her. In addition, she has been bleeding from her GI tract. First thing this morning, she had a gastroscopy to assist with the diagnosis, now she is quite drugged from the sedatives she was given. I can see her through the window of her room. She is not responding even slightly during the physical assessment by the renal physician and his team. She just lies there with her eyes closed breathing heavily. It looks bizarre like something from another world. The doctors heads are together. They are talking over her as if she is just a body to be inspected. They move their stethoscopes from point to point listening to her lungs, her breasts exposed for passers-by to see. This is unreal. We have a long way to go to acknowledge patients as feeling persons. Apparently, her lungs are quite congested— I was told in report that they are worried that she may develop pneumonia. She told the night nurse she was "fed up." I can see why. OK, get focused Marie, **STOP** editorializing. You have to get a handle on this woman's history fast since there's so much to do. First, check her drips and equipment. I'll put a warm blanket over her, cover her up.

written as a case story from the perspective of those living the experience such that the emotional dimension is included with a view to eliciting emotion in the reader by mirroring the holistic nature of illness experiences, and the relational nature of caring.

In reading about and speaking with educators who use CMT to prepare teachers for practice, I learned that a goal when writing a case is to write the social, political, and economic influences into a case to invite students to go ever deeper with their understandings. The cue for doing so is to ask learners to reflect on the big questions embedded in the case narrative (Wassermann, 1994). Examples of big questions that can be explored are:

- Is racism operating in the story?
- Is ageism operating in the story?
- Is sexism operating in the story?
- What power dynamics are operating in the story?

Thus, in the adapted PBL process, I included direction for learners to identify the big questions.

Learners were quite passionate that PBL was linear and what they experienced as nurses was circular and iterative. Thus the model moved beyond the question, "What is going on here?" to an interpretation of health-related patterns in the story, imagining nursing support, reflecting on learning and decisions. Re-engaging with the story anew closed the circle and marked the beginning of a new and different clinical decision-making process. Finally, to underscore the salience of caring to the entire process, caring was placed at the center of the model.[1] The final product was titled story-based learning, a student-centered strategy to guide nursing students' acquisition of clinical decision making skills. SBL is described below and illustrated in Figure 8.1.

STORY-BASED LEARNING: BLENDING CONTENT AND PROCESS TO LEARN NURSING

Throughout story-based learning, the learner's engagement with a clinical narrative is grounded in an ethic of caring: caring enough to compose or read a case story with attention to meanings and emotion; and caring enough to acquire theoretical, empirical, critical, personal, and interpersonal knowledge for practice. Engagement in the SBL occurs through a six-phase process of:

1. Attending to the story.
2. Determining what is going on in the story.
3. Identifying patterns of wholeness and disruption.
4. Envisioning nursing support.
5. Reflecting on learning and interpretations.
6. Returning to a "new" story.

Engagement with the SBL process calls for attention to detail, accessing and understanding new resources for learning, and dialogue. Thus, the learner builds substantive and disciplinary knowledge that is acquired through individual and group

[1] Dr. Anne Bruce, the research assistant on the project, contributed this insight.

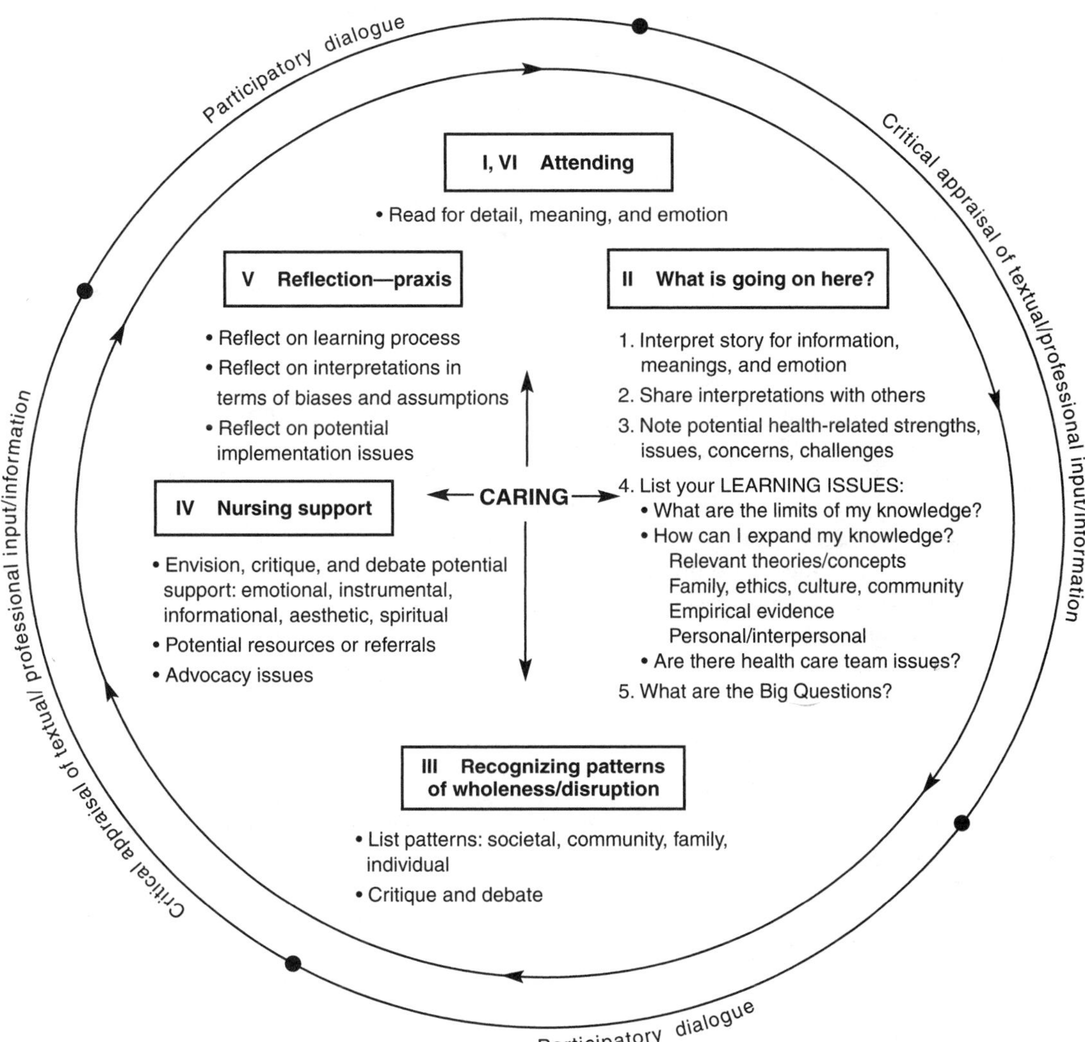

■ **FIGURE 8.1** Story-based learning model: Blending content and process to learn nursing.

work and through interactions with the instructor. The model guides students to critically appraise the materials, opinions, and interpretations encountered during the learning exercise. Thus, students rehearse clinical decision making in nursing guided by processes central to the caring curriculum.

Bevis and Watson (1989), architects of the caring curriculum, identify five positions central to the caring curriculum paradigm in nursing: first, the curriculum is interaction; second, active learning, held to be essential for the development of critical thinking, engages the intellectual efforts of students and faculty; third, students must assume leadership and responsibility for their own learning to mature; fourth, no one theory can account for the complexity of learning; fifth, curriculum development begins with faculty development. These five positions, they argue, converge into a whole entity that yields a curriculum that is educative rather than instructive in its essence. Bevis and Watson (1989) work from the assumption that "the cognitive processes that one teaches are as important as the content, and . . . most are more important than content" (p. 79). That interaction, active learning, taking responsibility for one's learning, and enabling the development of cognitive processes are at the heart of SBL suggests that this is a teaching strategy with potential for guiding learning within a caring curriculum.

The Story

As narratives of a health-related or health care experience, stories are designed to concurrently build on and integrate students' knowledge. Stories that inspire students' imaginations and elicit emotion thrust students into the moment. Narratives written to invite students to acquire more in-depth knowledge or draw attention to the constellation of factors that shape health experiences take students to new depths of understanding. Stories may be written by the educator or the students.

When students are invited to write stories, they tap into the aesthetic dimension of knowing thereby releasing creative energy. A story may allow a student to tap into the emotions elicited by nursing. Storywriting is an opportunity for students to use their imaginations to illustrate the innumerable factors that require a nurse's attention to decision making. Or, storywriting may introduce a student to previously hidden talent. Writing a story about a past experience may bring closure to a clinical experience left unfinished or unresolved.

Educators may write stories from current or past experience, or they may generate a story from a found source such as newspapers, magazines, books, films, or documentaries. For example, the story in Box 8.2 was based on a situation that I observed during a shadow experience in a CCU in a local hospital. To be consistent with the constructivist perspective on learning, educators would identify the themes of the stories they write through a consultative process with students so that the story addresses students' self-identified learning issues or knowledge gaps. For example, a focus on dialysis was selected for the Ranjit Sankrit narrative in response to students' requests to learn more about fluid and electrolytes. Educators may need to provide leadership in assisting students with identifying their learning issues since one does not always know what one does not know. For example, during an exercise in which students were asked to list ideas for case stories, no student requested a focus on neurological nursing. In discussion, I determined that this focus was absent from the list because neurological nursing was not on their radar screen. Educators also provide leadership with regards to how stories for SBL exercises are constructed. A SBL story incorporates physiological, social, ethical, political, ideological, and/or relational aspects of health experience. While some students can easily weave together these diverse threads of health experience in a story, other students need support from the instructor during one-on-one discussions about how to write a narrative in this way. I find that students can manage to address at least three diverse aspects of health-related experience in one story; for example, pathophysiology, family, and a social bias such as ageism. The story in Box 8.3 is an example of

BOX 8.3 JULIE'S STORY: THE IMPACT OF A HIGH-TECH BIRTHING EXPERIENCE

I thought I was prepared for this. I never dreamed that there would be so many procedures and this much pain. I am surrounded by noisy machines, and I seem to have tubes coming out of everywhere. I cannot even lie on my side because the fetal monitor is strapped to my belly, and these beds are so uncomfortable.

When I received the epidural they told me it would feel like a bee sting—maybe from a 300 pound bee. The past 48 hours have been exhausting. When they induced me yesterday it did nothing, except cause a lot of pain. Today they tried again, and still I have not dilated. The doctor and nurses are telling me not to worry because the baby's heart rate is fine. However, I still feel nervous. My husband has been supportive, but I need more reassurance from the staff. They seem so involved with the machines, and I cannot help but think something must be terribly wrong. I really do not want to have a C-section, but it looks like things are headed that way. I never thought that having a baby would be like this.

how three diverse aspects of care can be interwoven in a narrative; in this case, high risk childbirth; pain management; and, family nursing.

Storytelling rather than storywriting may focus SBL analyses. Storytellers may be a person with a chronic illness, a family member of someone with a mental illness, a narrator in a film or documentary, a story posted on the Internet, a story told by a student nurse, and so on. SBL stories can also be verbal accounts that are then written so that the details of the story can be scrutinized.

Educators play a crucial role in staging the storywriting or storytelling exercise by asking questions such as:

- Is the story adequately complex?
- Does it invite students to consider a wide range of problems, issues, and challenges from the physiological to the ideological?
- Does it build on students' existing knowledge base?
- Does the story elicit emotion?
- Is the presentation inviting, even dramatic?
- Does the story reflect the current realities of clinical practice?

Stories are generally written in first person, and involve few actors, often only one. The voice can be that of the nurse, the patient, or family member. However, stories may have more than one voice or be presented as a short play. Stories are generally a moment in time, but could be a series of stories presented in sequence to guide students through a more complex knowledge development process.

Students benefit from clear guidance for storywriting. I ask students to begin by thinking of a storyline or theme, and then to envision a beginning and an end to the story. Stories for SBL are best kept short, one page or less. While some students take great pleasure in storywriting, others find it to be a most challenging, almost impossible, exercise. Such students require considerable support from the instructor. When a student struggles, then succeeds, the student and instructor have much to celebrate.

Storywriting and storytelling as educational strategies are opportunities for students to develop **linguistic intelligence** by using words in new ways (Gardner, 1993). Directing students to prepare stories that elicit emotion is a way to provide opportunities for students to tap into their feelings, or to develop what Gardner (1993) calls **intrapersonal intelligence**. Overall, storywriting and storytelling open new and different spaces for expression and interaction such that dialogue in a SBL classroom is rich, enticing, and sometimes deeply meaningful.

Outer Circle: Participatory Dialogue

Participatory dialogue is one of two elements in the outer circle (Figure 8.1), a process central to creating a climate in which educators let students learn, for themselves and from each other. Participatory dialogue is a process that supports the development of students' capacities for authentic engagement, verbal expression, and logical argument. During case story analysis, learners practice the skill of engagement and experience what it is like to be authentically engaged. Practicing this skill during case story analysis may raise the learner's awareness to potential issues of engagement such as the challenges of attending to one's own and others emotions while listening for detail and meaning. Students have opportunities to learn from modeling as they experience the educator using skills necessary for participatory dialogue.

However, in a student-centered classroom the educator is no longer a content expert, rather an expert facilitator of learning, a role in which asking questions is the primary teaching tool. PBL evaluation research suggests that one of an educator's greatest challenges in working in a PBL classroom is developing skills to ask good questions (e.g., Kaufman & Holmes, 1996). Further, participatory dialogue requires a shift in power dynamics in the classroom. No longer is the educator in the role of expert knower whose power comes from possessing that knowledge. Now, the educator and students are colearners in power sharing relationships (Chinn, 2001). Therefore, if SBL is to be effective, faculty development will include support for acquiring the skill of questioning and capacity to share power.

Outer Circle: Critical Appraisal

Critical appraisal marks a shift from the transmission model of teaching that engenders rote learning and generally produces **received knowledge**. Critical appraisal as a requirement throughout the SBL process, underscores the salience of interpretive processes to surfacing and critiquing the assumptions operating in interpretations. Critical appraisal entails critical thinking to formulate questions such as:

- On what basis are truth claims being made?
- What is the scientific merit of the information?
- What is the practical value of the information?
- Is the science, information, or opinion sensitive to issues of race, culture, gender, age?

Critical appraisal during the case story analysis offers students the opportunity to rehearse this skill in a variety of conditions.

Inner Circle

PHASES ONE AND SIX: ATTENDING TO THE STORY

Attending to the story mirrors the real world act of listening to patients and clients. Students attend to the story for meanings, emotions, and detail while beginning to gather and synthesize information (Frederiksson, 1999; Kacperek, 1997). In so doing, they begin the relational, interpretive, embodied process that is necessary to enact caring as envisioned in a caring curriculum. Attending, as phase one and phase six, draws attention to the circular, iterative nature of the clinical decision making: the nurse begins by listening, engages in a professional decision-making process that concludes with listening. Clinical decision making is often a convoluted, iterative process that folds back on itself; however, such a nonlinear process is impossible to depict as a guide for teaching. Thus, it is recommended that when using the SBL, there is some discussion with students about the limits of depicting the clinical decision-making process relative to the merits of practicing the process in a systematic way to develop habits of mind that the learner may fall back on when clinical decisions must be made under duress in highly complex, deeply emotional situations.

PHASE TWO: WHAT IS GOING ON HERE?

Students begin to answer this question by identifying the health-related strengths, issues, and challenges evident in the story. Then, learners connect with the adequacy of their knowledge base to address this question distinguishing between what they know, and do not know, relative to clinical decision making while noting their knowledge gaps. During this process, learners may note that they require more knowledge about some aspect of the case story to make a good decision. These items may be noted in a section titled assessment issues. From the list of knowledge gaps, learners then articulate their learning issues. For example, a student may note that she has a knowledge gap related to fixed, dilated pupils in a case story about traumatic head injury. This learner may claim pathophysiology of fixed, dilated pupils and nursing care of a person with fixed, dilated pupils as learning issues. Learning issues, then, are those issues that if addressed will fill knowledge gaps toward more professional clinical decisions. For example, in the case story in Box 8.2, a nursing student may identify dialysis as a knowledge gap. The learning issues might include: fluid and electrolyte imbalances and renal failure; hemodynamics of dialysis; dialysis technology; complications of dialysis; nursing care of persons on hemodialysis; sleep deprivation in ICU patients; East Asian perspectives on healing, and, so on. Reflecting on the narrative in this way draws students' attention to the value of building a solid knowledge base to guide clinical decision making.

To challenge students to reflect on ideological influences on health experience, the SBL asks students to reflect on: "What are the big questions?" Learners are asked to articulate one or two questions that point to the influence of dominant ideologies on health experience, with a particular focus on issues of race, gender, socioeconomic status, and age. Students are asked to do no more than ask the big question. This provides evidence of their growing awareness of contextual influences on health experiences. Deconstructing those influences is beyond the scope of the SBL exercise when used with undergraduate nursing students. Turning again to the story in Box 8.2, big questions might include: Is the lack of attention to the woman's privacy related to power inequities between physicians and patients referred to in the literature in terms of the medical gaze? Would the health care team be as likely to expose the naked upper body of a young, Caucasian woman of high social standing?

SBL guides students to identify search strategies and list resources that were accessed to address their learning issues. Requesting that students note the search strategies used to acquire information opens a space for a discussion about information literacy skills. Learners will use textbooks, research articles, review articles, Internet resources, expert input, and so on to address their knowledge gaps. The constellation of resources selected by a student is an opening to discuss knowledge and information adequacy. When working in small groups, students bring their work back to the group for discussion. Comparing knowledge sources and understandings in small groups sensitizes learners to how much one can learn from others, an essential lesson for professional nurses. Further, reflecting on these discussions cues learners to such matters as: preferred learning styles; emotional reactions to group learning; how group discussion shapes opinion, and so on.

In this phase of the model, students acquire additional skills and knowledge for practice. Specifically, students acquire: the capacity to identify relevant health-related strengths, issues, and challenges evident in a case story; an appreciation for the interrelated nature of the physical, biological, behavioral, emotional, social, cultural, ethical, and interpersonal and personal influences on health; and, an appreciation that it is necessary to continually build knowledge for professional practice. This process cultivates skills with, and knowledge about, lifelong, self-directed learning (Crooks, Lunyk-Child, Patterson & LeGris, 2001; Jerlock, Falk, & Severinsson, 2003).

PHASE THREE: RECOGNIZING PATTERNS OF WHOLENESS AND DISRUPTION

When working with the case story, the student is required by this model to synthesize his or her analysis in terms of patterns of wholeness and disruption. These statements become the focus for what the nurse will do (or not do) in terms of action in the following phase. While professional practice across disciplines focuses on identifying and working with patterns, in professional nursing practice guided by a holistic philosophy of health, this skill is particularly salient (Cody, 2004; Cowling, 2000; Newman, 1999; Young, 2002; Young & Wharf-Higgins, 2004). As noted earlier, new paradigm nursing assumes a holistic stance toward patients and clients; this is a shift from the reductionist, systems view that is dominant in the biomedical view of health care (Young & Wharf-Higgins, 2004). Identifying patterns of wholeness and disruption is a way to synthesize that analysis of the first two phases of SBL (Newman, 1999). When applied to practice, such an engagement is held to be inherently transformative and health giving (Cowling, 2000; Young, 2002). Thus, practicing synthesizing health-related experiences in terms of wholeness and disruption is central to making decisions about meaningful action.

Because nursing is often practiced in situations in which main players define health as the absence of disease, synthesizing the analysis in terms of patterns of wholeness and disruption serves to distinguish the particular interests of nursing from the interests of others, such as medicine. Acquiring this acuity of discernment of purpose is vital for student nurses who will eventually practice in situations in which nurses' roles fuse with the roles of other professionals such that the vision for care that is particular to nursing may be lost. (See the case study in Chapter 9.) Providing students with an acute sense of the purpose of nursing through this analytical process empowers students to be confident about their clinical decision making. For example, a nurse confident in the importance of holding to the view of health as wholeness may be empowered to argue for a do not resuscitate (DNR) order to ensure that a patient's request to die with dignity is honored. Finally, it is through pattern recognition that nursing students bring prior knowledge to bear on a current situation in an integrated way. Thus, practicing pattern recognition as a pedagogical exercise is a way for students to develop flexibility, agility, and sophistication with knowledge use. Synthesizing the analysis in terms of these patterns is an important starting point for the student to envision what nursing actions are plausible.

PHASE FOUR: NURSING SUPPORT

Nursing support (Vandall-Walker, 2002) is envisioned as occurring within an ethic of caring and encompasses:

- Emotional support.
- Instrumental support.
- Informational support.
- Spiritual support.
- Aesthetic support.

While the focus of Vandall-Walker's (2002) typology is nursing support of the family, the categories she presents can be adapted for individuals, groups, populations and communities. Emotional support involves connecting authentically by demonstrating such qualities as empathy and respect and providing touch (as appropriate), explanations, and being present. Instrumental support involves being helpful by promoting comfort and understanding, drawing on expert knowledge, and taking on the role of advocate, for example. Informational nursing support is crucial to the empowerment of those in one's care, and occurs through teaching/learning interactions that are planned or in the moment. Spiritual nursing support involves discovering meaning, promoting hope, and enabling such spiritual practices as attending a religious service in the hospital. In addition to these dimensions of nursing support, I would add aesthetic support to this list. Nightingale (1860) wrote extensively on the impact of environmental factors on the healing potential of patients. Her writings are no less accurate today than 150 years ago. Attention to the aesthetic environment encompasses ensuring that the environment is aesthetically pleasing: Is the room clean and orderly? Are the colors of the unit relaxing? Is the air fresh? Is there attention to minimizing noise? Are there noxious odors and/or smells?

Clinical tools such as professional standards of care, for example, those developed by cardiovascular nurses (CCCU, 2000), and clinical pathways, can be used to draw attention to possible strategies for nursing support. Since SBL requires students to individualize these tools in application to a case story, thinking through how general ideas can be particularized in a specific context provides students with opportunities to rehearse this thinking process. In our work with students, we have found that students frequently have difficulty individualizing general ideas. Thus, providing opportunities for discussing this nursing challenge goes some way to prepare student nurses for practice where standards of care and clinical pathways are used. Noting possible short-term and long-term health-related outcomes assists students to organize their ideas about what care may be required over the long term. Rehearsing planning over an extended period is an opportunity to consider issues related to discharge planning, rehabilitation, or palliative care. Students are asked to identify potential referrals, such as to a community support group, an advanced practice nurse, or other health care professional. This broadens students' thinking about nursing care. Students may learn a great deal from each other in discussion about potential resources. Finally, since a nurse may need to assume the role of advocate to ensure those in his or her care receive the supports they require, the student is asked to envision one such possibility for each case story to rehearse this eventuality in his or her own practice.

PHASE FIVE: REFLECTION AND PRAXIS

Phase five of the SBL asks students to reflect in four ways on:

- What they learned when using the SBL.
- The adequacy of the empirical and theoretical sources they accessed in the analyses.
- Their reasoning relative to the meaning of health as wholeness.
- Biases operating in their interpretations.

Reflecting on learning provides students with opportunities to connect experiences, feelings, and knowledge, an important quality for professional nurses and a crucial dimension of critical thinking (Brown & Gillis, 1999; Brown, Matthew-Maich, & Royle, 2001; Murphy, 2004; Scheffer & Rubenfeld, 2000). Students are asked to reflect on what and how they learned, and to speak to various influences on their learning; for example, interactions with faculty and peers and their use of technology. The opening scenario for Chapter 1 of this book (page 3) is a student reflection submitted as part of a course assignment in which the student reflects on how her awareness was raised about her learning through assuming and reflecting on facilitating a small group learning activity. Reflecting on how one learns is a skill for lifelong learning, a highly valuable but relatively easy genre of reflection for undergraduate nursing students (Duke & Appleton, 2000). Not so for reflecting on the adequacy of the empirical and theoretical sources used in the analysis as this genre of reflection requires students to be knowledgeable about research methods and theory construction. Reflection that surfaces biases is a metacognitive skill that requires thinking about thinking; thus this genre of reflection develops students' capacities for metacognition.

When working across paradigms, such as is the case on acute care nursing units where medical thinking figures largely, reflection empowers learners to understand how particular ways of thinking shape practice. Such intellectual work develops learners' awareness of issues related to the fit between nursing practice envisioned as holistic care and the philosophy of care of the setting in which they are asked to provide care.

PHASES SIX AND ONE: ATTENDING TO THE STORY

Returning to the attending phase is figurative in SBL. This phase acknowledges the criticalness of attending carefully to the story of care as the last step in a completed process, and concurrently, the first step in a new process. Including phase six closes the circle of care, thereby symbolically representing the iterative, cyclical nature of caring.

SBL EVALUATION: STRENGTHS AND CHALLENGES

Story-based learning was evaluated during focus groups discussions and during individual interviews with faculty who had experience with it. Overall, students felt that the model was effective in assisting them to integrate the core content of the curriculum. Several students noted that the model was effective in shifting their focus beyond the biomedical. For one student the model "took away the medical focus . . . helped me understand the patient's situation, not me imposing my views . . . this person has a life, a history, other things are going on with them . . . at home, resources, family. . . . " Another student remarked that the model expanded her view: "You get to look at the person from a new angle." Such remarks were surprising given the holistic focus of the curriculum. Perhaps this points to a need for faculty to intentionally structure learning activities so that students can practice integrating the theoretical with the everyday practicalities of a nurses' world. While the SBL model has been used to guide learning about acute care nursing, it was also used once to teach a course on community health nursing. Following this application, one student noted, "I think the SBL is very relevant to community . . . it makes the whole process of community nursing not so overwhelming." The upper level students consistently commented, and with passion, that the model should be introduced much earlier in the program than its introduction in their final year.

Faculty had a range of experiences using the SBL model, with some finding the model relatively easy to use while others facing classroom management issues. Generally faculty appreciated the fit of the model to the caring curriculum. As one instructor observed, "It fits well with the curriculum, the aim is to get students thinking, to recognize their own strengths in terms of looking things up . . . develop as lifelong learners." Faculty members concurred with students' opinion on when the SBL should be introduced into the program. One faculty participant remarked: "This sort of analysis needs to come much earlier in a program."

Interviews with faculty and students suggest ongoing challenges with SBL. Regarding faculty, for those who use teacher-centered (transmission) approaches, shifting to student-centered teaching without preparation may be overwhelming. Selecting stories that are written at an appropriate level of complexity (not too complex and not too simple) is a challenge. Discussing the merits of particular stories with colleagues prior to use, and simple trial and error do much to refine instructors' storywriting skills. Regarding students, of all aspects of the model, they had the most difficulty grasping the idea of identifying the big questions; this despite having grappled with the influence of dominant ideologies on health experience in a course. To assist students with transferring this knowledge into application, a session devoted solely to this aspect of SBL may mitigate this problem. As mentioned earlier, another aspect of the model that challenged students was the process of individualizing care. When this issue arises, it is an opportunity for an educator to address the issue of individualizing care. Despite the challenges of using SBL, using this model to foster students' lifelong learning and clinical decision-making skills was generally received with enthusiasm by nurse educators.

STUDENT-CENTERED LEARNING: THE PARADOX

While theories, research, and logic suggest that student-centered learning would be a breath of fresh air in the academy, the paradox is that students and faculty may resist this approach, a phenomenon documented in the literature (e.g., Fichardt, Viljoen, Botma, & du Rand, 2000; Karlsen, Vik, & Westin, 2000; Pereira, Telang, Butler, & Joseph, 1993). Regarding students, introducing a student-centered approach moves students and faculty out of the safe zone (Azila, et al., 2001; Woods, 1994). Woods (1994) likens the resistance response of students' to a grieving process with eight stages: shock, denial, strong emotion, resistance, acceptance, struggle with frustrations, improved understanding, and integration. Several strategies can ameliorate students' anxiety about and resistance to the introduction of SBL. By way of anticipatory guidance for students, I introduce Wood's grieving process during class in the first or second week of term. Using stories from real practice ensures that the exercise has relevance for the learners; for example, asking students to write stories based on their own experiences, or inviting a peer who is in a practice placement to come to class with a story. Regarding faculty resistance, shifting from a teacher-centered classroom or lecture hall to a student-centered classroom is a major change for faculty. For example, student-centered classrooms make different demands on faculty members' knowledge and skills, such as knowledge about information literacy and skills with time management and group process (Bevis & Watson, 1989; Maudsley, 2003; Vernon & Hosokawa, 1996). Only with confidence will faculty risk using new and unfamiliar teaching strategies in academic contexts in which student evaluations figure so large in the tenure and promotion process. Student-centered teaching then is not a panacea, but rather, new territory for many students and educators for which models like SBL may be useful tools.

SUMMARY

Story-based learning (SBL) is a pedagogical model designed to support students' development as lifelong learners while practicing clinical decision making skills. SBL is an adaptation of the widely used, and rigorously evaluated, PBL. Its adaptation was informed by formative and summative evaluations with upper level nursing students in a caring curriculum and faculty members. This six-phase model is circular in contrast to the linear PBL. The six phases are: attending to the story; what is going on here?; recognizing patterns of wholeness and disruption; nursing support; reflection and praxis; and attending to the story. Evaluation of the model suggests that it is an effective pedagogical tool for supporting students' learning about clinical decision making in a caring curriculum. As a student-centered learning strategy, SBL is designed to foster the development of vital professional attributes: propensity for lifelong learning; critical thinking; reflection; using technology to access resources for clinical decision making; and the capacity for learning and working in a group. SBL reflects the foundational elements of the caring curriculum and therefore guides students through an imaginary application process that cues them to use the knowledge acquired during their nursing program. Thus, the SBL is designed to develop students' habits of mind such that their thinking about a caring process is consistent with the philosophical tenets of the curriculum. So applied, SBL is a way to develop tacit knowledge for practice.

Despite its attributes, like other student-centered strategies, all may not receive SBL warmly. Students and faculty may feel out of the safe zone when asked to shift from traditional teacher-centered learning to the less controlled classroom of student-centered learning methods. Faculty development and support for students in making such a shift are essential to successful applications of SBL. The final word goes to a student who when interviewed about her experience with SBL remarked: "I think this kind of helps put it all together . . . ."

LEARNING ACTIVITY

This learning activity is designed to prepare students to use the SBL model. The learning activity is designed to bridge between working in more conventional ways with cases and working with a story using the SBL. The questions are designed to provide students with a chance to practice distinguishing between what they know and do not know about details evident in a case story. The exercise introduces students to the idea of a case written as a story, demonstrating that more than one voice can be introduced into such a story to get at relational and ethical considerations that face nurses in everyday practice.

Sorting Out Sandy's Care: Nursing Station on a Medical Ward

It is my fifth evening shift in a row, a demanding set of evenings for sure with common medical problems primarily, nothing out of the ordinary. I arrive for report, a bit breathless as I chose to cycle to work today and it took a bit longer than I had planned, but it was such a gorgeous summer day . . . I couldn't resist. As I settle in, note the rooms that are my case load, I notice a familiar name, Sandy Spring. Hmmm, there was a Sandy Spring ahead of me in the nursing program. I wonder if it is the same person. She was pretty wild. . . .

Sandy Spring, Room 510, Bed 4, 32-year-old pediatric nurse, married, chest pain possible PE. She was just admitted, came through emergency today; on oral contraceptives (OCs); altered ABGs; V/Q scan with two mismatched bilateral defects; coagulation abnormalities; pain not controlled; on Morphine; on Heparin IV drip; really anxious; husband is with her; she has an 8-month-old infant at home who is breastfeeding; grandparents are with the baby; she hasn't eaten since early this am; and hasn't slept. . . .

Mmmmm, this is a different case, interesting. PE, pulmonary embolism, women on OCs are at risk. Are lactating women prescribed OCs? Ohhh, I am rusty on my Obs Gyne stuff and PE Tx; better do a quick check on the diagnosis and Tx before going into the room; have a look at the labwork and meds; nursing care. I wonder how I feel about handling her blood? breastmilk?

Locating Your Learning Issues: Can You Answer the Following?

1. What is the pathophysiology of pulmonary embolism (PE)? Symptoms?
2. Are women on OCs at risk for PE? Which OCs? Which women? Why?
3. What would you expect the arterial blood gases (ABGs) to be? Why?
4. What is a V/Q scan?
5. What do you know about IV Heparin? Dose? Care?
6. What is indicated with regard to rapid response for PE?
7. What about pain control? Blood/body fluid precautions?
8. How do you feel about caring for someone who you think may be at risk for HIV+?
9. How do you feel about caring for someone that you once knew professionally?
10. Can you assess the family needs and provide the required care?

RESOURCES FOR EDUCATORS

PLANNING THE TEACHING/LEARNING EXPERIENCE

Questions to Support a Thoughtful Reading

1. What experiences have you had with student-centered teaching? As teacher? As learner?
2. If you were a learner in a student-centered learning activity, tell us your story.
3. If you were a teacher in a student-centered learning activity, tell us your story.
4. How would you respond to the comment that teachers who do not lecture do not teach?
5. How would you react to a directive to use only student-centered teaching in your classroom?
6. What do you think would be your primary challenge with student-centered teaching? Managing the classroom? Managing questioning? Or managing time?
7. Do you believe that the teacher needs to be a content expert when working with the SBL? Explain please.
8. If you were dean within your faculty, how would you promote the development of questioning and sharing power in faculty members?
9. Brainstorm ways that SBL could be applied in teaching a class or a course.

Instructions for Educators

Evaluation of learning using student-centered strategies challenges the educator to incorporate self-evaluations and peer evaluations into the evaluation process, since student-centered teaching is not complete without including learners in the evaluation process. Evaluating students' learning using the story-based learning model is conducive to making such a shift. Following are examples of the evaluation components used in one course in which SBL was used.

Assignment 1: Case Study Facilitation

As case study facilitator (CSF), your role will be to facilitate group work on a case story assigned by the instructor. In the role of facilitator, you will have an opportunity to further integrate your knowledge about, and skills with, group process acquired throughout the BSN program. As group facilitator, you will: facilitate the task-related work of the group; guide students' acquisition of substantive knowledge by facilitating their use and sharing of resources; facilitate the morale component of the group; and, stimulate critical analysis by posing questions. You will receive the case story that you will facilitate one week prior to your scheduled facilitation date. This will allow you to work up the case on your own using the story-based learning model as a guide prior to enacting your role as CSF.

Group facilitation will occur over two classes. There will be time allotted during the first of these two classes to engage students in a discussion of the case, facilitate group members in identifying their learning issues, and the resources that they might access to fill their knowledge gaps. During this first class, you will organize which student will be responsible for going away and gathering information to bring back to the group for the final work-up of the case. During the second class, time will be allotted for you to facilitate the group in the task of putting together a comprehensive analysis.

Self-Evaluation of Case Story Facilitator Role (5%)

Self-evaluation is a critical component of professional practice. While this course has been designed to provide you with an opportunity to exercise skills and qualities that you can build on in your professional life, it would not be complete without providing you with an opportunity for self-evaluation. In this assignment, you are asked to comment on how you developed group facilitation skills during this group facilitation exercise. In a 1 to 2 page (12-point, single spaced) summary, reflect on your skill and knowledge development according to the criteria established for the role: (a) facilitating the task-related work of the group; (b) facilitating students' use and sharing of resources; (c) facilitating the morale component of the group; and (d) stimulating critical analysis by posing questions. Please provide examples. Assign yourself a mark out of 5.

Instructor Evaluation (5%)

You will receive a mark out of 5 from the instructor according to the following criteria and university grading guidelines: (a) facilitating the task-related work of the group; (b) facilitating students' use and sharing of resources; (c) facilitating the morale component of the group; and (d) stimulating critical analysis by posing questions.

Peer Evaluation (5%)

You will receive a mark from your group members that is collated by Dr. Young for a final mark out of 5 according to the above criteria. Criteria relate to your facilitation skills noted in the instructor evaluation above.

Assignment 2: Peer Evaluation (10%)

You have an opportunity to evaluate the contributions of case story facilitators (CSF) on five different occasions. For each CSF peer evaluation submitted you will be assigned a mark out of 2 for a total of 10% for the course. The peer evaluation you submit for each CSF will inform 5% of the mark CSF's receive for their work.

The mark out of 2 that you receive for submitted peer evaluations will derive from the following criteria for grading noted in this course outline. Roughly, excellent to exceptional peer evaluations will receive marks of 1.5 to 2 respectively, average work will receive a mark of 1, and, barely adequate work will receive a mark of 0.5.

Assignment 3A: Case Story (10%)—Part 1 of a two-part assignment

Storywriting is a creative endeavor, an opportunity to illustrate the innumerable factors that require a nurse's attention. The idea of writing stories that will then be analyzed is to provide you with a chance to express the layers of factors that impinge on real or imagined situations that have confronted you or may confront you in professional practice. The goal of writing a case story is for you to expand your awareness of the myriad of factors influencing professional decision making.

You are asked to identify your learning issues (i.e., gaps in your clinical knowledge). Once these have been noted, you will select three learning issues that you will then address in writing a case story that is based on your past experience or your imagination. For example, if (a) orthopedic nursing, (b) family nursing, and, (c) substance abuse are learning issues, you would choose to write a case story that brings forward these three dimensions. A presenting case that could be written as a story might read as follows: Jacque, a 24-year-old male from Powell River, was admitted to the unit last night with a fractured femur, the consequence of what is believed to be an alcohol-related motorcycle accident. Jacque's partner Bob, who looks several decades older than Jacque, is sitting by Jacque's bed looking extremely anxious. As a group, you will choose diverse content areas so that a range of content will be covered in Assignment 3.

Recommended length for this assignment is 2 ½ to 3 ½ pages maximum, 1 to 2 pages for knowledge gaps and related knowledge categories, 1 page for the story, 1 page for citations and Web search strategy.

Mark Allocation

1. List of three learning issues and related knowledge gaps consistent with categories in the "What is going on here?" phase of the SBL model. (3)
2. Story (derived from learning issues). (4)
3. Citations for relevant research articles with abstracts. (2)
4. Literature search strategy. (1)

NOTE: This assignment is designed to provide you with an opportunity to integrate your knowledge of **pathophysiology**, **lab results**, **diagnostic and biomedical procedures** and **treatments**, and **medications to support your decisions about nursing care**. Hence, the story should allow for inclusion of these aspects of the clinical decision making process.

Assignment 3B (35%)

In this assignment, you will submit an edited version of the case story you prepared for Assignment 3A and an analysis of it. You will use the story-based learning model to guide the analysis. This assignment is designed to provide you with an opportunity to integrate your knowledge of **pathophysiology**, **lab results**, and **biomedical procedures** and **treatments**, and **medications with your knowledge of nursing care**. Hence, assignments should address all of these aspects of a story.

Mark Allocation

The assignment is evaluated according to the evaluation criteria for the course:

1. Edited case story. (1)
2. What is going on here? (10)
3. What are the big questions? (4)
4. Referrals and Advocacy. (3)
5. Nursing support. (10)
6. Evaluation plan. (5)
7. Reflection on learning. (2)

Please submit a completed assignment of no more than 12 pages (single spaced) using APA format for references. Charts may be used to organize your work to fit in 12 pages.

Case analyses will be copied and presented as a collection in a document that can be used as a clinical resource during the CPEs or as a study guide that you can use to prepare for the RN exams. This document will be available through the library on reserve for an extended period.

EVALUATING THE TEACHING/LEARNING EXPERIENCE

Questions to Elicit Feedback from Students on their Learning

1. Having read this chapter, what additional resources might you seek to facilitate the application of the SBL model?
2. What aspects of the SBL model are unclear?
3. What elements of the model are missing for you?
4. Do you agree with the author's claims about the components of a story? If not, why not?
5. What is your understanding of information literacy?
6. What aspects of the model resonate with how you now teach?

Reflective Questions for Educators

1. Did I use silence effectively?
2. When working with groups on the in-class case analyses, how was the discussion distributed? How much of the airtime did I take? Did each student have an opportunity to contribute to the discussion?
3. Was classroom management comfortable? Stressful? Why?
4. In today's class, can I recall a situation in which it is clear that I am developing skills with guiding learning through asking good questions?

References

Azila, N. M., Sim, S. M., & Atiya, A. S. (2001). Encouraging learning how to fish: An uphill but worthwhile battle. *Annals of the Academy of Medicine, Singapore, 30*, 375–378.

Bandura, A. (1986). *Social foundations of thought and action: A social cognitive theory*. Englewood Cliffs, NJ: Prentice-Hall.

Barrows, H. S., & Tamblyn, R. M. (1980). *Problem based Learning: An approach to medical education*. New York: Springer.

Bensing J. (2000). Bridging the gap. The separate worlds of evidence-based medicine and patient-centered medicine. *Patient Education and Counseling, 39*, 17–25.

Bevis, E. O., & Watson, J. (1989). *Toward a caring curriculum. A new pedagogy for nursing*. Sudbury, MA: Jones & Bartlett.

Brown, B., Matthew-Maich, N., & Royle, J. A. (2001). Fostering reflection and reflective practice. In E. Rideout (Ed.), *Transforming nursing education through problem-based learning*, (pp. 199–164). Sudbury, MA: Jones & Bartlett.

Brown, S. & Gillis, M. (1999). Using reflective thinking to develop personal professional philosophies. *Journal of Nursing Education, 38*, 171–175.

Bruner, J. (1966). *Toward a theory of instruction*. Cambridge, MA: Harvard University Press.

Bruner, J. (1996). *The culture of education*. Cambridge, MA: Harvard University Press.

Callister, L. C., Matsumura, G., Lookinland, S., et al. (2005). Inquiry in baccalaureate nursing education: Fostering evidence-based practice. *Journal of Nursing Education, 44*, 59–64.

Canadian Council of Cardiovascular Nurses. (2000). *Standards of care*. Retrieved October 3, 2005, from http://www.cccn.ca/info/standards.cfm.

Chinn, P. (2001). *Peace and power: Building communities for the future* (5th ed.). New York: NLN Publishing.

Christensen, C. R., with Hansen, A. J. (1987). *Teaching and the case method*. Boston: Harvard Business School.

Cody, W. K. (2004). Diversity and becoming: Implications of human existence as coexistence. *Nursing Science Quarterly, 16*, 195–200.

Cowling, W. R. III. (2000). Healing as appreciating wholeness. *Advances in Nursing Science, 22*, 16–32.

Crooks, D., Lunyk-Child, O., Patterson, C., et al. (2001). Facilitating self-directed learning. In E. Rideout (Ed.), *Transforming nursing education through problem-based learning* (pp. 51–74). Boston: Jones & Bartlett.

Cunliffe, A. L. (2002). Reflexive dialogical practice in management learning. *Management Learning, 33*, 35–61.

De Nicholas, A. (2000). *Habits of mind: An introduction to the philosophy of education*. Lightning Sources.

Dewey, J. (1963/1938). *Experience and education*. New York: Collier Books.

Dordrecht, M. S. (2002). *The different faces of autonomy: Patient autonomy in ethical theory and hospital practice*. Boston/London: Kluwer Academic Publishers.

Duke, S., & Appleton, J. (2000). The use of reflection in a palliative care programme: a quantitative study of the development of reflective skills over an academic year. *Journal of Advanced Nursing, 32*, 1557–1568.

Fichardt, A. E., Viljoen, M. J., Botma,Y., et al. (2000). Adapting to and implementing a problem- and community-based approach to nursing education. *Curationis 23*, 86–91.

Frederiksson, L. (1999). Modes of relating in a caring conversation: a research synthesis on presence, touch and listening. *Journal of Advanced Nursing, 30*, 1365–2648.

Gardner, H. (1993). *Frames of mind: The theory of multiple intelligences*. New York: Basic Books.

Garvin, D. (2003). Making the case: Professional education for the world of practice. *Harvard Magazine, 106*, 56. Retrieved February 23, 2005, from http://www.harvardmagazine.com/on-line/090322.html.

Grkovic, I. (2005). Transition of the medical curriculum from classical to integrated: Problem-based approach and Australian way of keeping academia in medicine. *Croatian Medical Journal, 46*,16–20.

Heidegger, M. (1968). *What is called thinking*. (F. D. Wieck, & J. G. Gray, Trans.) New York: Harper.

Hiemstra, R., & Brockett, R. G. (Eds.). (1994). *Overcoming resistance to self-direction in adult learning* (Vol. 64). San Francisco: Jossey-Bass.

Hudson, J. N. & Buckley, P. (2004). An evaluation of case-based teaching: Evidence for continuing benefit and realization of aims. *Advances in Physiology Education, 28*, 15–22.

Hughes, W. (1997). *Critical thinking: An introduction to the basic skills*. Toronto: Broadview Press.

Jerlock, M., Falk, K., & Severinsson, E. (2003). Academic nursing education guidelines: tool for bridging the gap between theory, research and practice. *Nursing & Health Sciences, 5*, 219–228.

Kacperek, L. (1997). Non-verbal communication: the importance of listening. *British Journal of Nursing, 5*, 275–279.

Karlsen, K. A., Vik, T., & Westin, S. (2000). [The problem based medical curriculum in Trondheim—did it turn out as planned?]. [Norwegian]. *Tidsskrift for Den Norske Laegeforening 120*, 2269–2273.

Kaufman, D. M., & Holmes, D. B. (1996). Tutoring in problem-based learning: Perceptions of teachers and students. *Medical Education, 30*, 371–377.

Knowles, M. S. (1975). *Self-directed learning: A guide for learners and teachers.* New York: Cambridge Book Co.

Lee, W. M., Wong, F. K., & Mok, E. S. (2004). Problem based learning: Ancient Chinese educational philosophy reflected in a modern educational methodology. *Nurse Education Today, 24*, 136–144.

Lindemann, C. (2000). The future of nursing education. *Journal of Nursing Education, 39*, 5–12.

Malterud, K. (2000). Symptoms as a source of medical knowledge: understanding medically unexplained disorders in women. *Family Medicine, 32*, 603–611.

Malterud, K. (2001). The art and science of clinical knowledge: Evidence beyond measures and numbers. *Lancet, 358*, 397–400.

Maudsley, G. (2003). The limits of tutors' comfort zones with four integrated knowledge themes in a problem-based undergraduate medical curriculum (Interview study). *Medical Education, 37*, 417–423.

Morse, G. G. (1995). Reframing women's health in nursing education: A feminist approach. *Nursing Outlook, 43*, 273–277.

Murphy, J. I. (2004).Using focused reflection and articulation to promote clinical reasoning: An evidence-based teaching strategy. *Nursing Education Perspectives, 25*, 226–231.

Neufeld, V. R. & Barrows, H. S. (1974). The "McMaster Philosophy": An approach to medical education. *Journal of Medical Education, 49*, 1040–1050.

Newman, M. A. (1999). The rhythm of relating in a paradigm of wholeness. *Image: The Journal of Nursing Scholarship, 31*, 227–230.

Nightingale, F. (1860). *Notes on nursing: What it is, and what it is not.* New York: D. Appleton and Company. [First American Edition] Retrieved November 15, 2005, from http://digital.library.upenn.edu/women/nightingale/nursing/nursing.html.

Pauli, H. G., White, K. L., & McWhinney, I. R. (2000). Medical education, research, and scientific thinking in the 21st century. *Education for Health (Abingdon, England)13*, 173–186.

Pereira, L. M., Telang, B. V., Butler, K. A., et al. (1993). Preliminary evaluation of a new curriculum—incorporation of problem-based learning (PBL) into the traditional format. *Medical Teacher, 15*, 351–364.

Rideout, E. (2001). *Transforming nursing education through problem-based learning.* Sudbury, MA: Jones & Bartlett.

Rideout, E., England-Oxford, V., Brown, B., et al. (2002). A comparison of problem-based and conventional curricula in nursing education. *Advances in Health Sciences Education 7*, 3–17.

Scheffer, B. K., & Rubenfeld, M. G. (2000). A consensus statement on critical thinking in nursing. *Journal of Nursing Education, 39*, 352–359.

Schmidt, H. G. (1993). Foundations of problem-based learning: Some explanatory notes. *Medical Education, 27*, 422–432.

Slusarski, S. B. (1994). Enhancing self-direction in the adult learner: Instructional techniques for teachers and trainers. In R. Hiemstra & R. G. Brockett (Eds.), *Overcoming resistance to self-direction in adult learning* (Vol. 64, pp. 71–80). San Francisco: Jossey-Bass.

Smith, M. J. (2003). Michael Polanyi and tacit knowledge, the encyclopedia of informal education. Retrieved October 18, 2005 from www.infed.org/thinkers/polanyi.htm. Last updated June 4, 2005.

Taylor, C. (1991). On the way to teaching as letting learn. *Phenomenology + Pedagogy, 9*, 351–355.

Taylor, M. (1986). Learning for self-direction in the classroom. *Studies in Higher Education, 11*, 55.

Thompson, F. E. (2003). The practice setting: Site of ethical conflict for some mothers and midwives. *Nursing Ethics, 10*, 588–601.

Tomey. A. M. (2003). Learning with cases. *Journal of Continuing Education in Nursing, 34*, 34–38.

Vandall-Walker, V. (2002). Nursing support with families of the critically ill: A framework to guide practice. In L. Young & V. Hayes (Eds.), *Transforming health promotion practice: Concepts, issues, and applications*, (pp. 162–173). Philadelphia: F.A. Davis.

Vernon, D. T., & Hosokawa, M. C. (1996). Faculty attitudes and opinions about problem-based learning. *Academic Medicine, 71*, 1233–1238.

Vinicor, F. (1995). Interdisciplinary and intersectoral approach: A challenge for integrated care. *Patient Education and Counseling, 26,* 267–272.

Wassermann, S. (1994). *Introduction to case method teaching: A guide to the galaxy*. New York: Teachers College.

Weaver, S. M. (1993). Information literacy: Educating for life-long learning. *Nurse Educator, 18,* 30–32.

Woods, D. (1994). *Problem-based learning: How to gain the most from PBL.* McMaster University: Donald Woods, Hamilton, ON.

Yamada, S. & Maskarinec, G. (2004). Strengthening PBL through a discursive practices approach to case-writing. *Education for Health, 17,* 85–92.

Young, L. (2002). Transforming health promotion practice: Moving toward holistic care. In L. Young & V. Hayes (Eds.), *Transforming health promotion practice: Concepts, issues, and applications,* (pp. 3–21). Philadelphia: F.A. Davis.

Young, L. E., & Wharf-Higgins, J. (2004). Concepts of health: discourses, determinants, lay perspectives, and the role of the community health nurse. In L. Stamler & C. Yiu (Eds.). *Community Health Nursing: A Canadian Perspective,* (pp. 73–85). Don Mills, ON: Pearson Education Canada.

Additional Resources

Hirst, S. P., & Raffin, S. (2001). "I hated those darn chickens . . .": The power in stories for older adults and nurses. *Journal of Gerontological Nursing, 27,* 24–29; quiz 55–56.

McMaster University Problem based Learning in the context of large classes. Available at: http://chemeng.mc 7aster.ca/pbl/pbl.htm. Last accessed on October 22, 2005.

Queen's University (Kingston Ontario, Canada,) School of Medicine Problem-based Learning Home Page. Available at http://meds.queensu.ca/medicine/pbl/pblhome.htm. Last accessed on October 22, 2005.

Thomas, S., & Polio, H. (2002). *Listening to patients: A phenomenological approach to nursing research and practice.* New York: Springer.

Tuyn, L. K. (2003). Metaphors, letters, and stories: Narrative strategies for family healing. *Holistic Nursing Practices, 17,* 22–26.

Chapter 9

Teaching the McGill Model of Nursing and Client-Centered Care: Collaborative Strategies for Staff Education and Development

Catherine Pugnaire Gros
Lynne E. Young

It just so happens that learning by discovery and experience—through a process of critical reflection, question-raising, researching, and dialoguing—was the main focus of an "experimental" graduate program for non-nurses that I attended when it first opened at McGill in the mid-1970s.[1] I entered the program with no previous preparation in nursing and graduated three years later with a master's degree. I was in a class of 10. Within the first week or two of the program, each student was given the name and phone number of two healthy families. We were asked to contact these "clients" and begin weekly home visits that would continue for the entire school year. I remember asking myself lots of questions: I have to call these people and visit them on my own? Why isn't a teacher coming with me to show me what to do, or at least to introduce me to the family? Shouldn't someone be there to make sure I don't make a mistake? What if I say something wrong? Apart from a few basic concepts discussed in seminar, what do I know about nursing or how to be a nurse?

Well, at least I wasn't alone. My classmates were asking the exact same questions, and more. What is it with these teachers?, we wondered. Most of us were from pure science backgrounds. Our undergrad courses were loaded with material. As far as we could tell, we weren't being taught much of anything in this program. . . .

For me, learning to be a nurse meant the professors should simply sit us down and tell us what to do. But they never did. They just said things like: "Observe your client and family." And they asked questions like: What do you see and hear? What is Nursing? What is Health? What are you learning from this person and family? I just didn't get it. First, I already knew how to observe—or so I believed at the time. Second, what was so difficult about learning from the client and family? Anybody could do that! I wanted the client and family to learn from me, the nurse.

So what was I doing in this program? Well, I was definitely doing a lot of observing, listening, reflecting, discussing, and describing. Questions were always being raised like: Who is this person/family? What is your assessment? How are you responding? What do you need to know about this situation? Even the most general

[1] The first-person "I" is that of author C. Pugnaire Gros. She also acknowledges the leadership of Robyne Kershaw Bellemare and Danielle Corbeil, Department of Nursing, Douglas Hospital; the support of Nurse Managers Solange Urbain and Dolly Dastoor; the enthusiastic participation of the nursing team from the demonstration units; and, in particular, the dedication and involvement of Primary Nurse Jacqueline Murdoch. We are grateful to our clients and families for the privilege of learning from them and with them.

questions would get me thinking and reading and wondering. But I was itching to get on with it. I wanted to do the nursing. Please assign me to a real patient. Someone who's sick and in the hospital so I can DO something. Why weren't we being taught how to do the nursing? What was the big mystery? It was all terribly elusive to me at the time...

INTENT

In this chapter, a case from teaching practice is used to illustrate how a nurse educator can blend what is taught with how it is taught. The case is drawn from a staff education project carried out by author, nurse educator, and clinical consultant, Pugnaire Gros. The aim of the project was to teach the McGill Model of Nursing to staff nurses working in a hospital setting. The McGill Model is a collaborative, client- and family-centered approach to health care first developed by F. Moyra Allen at McGill University School of Nursing in the 1970s (Allen & Warner, 2002; Gottlieb & Rowat, 1987; Kravitz & Frey, 1989). The approach is consistent with contemporary frameworks of health promotion (Allen & Warner, 2002; Young, 2002) and reflects the perspective of learning advanced in this book. More specifically, the McGill Model of Nursing contends that health promotion is linked to a continuous process of learning; that learning occurs in social interaction and through daily experience; and that it involves reflection and problem solving around real life situations. The chapter provides a practice-based example of how this approach to learning and health care was applied in the context of a staff education project carried out with staff nurses practicing in the field of mental health. The authors describe the implementation and evaluation of the project. Selected teaching and learning strategies are presented, examples of innovative teaching and learning tools are provided, and clinical and educational outcomes are discussed. The chapter closes with reflections on lessons learned.

OVERVIEW

INTRODUCTION

Nursing staff education maintains and improves the quality of patient care in hospital and community settings and is important for the development of quality clinical learning sites for students. In this chapter, we present an example of an innovative education project for staff nurses initiated by the Nursing Directorate at the Douglas Hospital—a University-affiliated, 300-bed mental health facility located in a Metropolitan area. This hospital-based project began in 2002 and evolved in collaboration with the School of Nursing at McGill University. It was carried out by an experienced faculty member and nurse clinician specialist at the hospital. The overall aim of the project was to introduce the McGill Model of Nursing to staff nurses and to assist them to apply it in their everyday practice.

A number of factors influenced the decision by hospital nursing administrators to adopt the McGill Model as the framework for guiding nursing practice throughout the institution. These included a shared goal on the part of the department of nursing at the hospital and the University School of Nursing to strengthen existing ties and to work collaboratively to develop nursing through joint initiatives in clinical practice and education. From the university's point of view, developing practice settings in which collaborative, family-focused nursing is being applied would ensure consistency between what is taught in the classroom setting and what students experience in their clinical courses. From the hospital's perspective, this initiative had the potential to enhance recruitment and retention of graduates from the university program. For example, graduates would be inclined to seek employment in settings in which there was congruence between the approach to nursing studied in their education program and the approach being practiced in their work environment as nurses.

Finally, research on the McGill Model and similar approaches suggests that client-centered care leads to important physical and psychosocial health outcomes for patients, including reduced anxiety, symptom resolution, increased self-worth, and increased physiological and functional status (Pless, et al., 1994; Stewart, 1995; Stewart, et al., 1999). Increased satisfaction for patients, as well as clinicians, has also been associated with the practice of collaborative, client-centered care (Horowitz, Suchman, Branch, & Frankel, 2003; Suchman, Roter, Green, & Lipkin, 1993). Thus, the McGill Model was officially adopted as the approach that would be used to guide the future practice and development of nursing in this hospital setting.

THE McGILL MODEL OF NURSING: AN OVERVIEW

"This new perspective on nursing is a learning perspective; a learning model. I am not saying a teaching model or a teaching perspective, but a learning perspective."
(Allen, 1981, p. 1)

Within the McGill Model of Nursing, a philosophy of collaborative learning underpins how the main concepts of *health, family,* and *nursing* are defined. For example, health is viewed as a phenomenon that involves learning (Allen, 1981); and "learning to be healthy" is an ongoing process that occurs through experiences of daily living in the context of the family and social network (Allen, 1981; Warner, 1997). Thus, the family represents the context and focus of intervention. The concept of nursing within the McGill Model is defined as a collaborative, health-promoting interaction that involves a process of ongoing learning and continuous change for client and family as well as for the nurse (Pugnaire, 1981). Moreover, the nurse's role is envisioned as collaborator, facilitator, and stimulator of client and family learning (Gottlieb, 1997). Together, the nurse and client/family participate in a continuous process of learning that involves exploration, inquiry, experimentation, and evaluation (Allen, 1981). Specific health promoting strategies carried out in collaboration with individuals and families include: making and sharing observations; raising questions; talking and listening; gathering and sharing information; setting goals; making decisions; formulating plans; testing out ideas; and evaluating together the outcomes of the actions and decisions taken (Allen 1981; Ezer, Bray, & Gros, 1997; Gros & Ezer, 1997). Additional strategies implemented by the nurse include: listening to the client's story; tailoring care to fit the client's needs and perspectives; starting where the client is at; pacing and timing interventions according to the client's readiness; being available; being kind and caring; identifying and mobilizing strengths; and working as client advocate and health care coordinator (Allen, 1977; Ezer, et al., 1997; Feeley & Gottlieb, 1998; Gottlieb & Feeley, 2005; Kravitz & Frey, 1989).

While the McGill Model was originally developed as an approach to guide clinical nursing care, the principles of collaborative learning and client centeredness described in the model can also be used to guide nursing education and research (Allen, 1981). Thus, in the current project, principles of collaborative, client-centered practice guided the interactions between nurse educator and nursing staff. Overall, the approach to teaching and learning taken in this project involved applying the above strategies, which are consistent with student-centered philosophies of education described elsewhere and discussed throughout this book (Bevis & Watson, 1989; Freire, 1970; Meyers & Jones 1993; Woods, 1994).

THE McGILL MODEL OF NURSING: TEACHING CLIENT-CENTERED CARE TO PRACTICING NURSES

Teaching the McGill Model of Nursing to staff nurses involved working over time to develop a flexible, multifaceted learning program. The program evolved in response to the learning goals and interests of staff with a focus on addressing the issues and challenges encountered by the nurses in their clinical practice. Consistent with principles of student-centered teaching and health-promoting nursing, a main goal was to build collaborative working relations among staff, educator, patients, and families. Within this relational context, the learning activities offered included: delivering relevant content, providing innovative teaching exercises, and facilitating group discussions. In addition, teaching by example and through real-time experience were two powerful sources of learning. Teaching by example occurred across clinical and classroom settings and included using a learning together approach in which collaborative strategies were role modeled by the educator in nursing practice with clients and families as well as in teaching practice with the nurses. Learning through experience occurred by testing out interventions with clients and families. In addition, entering into a collaborative working relationship with the nurses served to reinforce the collaborative process being taught.

Within this project, the nurses' learning was also fostered by: offering classroom lectures, presentations, and workshops; distributing written reference materials; developing clinically based learning exercises and teaching tools; providing ongoing coaching; facilitating small group discussions; and promoting experiential learning through clinical application, reflective dialogue, and retrospective analysis. Although the program discussed in this chapter was specifically designed for staff nurses, similar strategies and approaches have been implemented with graduate and undergraduate students in the university setting.

In this staff education program, some traditional teaching approaches were used to introduce the McGill Model to the nurses. Given the educator's experience as a learner within the nursing program featured in the opening scenario of this chapter, a main goal was to present the model clearly and explicitly. Since the mid-1970s, significant increases in empirical knowledge and advances in our understanding of collaborative, client-centered practice have occurred, thus making it possible to present in more depth today, what were new and emerging concepts over two decades ago.

Thus, basic theory relating to the McGill Model was delivered to staff throughout the hospital using a traditional teaching approach. Introductory one-hour lectures, held on a repeated basis in a central location, were open to day and evening staff from across units and service divisions. In addition, a few full-day and half-day workshops were offered. The classroom lectures and workshops served as a venue to provide basic theory and concepts, to present empirical evidence supporting the approach, and to distribute written resources and reference materials. Written materials made available for distribution included copies of presentations and lecture notes and references for books and crucial articles. Each nurse was also given a practical pocket guide on the model. In addition to providing information and learning resources, the classroom sessions were intended to stimulate interest and to increase motivation regarding the development of nursing and the practice of collaborative, client/family-centered care.

Unlike teaching students in the academic setting, educators charged with nursing staff development are faced with the added challenge of designing learning activities that can be successfully integrated into the stressful and demanding work environments of practicing nurses. Moreover, these educators must also develop teaching strategies that are compatible with factors such as high staff turnover, rotating schedules, and shift work. In response to these challenges, three types of innovative learning tools were created. In terms of structure, all three tools were practice based, user-friendly, and appropriate for individualized learning. The tools were designed as mini learning exercises that focused on the application of knowledge to practice, in contrast to the acquisition of rote content alone. A secondary learning objective of these tools was to pique the nurses' curiosity and to stimulate their interest in learning more about collaborative nursing and the McGill Model. The three learning tools used in this project are described below.

The first tool, referred to as the "Client-Centered Care Quiz" (Box 9.1), was structured as a fun to complete self-assessment rating scale. It was designed to prompt reflection on various philosophical concepts and beliefs about health and professional practice. The quiz was distributed to individual nurses throughout the hospital via a kiosk on the McGill Model that was mounted in a central location during Nurses' Week. In this way, the tool was used as a self-administered reflective exercise. A modified version of the same tool has also been used in the classroom setting. In this context, the quiz serves to stimulate discussion among nurses or nursing students regarding their attitudes and beliefs about health care and the clinician's role in health promotion.

The second tool, "Nursing Practice Guidelines for Family Intervention" (Box 9.2), was designed to encourage nurses to apply theory to practice. It evolved out of two satellite projects that were coordinated by the educator and carried out with graduate students, staff nurses, and nurse managers on two separate units. The tool takes the form of a clinical practice guide to promote the concept of families as partners in care, an idea consistent with those advanced in the McGill Model and one that the nurses on both units were interested in developing. The specific focus and content of the tool was adapted to meet the expressed learning needs of the nurses in relation to their clinical practice. For example, nurses on one unit were facing difficult challenges related to discharge planning. Important concerns included lack of continuity in caregiving relationships and gaps in patient services during the transitional period from hospital to home, issues advanced elsewhere in the literature (e.g., Forchuck, Jewell, Schofield, Sircelj, & Valledor, 1998). From the perspective of the McGill Model, sustained family involvement and support during hospitalization is viewed as a source of continuity and stability for the client postdischarge. Thus, practice guidelines were developed with a focus on building collaborative working relationships with family members during visits to their hospitalized relative. The guide includes examples of specific strategies aimed at exploring and supporting family involvement in care during the hospital period toward the goal of promoting continuity of care postdischarge. The tool was disseminated to the nurses on each unit and distributed to individual nurses hospitalwide via the kiosk.

A third learning tool, composed of a series of written clinical scenarios, was also aimed at promoting the application of knowledge and concepts to practice. The tool is composed of various clinical situations. Each situation is followed by a variety of possible nursing responses. The learner is asked to rate the extent to which the proposed responses to the scenario are consistent with client-centered practice. The tool was originally developed by the educator as part of a previous study on interprofessional educa-

BOX 9.1 CLIENT-CENTERED CARE QUIZ

COLLABORATIVE PERSON/FAMILY-CENTERED NURSING: TEST THE CONCEPTS THAT GUIDE YOUR PRACTICE

Directions: Read each of the 19 statements in the column to the left. Determine the extent to which you agree or disagree with each statement and circle the corresponding number in the column to the right. Determine your final score by adding all the numbers together.

	STRONGLY AGREE	AGREE	NEITHER AGREE NOR DISAGREE	DISAGREE	STRONGLY DISAGREE
1. People's ability to access essential medical services (e.g., hospitals, clinics, health professionals) is the most important determinant of health.	5	4	3	2	1
2. When working with patients and families, nurses should always provide their expert advice on what the patient and family needs to do.	5	4	3	2	1
3. Not being able to solve a patient's problem or answer a patient's question prevents the nurse from giving effective care.	5	4	3	2	1
4. Collaboration is not possible in situations where patients and families are not able to make sound decisions for themselves.	5	4	3	2	1
5. Collaborative models of health promotion are not relevant in the acute phase of hospitalization before the patient's situation has stabilized.	5	4	3	2	1
6. Approaches aimed at promoting patient autonomy are being developed as a way to cope with shrinking health care budgets. ➔	5	4	3	2	1

■ BOX 9.1 Client-Centered Care Quiz (continued)

	STRONGLY AGREE	AGREE	NEITHER AGREE NOR DISAGREE	DISAGREE	STRONGLY DISAGREE
7. Promoting the patient/family's sense of mastery and control should not be a primary focus of nursing care in the hospital setting.	5	4	3	2	1
8. When working in situations of acute and chronic illness, maintaining physical health and safety should take priority over the psychosocial dimension of patient care.	5	4	3	2	1
9. Health education is the process whereby clinicians use their knowledge and expertise to teach the patient and family what to do and how to do it.	5	4	3	2	1
10. Freedom from illness, discomfort and pain is required before a patient can be considered healthy.	5	4	3	2	1
11. The nurse's most important role is to identify and solve health problems for the patient and family.	5	4	3	2	1
12. When providing factual information to clients and families, the timing and pacing of the intervention is less important than the accuracy of the content being delivered.	5	4	3	2	1
13. While having a sense of mastery and control may affect a person's quality of life, these outcomes have little or no impact on the person's actual health. →	5	4	3	2	1

■ BOX 9.1 Client-Centered Care Quiz (continued)

	STRONGLY AGREE	AGREE	NEITHER AGREE NOR DISAGREE	DISAGREE	STRONGLY DISAGREE
14. Learning from patients and families is not considered a critical aspect of professional nursing practice.	5	4	3	2	1
15. While patient perceptions may be important, objective measures are the best way to evaluate the effectiveness of care.	5	4	3	2	1
16. The ability of clinicians to provide collaborative, patient-centered care depends more on the clinician's natural personality than on the clinician's knowledge and skill.	5	4	3	2	1
17. Meaningful health outcomes take longer to achieve when nurses take the time to include patients and families in the decision-making process.	5	4	3	2	1
18. Evidence-based practice gives health professionals the knowledge and expertise to decide what is the best treatment approach for a particular patient.	5	4	3	2	1
19. The physical status of a person is the most important determinant of health.	5	4	3	2	1

TOTAL SCORE

19–21 points: A true collaborator. Congratulations!

22–38 points: A solid foundation. Great potential!

39–57 points: A shaky foundation. Reinforcement required. . .

58–95 points: Time to beef-up your knowledge base and reconsider your ideas. Learning to collaborate could increase your job satisfaction!

BOX 9.2 NURSING PRACTICE GUIDELINES FOR FAMILY INTERVENTION

OBJECTIVES

To facilitate patients' transition from hospital back to community through focused interventions with family members during hospital visits. The specific objectives for promoting collaborative care with families during hospital visits include:

1. To form working partnerships with family members and significant others beginning in the early phase of hospitalization.
2. To assess family visitors' availability and level of involvement during the hospitalization and in the postdischarge period.
3. To observe and monitor interactions among family members and between patient and family during hospital visits.
4. To identify and address the needs priorities and concerns of patient and family as they arise during hospital visits.
5. To identify and reinforce the patient/family strengths and resources that emerge during hospital visits.
6. To support, maintain and sustain continued family involvement and to develop the family's care giving capacity by promoting patient/family learning, coping, and problem solving during hospital visits.
7. To work in partnership with patients and family members on issues related to discharge planning and preparation (e.g., outings, passes, home visits) and to continue to remain available to patients and families throughout the first few days posthospitalization.

The following examples serve as a beginning point for the development of family interventions that can be useful in meeting the above objectives. They provide a common basis for reflection, experimentation, critique, and further development. These and other strategies can be integrated into your daily practice as you interact with patients and families during visitation. Consider the following:

- What strategies have you implemented in your previous interactions with visiting family members?
- What new strategies could assist you to meet the above objectives?

PRACTICE RECOMMENDATIONS

Questions to ask the patient:

- Which family members/friends are most involved in your care?
- Which family members/friends will visit you regularly during your hospitalization?
- Who among these visiting family members/friends should we work more closely with and who not?
- What do you think we can do to support and promote the involvement of these family members/friends?

Based on the above data, begin by approaching a family member during visitation. Introduce yourself and let the family know that you are interested in learning more about their experiences as caregivers to their hospitalized relative. Highlight your availability to them as a primary resource and support person during their visits as well as your desire to work together over the course of hospitalization and into the early postdischarge phase.

- Assess the family structure and social support resources by involving the patient and family in the development of a genogram and ecomap.
- Consider exploring the family visitors' availability and level of involvement during the hospitalization and in the postdischarge period. →

■ BOX 9.2 Nursing Practice Guidelines for Family Intervention (continued)

Questions to ask:

- How often and when do you plan to visit?
- How would you describe the nature and level of your involvement in your relative's care:
  - Prior to admission?
  - During the hospital period?
  - Following discharge from hospital?
- Whenever possible, take the time to check in with the patient and family before, during, and after their visits.
- What other questions would be important to ask?

BEFORE THE VISIT

Questions to ask the patient and visiting family members:

- How do you feel about visiting with your relative?
- What are your expectations?
- What are your concerns?
- What would you like to achieve?
- What would help you to achieve this?

DURING THE VISIT

- Remain available and provide support. Be there for the family. Express interest. Consider asking the following questions:
  - How are things going?
  - What are your concerns and priorities at this time?
  - What would be most helpful to you [patient and family] during this visit?
  - How might you benefit most from your time together?
- Observe and monitor interactions among family members and between patient and family. Reflect what you see and hear. In particular, observe for family strengths and involvement in care and reflect these back to the patient and family members.

AFTER THE VISIT

- Review the patient and families' experiences together. The following questions are designed to promote reflection and reinforce learning:
  - What is the biggest challenge you faced during the visit?
  - What helped you meet this challenge?
  - What was the best thing about your visit? What was the most difficult thing?
  - What did you learn from this visit?
  - How can you build on this learning in subsequent visits?
  - How can this learning be useful to you and your relative following discharge from hospital? →

■ BOX 9.2 Nursing Practice Guidelines for Family Intervention (continued)

Questions to ask patient and family at opportune times throughout the course of hospitalization:

- In what way(s) do see your visits as contributing to your relative's care and therapy?
- What would help you to maintain your involvement during your relative's hospitalization? Following discharge?
- What else do you think would be helpful to you and your relative at this time?
- How would you describe your ideal role and level of involvement in the planning and delivery of your relative's care?
- What specific ideas or concerns do you have regarding your relative's eventual discharge from hospital?
- How might we work together during subsequent visits to address these issues?

tion (Gros, Purden, & Ezer, 2000; Gros, Purden, Ezer, Belanger, & Naismith, 2002). Various scenarios were created based on firsthand observations of health care practice in the clinical setting. In this way, the tool includes typical situations encountered by health professionals and incorporates the type of language observed to be used by clinicians in their everyday interactions with patients and families. The tool was designed to promote critical thinking by helping learners examine collaborative practice in the context of a particular nurse–client situation. Interactive phenomena, such as the use of strengths-based language and the timing and fit of various strategies, are captured by the tool which has a number of potential applications. In the current project, the clinical scenario tool was used mainly to trigger discussion when working with small groups of nurses. Examples of various scenarios were also incorporated into the hospitalwide introductory lectures as a way to illustrate the application to practice of key concepts. (See the Learning Activity at the end of the chapter for an example of this.)

Variations of this tool have been used with university students in graduate and undergraduate nursing courses. In addition to serving as a stimulus for group discussion and analysis, various scenarios have been created and converted into a multiple choice exam format. In this way, the clinical scenarios tool has been adapted as an evaluative measure to assess students' ability to apply client-centered concepts to practice. The task of systematically evaluating the interpersonal and interactive dimension of nursing is essential yet tedious and time-consuming work for educators. This is particularly true when teaching large groups of nurses or nursing students. Thus, the development of objective, standardized tools to evaluate learning in the field of collaborative, client-centered care remains an ongoing challenge and an important focus for nurse educators.

Concurrent with the above strategies offered to staff within the hospital, two separate in-patient units were selected randomly and targeted to receive ongoing coaching and weekly contact with the nurse educator over the period of one year. The teaching methods used when working with the nurses on these demonstration units included small

BOX 9.3 STUDENT-CENTERED TEACHING AND COLLABORATIVE LEARNING: GUIDING PRINCIPLES AND PRACTICES

- Start where the student is at (e.g., identify attitudes, priorities, knowledge, skills, etc).
- Be available.
- Create and maintain a caring and supportive learning environment.
- Identify and work with the student's strengths.
- Listen to understand the student's story, feelings, beliefs, and perspectives.
- Tailor teaching/learning activities to fit the student's interests, needs, and priorities.
- Pace learning according to the student's readiness; time activities for best fit with learner's schedule.

group discussion sessions, one-to-one consultation, **case analyses**, and **role modeling** by actively applying vital concepts of the McGill Model in clinical practice (Meyers & Jones, 1993). The above activities were carried out according to a set of principles and practices consistent with student-centered teaching and collaborative learning. Examples of guiding principles are included in Box 9.3.

Discussing Nursing Practice

Throughout all facets of this project, participating in reflective dialogue with practicing nurses in small groups and on a one-to-one basis was a pivotal learning activity. A series of weekly small group clinical discussion sessions were held on each targeted nursing unit over the course of the year. These 60 to 90 minute sessions were open to all staff and nursing managers as well as to nursing students completing clinical rotations on these units. A flexible, open, informal, and relaxed learning atmosphere was created to promote staff engagement and to ensure a fit with the practical demands of the clinical working environment. For example, attendance was voluntary and nurses were encouraged to join the group whenever they could. The clinical discussion sessions were opportunities for the educator to provide ongoing coaching and support for staff learning. In addition, they enabled the educator to participate with staff in the process of learning together through open dialogue, question-raising, critical reflection and analysis, brainstorming, and problem solving.

Asking Questions

Question-raising was a crucial teaching strategy used by the nurse educator to stimulate reflection and to promote thinking out of the box. Questioning techniques were used in conversations with individual nurses as well as within small and large group teaching sessions. Examples of open-ended, reflective questions that are consistent with principles of student-centered learning and that were used in small group teaching include:

- What are the greatest challenges you face in your interactions with clients and families at this time? How are you responding?

- Describe a situation from your clinical practice that you find challenging in terms of establishing a collaborative working relationship with a client or family. What is the greatest challenge for you in this situation? How are you intervening? How is the client responding?
- Are you aware of the goals envisioned by the client and his or her family? How might you determine and clarify client and family goals? Are there tensions between the client's goals and the goals of the family? How might you intervene to help the family and individual members meet their goals and resolve their tensions?
- Are there tensions in your relationship with the client and family? What is your role in working through such tensions? What nursing interventions have you tried to resolve such tensions?
- What alternate strategies and approaches can we test out in the current situation through collaboration: with the client/family; with one another; with other health professionals?
- What are we learning from this situation? about the client/family? about ourselves? about our relationship with the client and family? about our role as nurses within the interprofessional team?
- What situations have you encountered in the past that were similar to this one? How did you respond? What was the outcome?

Questions such as these incited staff to participate actively in discussions and created a climate in which there was rich, energized learning. The strategy of incorporating current practice experiences into small group teaching sessions ensured relevancy, since the discussions centered on actual clinical cases that posed real dilemmas for the nurses, as well as for the teacher.

Learning Through Example and Experience: Role Modeling and Clinical Application

As implied above, current clinical experiences were powerful sources of learning for the staff, as well as for the educator. Emphasis was placed on learning from clients and families about their perspectives, goals, and needs. In addition, learning with clients and families took place by working out plans of action together and discovering over time what the clients and families were finding helpful and not helpful.

In order to promote this approach to practice, individual and small group meetings with the nurses focused on sharing and analyzing clinical data, and on discussing plans for collaborative intervention (e.g., developing strategies for exploring client/family perspectives, setting mutual goals, etc.). In addition, learning through clinical experience was promoted by applying in practice the ideas and strategies generated through the discussion sessions and then debriefing by sharing clinical findings and experiences in follow-up meetings. As the educator, I was an active participant in this process; sharing with staff what I was learning through our interactions with clients and families, as well as what I was learning from the nurses through our discussions together.

In the next section, we illustrate this process in detail by presenting an example of one particularly challenging case introduced by the nurses on one unit and discussed over time in the small group sessions.[2] The experience was a powerful source of learning for all involved, and we believe it captures the blending of content and process within the context of collaborative, student-centered nursing education.

COLLABORATIVE LEARNING THROUGH CASE ANALYSIS: NURSING THE D FAMILY

Katie D is a 28 year old woman of Greek origin. She immigrated to Canada with her parents when she was 6 years old. Her father committed suicide the year after. At age 16, she was diagnosed as having schizoaffective disorder with bipolar features .Over the years, Katie was hospitalized repeatedly with delusions, irrational thinking, manic episodes and substance abuse. At the time of the current admission, she was also 3 months pregnant. This was the fourth pregnancy for Katie and her partner, Bob. The first two pregnancies ended in miscarriage. The third pregnancy ended tragically in the final month of gestation when baby Sam was stillborn, following Katie's involvement in a serious car accident.

Katie and Bob have been together for 8 years. Bob lives on the street and has a long-standing history of addiction to alcohol and crack cocaine. The couple's relationship has included episodes of violence, such as past verbal abuse and possible physical aggression by Bob toward Katie. Consequently, a restraining order preventing Bob from entering the D Family home was invoked by Katie's mother, Mrs D., and her husband, Ray. Katie smokes one pack of cigarettes per day and has tried a wide variety of street drugs including crack cocaine. She is unemployed and receives social assistance.

Guided by principles of student-centered teaching and collaborative learning, the educator began where the nurses were at. This involved asking questions, discussing the case, and identifying practice dilemmas. Small group discussions provided an opportunity for nurses and the educator to explore the case together and, in the process, to review together the plan of care for Katie that had been set by the interprofessional team.

The current plan of care diverged from the concepts of collaborative, client-centered and family-centered practice along several crucial dimensions. For example, Katie's care plan focused on the individual client, versus the family; and it was oriented toward identifying and eliminating risks and deficits, as opposed to finding and building strengths. Thus, the plan highlighted many current and potential problems and Katie's situation was labeled as very high risk. In addition, the existing plan of care for Katie was developed by the professional team without active client and family involvement. Assessments were based on the clinicians' previous experiences and decisions were made according to the judgment of the professionals, who acted as the sole experts. Thus, the plan was set according to what the team believed to be in the client's and family's best interest and reflected the way in which other high risk situations of this nature were typically managed. More specifically, the long-term plan was for Katie to stay in hospital throughout the remainder of the pregnancy and for her baby to be placed in foster care at the time of birth. The short-term plans established for Katie included: stabilizing and

---

[2] This case description has been fictionalized to ensure complete anonymity of individual clientele. Small group discussion sessions represent an educational initiative offered across service units for the purpose of developing nursing practice. The nurses, students and other staff participating in the sessions are all involved in various capacities as care providers in the actual clinical situations being discussed.

managing her psychiatric symptoms; preventing her use of alcohol, tobacco, and street drugs; monitoring her interactions with Bob; monitoring the pregnancy; and promoting compliance with prenatal care appointments.

The nurses appreciated having a forum to discuss their thoughts and feelings surrounding their work with Katie. Asking them to describe the case to me prompted reflection on the situation and their responses to it. Thus, the nurses were able to take stock of the situation and to identify two main challenges they were facing in this situation: Katie's cigarette smoking and the removal of Katie's child from her care at birth.

Katie's smoking was an issue for the nurses since she was continuing to smoke heavily during the pregnancy despite the nurses' ongoing efforts to prevent her from doing so. Questions posed by the educator to the nurses to stimulate reflection and analysis included: How are you responding in this situation? How is the client responding to your interventions? The nurses' replies indicated that they were focused on taking control in order to achieve client outcomes. This focus was reflected in statements such as the following: "We have to protect the baby." "We have to get Katie to stop smoking, but she's not listening. She's not responsible. . . . I wish we could just take the cigarettes away." Thus, current nursing interventions were aimed at achieving specific outcomes such as getting Katie to quit or cut down smoking and included: reminding her that she shouldn't smoke; setting and reinforcing limits; and trying to persuade her to quit by providing information on the detrimental effects of smoking on fetal health.

Turning to client data as a way to evaluate current strategies, it became clear that these strategies were not working. According to the nurses, Katie's smoking was showing no signs of improvement. In addition, merely broaching the smoking issue with Katie would provoke a strong and angry reaction from her. For example, she would yell and swear at staff, then storm off to the smoking lounge calling out: "Leave me alone! I need a cigarette!" Reflecting on this we asked: By focusing efforts and energies on getting Katie to quit, could we inadvertently be making things worse? Through our discussions, it became evident that spending time struggling to get Katie to quit smoking had become a negative pattern of interaction and a constant source of conflict in the nurse–client relationship. This battle of wills also shaped the professionals' perceptions of Katie as a person. She came to be understood as noncompliant, not listening, and not responsible. In addition, questions about her capacity to be a good mother were raised in remarks such as: "How could she possibly care about her unborn child if she refuses to listen and continues to smoke?"

Negative perceptions such as these were incompatible with the practice of collaborative, client-centered care and needed to be reframed. As the educator, I role modeled the collaborative process in my interactions with the nurses by starting where the nurses were at and by looking for strengths in what they were saying and experiencing. This involved listening and describing what I was hearing using words and labels that were consistent with the concept of collaborative care. Sample responses phrased to accomplish this objective included: "This is a really challenging and complex situation; I hear your frustration; I can see how involved you are and how much you want to help; Wanting to take away the cigarettes is an expression of your caring; You have brought the case up for group discussion, and we're talking a lot about it. I can see how important this is to you, so we will take the time to work through this together." Strategies such as these helped to find common ground between the nurses and the educator, helped to establish shared goals, and provided a basic foundation for developing a collaborative working alliance.

Through the process of describing the situation to me, the nurses were able to pinpoint areas of difficulty, to review the effectiveness of current strategies, and to begin considering alternate approaches. As it became clear that Katie had no intention of quitting smoking at this time, discussion and debate centered on addressing the affective dimension of nursing practice. For example, Katie's resistance to the nurses' attempts to help her quit left the nurses feeling angry, frustrated, and powerless. Group discussions enabled participants to identify, accept, and gain insight into their feelings and to offer mutual support to one another. Provocative questions raised by group members guided our discussions and invited participants to share emotional responses and perspectives. For example, the nurses asked: How can we, as nurses, just sit there and watch Katie inhale cigarette after cigarette? As a nurse and educator, I shared my own distress. Bearing witness to Katie's smoking was extremely difficult. However, I also offered the perspective that remaining by Katie's side, unconditionally, was a true expression of caring (Mayeroff, 1971). From this perspective, being in attendance while Katie smoked demonstrated respect for the client's choices, conveyed acceptance of where she was at, and represented the starting point of the collaborative relationship. Thus, in the context of this clinical situation, silent presence and accompaniment could be viewed, not as passive strategies, but as deliberate interventions whose implementation required a great deal of patience and restraint. This situation also sparked lively debate around the legal and ethical aspects of care. For example, our discussions served to review and reinforce staff's current knowledge of and respect for clients' rights; and to highlight the congruence between The McGill Model of Nursing and the legal and ethical principles of professional practice.

Turning now to the second challenge the nurses faced: How to address the pregnancy knowing of the team's plan to have the child placed in foster care at birth. The situation was particularly difficult since Katie had not yet been informed of the plan and decisions regarding when and how to inform her remained uncertain. In the interim, Katie was bonding with her unborn child and was looking forward to the prospect of motherhood. "It's a girl! Her name is Jenny Marie. Look! She's kicking!" Ironically, the joy in Katie's face when she talked about the baby strained our interactions with her and made us feel uncomfortable in that reinforcing Katie's growing maternal attachment seemed inappropriate knowing what lay ahead. At the same time, open and honest discussions about Katie's future relationship with the baby were not possible given that the decision by professionals to place the baby in foster care had not yet been revealed to her. The situation raised lots of questions like: "How should we respond when Katie talks about the baby? Should we refocus the conversation or let her go on and act like everything's normal?" Unfortunately, under these circumstances, the most comfortable alternative seemed to be to keep encounters with Katie brief and superficial. However, the nurses in this group recognized that avoiding the issue of the pregnancy was not a viable solution. As one nurse stated, "I don't feel good about this case. We're not doing anything to help Katie by avoiding her and the pregnancy. We're just keeping her here [in hospital] until she gives birth. Something must be done. We need to find a way to help."

The process of raising questions, and sharing feelings, perspectives, and ideas through group discussion led to new realizations. These pivotal turning points in the group's learning opened a space for shifting thinking and reorienting current practices. Changes in the nature of the questions being posed in group discussions indicated the group's readiness to begin considering alternate ways of responding to Katie and her family. Examples of these sorts of questions in-

cluded: How can we meet Katie's needs for support during this pregnancy? Is it possible to help Katie make a healthy transition to parenthood under the current circumstances? If so, how?

Turning to the principles of collaborative, client-centered health care put forward in the McGill Model of Nursing, the process of developing a collaborative plan of care for Katie began by considering the following possibilities: Perhaps in our role as nurses we need to let go of the need to control client decisions and outcomes and accept that Katie is not ready to quit smoking at this time? Rather than focusing on trying to get Katie to stop smoking, perhaps we need to refocus our time and energy onto developing a collaborative nurse–client relationship? Perhaps we need to explore the meaning of the pregnancy from Katie's perspective, and to determine her present and future goals? Thus, the group began to shift their view of nursing from one based on illness, deficits, risks, and a priori decision making aimed at taking over responsibility for the client's health and controlling outcomes, to one based on health promotion, strengths, and potentials, that involved understanding and respecting the client's goals, that focused on learning to trust and accept where the client was at, that valued learning from the client and working together over time, and that was process oriented versus outcomes oriented.

In sum, learning through question-raising, reflective dialogue, and analysis of actual clinical practice situations was part of a continuous process of building group cohesion, finding common ground, establishing common goals, and developing collaborative working alliances between educator, staff, and client. The case discussion sessions enabled the nurses to rethink their professional role and responsibilities, to reframe their negative perceptions of the client, to rekindle their sense of empowerment, and to reinforce their ability to make a difference. Through this interactive process, staff were helped to redirect current caring behaviors away from trying to change client behavior and control client outcomes, and onto developing a collaborative nurse–client relationship.

Vital questions raised by the educator and used as a guide to further the development of collaborative practice in this situation include the following:

- *How can we form a collaborative, working relationship with Katie and her family? What strategies should we implement in order to do so?*
- *What are the strengths of Katie and her family?*
- *How do Katie and family perceive their situation?*
- *What are their goals?*
- *How can nurses support this family in meeting their goals?*
- *What would happen if we focus on answering the above questions rather than focusing on outcomes, such as smoking cessation or the placement of the child foster care postpartum?*

Guided by the above questions, the primary nurse and the nurse educator spent time with Katie and her family. The goal was to start where the client and family were at by exploring the situation from their perspective with a focus on learning from them by listening, observing, and asking open-ended questions.

Through the process of exploring Katie's perceptions with her, we learned many things. First, we were able to confirm that Katie agreed with the team's plan that she should remain in hospital until the birth of the baby. However, we also discovered significant differences in how Katie perceived the pregnancy compared to how the health professionals saw it. For example, we learned from Katie that, for her, the pregnancy was a wonderful event and to be a mother was something she had wanted all her life. In contrast, for the professionals, the pregnancy was viewed as a terrible problem. We also discovered that Katie had a sense of the team's recommendation to place the child in foster care: "I'm not stupid," she remarked,."I know you people want to take Jenny away from me, but I won't let that happen. Jenny is my baby. I want to keep her and I want to take care of her." Thus, it became clear that Katie's long-term goal to keep the baby was inconsistent with the care plan put forth by the interprofessional team.

In addition to exploring the goals and perceptions of Katie and family, interventions aimed at starting where the client was at included sitting with Katie while she had a cigarette. The strategy of silent presence was consistent with crucial concepts within the McGill Model of Nursing in that it was intended to foster Katie's overall sense of control over her life, and to communicate to her that, she was ultimately responsible for her own actions, that she had ownership over her decisions, and that she was in charge of determining the nature and timing of our care which would be tailored to suit her own needs and readiness. Through the use of silent presence, Katie eventually brought up the issue of smoking by herself, in her own time. Thus, we began to understand what was behind her reluctance to quit smoking. In Katie's own words: "I need to smoke because smoking is good for the baby. I know it is. I quit smoking last pregnancy, and Sam was born dead. I need Jenny to live. I have to smoke so she won't be born dead like Sam. I couldn't handle having another dead baby."

Client data such as these were shared in small group discussion sessions. Introducing Katie's perspective in this way shed new light on the nurses' previous questions regarding whether or not Katie was a caring mother. At the same time, the nurses' negative views of Katie began to change, and their anger and frustration toward her diminished. Helping the nurses to understand the situation from the client's perspective fostered in them a sense of caring and empathy for Katie as a person and motivated them to begin advocating on her behalf.

By spending time with Katie's mother, Mrs. D, and her partner, Ray, we gained an understanding of the family's perceptions of Katie's situation and came to view family members as important partners in Katie's care. For example, Mrs. D shared her views and concerns about Katie in remarks such as the following: "Katie absolutely wants this baby. It was really hard for her when Sam died. . . . if this baby gets taken away, I'm scared she'll go right down mental healthwise and we'll lose her. I hope to God she'll be given a chance." Inviting Mrs. D to tell her story opened a space for considering the family as client, and prompted us to begin working collaboratively with family members, ideas salient to the McGill Model. In addition, through the process of listening and learning from the family, a number of important client and family strengths were identified which contributed to the development of a strong nurse–family partnership. Examples of family strengths included the following:

- *Katie's mother, Mrs. D, stood by her daughter consistently through the long and difficult course of Katie's illness.*
- *Mrs. D remained present for Katie and was willing to help her reach her goal of keeping the baby by providing ongoing support, supervision, and child care.*
- *Mrs. D was the full-time caregiver to her 4-year-old nephew, John, indicating her experience as a parent figure and her ability to care for small children.*

- *Mrs. D's partner, Ray, was sensitive to Katie's needs. He was supportive of Mrs. D's desire to help her daughter. Ray agreed that Katie and her baby could live with them following the baby's birth.*
- *Mrs. D and Ray welcomed outside help and were open to home visits by the Department of Youth Protection.*

Interventions to engage the baby's father, Bob, in a collaborative relationship were less successful. These interventions included expressing our interest in him as a person and as a father-to-be. As was the case for all family members, we conveyed our desire to spend time with him in order to get to know him and to support him in his goals. However, Bob's visits to the unit were infrequent and sporadic. He declined the opportunity to be involved in interprofessional family meetings and was consistently absent for our planned meetings with him. Thus, limited contact time with Bob interfered with our ability to identify and support his strengths, and to engage, explore, and follow up on any concerns he might have. We hypothesized that his current drug and alcohol addiction was likely at the root of the problem, that he was neither able nor ready to discuss this issue with us, and that he was not prepared to give up the drugs at this time. Thus, his current choice not to engage with us was respected. In the interim, we took every opportunity to convey our availability to him and left the door open with the hope that he would be ready to work with us in the future. However, Bob's visits to the unit continued to diminish over time, as did his connection with Katie, and eventually we lost all contact with him.

Together, in weekly small group meetings, the nurses discussed client/family perspectives and goals; shared information concerning their strengths and resources; and considered approaches that might enable Katie, Mrs. D, and her partner, Ray, to meet their goal of keeping the baby in the family. So now, as the family's goals became clear to us, we were faced with yet another dilemma: What could be done to help this family meet their goals? What interventions would help them succeed? Our discussions were lively and engaging, but skepticism and a continued focus on outcome achievement prevailed. This orientation was evident in comments such as, "This will never work" or "We're wasting our time." The belief was that, sooner or later, Katie's baby would end up in foster care. The nurses were unanimous in this regard. From their perspective, not achieving the target outcome would mean that the effort was useless. But was it? The educator challenged the nurses' current beliefs: Were we really wasting our time? What other sorts of outcomes, besides the attainment of this goal, could be achieved by practicing collaborative, client-centered nursing as described in the McGill Model?

Acknowledging the pessimism expressed by all of the nurses in terms of whether or not the outcome of keeping the baby in the family could ever be attained, the educator proposed that we elaborate and carry out a plan of care guided by the McGill Model of Nursing. This plan would focus on the process of continuing to build collaborative working relationships with Katie and her family. It would be aimed at assisting the family to reach their goal of keeping their child in the family; regardless of whether or not this goal would actually be attained.

Thus, the original plan of care included getting Katie to quit smoking and removing the child from the mother at birth, focused on eliminating risks and was derived from clinicians' expertise, previous experience, and professional judgment about what was in the client and family's best interest. In contrast, a collaborative, family-centered plan would focus on identifying and promoting the family's strengths and capacities. The new plan would evolve from client and family expertise and experience, and it would be derived from client and family goals, perceptions of needs and beliefs about what might be helpful to the family in the face of this transition. The consensus among the nurses was clear: "We have nothing to lose." Thus, Katie's primary nurse agreed to take a lead role in working with the educator to develop a new plan of care (Box 9.4). Unit staff and the nurse manager offered their support and individual nurses would continue their ongoing participation. Consistent with the tenets of the McGill Model of Nursing, the new plan not only addressed care for Katie, but included collaborative, strengths-based intervention with family members.

PROJECT EVALUATION AND OUTCOMES

The outcomes of this project were evaluated using formal and informal methods. Throughout the project, feedback was sought from nurses, clients, and families on a regular basis. Thus, evaluative data were collected in an ongoing way through strategies such as listening, making observations, and inviting comments and suggestions. In addition, nurse participants completed written evaluation forms which invited feedback on various learning activities including presentations, workshops, and clinical teaching tools.

The outcomes of the small group teaching and learning interventions with nurses were evaluated using a comprehensive evaluation form (Box 9.5) distributed to the participants at the end of the project. The questionnaire assessed the nurses' satisfaction

BOX 9.4 REVISED CARE PLAN FOR THE D FAMILY

NURSING STRATEGIES AND INTERVENTIONS

- Develop and maintain a collaborative relationship with Katie and family.
  - Remain available, offer supportive presence. Be there unconditionally.
  - Spend time listening, exploring.
  - Demonstrate interest, openness, kindness, respect; use touch (Katie likes hugs).
- Start where Katie is.
  - Celebrate the pregnancy.
  - Support Katie's preparation for childbirth and parenting.
- Identify strengths and build on the positive.
  - Katie's sense of humor.
  - Katie's decision to remain in hospital during her pregnancy.
  - Katie's love and attachment toward her unborn child.
  - Family's presence, love, concern, and commitment to helping Katie.
- Provide continuity of care over time and across settings.
- Work with interprofessional team members.
  - Act as a support and advocate for Katie and her family.
    - Share the client's story.
    - Speak to the perspectives, strengths and goals of the client/family.
  - Articulate nursing's perspective and commitment to collaborative, client-centered care.
  - Work with the interprofessional team on developing a plan of care that would promote the health and safety of the child *and* enable the client and family to work toward their goals.

BOX 9.5 PROJECT EVALUATION FORM

THE McGILL MODEL OF NURSING: A COLLABORATIVE, FAMILY-CENTERED APPROACH TO CARE STAFF FEEDBACK AND EVALUATION

Over the past year, various learning activities on the McGill Model were offered to nursing staff on your unit. These included: small group discussions, live/videotaped presentations, written reference materials, and individual case consultation.

Your comments and feedback will be used to evaluate the usefulness of these activities as well as to develop learning opportunities in the future.

Please complete the following questionnaire and return it to the labeled box project in the nursing station. All information received will remain anonymous. Your feedback will inform future planning.

A. Small group clinical discussion meetings

1. Approximately how many clinical discussion meetings did you attend?

   None ☐ 1–2 ☐ 3–6 ☐ 7–10 ☐ >10 ☐

   (go to question 8)

2. These discussions helped me reflect on my nursing care from a collaborative, person/family-centered perspective.

1	2	3	4	5
strongly disagree		neutral		strongly agree

3. These meetings were a source of support and guidance that reinforced my efforts to care for clients in complex situations using a collaborative, family-centered approach.

1	2	3	4	5
strongly disagree		neutral		strongly agree

4. These meetings reinforced the strengths and potentials of the patient/family as well as those of the nurse.

1	2	3	4	5
strongly disagree		neutral		strongly agree

5. The issues and topics discussed in these meetings were relevant to my clinical practice and were consistent with my professional needs and goals.

1	2	3	4	5
strongly disagree		neutral		strongly agree

6. To what extent were the clinical discussion meetings useful in terms of contributing to the development of your clinical practice?

1	2	3	4	5
not useful at all		moderately useful		most useful

7. What effect did participation in these discussions have on you and your nursing? (please include specific examples):

   Your suggestions for improving these meetings:

8. Would you be interested in attending clinical discussion meetings in the future?

   No ☐ Possibly ☐ Yes ☐

   What factors would facilitate your attendance? ➔

■ BOX 9.5 Project Evaluation Form (continued)

B. Live and videotaped presentations on the model

9. I attended at least one general presentation or workshop on the McGill Model of Nursing (offered throughout the hospital at various times and locations over the past 24 months).

   No ☐ Do not recall ☐ Yes ☐

10. I viewed the videotaped presentation on "Nurse–Family Collaboration."

   No ☐ Do not recall ☐ Yes ☐

(if no, go to question 14)

11. To what extent were the presentations/workshops useful in terms of helping you develop your nursing practice?

1	2	3	4	5
not useful at all		moderately useful		most useful

C. Written reference materials

12. I received a copy of written materials from the above presentations/workshops I attended.

   No ☐ Do not recall ☐ Yes ☐

(if no, go to question 14)

13. To what extent were presentation materials useful in terms of helping you develop your nursing practice?

1	2	3	4	5
not useful		moderately useful		most useful

Please comment on reference materials.

D. Individual case consultation

14. I had the opportunity to work directly with the clinical consultant on one or more of my assigned clients/families.

   No ☐ Do not recall ☐ Yes ☐

(if no, go to question 16)

15. Please indicate the strategies you found most helpful (check all that apply).

   Supportive involvement ☐
   Providing direct assistance (perspective sharing, help with assessments/care planning/documentation, etc.) ☐
   Coaching and encouragement ☐
   Participating in client/family meetings/home visits ☐
   Role modeling ☐
   Providing feedback ☐

E. Other:

16. Overall, I am interested in continuing to develop my knowledge and skills related to collaborative, family centered nursing and the McGill Model.

1	2	3	4	5
strongly disagree				strongly agree

Please include your suggestions about other kinds of learning activities and supports that would help you in this process. →

■ BOX 9.5 Project Evaluation Form (continued)

17. Overall, how would you rate your experience as a participant in the above learning activities?

1	2	3	4	5
poor				excellent

18. What, if anything, *has changed in your clinical practice* as a result of your participation in the above learning activity(ies)? Provide specific examples where possible:

with the overall project, and the usefulness of the various learning activities offered, such as the small group discussion sessions. Feedback about the various teaching strategies used by the educator, such as coaching and role modeling, was also sought. Finally, self-reported learning outcomes such as perceived changes in clinical practice as a result of the project were obtained based on the nurses' written responses to open-ended questions.

Clinical Outcomes: Client and Family

Using client/family feedback to evaluate the clinical outcomes of care is an integral part of collaborative, client-centered nursing as defined within the McGill Model (Allen, 1977). Thus, throughout the project, the impact of our nursing was assessed by inviting clients and families to share their feedback with us. Additional measures used to assess client/family outcomes included clinical observations and documented changes client/family in status. The following clinical outcomes were identified in relation to the case example of the D family presented above:

- Katie remained in the hospital voluntarily throughout pregnancy.
- Katie continued to smoke cigarettes.
- Katie tested positive for marijuana and there was no evidence that she used alcohol or other drugs.
- A healthy 7-pound baby girl, Jenny Marie, was born at term.
- Family involvement and support was sustained throughout the prenatal and perinatal period; with the exception of Bob, whose contact and involvement within the family and with the nurses decreased steadily over time.
- Maternal–infant interactions were loving and caring.
- There was no change noted in Katie's baseline mental status.
- Clinical and community partners agreed to support a collaborative plan of care aimed at keeping the child with the family, as proposed by the nurses.
- Katie and her baby were discharged home to live with Mrs. D and Ray with the provision of adequate community follow up and support services.
- Client/family feedback to the nurses: "Thank you. Thank you for letting us have this chance. This wouldn't have been possible without you [the nurses]. You were on our side."

The client/family outcomes achieved through the nurses' interventions were a powerful reinforcer of nurse learning and an invaluable source of professional development for the participants in this project. Additional learning outcomes for nursing staff and nurse educator follow.

Learning Outcomes: Nursing Staff and Nurse Educator

Analysis of the nurses' responses to the written evaluation questionnaire indicated general satisfaction with the program. The ratings of learning activities such as presentations and workshops ranged from "very good" to "excellent" for most participants. The feedback on the clinical scenarios tool indicated that this exercise helped the nurses reflect on their clinical practice. Additionally, the great majority of nurses reported that they were interested in learning more about the concepts and ideas presented in the tools.

However, not all nurses reported high levels of satisfaction with the program. The data indicate that the level of nurse satisfaction was positively correlated with factors such as nurse attendance and level of participation in various learning activities. This trend is consistent with findings from a previous learning program carried out with practicing nurses and physicians (Gros, et al., 2002). It is clear that increased efforts need to be targeted toward increasing the motivation and involvement of staff members with low levels of participation in learning activities.

Evaluating the unit-based clinical discussion sessions, the nurses on the demonstration units clearly enjoyed our small group meetings, as did the educator. Over time, for the group of nurses on each unit, initial reluctance to take part in the project gave way to enthusiastic participation. In reference to the weekly discussion sessions, one nurse commented: "I love our meetings. I've worked in nursing for over 20 years and I've never had meetings where we talk about these kinds of things." Thus, it was clear that the chance to discuss nursing was a novel experience for the staff and that they benefited from the opportunity to work through complex cases such as the one presented above. While the results of this project suggest that open discussions about nursing are essential for professional development, these types of meetings are not routinely offered in practice settings. In effect, the discussion forums traditionally available to staff, such as ward meetings and interprofessional team meetings, tend to be procedurally oriented with a set agenda. Thus, current forums would need to be restructured to allow for more open exchange and their objectives redesigned in order to offer the type of support for nurses and nursing practice that staff value and require.

In sum, despite their heavy workloads, the nurses on the demonstration units made time for the small group clinical discussion sessions and looked forward to them. In contrast, low staff attendance at centrally located, hospitalwide didactic presentations was an ongoing concern. Based on these data, traditional lecture type presentations have been discontinued. The educator is now presenting introductory information on the McGill Model to small groups of nurses on individual units. A plan to offer small group clinical discussion sessions with nurses from various service divisions is also being instituted. It is hoped that these outreach strategies will help to engage nurses whose level of participation in learning thus far has been low.

Reflecting back on this project, the focus on learning together with the nurses through real-time experience and clinical application is what I believe to be the single most important teaching strategy of all. As an educator, it is one thing to present theory and content; to tell students or clinicians that collaborative, client-centered care makes a difference; to profess that we, as nurses, have the power to influence change in client/family's health; and to suggest that the voice of the nurse in the interdisciplinary team is invaluable. However, it is another thing altogether for an educator to structure learning and to accompany students and staff through a process whereby we are able to experience this process and the resulting outcomes firsthand.

As described in previous sections, several main areas of focused intervention were addressed through the process of clinical application and experiential learning. These activities led to shifts in thinking that are essential for the practice of collaborative nursing. Throughout this process, support and encouragement offered by the educator was oriented toward helping the nurses learn to:

- Trust the client and family (versus trying to get the client to trust the nurse).
- Let go of the need to control outcomes.
- Take risks and accept uncertainty.

In the context of the clinical situation described above, these were salient features in the nurses' learning just as they were in my own. Together, the nurses and I tested ideas and took risks. While uncertain of the outcomes, we were united as a group. Waiting, watching, wondering, and discovering together through this and other clinical situations created a sense of cohesion and mutual support within the team, an important outcome reported by the nurses themselves.

Regarding changes in clinical practice catalyzed through their participation in this project, the nurses reported that they discovered and used new ways of relating with patients and families, that they were involved differently in their practice compared to before the program, and that they experienced an enhanced sense of professional self-worth and team cohesion.

In terms of clinical practice, the nurses reported that through this project, they experienced more genuine and humane interactions with their clients, and this was linked to increased satisfaction in the nurse–client relationship. For example, one nurse wrote: "Communication has become less strenuous. Talking, laughing, and shaking off artificialities, the relationship is more satisfying for all." The nurses' written comments also suggested that they became more empathic and less detached as a result of their involvement program. The following quote captures this kind of change: "Before, I wished for a 100% detachment from a birth. Now I find myself rejoicing and praying for this child." Changes in professional self-worth included statements such as the following: "This [the program] made me feel like . . . I'm a good nurse . . . being a valuable part of my patient's progress brought back this sense of self-esteem." This sense of pride and enthusiasm for nursing was observed and reported by the nurses on both units. Finally, a renewed sense of working together with nursing colleagues was also reported. As one nurse wrote: "The group discussions reinforced a sense of team spirit."

POSTSCRIPT: LESSONS LEARNED

It took a while, but eventually, as I wound up my first year of study as a nursing student in the McGill program, I began to see the light. Eventually, I learned to see method in the madness. There was a beginning sense of structure to what felt like the most unstructured educational experience on earth. Eventually, I came to appreciate the great vision and sense of knowing in those nursing leaders and former teachers of mine.

In retrospect, it is clear that the ideas faculty presented to students back then were truly revolutionary. However, only later—much later—did I recognize and come to value what I was learning. I was learning to view nursing as a complex process that encompassed a rich variety of knowledge, concepts, and skills. I was learning how to think, how to raise questions and how to describe what I was seeing and hearing. I was learning to critically reflect on what I was doing in my interactions with clients and families and how to evaluate their responses. I also came to understand how different and new this perspective was, and how my education had helped me learn to think out of the box. I learned that everything was open for questioning and that thinking out of the box involved considering the obvious and asking why or why not? This type of learning involved tuning in to the everyday things nurses do and asking: Why is this important? What difference does this make? What is the rationale for this? Only later did I come to understand that this was it. At its foundation, this was what learning to nurse was all about.

Over time, as a student, a shift in my thinking began to occur as my understanding of what my teachers were trying to do became clearer to me. What was responsible for this change? Unlike learning facts, understanding complex phenomena like nursing and health promotion is a multifaceted process. It was not one thing that the teachers did or said. It was not one single interaction with the client and family or one class or seminar discussion that was responsible. It was all of these things, and more, working in concert that made the change happen.

Now I wonder: What if the teachers had given us answers? What if they had told us what to do? Perhaps we would have been left with the impression that there was one right way of doing things. Perhaps we would have learned that nursing was simple and straightforward. However, nothing could be further from the truth. Nursing is full of surprises. It is fraught with uncertainty, but rich in discovery. In the end, I came to understand the reason why my teachers did not provide the answers. While doing so would have decreased the uncertainty, albeit temporarily, it would have closed off infinite possibilities for learning. What if my teachers had accompanied me on those first visits to my client's home? My learning probably would have focused on observing the teacher instead of the client. I probably would have tried to imitate what the teacher was doing versus looking to the client and family for cues about what I should or should not be doing. I would have focused on trying to figure out what the teacher expected of me versus trying to figure out what the client and family wanted or needed from me. What if the teachers had supplied me with reams of information and coursework prior to meeting my clients? This would have left me with the impression that I should enter into the client's world as an expert, not as a learner. I have since come to understand that a traditional approach to teaching such as this would have been inconsistent with a curriculum aimed at promoting collaborative, client/family-centered nursing. Indeed, it was all terribly elusive to me at the time. Now, some 25 years down the road, it is getting clearer, but I am still questioning and I am still learning.

SUMMARY

In this chapter, we described an educational project in which staff nurses participated in a collaborative learning process in which the McGill Model of Nursing was introduced. The educator's approach ensured that what was taught was modeled through how it was taught; thereby creating synergy between nursing education and nursing practice. The outcomes of this project suggest that a collaborative, learner-centered approach to education used in a staff development context is a time-consuming, intense way to bridge the gap between nursing theory and practice and that it reaps important benefits for nurses as well as for clients and families. Further, the collaboration between hospital nursing administration and university faculty through this initiative represented an important step toward strengthening the ties between academic and practice settings.

LEARNING ACTIVITY

This activity can be used with students at all levels, as well as with practicing nurses.

- Distribute a copy of a clinical scenario such as that offered below to learners. Allow approximately 10 minutes for learners to read and respond to the scenario. If the group is organized in small groups, allow ample time for group discussion and debate.
- Using the following questions as a guide, review each strategy proposed on the accompanying list asking learners to share their responses with the rationale underlying their decisions.
    - In what way(s) does the proposed strategy reflect the principles of collaborative, client-centered care?
    - In what way(s) does the strategy conflict with those principles?
    - Is such a strategy ever useful in clinical practice?
    - If so, under what circumstances?
- Complement the learners' decisions and rationales with the educator's reflections. (See examples of educator's responses and comments below.)

Directions: A patient situation is described below. The clinical scenario is followed by a set of possible nursing responses. Please indicate the extent to which you agree or disagree with each of the proposed responses by marking your answer along the 5-point scale. The extent to which you agree or disagree with an option should be determined by considering whether or not *you believe* the response is consistent with the practice of a collaborative, client-centered approach to nursing as described in the McGill Model. Enter your rationale and comments in the space provided.

Clinical Scenario

Mr. F was admitted to the hospital two weeks ago with a diagnosis of depression. Up until this time, Mr. F has followed his treatment plan and seems to have made good progress. However, in the past few days, Mr. F has refused to participate in individual therapy and group activities. Increasingly, he is isolating himself in his room, where he can be found sitting on his bed repeating, "I want to get out of here. I want to go home." Based only on this information, your approach to working with Mr. F at this time would include the following strategies:

	STRONGLY AGREE	AGREE	NEITHER AGREE NOR DISAGREE	DISAGREE	STRONGLY DISAGREE
1. Ask Mr. F to tell you more about his desire to go home.	5 XXX	4	3	2	1

Educators' Comments:
Strongly agree. *Asking open-ended exploratory questions will help the nurse understand the situation from Mr. F's perspective. Learning from Mr. F about his feelings, perceptions and priorities will result in valuable insights to guide intervention.*

	STRONGLY AGREE	AGREE	NEITHER AGREE NOR DISAGREE	DISAGREE	STRONGLY DISAGREE
2. Provide information to get Mr. F to recognize the health benefits of individual psychotherapy and group activities.	5	4	3	2	1 XXX

Comments:
Strongly Disagree. *The timing of this strategy does not fit the situation. The nurse needs to explore Mr. F's decision not to attend therapy rather than to assume that his behavior is related to a lack of information about the health benefits of this activity. Also providing this information at this time implies that the nurse is focused on the outcome of getting Mr. F to resume his previous activities, rather than focusing on what Mr. F is currently experiencing. Additionally, by providing information to try and convince Mr. F of the health benefits of these therapies, the nurse is not acknowledging what Mr. F has learned from his previous experience and involvement in these activities. What health benefits, if any, has he experienced through his participation in these therapies thus far? Has he found theses activities helpful or not?*

	STRONGLY AGREE	AGREE	NEITHER AGREE NOR DISAGREE	DISAGREE	STRONGLY DISAGREE
3. Remind Mr. F of his upcoming discharge and suggest that he won't be able to go home if he continues to be uncooperative and fails to make progress.	5	4	3	2	1 XXX

Comments:
Strongly Disagree. *Here, the nurse is using a form of coercion to get the client to do what she thinks is in his best interest. The nurse needs to let go of trying to "get the client to cooperate" and shift the focus off of the need to make progress and onto the process of exploring the situation further. The goal at this time is to develop an understanding of what is going on from the client's perspective. Additionally, the language used is not consistent with a collaborative approach. The person is labeled as uncooperative and setbacks in client health are judged as personal failures.*

	STRONGLY AGREE	AGREE	NEITHER AGREE NOR DISAGREE	DISAGREE	STRONGLY DISAGREE
4. Empathize with Mr. F's feelings, while maintaining that attendance at group and individual therapy is not a negotiable part of his care plan.	5	4	3	2	1 XXX

Comments:
Strongly Disagree. *Care plans are formulated in collaboration with the client. If the client is "noncompliant", then the plan needs to be reviewed with the client and possibly renegotiated. The nurse should not be in a position of having to enforce the client's plan of care (unless it has been previously established by the client that the nurse should take charge in this way).*

5. Intervene to prevent further decline by suggesting that Mr. F's medication be increased.	5	4	3	2	1 XXX

Comments
Strongly Disagree. *Insufficient data. The nurse is focusing on a quick fix. The nurse needs to explore with the client further before deciding that the dose of Mr. F's medication needs to be adjusted.*

6. Make yourself available to Mr. F by offering to spend time alone with him in his room.	5 XXX	4	3	2	1

Comments:
Strongly agree. *Start where Mr. F is at. He is staying in his room. Offering your presence by joining him in his room (as opposed to coaxing or trying to convince him to come out) is consistent with a collaborative approach. Spending time and staying connected with Mr. F as per his needs, does not mean that the client is seeking attention and that the nurse is being manipulated into meeting his needs; nor should the nurse be concerned that this action will positively reinforce Mr. F's desire to remain isolated .*

7. Inform Mr. F that he will begin to lose his ward privileges if he continues to isolate himself.	5	4	3	2	1 XXX

Comments:
Strongly Disagree. *Mr. F's behavior suggests he is experiencing difficulty at this time. He needs to know that he will be helped, not punished. Additionally, the nurse is implying that Mr. F's isolation is bad for him. Instead of acting on this assumption, the nurse needs to consider that Mr. F knows best and to recognize that spending time in his room by himself may be the most therapeutic intervention for Mr. F at this time.*

RESOURCES FOR EDUCATORS

PLANNING THE TEACHING/LEARNING EXPERIENCE

Questions to Support a Thoughtful Reading

1. Think about a time that you were frustrated in your health promotion work with families. Reflecting back on this time, what aspects of your practice do you think were not helpful in resolving the issue? Why? What aspects of your practice were helpful?
2. How do policies, either hospital based or community based, interfere with your family health promoting nursing practice? What policies support these practices?
3. How do beliefs and assumptions of physicians and other professional colleagues support or interfere with your family health promoting nursing practice?
4. How could the stories of nurses about their family health promoting nursing practice be used to support nurses' learning about family health promotion?

EVALUATING THE TEACHING/LEARNING EXPERIENCE

Sample Evaluation Tool

See Box 9.5

References

Allen, F. M. (1977). Comparative theories of the expanded role in nursing and implications for nursing practice: A working paper. *Nursing Papers, 9*, 38–45.

Allen, F. M. (1981). A new perspective on nursing. Learning to be healthy: Where do nurses fit? Paper presented at Nursing Explorations Conference, February 2, 1981, McGill University, Montreal.

Allen, F. M. & Warner, M. (2002). A development model of health and nursing. *Journal of Family Nursing, 8*, 96–135.

Bevis, E. O., & Watson, J. (1989). *Toward a new curriculum: A new pedagogy for nursing*. New York: NLN.

Ezer, H., Bray, C., & Gros, C.P. (1997). Families' description of the nursing intervention in a randomized control trial. In L. N. Gottlieb & H. Ezer (Eds.), *A perspective on health, family, learning and collaborative nursing: A collection of writings on the McGill Model of Nursing* (pp. 271–276). Montreal: McGill School of Nursing.

Feeley, N., & Gottlieb, L. N. (1998). Classification systems for health concerns, nursing strategies, and client outcomes: Nursing practice with families who have a child with a chronic illness. *Canadian Journal of Nursing Research, 30*, 45–59.

Forchuck, C., Jewell, S., Schofield, I., et al. (1998). From hospital to community: Bridging therapeutic relationships. *Journal of Psychiatric and Mental Health Nursing, 5*, 197–202.

Freire, P. (1970). *Pedagogy of the oppressed*. New York: Herder and Herder.

Gottlieb, L. N. (1997). Health promoters: Two contrasting styles in community Nursing. In L.N. Gottlieb & H. Ezer (Eds.), *A perspective on health, family, learning and collaborative nursing: A collection of writings on the McGill Model of Nursing* (pp. 87–100). Montreal: McGill University School of Nursing.

Gottlieb, L. N., & Feeley, N. with Dalton, C. (2005). *The collaborative partnership approach to care: A delicate balance*. Toronto: Elsevier-Mosby.

Gottlieb, L. N., & Rowat, K. (1987). The McGill Model of Nursing: A practice derived nodel. *Advances in Nursing Science, 9*, 51–61.

Gros, C., & Ezer, H. (1997). Promoting inquiry and nurse-client collaboration: A unique approach to teaching and learning. In L. N. Gottlieb & H. Ezer (Eds), *A perspective on health, family, learning and collabora-*

tive nursing: A collection of writings on the McGill Model of Nursing (pp. 219–225). Montreal: McGill University School of Nursing.

Gros, C., Purden, M., & Ezer, H. (2000). Final Report Phase I. Promoting a self-care approach in clinical practice: A demonstration project. Unpublished Report. Ottawa: Health Canada.

Gros, C., Purden, M., Ezer, H., et al. (2002). Final Report Phase II. Developing and implementing strategies that promote a collaborative, self-care approach in the practice of nurses and physicians. Unpublished Report. Ottawa: Health Canada.

Horowitz, C. R., Suchman, A. L., Branch, W. T., et al. (2003). What do doctors find meaningful about their work? *Annals of Internal Medicine, 138,* 772–775.

Kravitz, M., & Frey, M. A. (1989). The Allen Nursing Model. In J. Fitzpatrick & A. L. Whall, (Eds.), *Conceptual models of nursing: Analysis and application* (2nd ed., pp. 313–329). Norwalk, CT: Appleton & Lange.

Mayeroff, M. (1971). *On caring.* New York: Perennial Library.

Meyers, C., & Jones, T. B. (1993). *Promoting active learning: Strategies for the college classroom.* San Francisco: Jossey-Bass.

Pless, I. B., Feeley, N., Gottlieb, L. N., et al.(1994). A randomized trial of a nursing intervention to promote the adjustment of children with chronic physical disorders. *Pediatrics, 94,* 70–75.

Pugnaire, C. (1981). *Nursing: The science of health-promoting interactions.* Unpublished Thesis. Montreal: McGill University School of Nursing.

Stewart, M. (1995).Effective physician-patient communication and health outcomes: A review. *Canadian Medical Association Journal, 152,* 1423–1433.

Stewart, M., Brown, J. B. Boon, H., et al. (1999). Evidence on patient–doctor communication. *Cancer Prevention and Control, 3,* 25–30.

Suchman, A. L., Roter, D., Green, M., et al. (1993). Physician satisfaction with primary care office visits. Collaborative study group of the American Academy on physician and patient. *Medical Care,* 31, 1083–1092.

Woods, D. (1994). *Problem-based learning: How to gain the most from PBL.* Waterdown, ON: Donald R Woods.

Young, L. (2002). Transforming health promotion practice: Moving toward holistic care. In L. Young & V. Hayes, (Eds.), *Transforming health promotion practice: Concepts, issues, and applications,* (pp. 3–21). Philadelphia: F.A. Davis.

Additional Resources

1. Nursing Best Practice Guidelines. Client-centered care, Appendix A: Educational Program Outline, pp. 43–66. Retrieved October 7, 2005, from http://www.rnao.org/bestpractices/PDF/BPG_CCCare.pdf.
2. Feeley, N. Gottlieb, L. N., Dalton, C. et al. (2005). *Instructor's manual for a collaborative partnership approach to care: The delicate balance.* Toronto: Elsevier.

Chapter 10

Context-Based Learning

Beverly Williams
Rene A. Day

During a recent visit to an undergraduate nursing tutorial, it was difficult to identify the faculty member amid the lively discussion. However when learners were asked after tutorial what they were learning, they provided the following startling response: "We taught ourselves—the professor made us do it ourselves and we don't know if we are learning what we need to and we don't know if we will pass the course exam." Learners did acknowledge that the faculty was actively involved in the discussion, particularly in asking questions that required deeper thinking and clarifying information that was shared by other learners.

In reflecting on this situation, we felt that this comment might suggest that when learners are responsible for directing their own learning, they feel uncertain that they are learning what they need to. They might also feel unprepared for evaluation. However, these learners also seemed to be suggesting that if faculty provides the information, they, as learners, would know what to learn. Furthermore, if evaluation were to focus on information that had been presented by faculty, and learners did well, they could be assured that they had learned what was expected. Do you think a learner-centered or teacher-centered approach to learning is most effective in preparing nurses for the complexity of current nursing practice?

INTENT Educating nurses for professional practice during an era of unprecedented worldwide change is a challenge for nurse educators. With the health care system also in the midst of revolutionary change, nurses are increasingly expected to think critically about practice, reflect on practice, collaborate in interdisciplinary teams, and continue learning. **Context-based learning** (CBL) as a philosophical variation of problem-based learning is one strategy that nurses have developed for undergraduate nursing education. CBL facilitates the development of competencies for practice in a rapidly changing health care environment in an increasingly global community. The basic tenets of CBL and evidence for its effectiveness as a teaching/learning strategy in undergraduate nursing education are described in this chapter.

OVERVIEW

INTRODUCTION

University and college professors often base their instructional practices on models they have observed in their own experience as learners. This might explain why teaching approaches have changed so little over many decades. The lecture as a teaching strategy emerged during a time when books were scarce (Boyer Commission, 1998) and despite exponentially enhanced access to printed materials, lectures continue to be the mainstay of university and college education (Duch, Groh, & Allen, 2001). In the traditional approach to education the terms "student" and "teacher" are strongly associated with lectures, an emphasis on teaching and student as recipient of information. To a large number of learners, lecturing is considered to be an efficient way to transmit information, but its effectiveness in facilitating learning is questionable at best. In the final analysis, all learning is self-directed, in that no one can learn on the individual learner's behalf. As early as 1916, Dewey cautioned that the teacher should be the one who guides but does not interfere with the process of learning. The terms tutor and learner are more congruent with an approach to education that emphasizes learning through active involvement in seeking out and synthesizing information. Therefore, although the term student-centered teaching is the focus of this book, we have chosen to emphasize the student as learner and the teacher as tutor. Tutor and learner are the terms that will be used throughout this chapter.

WHY CHANGE THE WAY WE TEACH?

The goals of a university education have changed. With future knowledge explosion in mind, Hesburgh, Miller, and Wharton (1974) suggested that the most essential outcome of a postsecondary education is to inculcate learners with an understanding that learning is continuous and that they must be self-directed in their pursuit of learning. More recently, the Boyer Commission (1998) urged universities to facilitate learner inquiry with the expectation that faculty should be companions and guides to learners rather than transmitters of information. Faculty is strategically positioned to help facilitate learning by acknowledging prior learning; creating a curriculum that stimulates inquiry; providing guidance on learning strategies; and offering thoughtful, constructive feedback on learner performance and achievement.

In a frequently cited landmark conference (Wingspread Conference, 1994), policymakers, corporate leaders, university professors, and accreditation communities developed the following list of essential characteristics of quality performance for university graduates:

- High level skills in communication and information retrieval.
- An ability to arrive at informed judgments through defining problems, gathering information and developing solutions.
- An ability to function in a global community which requires flexibility, adaptability, an ability to deal with ambiguity and diversity, self-directedness, and an ability to be collaborative.
- An ability to address specific problems in complex real world settings.
- An ability to continue to learn.

Since health care systems are also in the midst of revolutionary change, the needs of nursing employers are consistent with those of general employers of university graduates (Tompkins, 2001). Valanis (2000) has succinctly captured the essential qualities of a competent 21st century nurse:

- An independent practitioner who critically reflects on practice.
- Self-directed and actively involved in continuous learning.
- Encourages colleagues to engage in continuous learning.
- Encourages patients/clients to actively engage in self-care.
- Manages care across facility boundaries through interdisciplinary collaboration.
- Promotes the health of the community through interdisciplinary collaboration.
- Ensures quality and cost-effective care.
- Exerts leadership in policy development from local to international levels.

And equally important, over the last few decades, theories about how people learn have also evolved. Early behaviorists claimed that it is observable behavior that indicates whether or not the learner has learned (Skinner, 1974). Later on, cognitive psychologists conceptualized learning as an internal process and suggested that the depth of learning depends on the learner's existing knowledge structure, how well the learner processes information, how much energy is expended during the process, and the depth of the processing (Craik & Tulvig, 1975). More recently, constructivist theorists claim that learners actively contextualize information according to their own reality through observation, processing, interpretation, and integration into their existing framework of knowledge (Duffy & Cunningham, 1996). According to constructivists, the active process of learning is triggered by engaging learners in meaningful activity which is often presented as a problem.

When the three schools of thought are analyzed, the utility of each becomes apparent in creating an optimal learning environment. Effective learning is based on guided discovery and active involvement of the learner who builds on what is already known. Learners learn best when they can discuss and contextualize what they are learning, ascribe personal meaning for application and demonstrate their achievement. Learner-centered, inquiry-based approaches to learning such as context-based learning (CBL) are based on all three schools of thought and help learners develop the skills and abilities that employers of university nursing graduates are seeking.

CONTEXT-BASED LEARNING (CBL)

Context-based learning (CBL) is a philosophical variation of problem-based learning (PBL). Recognizing that conventional classroom instruction was not completely preparing medical learners to transfer the knowledge and skills learned in school to the demands of medical practice, McMaster University School of Medicine faculty designed and implemented a PBL curriculum in 1969 (Barrows, 1996). Since that time, the use of PBL in post secondary institutions has been reported with increasing frequency in a variety of disciplines such as architecture (Kingsland, 1996), business (Stinson & Milter, 1996), elementary and secondary education (Jaramillo, 1999), engineering (Woods, 1996), mathematics (Seltzer, Hilbert, Maceli, Robinson & Schwartz, 1996), rehabilitation medicine (Saarinen & Salvatori, 1994), and science (Allen, Duch, & Groh, 1996). The Samford University PBL Web site lists over 300 institutions world wide that are using PBL.

Within the PBL approach, the term problem is intended to refer to any situation relevant to learning to become a professional practitioner. The problem becomes the stimulus and focus of all learning activity. However, the use of the term problem in the discipline of nursing can be interpreted to suggest that nursing practice consists of helping people with problems. Focusing on patient/client problems tends to overemphasize illness, difficulties, and problem solution. It is important to remember that not everything that patients/clients experience is a problem and not all problems can be solved. Today, professional nursing practice increasingly focuses on health, strengths, situation exploration, and support. Using the term context-based learning is a conscious attempt to select a term that more effectively reflects the holistic nature of professional nursing practice.

Learners in CBL acquire knowledge and skill in nursing by encountering authentic professional practice situations as the initial stimulus and focus of their learning activity (Barrows, 1996; Boud & Feletti, 1998). This varies from conventional instructional practice that relies on the use of professional practice situations as a culminating activity following faculty presentation of nursing content. Typically, a nursing course in a CBL program would consist of several real nursing practice situations. Each situation (example on page 226) is accompanied by overall learning goals that identify essential concepts embedded in the situation. The situation should be complex enough that the possible

BOX 10.1 PHASES OF CBL

PHASES OF CBL

1. The situation is examined; learning issues and possible information sources are identified.
2. Information is gathered and independent/colleagial study occurs.
3. New information is discussed and applied to the situation in a practical way.
4. Context and process of learning is reflected upon.

outcome(s) for the individuals in the situation can best be identified and debated through the cooperative efforts of the tutorial group. A CBL situation is considered effective if learners are engaged and motivated to probe ever more deeply for understanding.

Generally, in a small **tutorial** group of 9–12, guided by a faculty member (**tutor**), learners grapple with the complexities of each practice situation. They search for connections across disciplines drawing on existing and newly acquired knowledge to generate possible outcomes for each situation. The learners present, justify, and debate each possibility, searching for the best possible outcome for a particular situation. Through collaborative investigation with classmates, learners refine and enhance their disciplinary knowledge and skills. Each situation occupies learners for a minimum of two sessions and the process consists of four phases as shown in Box 10.1.

Phases of CBL

PHASE ONE: EXAMINING THE SITUATION

In phase one of the CBL process, a tutorial group of nursing learners and a faculty tutor begin discussion of an authentic nursing practice situation that has been generated by practicing nurses. Each situation is constructed to be less detailed than a case study. In some cases, not all of the information in the situation is relevant and not all of the relevant information is actually in the situation—just like the real world. The situation may be presented as a video, an audio tape, or a written scenario complete with photos. Learners are encouraged to explore the situation with a focus on health (defined as a resource for everyday life), strengths of the client (person, family, aggregate, community), and their role as nurse in the situation.

During a tutorial session, nursing learners begin by reasoning aloud through discussion of the nursing situation, identifying what they do know based on their previous experience, what they do not know, and what they need to know in order to interact as a nurse in the situation. Learners formulate explanations, clarify understanding through negotiation, critique classmates' comments, establish learning goals, and create an action plan to meet those goals. With tutor coaching and by using their own thinking processes, learners develop the **self-monitoring** skills they need to identify and meet their learning goals. Developing self-monitoring skills is an important part of **metacognition** (Barrows, 1996). These skills contribute to each learners' ability to be critically reflective. For example, learners might be presented with the situation described in Box 10.2.

BOX 10.2 SAMPLE LEARNING PACKAGE

LEARNING GOALS

Through this learning package the student will be introduced to the care of clients with alternative lifestyles. Issues related to inner city culture will be explored. The focus is on health promotion and primary prevention with vulnerable populations. Positive aspects of inner city culture and strategies for confidence building, reinforcement, and sharing values will be discussed.

CONCEPTS

Essential concepts are identified and might include women's health, intimate partner violence, stereotypes, vulnerability, empowerment.

SCENARIO

Angie, a 20-year-old woman, visits the inner city health clinic where you work as an RN. She has been to the clinic previously and the last time was diagnosed with vaginitis. This time she presents with a swollen nose and left eye. There is blood on her face and she says she had an argument with her boyfriend.

PHASE ONE

Through initial discussion, learners might identify the following learning issues or examples of areas for further learning:

- Developmental tasks of young adulthood.
- Inner city demographics, culture, and health.
- Health clinic nursing.
- Sexually transmitted disease, abuse, poverty.
- Sex trade workers, stigma, stereotypes.
- Working with vulnerable populations.
- Empowerment.
- Physical examination of the nose, eyes, genitalia.

Tutors can challenge learners to critically analyze the situation, identify gaps in their knowledge and pose questions on areas they may lack understanding. For example: What do you think is going on here? What are some of the possible outcomes of being hit on the head? What makes you think that Angie may be in the sex trade? What are some of the risks associated with being in the sex trade? How do you feel about interacting with Angie? How do we as nurses support Angie? What community resources are available for Angie to use?

PHASE TWO: SELF-DIRECTED STUDY

In the second phase of CBL, learners activate their plans to meet their learning goals by engaging in self-directed study either by themselves or in pairs. Learners determine how they will learn the knowledge and skills they have identified and what credible resources they will use to assist them. This process helps learners develop the reflective skills and self-directed learning skills critical to learning. While engaged in self-directed learning activities (reading, consulting resource/people), learners may identify discrepancies in their beliefs, values or assumptions. Learners may begin to ask, "Why? What makes me ——? Or what will happen if ——?"

PHASE THREE: INTEGRATING NEW INFORMATION

During this phase learners reconvene and continue to explore the situation, sharing what they have learned and integrating new information into the context of the situation. Learners are encouraged to connect new concepts to old ones and may continue to identify new learning issues. This process is critical to ensure retrieval of what has been learned when a similar situation is encountered in the future. During this phase the tutor might ask the following questions: "Why do you think Angie might have become associated with the sex trade? How do you think being a sex trade worker is connected to self-esteem? Why do you think Angie might stay in an abusive relationship? How has media portrayal of abuse of women influenced your view of Angie? As nurses, how can we facilitate Angie's empowerment? What are the similarities between activity limitations with a situation of increased intraocular pressure and one of increased intracranial pressure?" Over a period of time learners will begin to challenge themselves and each other with "What? How? Why? What makes me/you ——? What do you think would happen if ——?" types of questions. When this happens learners exhibit increased autonomy in **critical reflection**.

During this phase of learning, nursing learners summarize what they learned and discuss how their knowledge and skills might be used in future nursing practice situations. Ultimately, learners should feel confident interacting in this or a similar situation. A final check from the tutor could include the following comment: "You are the nurse and you walk into the examining room where Angie is waiting. Let's role play your initial interaction and health history interview." If the CBL process has been successful, learners consciously recall and reflect on learning that occurred, elaborate on the learning and integrate it into their **existing cognitive structures** (Lefrancois, 2000).

PHASE FOUR: REFLECTING

During the fourth phase of each situation discussion, learners critique resources and research methods utilized by themselves and their peers during self-study. When critiquing methods and resources for value and effectiveness, learners consider alternatives to their choices. Continuous evaluation of research methods and resources is critical to the process of reflective learning. Another critical component of the CBL process is reflection on group process. Learners identify what worked well and what they would like to change before going on to the next situation. Each learner also has an opportunity to assume the leadership role of the group for some designated period of time.

Through the CBL process, learners have opportunities to develop skill in giving constructive feedback to peers and their tutor. At the end of each situation discussion, learners and the tutor provide constructive criticism to each other about individual contributions to learning and to the group process. Through these feedback sessions, learners learn to develop and critically reflect on their research, communicative, collaborative, and leadership abilities.

The ability of learners to be self-directed and critically reflective in their learning is developed through critical questioning by the faculty tutor during situational analysis, learning needs determination, application of knowledge, critiquing of resources/personal problem-solving processes, and summarizing what was learned. The CBL process engages learners in activities that:

1. Reveal their thinking processes so that they can monitor the effectiveness of their ability to analyze, reason, and acquire knowledge.
2. Facilitate the development of interpersonal collaborative skills—particularly listening, questioning, and summarizing.
3. Enable them to assume increasing autonomy, responsibility, and control for their own reflective learning.

THEORETICAL FOUNDATIONS OF CBL

The rationale for choosing CBL is often based on recognition that conventional classroom lectures do not completely prepare nursing learners to apply the knowledge and skills learned in the classroom to the demands of the clinical setting. According to modern learning theorists, lecture content that is learned without a context for application is more difficult to recall when needed for application in the clinical area (Savery & Duffy, 1995). While choosing CBL is often based more on ramifications for professional practice than on any specific existing theoretical support, the decision does reflect the theoretical perspectives of such cognitive scientists as Dewey, Bruner, and Piaget (Norman & Schmidt, 1992; Schmidt, 1983, 1993; Wilkerson & Feletti, 1989). Within the cognitive science domain, CBL reflects both the rationalist (Albanese & Mitchell, 1993; Norman & Schmidt, 1992; Schmidt, 1983, 1993) and the constructivist view of learning (Savery & Duffy, 1995).

Rationalist Perspective

A rationalist perspective of learning assumes that knowledge acquisition is primarily a result of individual cognitive activity in processing information (Schmidt, 1993). As early as 1938, Dewey suggested that knowledge could not be transferred simply from one individual to another but could only be acquired through active cognitive engagement. According to a rationalist perspective, existing cognitive structures within the individual will influence the extent to which new information will be understood. In 1960, Bruner suggested that material organized according to the individual's own interests and cognitive structures is material that has the best chance of being accessible to the individual's memory. The information processing perspective also reflects Piaget's description of cognition and the notion that thinking skills can be directly taught (Slavin, 1994).

Schmidt (1993) presents several principles that can be used to guide the design of CBL based on the rationalist perspective of cognition. A CBL activity employs the following instructional strategies and tactics:

1. Relevant prior knowledge is activated by engaging learners in practical situational analysis initiated with articulation about what they do, and do not, know about the situation.

2. Elaboration on prior knowledge occurs through engagement of learners in small group discussion, generation and critique of hypotheses, and peer teaching. During the review process that occurs at the completion of each practical situation discussion, learners elaborate further on the relationship of new knowledge to prior knowledge.
3. Because the practical situation drives the learning of content and skills, learners are continuously restructuring their knowledge as they work toward the best outcome.
4. Authentic practical situations that reflect the types of situations learners will face as professionals serve as the framework for storing contextual cues, and improving learners' abilities to retrieve relevant knowledge when faced with similar situations in the future. As one first-year student stated, "Years from now we will still remember the concepts from this scenario."
5. Learners are motivated and spend more time processing information when they are discussing authentic practical situations which they perceive as relevant and meaningful. Increased time spent processing information results in a more complete cognitive structure from which to retrieve information.

From a rationalist perspective of learning, CBL utilizes instructional strategies to assist learners to process and store knowledge in such a way that it can be retrieved easily when required in the future. The process of CBL helps learners to activate prior knowledge and connect new knowledge to prior knowledge. It also facilitates the process of knowledge elaboration by structuring knowledge with contextual cues. This results in the creation of strong multiple connections in memory. Through the CBL process, learners are prompted to reflect on what they have learned and how they might apply what they have learned to similar situations that they may encounter in the future.

Constructivist Perspective

The constructivist perspective of learning assumes that knowledge acquisition is a continuous process of building and reshaping understanding as a natural consequence of experience in the world (Savery & Duffy, 1995). Learning is not only about the acquisition of new knowledge but also the ongoing reconstruction of what an individual already knows. The stimulus for learning is a cognitive conflict or puzzle (Dewey, 1938; Savery & Duffy, 1995). Learners must constantly check new information against existing information and adjust accordingly. In addition to being a continuous process, learning is also described as a collaborative process in which individual understanding is rooted in social interaction. Knowledge acquisition is firmly embedded in the social and emotional context in which learning takes place. Conceptual growth arises from sharing perspectives and testing ideas with others. Such negotiation culminates in modifications in cognitive structure. See Chapter 1 for a full discussion.

Savery and Duffy (1995) present principles that can be used to govern the design of CBL based on the constructivist perspective of cognition. The principles are derived from the constructivist concepts of cognitive conflict, understanding through interaction, and social negotiation. Based on the assumptions of a constructivist perspective of cognition and learning, CBL activity employs the following instructional strategies and tactics:

1. Learning is essentially an act of active construction on the part of the student (Savery & Duffy, 1995). By requiring learners to assume the role of professional

and engage in self-directed learning, learners experience the knowledge construction process.
2. Through collaborative group work and accessing a wide variety of resources, learners experience and develop an appreciation for multiple perspectives.
3. Learning is embedded in authentic contexts so learners acquire content and skills through the discussion of actual professional practice situations. This strategy enhances the retrievability of knowledge and skill when it is needed.
4. Learners assume responsibility for their own learning and practice through self-directed learning and leadership activities inherent in every CBL activity.
5. Self-awareness of the knowledge construction and skill acquisition process is encouraged during the reflective activities embedded in each CBL activity and during the review process that occurs with the completion of the situation.

From a constructivist perspective, CBL prepares learners for professional practice by engaging them in authentic activities during their learning for that practice. Knowledge and skills are learned within a context that reflects the environment that graduates will practice in as professionals. Contextualization of learning and the social support and interaction during learning help prepare learners to transfer what they have learned to new situations and avoid the pitfalls of inert knowledge. Specific instructional strategies proposed by proponents of both rationalist and constructivist perspectives include aspects of student self-awareness, autonomy and responsibility, interaction and collaboration, reflection and review, and leadership.

ASSESSING LEARNING OUTCOMES

Assessment of learning outcomes is a central feature of the CBL process and includes assessment of individual achievement and tutorial effectiveness. The ways in which assessment is structured will have an impact on how learners learn. Because assessment is an indication of what learners will be rewarded for doing, assessment strategies must convince learners that critical thinking, self-direction, collaboration, leadership, and reflection are valued. Although a variety of evaluation strategies can be used with CBL courses, the following components are usually included in the evaluation process:

1. Tutorial participation.
2. Content examination.
3. Critical thinking through scholarly writing.

To arrive at a tutorial participation grade, learners usually rank themselves and are ranked by the tutor in the following areas: critical thinking, communication and respect, self-direction, and group process. Through peer and self-evaluation, learners gather data in each of the areas in order to provide specific examples of their tutorial behavior as evidence of having met the participation criteria. The tutor also compares the performance of each learner to the criteria outlined for tutorial participation. An example of criteria that learners and faculty might use to evaluate tutorial participation is outlined in Box 10.3 (University of Alberta Collaborative Baccalaureate Program, 2003). Learners are provided with further guidelines (Box 10.4) related to completing an accurate and effective self evaluation (University of Alberta Collaborative Baccalaureate Program, 2003).

BOX 10.3 GUIDE FOR EVALUATION: LEARNER PERFORMANCE IN TUTORIAL

STUDENT PERFORMANCE ABILITIES

Critical Thinking and Problem Solving

1. Shares evidence-based content in each scenario that:
   a. is obtained from a variety of references including: textbooks, other-than-text books relevant to research area, peer-reviewed journals, agency materials, and the Web.
   b. is relevant to the learning goals and course objectives.
   c. addresses the area to be researched in depth.
2. Facilitates discussion to promote an understanding of the content area by:
   a. being able to explain, explore, and utilize key concepts with precision and supporting rationale.
   b. developing the topic under exploration by asking the group critical thinking questions.
   c. demonstrating creativity in sharing information.
3. Independently promotes deeper understanding of subject within a group discussion by:
   a. verbally reflecting on content.
   b. raising significant points and/or asking relevant questions.
   c. proposing related concepts/ideas.
   d. using information that supports claim; considers alternative information that offers contradictory evidence.
   e. openly examining own and alternate points of view for strengths and weaknesses in addressing the subject, problem, or question at hand.
4. Uses an obvious decision-making process to verbally:
   a. identify, justify, and/or discard assumptions, myths, and differing points of view.
   b. make reasonable inferences and conclusions and explore possible strategies to address question or issues.
   c. differentiate between opinion and fact.
5. Participates in discussions of professional/ethical/moral issues.

Self-Direction

1. Independently identifies ways to promote personal development in tutorial setting, i.e.:
   a. identifies own strengths and limitations that affect group and individual learning.
   b. sets goals and objectives.
   c. follows through with personal development plans.
   d. evaluates progress with examples.
2. Collects and validates information gathered to conduct self-assessment throughout tutorial process, at midterm and final evaluation of tutorial.
3. Explores how own behaviors affect ability of group to function during evaluation of group process.
4. Responds to fair evaluative comments from others in accepting manner without becoming defensive, blaming others, or being negative.
5. Demonstrates understanding of differences between tutor-directed and self-directed learning; views tutor as facilitator and additional resource.
6. Identifies self-assessment of learning and possible gaps in knowledge.
7. Completes assigned tasks as presented in course outline.
8. In the event of an absence, notifies tutor prior to tutorial or lab. ➔

■ BOX 10.3 Guide for Evaluation: Learner Performance in Tutorial (continued)

Communication and Respect

1. Shares information clearly.
2. Is alert to cues of lack of understanding in others and responds.
3. Verbal/nonverbal behavior recognizes presence of all others in tutorial group, i.e.:
   a. speaks directly to group members.
   b. actively listens and responds to others with respect.
   c. waits for others to finish speaking before beginning to speak.
   d. gives others the opportunity to speak as much as self.
4. Utilizes a variety of strategies for effective communication within the group such as: asking open-ended questions, paraphrasing, clarifying assumptions/misunderstandings, focusing, summarizing, etc.
5. Verbal/nonverbal behavior recognizes the rights of others to express own views without being put down.
6. Maintains confidentiality of information and experiences shared in tutorial, lab, and fixed resource sessions.

Group Process

1. Approaches all components of course as a professional workplace by:
   a. consistently demonstrating professional behavior.
   b. demonstrating professional verbal and written communication including e-mail and telephone messages.
   c. following Professional Code of Ethics.
   d. following Code of Student Behavior as outlined in the U of A calendar.
   e. being punctual, present, and participating in all tutorials and labs.
2. Contributes to the development/maintenance of group objectives/norms.
3. Assumes an active, functional role in group discussions, both verbally and nonverbally.
4. Relates to peers collaboratively and as resources for learning.
5. Assumes a leadership role in CBL both formally and informally by:
   a. helping to keep the group task oriented.
   b. encouraging/facilitating participation of others.
   c. fostering group discussion.
   d. assisting group members in their learning.
   e. recognizing and responding to verbal and nonverbal communication that impedes group process.
   f. taking constructive action to resolve individual and group concerns and conflicts.
6. Takes part in the evaluation of CBL group process work that involves self and other group members. Gives both verbal and written feedback to others that is:
   a. constructive (positive and developmental in nature).
   b. in-depth, meaningful.
   c. honest and direct.

University of Alberta Faculty of Nursing (2003).

BOX 10.4 SELF-EVALUATION IN CBL TUTORIALS

Please complete a written midterm and final self-evaluation commenting on the criteria outlined in each of the four areas listed in the Guide for Evaluation: Learner Performance in Tutorial (Box 10.3): Critical Thinking and Problem Solving; Self-Direction; Communication and Respect; and Group Process. Take time to reflect on your performance in each category utilizing specific examples from self-observation and peer feedback. Make reference to peer feedback and attach the peer feedback evaluations. Please attach your written peer feedback evaluations.

Self-Scoring: To guide you in accurately evaluating (scoring) yourself, here are some guidelines. An "Excellent" 5 learner would *consistently* demonstrate:

- Synthesis of information from a variety of references for each topic investigated.
- Integration of research findings from peer-reviewed nursing journals into handouts and discussion of each topic investigated.
- Enough familiarity with the information to be able to identify key concepts and facilitate discussion and application of the information without reading.
- Creative sharing of information (role play, use of model, visual representations, quizzes, matching activities, etc.).
- Creating of critical questions that facilitate application of the information to the situation but also extend discussion beyond the scenario to similar situations.
- Active facilitation of group discussion of assigned topic that includes all members utilizing a variety of communication strategies.
- The ability to provide honest, direct, constructive peer/tutor feedback during evaluation sessions.
- Thoughtful consideration of the logic underlying alternate points of view.
- Strong formal and informal leadership skills and abilities.

A "Very Good" 4 learner would *consistently* demonstrate the *majority* of these behaviors, and an "Expected" 3 learner would exhibit fewer behaviors and with less consistency, and so on.

One effective mechanism to ensure that feedback is specific and constructive is to have learners draw names at the beginning of a learning package discussion. All tutorial group members, including the tutor, are involved in the name drawing. Each learner then observes the individual whose name they have drawn and provides them with examples of how they have or have not met the criteria for learner performance in tutorial during each learning package discussion. Feedback is provided verbally in the tutorial setting and each tutorial group member is also provided with written feedback that they can use in supporting their individual midterm and final self-evaluation. Generally the tutorial participation marks within a single group reflect a range of skill and ability.

In some models of CBL a tutor may facilitate several tutorial groups at the same time. Opportunities for consistent observation of individual learners and overall group effectiveness may be limited. If this is the case, an **objective structured tutorial evaluation** (OSTE) may be useful (Box 10.5). An OSTE is another way to assess knowledge and skill of individual learners as well as tutorial group effectiveness. The OSTE usually occurs at the end of term. It is an abbreviated (30-minute) tutorial session that occurs without the

BOX 10.5 OBJECTIVE STRUCTURED TUTORIAL EVALUATION (OSTE)

Note: This is an individual mark.

- Each evaluation session is 30 minutes long.
- Please sit according to the specified seating plan.
- As soon as you arrive, you will draw from a hat to determine group member roles.
- Each learner in the group will receive the same short scenario and as a group, you will need to identify the client's priority need(s), develop nursing diagnoses, select the priority nursing diagnosis, and develop a relevant nursing action plan.
- The group needs to conclude by having each learner conduct a brief self-evaluation of their contributions to the discussion.
- You will each be marked by your tutor and an objective second person according to the following criteria taken from the Guide for Evaluation: Learner Performance in Tutorial:
  - Critical thinking/problem solving (# 3, 4, 5)
  - Communication/respect (# 1, 2, 3, 4, 5)
  - Group process (# 1, 2, 4, 5, 6)

guidance of a tutor (University of Alberta Collaborative Baccalaureate Program, 2003). The tutor becomes an evaluator during the OSTE session.

As learners arrive for the OSTE, they draw from a hat the role that each of them will assume during the OSTE. Roles might include: leader, recorder, timekeeper, clarifier, summarizer, etc. Each learner in the tutorial group receives the same short scenario. As a group, learners are asked to reach verbal consensus in identifying priority client needs, formulating a nursing diagnosis, and developing a relevant plan of action. The OSTE concludes with each learner conducting a brief self-evaluation. The faculty tutor and the objective individual, often the course coordinator, observe the learners during the OSTE. They independently evaluate the individual learners based on specified tutorial participation criteria. Occasionally some negotiation is required between the two faculty members in order to arrive at a final mark for each learner who participates in the OSTE. The tutor and objective observer also comment on the overall effectiveness of the tutorial group.

The OSTE is an effective strategy for evaluation even when the tutor has only one or two tutorial groups at the same time. It is congruent with the experience that learners engage in throughout a CBL course. In preparation for the OSTE, quieter learners are challenged to speak up more during tutorials and all learners are challenged to practice taking on roles in tutorial that they might not be comfortable with. The OSTE provides a clear portrayal of both individual and group effectiveness in CBL.

An important goal of CBL is to help learners integrate concepts from different disciplines of knowledge. Assessment strategies that encourage learners to integrate concepts from nursing, the sciences, and humanities are desirable. Scholarly writing is one strategy that facilitates learner integration of knowledge from different disciplines. Scholarly paper topics can focus on a current issue related to health care and the implications of the issue for professional nursing. For example, learners may be asked to "discuss the effects of privatization on healthcare for Canadians" or "argue that employing baccalaureate nurses is beneficial to the health of Americans." Both of the suggested topics require learners to think about concepts from nursing, philosophy, and political science. When marking scholarly papers, attention should be paid to presentation, creativity and how well learners use supporting evidence to argue their point of view. Box 10.6 is an

BOX 10.6 SCHOLARLY PAPER-MARKING GUIDELINES (25 = 100%)

Outstanding (24, 25)	Extraordinary and creative writing ability demonstrated in development and presentation of ideas. Outstanding integration of theoretical and/or empirical knowledge. Consistent identification of salient argument(s) throughout. Objective application of evidence and reasons to support warranted, justified conclusions and appropriate generalizations in relation to the topic. Grammatical presentation and APA format require minimal revision.
Excellent (21, 22, 23)	Excellent writing ability demonstrated. Paper has structure and is well organized. Identifies relevant ideas. Creative and thorough integration of theoretical and/or empirical knowledge with own ideas. Thoughtfully evaluates alternative points of view. Draws warranted conclusions. Grammatical presentation and APA format require minimal revision.
Very Good (18, 19, 20)	Sound writing ability evidenced. Structure and organization of paper is appropriate Integration of theoretical and/or empirical knowledge is evident. Accurate interpretation of evidence, statements, graphics, and questions related to the topic, allows for identification of most vital ideas. Thoughtfully evaluates major alternative points of view. Justifies conclusions appropriately. Grammatical presentation and APA format require a few revisions.
Good (15, 16, 17)	Generally well written with a few specific areas regarding structure and/or organization requiring improvement. Integration of theoretical and/or empirical knowledge with own ideas is evident in the identification of vital ideas. Identifies some alternative points of view. Offers some relevant supporting evidence for ideas. Draws conclusions. Explanation of assumptions and reasons for conclusions is attempted. A few incorrect grammatical structures and spelling errors evident. APA format requires some revision.
Satisfactory (13, 14)	Acceptably written with several specific areas regarding structure and organization needing improvement. An attempt to integrate theoretical and/or empirical knowledge with own ideas is evident. Identifies a few vital ideas, however information is incomplete and/or superficial. Little evidence of analysis or evaluation of alternative points of view. Draws a few conclusions. Explanation of assumptions and reasons for conclusions is inadequate. Several incorrect grammatical structures and spelling errors are present. APA format is inconsistently followed throughout the paper.
Fail (0)	Paper not handed in or paper plagiarized.

University of Alberta Faculty of Nursing (2003).

example of a guide that can be used to mark scholarly papers in a CBL program (University of Alberta Collaborative Baccalaureate Program, 2003).

Traditional examinations can be used in CBL to assess content understanding. A typical CBL course examination often includes multiple choice questions (MCQs), as well as short and long answer questions. Learners relate better to MCQs if each series of questions is preceded by a short description of a client/patient situation to which the questions relate. This form of examination construction reflects the tutorial process and is consistent with how learners learn the information and also prepares learners to write a Professional Nurse Registration Examination. The questions can be designed in such a way that higher levels of thinking (application, analysis, evaluation, synthesis) are required in order to correctly answer the questions. The goal is to avoid multiple choice questions that focus on minute detail but rather focus on understanding of essential concepts. In CBL, learners will attend to detail but the goal of examination is to assess the learner's ability to apply the knowledge to real nursing practice situations.

Short answer questions and longer essay style questions can also be included. A sample long answer question is included in Box 10.7.

Since group work is so predominant in CBL tutorial, having CBL learners write out answers to questions provides the faculty with a clearer indication of the individual learner's level of thinking and understanding. Written answers to examination questions also provides an assurance that this is the learner's own work, an assurance that is more difficult to achieve when evaluating scholarly papers.

Learners in CBL often express concern that what they studied was not on the examination. One novel way to address this concern is to have a short answer question asking learners to identify a specific number of concepts that they learned about that were not tested on the examination and provide an example from practice that exemplifies the importance or application of each concept.

BOX 10.7 SAMPLE ESSAY-STYLE QUESTIONS

Silvercrest Health Clinic serves an area of the city where 20% of the population is elderly. Many senior citizens live alone and there has been a high incidence of break-ins in the area. As a community health nurse you are also concerned about the likelihood of depression, hypertension, and falls.

- Suggest strategies that you could use to assess whether your concerns are justified. Include discussion of legal, ethical, and practical implications of collecting data that you will need.

Your assessment data confirms your concerns. Findings suggest a high incidence of hypertension, falls, and depression related to fears of possible break-ins. You decide to respond by developing a program to address priority issues.

- How will you determine priority issues for initiating a health promotion program?
- Select three priority issues that relate to this scenario. State your rationale for choosing them and rank them in order of priority.
- Outline a program to address one priority issue. You should include an overall goal, objectives, strategies, resources required, barriers that might be encountered, and evaluation criteria.

MODELS OF CBL CURRICULA

There are a variety of ways to integrate CBL into undergraduate nursing curricula. The model that has been discussed in this chapter would be classified as a total curriculum approach to CBL. Each course is comprised of a series of scenarios. Tutorial time is spent in interaction and time between tutorials is spent in self-directed study. There is little or no formal class time, although, on occasion guest speakers may be invited to interact with all of the learners during an established fixed resource session. The ratio of tutors to tutorial groups may be one-to-one or one-to-several. If the ratio is one-to-several, the tutor spends a designated amount of time with each of the tutorial groups during specified class time. The one-to-several ratio is particularly valuable with senior learners who have learned how to effectively lead and manage group interaction and learning. Laboratory learning still occurs but usually with much less faculty presentation/demonstration and more learner interaction and practice.

CBL can also be utilized in a single course. The course can be designed as a series of scenarios. Learners can bring various resources to class. Working in small tutorial groups, learners might spend about half of the time working on learner-generated questions related to the scenario and they spend the remaining time sharing their responses. The learner/faculty ratio might be one tutor per class if it is a relatively small class or one tutor and one or more teaching assistants per class if the class is larger.

A third model of CBL could involve using the principles of CBL in a single class. The faculty might begin the class with a scenario. Again learners might spend about half of the time working on learner-generated questions related to the scenario and the other half of the time sharing their responses. With single-course and single-class models of CBL there tends to be less emphasis on self-directed learning, critiquing of resources and methods of searching for information, constructive criticism of individual learners, leadership, and reflection on the group process. The learning activity at the end of the chapter will help you to think about how you might use CBL in your own teaching practice.

CHALLENGES TO USING CBL

Making the transition from a traditional to a CBL curriculum is not an easy process. CBL requires simultaneous changes in philosophy, curriculum, faculty development, faculty-learner interaction, learner orientation, and assessment practices in order to ensure success (Barron et al, 1998; Williams, 2002). Both faculty and learners take time to adjust to CBL. Most of the published research relates to the effectiveness of PBL in facilitating the learning of undergraduate nursing learners.

Learners frequently express concerns about the amount of time it takes to adjust to the roles of faculty and learners in a PBL program (Ishida, 1995; Rideout, 1998; Solomon & Finch, 1998; Williams, 2002). They identify concerns about group process issues and the inconsistency among faculty tutors (Ishida, 1995; Rideout, 1998; Williams, 2002). Learners express insecurities about the accuracy of the information that their colleagues are sharing with them (Ishida, 1995; Solomon & Finch, 1998; Williams, 2002) and are often uncertain about the breadth and depth of knowledge that they are acquiring (Rideout, 1998; Solomon & Finch, 1998; Williams, 2002). Many of these issues can be minimized with effective faculty development and learner orientation to the roles of each in PBL.

Faculty tutors identify fewer concerns with PBL. They are primarily concerned with the perceived lack of efficiency of PBL (Vernon, 1995). In addition, faculty tutors are often concerned about the amount of time it takes learners to adjust to PBL and their own loss of control (Vernon, 1995; Williams, 2002).

EVIDENCE THAT CBL WORKS

While there is a significant body of research about PBL, there is limited research related to CBL. Recent research indicates that there is no significant difference on standardized examinations between nursing learners from conventional programs and those from PBL Programs (Newman, 1995; Rideout, et al., 2002). Williams (2006) reported that when learners from a CBL program were compared to learners in a traditional nursing program on the same multiple choice questions, the mean range for learners in the traditional course was 66 to 68% and the mean range for CBL learners on the same questions was 68 to 77%. In addition, 100% of the first CBL class passed the National Professional Nurse Registration Exam, an unprecedented event in the history of this particular undergraduate nursing program. These results suggest that these CBL learners were learning content that faculty and the National Association considered relevant to nursing practice.

PBL nursing graduates tend to be rated higher on their clinical performance than their conventional program counterparts (Rideout, et al., 2002). Williams (2006) reported that when compared to their traditional program peers, CBL learners at the end of the third year in one CBL program scored "strong" in clinical decision making as often as the end of year four learners in the traditional program. A summary of unsolicited comments from employers of senior nursing learners included the following: "These learners are different. They are confident and well-grounded in practice, resourceful, doing research to verify questions about nursing practice, are aware of their limitations and can also identify how to remedy any deficiencies."

By the end of the first year in a CBL program, learner achievement of specific level outcomes and the documented outcomes of CBL was evident. In a small pilot study, Day and Williams (2000) reported an increase in the critical thinking skills and dispositions of CBL learners from the program entry to the end of the first year. Williams (2004) also reported that although learners did not demonstrate any increase in self-directed learning, as measured by a standardized scale, at the end of one year in a CBL program, they were able to describe themselves as having developed many of the documented characteristics associated with self-directed learners. In their self/course evaluations, learners provided evidence to support their descriptions of themselves as developing the characteristics of self-directed learners as outlined in the literature. They recognized the sense of responsibility they were developing in being able to work with others. Learners indicated they were confident in their ability to identify their learning needs, select and use a variety of resources, choose relevant information, and share their information in creative ways. They acknowledged that they were learning how to effectively question each other, deal with ambiguity, and value a diversity of viewpoints. Learners commented that through regular self-evaluation and peer evaluation they were developing a deeper awareness of themselves and others and were increasingly able to communicate their observations of each other. Finally, learners indicated that they were developing the skills that would enable them to continue to learn once they were practicing professionals.

SUMMARY

Promotion of learner-centered strategies in nursing education is essential if the profession of nursing wants practitioners who are able to think critically, practice reflectively, collaborate in interdisciplinary teams and continue to learn throughout their professional careers. Through the CBL process learners continually focus on learning how to identify their learning needs; accessing and applying current evidence-based knowledge; and developing leadership, collaborative, and reflective skills/abilities within the context of real nursing practice. Context-based learning is one learner-centered strategy that can facilitate learner development of the essential qualities of a competent 21st century nurse working in a rapidly changing health care system in an increasingly global community.

LEARNING ACTIVITY

Developing a CBL Learning Package

Think about one of the courses that you currently teach.

1. Identify the essential concepts or principles that you would like your learners to be able to apply to nursing practice when they finish your course.
2. Now, think of a real nursing practice situation in which some of those concepts are relevant.
3. Identify a nurse in practice who might be able to provide you with a real situation to use as a prototype.
4. After you collected enough information, briefly recreate the situation as it happened—but not in too much detail.
5. Outline learning goals and objectives for the situation—ensure objectives challenge the learners to develop higher order thinking skills (synthesis, evaluation, analysis).
6. Think about questions that you might ask to help learners extend this knowledge to other nursing situations—"what if" kinds of questions.
7. Repeat the process until all essential concepts have been addressed and you will have the content structure of a CBL course.

RESOURCES FOR EDUCATORS

PLANNING THE TEACHING/LEARNING EXPERIENCE

Questions to Support a Thoughtful Reading

1. What does it mean to "learn about nursing"?
2. Who is responsible for learning?
3. What does it mean to teach about nursing?
4. Do some forms of teaching foster learning more effectively than others?
5. Do I believe that learners can learn without me telling them the information?
6. Could I be comfortable with the role of tutor?

7. Can I ask questions beyond the level of knowledge recall?
8. How comfortable am I in providing constructive criticism to learners in a public forum?
9. How comfortable am I in receiving constructive criticism from learners in a public forum?

EVALUATING THE TEACHING/LEARNING EXPERIENCE

Questions to Elicit Feedback from Students on Their Learning

On a scale of 1 to 5 where 1 = strongly disagree and 5 = strongly agree, rate yourself on the following:

1. I am able to identify the essential concepts in this chapter.
2. I am motivated to learn more about these concepts.
3. I increased my knowledge about these concepts.
4. I can describe how I will use these concepts in my teaching practice.
5. I am stimulated to discuss topics raised in this chapter with other faculty.
6. I have a better understanding of the evidence that underpins CBL.
7. I have developed greater confidence in my ability to use CBL principles in my teaching practice.
8. I have developed a clearer sense of professional identity as a facilitator of learning.

References

Albanese, M., & Mitchell, S. (1993). Problem-based learning: A review of the literature on its outcomes and implementation issues. *Academic Medicine, 68*, 52–81.

Allen, D., Duch, B., & Groh, S. (1996). The power of problem-based learning in teaching introductory science courses. In L. Wilkerson & W. Gijselaers (Eds.), *Bringing problem-based learning to higher education: Theory and practice*. San Francisco: Jossey-Bass.

Barron, B., Schwartz, D., Vye, N., et al. (1998). Doing with understanding: Lessons from research on problem-based and project-based learning. *Journal of the Learning Sciences, 7*(3–4), 271–311.

Barrows, H. (1996). Problem-based learning in medicine and beyond: A brief overview. In L. Wilkerson & W. Gijselaers (Eds.), *Bringing problem-based learning to higher education: Theory and practice*. San Francisco: Jossey-Bass.

Boud, D., & Feletti, G. (1998). *The challenge of problem-based learning*. London: Kogan Page.

Boyer Commission on Educating Undergraduates in the Research University for the Carnegie Foundation for the Advancement for Teaching. (1998). *Reinventing undergraduate education: A blueprint for America's research Universities*. Retrieved on May 15, 2003 from http://notes.cc.sunysb.edu/Pres/boyer.nsf.

Bruner, J. (1960). *The process of education*. Cambridge, MA: Harvard University Press.

Craik, F., & Tulvig, E. (1975). Depth of processing and the retention of words in episodic memory. *Journal of Verbal Learning and Verbal Behavior, 11*, 671–684.

Day, R., & Williams, B. (2000). Development of critical thinking through problem-based learning: A pilot study. *Journal of Excellence in College Teaching, 11*(2–3), 203–226.

Dewey, J. (1916). *Education and democracy*. New York: Macmillan.

Dewey, J. (1938). *Logic: The theory of inquiry*. New York: Holt.

Duch, B., Groh, S., & Allen, D. (2001). *The power of problem-based learning*. Sterling, Virgina: Stylus.

Duffy, T. & Cunningham, D. (1996). Constructivism: Implications for the design and delivery of instruction. In D. Jonassen (Ed.), *Handbook of research for educational communications and technology* (pp. 170–198). New York: Simon & Schuster Macmillan.

Hesburgh, T., Miller, P., & Wharton, C. (1974). *Patterns for lifelong learning*. San Francisco: Jossey-Bass.

Ishida, D. (1995). *Learning preferences among ethnically diverse nursing learners exposed to a variety of collaborative learning approaches including problem-based learning*. Unpublished doctoral dissertation, University of Hawaii.

Jaramillo, F. (1999). We got our kicks on route 66: A PBL case study. In J. Conway, D. Melville, & A. Williams, (Eds.), *Research and development in problem-based learning*. Callahan, Australia: PROBLARC.

Kingsland, A. (1996). Time expenditure, workload, and student satisfaction in problem-based learning. In L. Wilkerson & W. Gijselaers (Eds.), *Bringing problem-based learning to higher education: Theory and practice*. San Francisco: Jossey-Bass.

Lefrancois, G. (2000). *Psychology for learning*. Belmont, CA: Wadsworth.

Newman, M. (1995). *A comparison of nursing learners in problem-based and the lecture method*. Unpublished masters thesis, University of Alberta.

Norman, G., & Schmidt, H. (1992). The psychological basis of problem-based learning. *Academic Medicine, 67*, 557–565.

Rideout, E. (1998). *The experience of learning and teaching in a non-conventional nursing curriculum*. Unpublished doctoral dissertation, University of Toronto.

Rideout, E., England-Oxford, B., Brown, B., et al. (2002). A comparison of problem-based and conventional curricula in nursing education. *Advances in Health Sciences Education, 7*(1), 3–17.

Saarinen, H., & Salvatori, P. (1994). Education of occupational and physiotherapists for the year 2000: What, no anatomy course? *Physiotherapy Canada, 46*, 81–86.

Savery, J., & Duffy, T. (1995). Problem-based learning: An instructional model and its constructivist framework. *Education Technology, 35*, 31–38.

Schmidt, H. (1983). Problem-based learning: Rationale and description. *Medical Education, 17*, 11–16.

Schmidt, H. (1993). Foundations of problem-based learning: Some explanatory notes. *Medical Education, 27*, 422–432.

Seltzer, S., Hilbert, S., Maceli, J., et al. (1996). An active approach to calculus. In L. Wilkerson & W. Gijselaers (Eds.), *Bringing problem-based learning to higher education: Theory and practice*. San Francisco: Jossey-Bass.

Skinner, B. F. (1974). *About behaviorism*. New York: Knopf.

Slavin, R. (1994). *Educational psychology*. Boston: Allyn & Bacon.

Solomon, R., & Finch, E. (1998). A qualitative study identifying stressors associated with adapting to problem-based learning. *Teaching and Learning in Medicine, 10*(2), 58–64.

Stinson, J., & Milter, R. (1996). Problem-based learning in business education. In L. Wilkerson & W. Gijselaers (Eds.), *Bringing problem-based learning to higher education: Theory and practice*. San Francisco: Jossey-Bass.

Tompkins, C. (2001). Nursing education for the twenty-first century. In L. Rideout (Ed.), *Transforming nursing education through problem-based learning* (pp. 1–19). Toronto: Jones & Bartlett.

University of Alberta Collaborative Baccalaureate Program. (2003). NURS 394 Course Outline: Edmonton, AB: University of Alberta.

Valanis, B. (2000). Professional nursing practice in an HMO: The future is now. *Journal of Nursing Education, 39*(1), 13–20.

Vernon, D., (1995). Attitudes and opinions of faculty tutors about problem-based learning. *Academic Medicine, 70*(3), 216–223.

Wilkerson, L., & Feletti, G. (1989). Problem-based learning: One approach to increasing student participation. In A. Lucus (Ed.), *The department chairperson's role in enhancing college teaching. New directions for teaching and learning* (pp. 51–60). San Francisco: Jossey-Bass.

Williams, B. (2002). *The self-directed learning readiness of baccalaureate nursing learners and faculty after one year in a problem-based undergraduate nursing program*. Unpublished doctoral dissertation, University of Alberta.

Williams, B. (2004). Self direction in a problem based learning program. *Nurse Education Today, 24*(4), 277–285.

Williams, B. (2006). Demonstrating the scholarship of teaching: A sample teaching portfolio. In L. Young & B. Paterson (Eds.), *Teaching nursing: Student centered theories, models, and strategies for nurse educators*. Philadelphia: Lippincott Williams & Wilkins.

Wingspread Conference. (1994). *Quality assurance in undergraduate education: What the public expects*. Denver: Education Commission of the States.

Woods, D. (1996). Problem-based learning for large classes in chemical engineering. In L. Wilkerson & W. M. Gijselaers (Eds.), *Bringing problem-based learning to higher education: Theory and practice*. San Francisco: Jossey-Bass.

Chapter 11

Tutoring Problem-Based Learning: A Model for Student-Centered Teaching

Angela Wolff

As a graduate of a problem-based learning baccalaureate nursing program, I never truly understood the difference between student-centered and content-centered teaching until I became an educator myself. I clearly remember standing in front of the classroom delivering a lecture on communication theory to a group of 30 students. I realized that the "chalk and talk" method delivery was not rewarding to either the students or myself. I remember thinking while lecturing: Why am I the one doing all the work? Preparing for the class? Deciding what should be learned? Telling the students what to read? Why, I wondered, are the students happy just listening to me?

When the dean of the nursing program announced a shift toward problem-based learning, I was ecstatic to have the opportunity to teach in a program based upon a student-centered model of education. However, many of my colleagues did not share my enthusiasm. Attending a professional development session on becoming a problem-based learning tutor, I observed some of the anxieties and apprehensions my colleagues were experiencing as they adopted a more student-centered approach to learning. Specifically, those new to problem-based learning were apprehensive about how the proposed model of learning would alter their current ways of teaching such as sharing control in the classroom, relinquishing their status as expert, and forming learning partnerships with students. At the same time, other faculty members were concerned about whether students would learn what was needed to practice competently. Those open to adopting the new teaching model showed concern about how to build their expertise as a tutor. Through these discussions, I began to appreciate the uncertainty my colleagues were experiencing having to teach in an entirely new way.

INTENT In this chapter, tutoring in a particular student-centered learning model, problem-based learning, is described and discussed. The **competencies** required of educators in a faculty tutor role are explored. Requisite group facilitation skills of the **faculty tutor** are addressed, in particular, guiding the student group toward deeper understandings by resolving specially prepared problems. To illustrate the competencies required of faculty tutors, the author describes various **facilitation** techniques and questioning strategies used to support student learning. Challenges faced by faculty tutors are raised including those that relate to debates about content versus process expert, type and frequency of interventions, and pedagogical shifts.

OVERVIEW

INTRODUCTION

Problem-based learning (PBL) is one educational model that drives curriculum design, educational culture, instructional delivery, and student assessment. The rationale for, and philosophy of, PBL are consistent with the changing epistemology of professional nursing practice. PBL shifts the center of the teaching/learning enterprise from teacher to student. Similarly, emerging models of nursing practice shift the center of nursing from nurse to patient or client. Further, PBL is designed to move beyond educational models that deliver content and technical knowledge. Rather, it is designed to prepare prospective registered nurses to manage rapid changes in health care, access, organize, and interpret the wealth of knowledge available and its diminished lifespan, and respond to the increasing complexity of practice. In many nursing programs, PBL plays a vital role in helping student nurses to develop the competencies required of beginning practitioners and the lifelong learning skills that can be transferred into clinical practice. Educators who are asked to shift from delivering content and technical skills to facilitating students' acquisition of knowledge-related competencies are required to make dramatic shifts in how they understand and implement their role.

Central to a PBL curriculum is small group learning. In the context of small groups, educators adopt a role as tutor, a role that is not common in traditional educational models. The values underlying the culture of small group work in PBL are **partnership**, honesty, openness, respect, and trust (Baptiste, 2003). Educators are full partners in the learning process, not the primary holders of knowledge. Within this partnership, educators strive to enable students to develop skills such as problem solving, critical thinking, group process, creativity, information literacy, and reflection that are of no particular concern to educators using the lecture as a primary teaching strategy. Since PBL actively engages students, it requires adherence to ethical principles, it promotes **inquiry-based learning**, and it is concerned not only with what students learn, but also how they learn it in a collaborative context.

CONCEPTUALIZATION OF PROBLEM-BASED LEARNING

Problem-based learning is a small-group educational philosophy characterized by goal-oriented sessions that follow a systematic process (Table 11.1) to work through a problem situation as a means of accomplishing the learning objectives. The use of an **authentic problem**, derived from clinical experience, serves as the context for students to learn clinical reasoning skills, to acquire nursing knowledge, and to integrate and apply concepts of nursing in a clinical context (Rideout & Carpio, 2001). Each specially prepared problem is presented in the form of a **scenario** that becomes the stimulus for learning and a focus of the groups' purpose for a minimum of two tutorial sessions.[1] Each scenario may be composed of three to seven parts, in which each part is printed on a separate piece of paper for distribution at different times of the PBL session.

Another unique characteristic of PBL is the people involved. Typically a group consists of five to ten learners who meet weekly or biweekly with a faculty tutor. A faculty tutor provides guidance to ensure that appropriate learning objectives (i.e., course and curriculum) and essential content are met, and to facilitate the learning process. Table 11.1 reflects the tutor's active role in facilitating group process and enhancing learning.

Furthermore, a learning environment that is student-centered characterizes PBL. As such, the acquisition and understanding of new information occurs through **self-directed learning**. Students' self-directed learning time is the period between the problem presentation and the problem discussion meetings. An allocated amount of time for **independent learning** is distinctive to PBL. Evaluation of learning outcomes

[1] In most instances, each PBL problem situation consists of three to five tutorial sessions to allow sufficient time for presenting the problem situation, discussing the new information sought to satisfy the identified learning issues, and evaluating the session.

TABLE 11.1 TUTOR ROLES BY THE STEPS OF THE PBL PROCESS

STEPS OF THE PBL PROCESS	TUTOR ROLES
1. Present the problem situation to the group. Interact with each other to explore existing knowledge as it relates to the problem and to clarify and review terms.	Urge application of prior knowledge, provide corrective feedback, and facilitate group process.
2. Brainstorm to generate hypotheses and identify issues. Use prior knowledge and experience. List the phenomena to be explained.	Stimulate inquiry and critical thinking through the use of thought-provoking open-ended questions. Facilitate group process and encourage participation.
3. Identify learning gaps, prioritize learning needs, set learning goals and objectives, and identify possible resources to utilize.	Facilitate the identification of learning gaps and learning goals. Question plans for seeking information and suggest alternatives. Ensure students leave with a clear direction.
4. Undertake self-study between group meetings and gather information.	Be accessible for consultation.
5. Critically discuss and debate the information acquired with your group. Share new knowledge.	Judge adequacy of information sources. Debate the information being presented and compare it with prior knowledge of the subject. Ensure discussion is at a level of rigor, depth, and breadth appropriate for the stage of the group. Challenge students by asking for fuller explanations, for clarification of points made, and for links with other new and prior knowledge.
6. Apply knowledge to the problem in a practical way.	Facilitate integration of knowledge obtained and appraise clinical reasoning. Ask metacognitive questions to ensure that the problem is examined in sufficient depth and breadth. Pursue hypotheses acceptance or rejection.
7. Repeat steps 2 to 6 as necessary (or with the introduction of additional parts of the scenario).	Facilitate integration of expanded problem and evaluate plans for seeking information.
8. Reflect on the content and process of learning.	Initiate evaluation and model self-assessment. Reflect on the content and process of learning. Summarize and integrate learning into the student's existing knowledge, skills, and attitudes. Review what has been learned from the exploration of the problem.

for both individuals and the group is an integral part of each PBL session (Benson, Noesgaard, & Drummond-Young, 2001). For further information about the educational objectives of PBL and the evidence for determining the effectiveness of the PBL model refer to Chapter 10.

SMALL GROUP LEARNING IN PROBLEM-BASED LEARNING

The PBL model of small group learning places students at the center of the learning experience by giving them a framework to find and evaluate information, discuss and debate it, and determine its applicability to the problem situation. Within the small group learning environment, group members consciously and conscientiously strive to achieve particular learning outcomes. Students examine meaningful problem situations with other learners under the guidance of a faculty tutor. Learning in a small group provides a simulated environment for group problem solving allowing the learners to:

- Compare learning performance with peers.
- Develop a sense of responsibility for their learning progress.
- Learn more about human interaction, develop interpersonal skills, and become aware of one's own emotional reactions.
- Develop maturity and **decision-making skills** as a function of independent learning.
- Learn how to listen, receive criticism, and give accurate and candid feedback to each other; and facilitate self-evaluation (Neufeld and Barrows, 1974 as cited by Benson, Noesgaard, & Drummond-Young, 2001).

Cognitive mind mapping, a creative method of visually displaying prior knowledge and group learning issues, is a more recent educational strategy adopted by tutorial groups to facilitate small group learning (Box 11.1). For more information on integrating mind mapping techniques in small group learning situations, and their differentiation from concept mapping, refer to Buzan and Buzan (1998), All and Havens (1997), and Daley (1996). See Chapter 2 for a visual example of a mind map.

Differences between PBL and other small group learning approaches (e.g., case method) relate to the:

- Problem being presented prior to the students having learned basic knowledge.
- Problem being presented in progressive stages stimulating the students to seek additional information.
- Construction of knowledge within a specific context.
- Collaborative student-centered learning environment.
- Tutoring role of the educator (Baker, 2000).

BOX 11.1 COGNITIVE MIND MAPPING

Mapping techniques are used to provide a visual display of the students' ideas and their interpretation of the concepts pertaining to the problem situation. The emphasis is placed on the understanding and linking of ideas, as opposed to memorization. This technique helps people learn and builds on the prior knowledge of the learner. Mapping techniques can be used at any step of the PBL process in addition to note taking, studying, and project planning.

Adapted from Buzan, T., & Buzan, B. (1998). *The mind map book*. London: BBC Books.

PHILOSOPHICAL UNDERPINNINGS OF PROBLEM-BASED LEARNING

Constructivist views on learning theory underpin the PBL model of education in that knowledge is constructed by the learner based on previous knowledge and worldview. The center of teaching is shifted from the teacher to the student by adopting an andragogical philosophy of adult learning[2] that focuses on student-directed or self-directed learning. As such, the educator is not viewed as the primary holder of knowledge but rather a partner in the learning process. Since small group work is the cornerstone of the PBL model, the educator takes on a tutor role. The educator fulfilling the tutor role begins with the experience of the student and together they build competencies necessary for professional practice. In this role, the educator actively engages the learners to develop lifelong learning skills. Based on the tenets of constructivism, the faculty tutor of these small groups facilitate learning by providing students with opportunities to construct knowledge in the context of social environments, not simply facilitating them to obtain it (Brooks & Brooks, 1993).

Consistent with cognitive and social constructivist epistemology, the theoretical underpinnings of PBL are based on four principles:

1. Activating prior knowledge, elaborating knowledge, and restructuring knowledge are requisites for the processing of new knowledge.
2. Students interact with the environment which mirrors that of clinical practice to gain a better understanding of a particular situation.
3. Meaningful learning experiences foster the development of creative intelligence.
4. Activities and experiences of the learner are guided by more capable or knowledgeable persons (David & Patel, 1995; Rideout & Carpio, 2001; Savery & Duffy, 1995).

For more information about these principles the reader is referred to Chapter 10. Based on the constructivist propositions, Table 11.2 provides a list of instructional principles that can guide the tutor's teaching practices and set the tone for the learning environment.

THE FACULTY TUTOR ROLE IN PROBLEM-BASED LEARNING

The faculty tutor role is central to PBL. As such, there is consensus that adoption of that role requires a profound reframing of the assumptions and fundamental beliefs about learning and teaching. To be effective, faculty enacting the PBL tutor role must depart from the more didactic 'chalk and talk' approach to the classroom that emphasizes the dissemination of information, and become facilitators of learning. The role of the facilitator varies within the literature from a practical, task-driven role of "doing for others" to a more complex, multifaceted role of "enabling others" (Burrows, 1997). These role definitions depend on the underlying purpose and interpretation of facilitation in the context in

[2] Based on the work of Knowles (1975), who proposed the term androgogy in reference to the philosophy of adult education as the art and science of helping adults learn.

TABLE 11.2 CONSTRUCTIVISM AND ITS IMPLICATIONS FOR PBL TUTORS

INSTRUCTIONAL PRINCIPLES BASED ON CONSTRUCTIVIST PROPOSITIONS	IMPLICATION FOR PBL TUTORS
Purposefully connect all learning activities to a larger problem situation (context).	• During the eight-step PBL process, the tutor provides assistance to the students, as needed, to connect their learning activities to the specific problem situation. The tutor assists students to understand the relevance of the specific learning activity in the context of the bigger picture. • Tutors need to design authentic problems embedded with triggers to achieve the specified course and program learning objectives.
Guide and support the learner to accept responsibility for the overall problem situation.	• Assist students to see the relevance of the paper problem to nursing practice. • Allow students to develop their own learning goals and outcomes within the context of the course objectives. • As a stimulus for learning, collect problem situations from the learners or establish authentic problems in such a way that the students are motivated to adopt the problem as their own.
Design authentic problem situations.	• Problems designed by curriculum-developers for students in the learning environment should mirror those that the students will encounter in professional practice. Real problems engage the learners and create personal relevance.
Design the problem situations and learning environment to reflect the complexity of the practice environment that they should be able to function in at the end of learning.	• The tutor supports the students to work in the complex environment of professional practice. Using appropriately complex problem situations the tutor assists the students to develop their metacognitive skills and directs their decision-making skills (Wee, Kek, & Sim, 2002). • Following the steps of the PBL process requires the students to go through the same activities during learning that are valued in the real world. As such, educators need to craft problems situations that are current, relevant, and assist students to attain the exit outcomes expected of graduates (Wee, et al., 2002).
Provide an opportunity for the learner to take ownership of the process used to develop a solution to the problem situation.	• Tutors must strike a balance between directing the learning and allowing for experiential learning. • To surrender authority, the PBL tutor allows students to take ownership of the PBL process and resolution of the problem situation itself. • The students are freely encouraged to identify the learning resources they wish to use to achieve the identified learning goals.
Create a learning environment to support and challenge the learner in becoming a critical thinker.	• The tutor, as consultant and coach, provides support to the students by posing inquiring questions that challenge the students' thinking. • The students generate learning issues or objectives based on their analysis of the problem situation. Also, they decide which information resources to access to support their inquiry. Returning from self-study, students reflect upon the usefulness of the accessed resources. • The tutor establishes a group climate that allows for a cognitive apprenticeship of critical thinking skills.

(continued)

■ TABLE 11-2 Constructivism and its Implications for PBL Tutors (continued)

INSTRUCTIONAL PRINCIPLES BASED ON CONSTRUCTIVIST PROPOSITIONS	IMPLICATION FOR PBL TUTORS
Provide an opportunity for the testing of ideas against alternative views and alternative contexts.	• During a group session, each student needs to have an opportunity to verbally reflect on his or her beliefs about the problem situation and assume responsibility for particular learning issues that are identified. • Tutors facilitate the learning process in such a way that other points of view are considered relative to the students understanding. Each student's ideas are heard and considered in the resolution of the problem situation. Similar and conflicting opinions among group members are encouraged and debated.
Allow time for, and encouragement of, reflection on both the content learned and the learning process.	• Throughout the learning process the tutor models both reflection on action and reflection in action. As well, the tutor supports the students in reflection on the group process in addition to what was learned. Time is dedicated to both peer and self-evaluation of the overall process.

Adapted from Savery, J. R., & Duffy, T. (1995). Problem-based learning: An instructional model and its constructivist framework. *Educational Technology, 33*(5), 31–38.

which it is applied. In PBL, the purpose of facilitation is to enable students (within tutorial groups) to analyze, reflect, and change their own attitudes, behaviors, and ways of thinking (Harvey, et al., 2002). To do this, PBL tutors implement actions such as:

- Questioning student logic, values, and beliefs.
- Assisting students to clarify their learning needs and to select resources for self-study.
- Facilitating student discussion, group process, and evaluation.
- Nurturing students' ability to think critically.
- Encouraging inquiry and decision-making skills.
- Fostering habits of continued learning.

Faculty tutors support students to think for themselves and to trust their own problem-solving skills. In contrast to a task-specific focus of facilitation, the enabling perspective is holistic in nature, seeking to address a problem in the context of the whole situation and the whole person (Burrows, 1997).

The transition from expert to facilitator requires the learning of new skills, making some important shifts in teaching behaviors, and a willingness to examine one's beliefs and values about authority, control, teacher–student relationships, and the ego rewards of teaching. While some faculty may find relinquishing their status as expert and sharing control in the classroom a cause for uncertainty, those who embrace PBL approaches discover a sense of freedom and relationships that are empowering to students and rewarding to faculty. As such, the adoption of PBL has profound implications regarding the educator role of faculty as facilitator. Faculty tutor roles discussed in this section are applicable to PBL and context-based learning as well as other forms of small group learning that involve the act of facilitation.

Meaning of Facilitation

The purpose of facilitation is to create an environment in which students are free to define and advance their own learning. To provide this type of learning experience, the PBL tutor engages in the act of facilitation. The dictionary definition of facilitation refers to the process of enabling or making things easier for others (Harvey, et al., 2002). In the context of PBL, this quote by a student illustrates the nature of facilitation:

> *Having a facilitator was a wonderful experience. Somebody who would support you but encourage you to be responsible for your own learning. Who encouraged reflection and ultimately personal and professional growth; who recognized all group members and promoted a functional group. (Katz, 1995, p. 52)*

For the purposes of this chapter, facilitation is defined as "a goal-oriented dynamic process, in which participants work together in an atmosphere of genuine mutual respect, in order to learn through critical reflection" (Burrows, 1997, p. 401). Many of the defining characteristics of facilitation (Box 11.2) are congruent with the principles of PBL and student-centered learning. Facilitated learning values process equally with content, emphasizing the development of self-direction and inquiry skills.

In keeping with the tenets of constructivism, facilitation then embraces the partnership between PBL tutors and students as they work together to learn personally and professionally (Burrows, 1997). Such partnerships should reflect the intentions of openness and honesty. Those involved in the learning partnerships need to view one another in a collegial and collaborative way. As learning partners, facilitators are part of the same system as the students; both have the same desired outcomes and both adopt various teacher and learner roles. Within the learning partnership, the facilitator fosters and encourages leadership behaviors among the students. Using a democratic form of group leadership, the tutor and student members negotiate their respective leadership roles. In some instances, the facilitator is quite clearly the leader, while in others they may not be (Katz, 1995). While the facilitator is centrally placed as the group leader in terms of making curriculum decisions, Williams (2004) reminds us that when students are guided to become self-directed, they may become overwhelmed, anxious, and frustrated. As a partner in learning, tutors need to gauge the type of guidance and support required of students. **Learning plans** are a tool that may be useful for assisting students to identify their learning goals (Burrows, 1997).

For facilitation to be effective, respect toward students must be authentic and reciprocal in nature. Mutual respect, in addition to shared power, reciprocity, and openness

BOX 11.2 FOUR DEFINING CHARACTERISTICS OF FACILITATION

1. Partnership.
2. Genuine mutual respect.
3. Dynamic goal-oriented process.
4. Critical reflection.

are essential in the development of the student–teacher relationship in PBL. The attitudes of all group members, students and tutors alike, must be congruent with their behavior. For tutors, genuine mutual respect can be achieved by establishing an open learning climate that provides a safe place for students to express their thoughts and feelings. Tutors create a respectful environment that allows for the sharing of tentative hypotheses and opinions, the acknowledgement of positive and negative contributions, the objective exploration of mistakes without demeaning the personal integrity of individual group members, the view that risk taking and errors are part of the learning process, and the expression of uncertainty or sudden insight (Burrows, 1997). In this type of learning environment, collaborative effort is valued and understood. How the informal rules of the group are created within an environment provides cues and clues to how the group will function. Establishing a respectful, trusting, and supportive learning environment is made easier if the facilitator approaches it with a basic understanding of group process and group dynamics. An understanding of the different types of groups, their structures and processes, is a requisite for effective facilitation (Katz, 1995). It has been the author's experience in working with students who have completed other PBL courses that time should be taken during the first session to discuss their previous experience, their likes and dislikes, and their expectations for this new course. This introductory session is also time for the faculty member to share expectations about respect toward you and their peers.

As a proactive and dynamic process, the practice of facilitation requires that tutors act as a catalyst to engage students in their learning (Burrows, 1997). Throughout the **goal-oriented process** of facilitation the tutor ensures that appropriate learning objectives (i.e., course and curriculum) are met and essential content is embedded in the students' plan for subsequent learning. Given the dynamic nature of facilitation, the skills utilized and roles enacted by tutors are situation and context specific. Some common actions used by facilitators to guide students through the PBL process include assisting with goal identification, encouraging investigation, establishing a climate conducive to motivating students, giving meaning to activities, challenging thinking, supporting the application of new knowledge, suggesting appropriate resources, and sharing their knowledge and experiences to enlighten the discussion.

Through critical reflection, the goals of scientific inquiry and experiential learning are achieved. In a supportive group environment that displays genuine mutual respect and trust, group members are comfortable to be challenged and to challenge each other. Acting as a role model, the tutor facilitates PBL sessions by promoting strategies of questioning, probing, and debating so that with increasing experience and confidence students are able to take risks and to question their own and other's assumptions, thoughts, and attitudes. For tutors and students alike, skills of self-evaluation and critical reflection enable growth, maximize learning, and promote self-direction (Burrows, 1997).

In addition to the four defining characteristics of facilitation, there are several prerequisites that need to be in place for the process of facilitation to occur: (a) two or more people are voluntarily participating[3] within a learning situation; (b) all

[3] The author acknowledges that while student participation is a requirement of PBL courses, it is the individual's decision as to when and how they participate within any given learning situation.

group members acknowledge that learning is not taught; (c) the tutor possesses effective interpersonal skills and has the ability to gain insight from his or her experiences; and (d) all participants of the group have a common understanding of what facilitation is and how it can be implemented. When starting with a new group, it is advantageous to spend some time establishing the ground rules, group expectations, and roles and responsibilities of all group members. All antecedents must be in place to ensure success of the facilitation process and to reduce student anxiety and frustration (Burrows, 1997).

Essential to the success of the PBL model is effective facilitation. Facilitation and the facilitated learning experience refer to a process of teaching/learning that requires a philosophical reframing of the role of the teacher and alters the student–teacher relationship (Katz, 1995). As the PBL tutor adopts an enabling role as facilitator he or she becomes a colearner within the group, delegating and sharing responsibility with the students. As such, control shifts to the students. Consistent with the goals of PBL, when a tutor is successful in facilitating a group, the students become active, motivated, and self-directed learners. With such successes within a group, there is a greater sense that optimal learning has occurred (Burrows, 1997). Overall, PBL facilitators of small group learning have a vital role to play in helping (enabling) students to integrate theory with practice. Moreover, the faculty tutor is responsible for providing clear task and goal structures, orientating students to group learning, allowing individual choice in group assignments, establishing a climate conducive to motivating learners, taking a personal interest in the learners, and influencing group work activities (Benson, et al., 2001; Rideout & Carpio, 2001). Table 11.3 outlines the roles the faculty tutor adopts in the act of facilitation within the PBL model.

Student and Faculty Perceptions of the Faculty Tutor Role

Both student and faculty perspectives have been explored regarding the importance of the faculty tutor role in the PBL model and strategies for successful enactment of the role. There is significant congruence between these two groups about the behaviors and strategies that are valued. Students describe the tutor role as crucial to effective learning in PBL tutorials. This was made abundantly clear in a study by Rideout (1999), where students in a PBL program provided the following comments on the role and influence of the tutor:

> *I think the tutors are vital in moving the group and having us cover things that are important because tutors know better than [we do] what is important and what we should be getting out of this. (p. 174)*
>
> *The tutors' role was certainly that of guidance for the group. (p. 174)*
>
> *The tutors' role is to make sure we don't miss the big things and to redirect us if we got off topic. (p. 174)*
>
> *The group was good because of the tutor. (She) helped us identify our own issues; if someone was standing back she would help us deal with it. She facilitated. (p. 175)*

TABLE 11.3 FACILITATOR ROLES

ROLE	DESCRIPTION
Modeling	Faculty tutors model the performance expected of students in PBL. For example, tutors model metacognitive thinking/problem solving by demonstrating questioning techniques that are used as part of the facilitative learning process. By guiding the students with questions, the tutor contributes to the productivity of the group. By modeling, the tutor's questions will give the students an awareness of what questions they should be asking themselves as they tackle the problem. During the evaluation process, tutors may take a more directive approach in modeling their ability to provide frank, open, and constructive feedback. The quality of the learning process in a small group is dependent on the quality of input of all members, including the tutor.
Challenger	As challenger, faculty tutors adopt a role similar to that of devil's advocate. Tutors use questioning skills to challenge students' beliefs and invite them to substantiate their points of view. Students are encouraged to analyze and question each other as well. When seeking responses from students, tutors must allow wait time to allow students time to develop their arguments.
Negotiator and mediator	Negotiation is referred to as "overcoming obstacles skillfully." Faculty tutors become guides who negotiate meaning and probe the limits of the students' understanding. During hypothesis generation, tutors moderate student debates and facilitate student–student interaction. Uncertainty and conflict are seen as important positive aspects of learning. When appropriate, tutors step in to mediate unresolved disputes.
Director	The role of the director is to coax student thinking in a focused and persevering manner so that the problem situation of study is explored in detail. Faculty tutors need to emphasize the depth of student learning by keeping students focused on a few central ideas while concurrently considering the breadth of the scenario. The identification of main ideas or concepts in relation to stated student-learning needs enables tutors to give direction to the learning sequence.
Learner	One of the major differences from the traditional lecture format is that faculty tutors and students both accept that neither has all the answers. However, faculty tutors have differing levels of comfort in admitting that they do not hold all the answers. While students tend to praise tutors for adopting an attitude of learning along with them, some tutors fear loss of their students' respect if their lack of content expertise is discovered. Realistically it is virtually impossible to find faculty tutors who are truly expert in all aspects of the course content.
Evaluator	Reflection and evaluation are a component of each PBL session. As such, faculty tutors are required to have the skills necessary to evaluate individual (i.e., student and tutor) and group functioning, and provide constructive feedback accordingly.
Activator and listener	A balance between activity and listening is essential. Both students and faculty tutors must remain active in the learning process. As an active participant, the tutor strives to provide an environment that is motivating to students and engages them through questioning. A vital point is not how much the tutor talks (within reason); but that the tutor makes a considered decision when to interject and when to hold back. At the same time, tutors listen to student concerns.

Adapted from: Barrows, H. S. (1988). *The tutorial process.* Springfield, IL: Southern Illinois University School of Medicine; Holmes, D. B., & Kaufman, D. M. (1994). Tutoring in problem-based learning: A teacher development process. *Medical Education, 28*(4), 275–283; Mayo, W. P., Donnelly, M. B., & Schwartz, R. W. (1995). Characteristics of the ideal problem-based learning tutor in clinical medicine. *Evaluation and the Health Professions, 18*, 124–136; Wilkerson, L., & Hundert, E. M. (1991). Becoming a problem-based tutor: Increasing self-awareness thorough faculty development. In D. Boud & G. Feletti, (Eds.), *The challenge of problem-based learning* (pp. 159–171). London: Kogan Page.

Similar comments are evident when students describe the tutor role as facilitating the group rather than leading it; for example helping to keep the group focused. The tutor does a considerable amount of silent work by attending to group process and assisting the group to keep the discussion focused on the problem situation. The faculty tutors direct involvement with the group discussion, and students find the tutors' presence comforting (Rideout, 1999).

Faculty tutors also described their role as that of guide and advocate. Fulfilling such a facilitative role, the faculty tutor is there to help students bridge their pre-existing knowledge with new information; challenge students to explore issues in depth; ensure students develop correct and current information; and set standards of achievement. To do this, tutors intervene in the PBL process by implementing actions such as: (a) asking questions to broaden the scope of investigation of issues, to ensure accuracy of information, or to steer the group in the right direction; (b) helping the group to establish standards and checking in with students when inconsistencies are noted; (c) dealing with problematic group dynamics; (d) acting as a resource to the group; and (e) encouraging group reflection to evaluate individual and group performance (Haith-Cooper, 2003; Rideout, 1999).

Faculty also described the importance of letting students know you know what they are talking about and challenging students if they have incorrect information. They also acknowledged that all this must take place within a supportive environment, in an atmosphere of trust and caring facilitated by the tutor. Similar descriptions were reported by authors such as Stinson and Milter (1996) who noted the teacher observes, corrects, and encourages the performance of students, and Gijselaers (1996) who described the role as "a balance between allowing the students to discuss issues and intervening to make sure that critical issues are identified" (p. 19). While it is generally agreed that it is the tutor's role to intervene in the PBL process, there are conflicting opinions regarding the level of intervention and the timing at which intervention is required (Haith-Cooper, 2000).

The need to adapt the role to the level of student has also been acknowledged (Haith-Cooper, 2000). Words like coaching, cajoling, and guiding were used to describe the role in interactions with beginning students, while collaborating, relinquishing control, and becoming more of a mentor were the role expectations in the senior year of the program. These role descriptions mirror those of Barrows (1988) who spoke of the role change as one that moved from modeling to coaching to fading. The words of students are perhaps most informative on this issue (Rideout, 1999):

> *I saw the tutor as a very strong role in guiding and learning. They coached and cajoled you, especially in first year. (p. 174)*
>
> *The tutor became more of a collaborator with the student. By fourth year the tutor totally backed off, they never told you what to do, it was more what did you do today and where do you want to go from here? (p. 174)*
>
> *In second year she took on leadership roles. In fourth year she was willing to relinquish control. She was a great role model. (p. 175)*

In addition to the roles that faculty fulfill within the tutorial group setting, they also adopt a number of other roles related to curriculum design and scenario development issues. To effectively fulfill the facilitative role, other faculty tutor qualities must be considered. Such qualities will be discussed in the following section.

Effective and Ineffective Faculty Tutor Behaviors

Various personal and professional qualities characteristic of helpful tutors, in addition to the type and degree of expertise, have been noted in the literature. Not surprisingly, the positive and negative tutor actions described are similar to those identified in the extensive literature that describes more or less desirable faculty behaviors in nonPBL curricula (Cust, 1996; Reilly & Oermann, 1999; Wong & Wong, 1987). Mayo, Donnelly, and Schwartz (1995) suggest that the effective or outstanding faculty tutors demonstrate the ability and patience to listen to students. Since tutors who intervene too quickly to provide direct answers can short circuit the entire learning process, effective tutors must possess the fortitude not to give the answers prematurely or force personal views when students fumble. Furthermore, skilled tutors support the group in choosing a course of action and guide them through the steps of the PBL process. They keep the dialogue focused, ask thought-provoking questions, provide constructive feedback that focuses on behaviors rather than personality traits, and act as role models by illustrating their ability to apply the principles of PBL.

Effective tutors relinquish control to the students by fostering a climate in which students actively learn in a manner that aims to motivate while liberating students to learn on their own. Another essential quality of effective tutors is the ability to engage in reflection to gain insight and improvement in their tutoring practices. PBL tutors recognize their success by the action of the PBL group; that is, the tutorial group can function independently or with minimal guidance (Barrows, 1988).

Two other desirable qualities of helpful tutors relate to clinical expertise and the student–teacher interactions. First, faculty tutors are considered helpful when they demonstrate knowledge and expertise, including being up-to-date clinically (Rideout, 1999). Williams (2004) found that students transitioning into PBL required tutors to be confident in their role, credible as a professional, and consistent in their tutoring behaviors. Pang, et al. (2002) also noted that students appreciated faculty tutors who shared their nursing experiences with them so they could better grasp clinical realities as they addressed the issues raised in the problem scenarios. Second, effective tutors interact with students enthusiastically. Such tutors take an interest in students and their learning; demonstrate empathy, patience, and flexibility; and provide ongoing support. Conversely, ineffective faculty tutors are described as being severe and harsh in their student–tutor interactions (e.g., being outspoken, abrupt, critical, and/or rigid) (Rideout, 1999).

Several writers have identified tutor qualities and behaviors that hindered the learning process. DesMarchais (1991) reported that students identified such tutors as those who did not intervene and/or those who seemed unconcerned with group process. Kaufman and Holmes (1996) recount tutor weaknesses in managing group process, including being too directive, letting the group get off topic, being disrespectful to students, and having no sense of humor. Similarly, Rideout (1999) described ineffective tutors as those who demonstrate a lack of sufficient engagement with students (e.g., being disorganized, wishy-washy, not punctual, too laid back, inconsistent and subjective; and not dealing with issues of group process). The situations described below exemplify the behaviors perceived by students as negative for learning:

> *She is very intense, and a lot of "you don't know this or that," a lot of constructive criticism and not very much that was good. I need to be told I am doing something well also. (Rideout, 1999, p. 175)*
>
> *We were very on edge, trying to figure out what she wanted. . . . The group was stressful and the whole atmosphere was very tense. (Rideout, 1999, p. 175)*
>
> *I have been in groups where the tutor was very directive and we ended up doing something we didn't feel was important. In that kind of environment we ended up feeling frustrated and dreading the next class. (Rideout, 1999, p. 175)*
>
> *We were left to do a lot on our own and not given much incentive to get moving. (Rideout, 1999, p. 175)*
>
> *She could have been a little more active, it took us so long to get going, and she could have given us a few more suggestions. (Rideout, 1999, p. 175)*

Content Versus Process Expertise

The voices of students and faculty tutors indicate that a broad range of behaviors and skills are required for effective and enjoyable learning to occur. While there is some support for the contention that tutors should have content expertise, the research comparing students' performance guided by content expert[4] and noncontent expert tutors reveals contradictory findings. As such, in the 1990s researchers shifted their attention on the differential influence of content and process expertise on the success of the tutorial/learning process (De Grave, Dolmans, & van der Vleuten, 1999; Eagle, Harasym, & Mandin, 1992; Kaufman & Holmes, 1996; Schmidt, van der Arend, Moust, Kokx, & Boon, 1993; Silver & Wilkerson, 1991).

In general, these studies demonstrated that tutors lacking content expertise tend to use their process facilitation expertise more to guide the tutorial group. Conversely, content expert tutors took a more directive role in the tutorials, speaking more often and for longer periods, and providing more direct answers. Moreover, groups led by content experts devoted more time to teacher-led activities and generated twice as many student-learning issues (Davis, Nairn, Paine, Anderson, & Oh, 1992; Eagle, et al., 1992). Consequently, students spent approximately twice as much self-study time per problem scenario to overcome identified learning needs (Schmidt, et al., 1993). Researchers in this field of study concluded that the use of content expert tutors resulted in more teacher-directed discussion, which is at odds with the educational philosophy and benefits of student-directed interaction on learning outcomes. Further evidence from process-oriented studies

[4] Content expert refers to a tutor who has a suitable knowledge base with regards to the discipline being studied by students which could be derived from education and/or experience.

also led researchers to conclude that that subject matter knowledge and process facilitation skills "are intimately intertwined in the behaviors of effective tutors and that both contribute to the learning of students" (Schmidt, et al., 1993, p. 790).

Given the complexity of the PBL learning environment, inconclusive findings from process-oriented studies led some researchers to investigate the dynamic influence of various contextual factors[5] on tutor behavior, regardless of content expertise (Dolmans, et al., 2002). Conclusions drawn from this body of research indicated, "a tutor's performance is not a stable teaching characteristic, but is rather situation specific . . . a tutor's performance may be partly tutor-specific and partly situation-specific" (Dolmans, et al., 2002, p. 177). This finding is consistent with the literature that describes the performance of neophyte clinical teachers (Wolff, 1998). As neophyte clinical teachers deal with the role change and develop expertise as an educator, they rely on their content expertise as clinicians. Conversely, expert clinical teachers utilize both content knowledge and pedagogical expertise in various ways depending on the contextual and situational factors.

Overall, the study findings and the related literature support the conclusion that a variety of group situations encountered by a PBL tutor requires a combination of expertise in content knowledge and group process to ensure optimal learning for students and satisfaction for tutors. Students learn best when tutors combined content expertise with personal qualities that created an atmosphere for learning, namely a commitment to students' learning and an ability to express oneself in a language understood by students (Schmidt & Moust, 1995). Moreover, the development and maintenance of a PBL tutor's **competence** is characterized as being a dynamic process that is influenced by a number of contextual and situational variables. As variables are altered within the learning context, the expertise required unfolds in a unique and complex manner. Given the complex nature of the PBL tutorial environment, further evidence is necessary to learn about the influence of contextual and situational factors on tutor behavior. Also absent from the literature is the investigation of the developmental process that faculty experience as they deal with the transition to the PBL tutor role.

COMPETENCIES REQUIRED OF EDUCATORS IN A FACILITATOR TUTORING ROLE

Two decades of research has provided inconclusive findings regarding the mix and relative importance of the core competencies needed for the successful performance of the PBL tutor. As previously established, a central function of PBL tutors is facilitation. Performing competently in this role the ideal tutor must possess the capabilities required to enable and support the learners. To function effectively, facilitators possess a range of **knowledge**, **skills**, **attitudes**, and **judgments** that are employed according to the needs of the context and environment in which they are working (Harvey, et al., 2002). Depending on the contextual and situational circumstances, faculty tutors use various resources that enable students to learn and groups to function. While some may

[5] For example, the quality of the problem scenario, the structure of the PBL courses, the link with students' level of prior knowledge, the structure of the curriculum, the functioning of tutorial groups, the length of time fulfilling the role as PBL tutor, and so on (Dolmans, et al., 2002).

mistakenly believe that the role of the facilitator is somehow reduced to that of a peripheral consultant, it is clear that the role of the tutor involves many skill sets (e.g., sound application of the principles and practices of PBL, knowledge of group dynamics, comfort with nontraditional forms of student assessment, the design of learning resources, and the management of group tasks to meet objectives within a given time frame) (Baptiste, 2003). A wealth of literature exists which highlight the specific strategies and skills used when starting a PBL session and in facilitating PBL groups (Rideout, 2001). Absent from the literature is the identification of the core competencies necessary for and demonstrated by competent PBL tutors. This section will present some tentative core tutor competencies alluded to in the literature. Specific facilitation techniques and questioning strategies related to these competencies will be further delineated. For the purpose of this chapter, competence is defined as the dynamic process of integrating and applying knowledge, skills, attitudes, and judgment required to perform safely within the scope of an educator's role (Wolff, 1998).

Core Competencies

The core competencies outlined in Box 11.3 provide a tentative list of the knowledge, skills, attitudes, and judgment required of educators to competently perform as PBL tutors. Experience has shown that the PBL tutor must possess knowledge and skills in three areas. The first area consists of knowledge and skill relating to the procedure of the PBL process. That is, how to establish the learning climate, how to plan a tutorial session, how to keep the learning process moving, and how to intervene when necessary. The ability to work through the steps of the tutorial process calls for the tutor to be able to involve all students in the discussion and keep the discussion focused on the problem. Second, the tutor requires a degree of knowledge and skill to help students acquire well-developed **metacognitive skills** to monitor, critique, and direct the development of their reasoning skills for professional practice. The tutor assists students to acquire metacognitive skills by encouraging them to hypothesize, justify, experiment, and question their reasoning process. To do this, tutors rely heavily on the use of nondirective, open-ended questions. The third set of tutor competencies that are cognitive and psychomotor in nature are those related to the managing of the interpersonal dynamics among group members. Being sensitive to cues of disharmony or ineffectiveness in a group is crucial to managing these problems. Strong interpersonal and communication skills are a prerequisite requirement of any facilitator (Barrows, 1988).

The attitudes guiding the behavior of PBL tutors are those consistent with student-centered learning and constructivism. The faculty tutor is not an authority on the information being learned; rather, the tutor takes on a facilitative role to guide student learning while adhering to the principles of the PBL process. As such, tutors focus on the learners, what they bring to the learning situation, and how their needs may be met in the context of small group learning. Shared power, reciprocity, trust, partnerships, openness, honesty, and respect are essential in the development of the student–teacher relationship in PBL. Not only do faculty tutors need to believe that PBL will work, they need to trust that their feelings of uncertainty that accompany the transition to PBL will result in a change for the betterment of the nursing profession.

BOX 11.3 COMPETENCIES REQUIRED OF PBL TUTORS

KNOWLEDGE AND SKILL

- Applies learning theory to establish a supportive learning environment.
- Promotes efficient group functioning by assisting the group to set goals, create a plan, and attend to group process.
- Understands the stage of group development and group roles.
- Applies the basic principles of therapeutic communication.
- Stimulates inquiry, problem-solving, and critical thinking through the use of questioning techniques, responding to cues, avoiding lecturing, and designing problem situations.
- Assists students to identify their strengths and weaknesses.
- Encourages students' expression of feelings, thoughts, opinions, and ideas.
- Explores students' understanding.
- Urges the application of prior knowledge and identifying gaps in prior knowledge.
- Stimulates elaboration by asking questions for clarification and aiding in-depth brainstorming.
- Assists with the identification of learning resources to consider and access.
- Challenges students to assist with the analysis, integration, and application of new knowledge to the problem situation.
- Stimulates students' integration of new acquired knowledge with knowledge acquired with previous problem situations with the same course.
- Assists with the critique of resources used by students during self-study period.
- Manages the group process and attends to issues that may arise.
- Coaches students to become self-directed in their learning.
- Helps students to become collaborative learners.
- Supports students to apply the knowledge gained during self-study to explain the phenomena described in the problem situation.
- Models the desired behaviors of students.
- Summarizes the discussion for the students.
- Provides constructive feedback on a continuing basis.
- Promotes learning of each student and encourages individual participation.
- Guides discussions to review the learning outcomes from the exploration of the problem situation.
- Fosters student interaction while they report back to the group about the findings from self-study.
- Ensures group member accountability.
- Coordinates formative and summative evaluations to assess performances of the student, the group, and the tutor.
- Initiates, maintains, and terminates professional student–tutor relationships.
- Utilizes a student-centered approach.
- Implements PBL principles.
- Probes the students' thinking to determine what internal metacognitive ideas drive the external activities of the students.
- Ensures that all students are involved in the group process.
- Implements conflict resolution skills. ➔

BOX 11.3 Competencies Required of PBL Tutors (continued)

ATTITUDE

- Students are active participants of the learning process; as such they are able to make decisions about their learning.
- Teaches according to the PBL principles and practices.
- Trust that PBL works.
- Responsibility for learning is shared; the teacher relinquishes control and authority.
- Students take responsibility for learning, creating partnerships with teachers.
- Nonjudgmental toward, and respectful of, students.
- Self-awareness of own beliefs, values, and reactions to PBL and students' learning choices.
- Values the diversity in others.
- Students themselves construct knowledge, rather than it being transferred from one individual to another.
- Students are active participants in identifying their own learning needs and pursuing the needed knowledge and skills.
- Knowledge is acquired and applied in a variety of contexts.
- Teachers relinquish control of teaching and join in partnerships with the learners in a mutual journey of exploration.
- Demonstrates awareness of strengths, areas for development, and personal preferences.

JUDGMENT

- Shares knowledge as appropriate to foster group productivity.
- Ensures that student discussions are at the level of rigor, depth, and breadth appropriate for the stage of the group.
- Helps students make informed choices about their learning plans.
- Determines when and how to assist with issue identification, refocus discussion, ensure knowledge accuracy, attend to process, and deal with group disruptions.
- Assists students to generate learning issues with sufficient depth and breadth. When necessary the tutor may be required to draw attention to gaps in prior knowledge.
- Identifies own knowledge gaps and finds information to support self-learning.
- Applies current evidence from research and other sources to make decisions.
- Evaluates attainment of learning objectives using valid and reliable measures.
- Establishes leadership role and negotiates with students the sharing of this role.
- Determines strategies for developing a student-centered approach.
- Identifies degree of support required of students.
- Monitors the educational process of each student in the group.
- Modulates the challenge of the problem situation at hand.

Having the knowledge and skills in the aforementioned areas is necessary to make appropriate judgments regarding the students' learning. Throughout the iterative PBL process, the faculty tutor critically analyzes a given situation to form a conclusion. Once a conclusion is drawn, a decision is made and plan of action is constructed. Box 11.3 lists the judgment competencies required of the facilitator to foster the PBL process and to develop the metacognitive skills of students. According to Haith-Cooper (2003), one of the most challenging aspects of the tutors' role is deciding when and how to intervene in the PBL process. The following section will provide some examples of techniques used by tutors to facilitate learning and to intervene as appropriate.

Techniques for Facilitating Learning

During the PBL process, the faculty tutor uses facilitation techniques and questioning strategies to facilitate the students' learning (Table 11.4). These techniques and strategies are applicable in a number of learning situations. For further guidance to the new and seasoned PBL tutor groups, the reader is referred to a wealth of literature on the topic of implementing the PBL model and group process (Alavi, 1995; Barrows, 1988; Corey & Corey, 1997; Rideout, 2001; Tiberius, 1990; Westberg & Jason, 1996; Wolff, 2000). A topic of far greater concern, for which a paucity of information exists, is about when and how a facilitator should intervene in the PBL process.

The central focus of the facilitator role has a corresponding influence on the level and amount of intervention provided by the faculty tutor. While it is generally accepted that tutors have a role to play in intervening in the learning process, challenges commonly encountered by tutors include knowing what types of issues constitute intervention on behalf of the tutor, how long to wait before intervening, and how to take corrective action. According to Barrows (1988), the ideal situation is "to let the problem go long enough for a student eventually to express a concern that there is a problem or that the group does not seem to be going anywhere or accomplishing anything" (p. 13). When it is not reasonable to let the group deteriorate while waiting for a student response, a rule of thumb is to assess group productivity. If the group is productive then the tutor should wait to intervene. Haith-Cooper (2003) identified four classifications of issues that require tutor intervention: unfocussed discussion, incorrect content, missing a step of the PBL process, and disruptive group dynamics.

Once a tutor has correctly identified the need to intervene, he or she then needs to determine the corrective action to take. Five possible types of interventions can be used in conjunction with the various facilitation techniques (Table 11.4). First, the faculty tutor uses metacognitive questioning techniques such as elicitation, re-elicitation, and prompting in response to an inadequate explanation, gaps in students' knowledge, or inconsistencies in their thinking (Gilkison, 2003). To probe the student's knowledge deeply the tutor must constantly ask questions such as "What do you mean by that?" or "What is the evidence to support that idea?" When a student addresses the tutor directly with a question or comment, the tutor could say, "Who has some thoughts about this comment/question?"

TABLE 11.4 TECHNIQUES AND QUESTIONS FOR PBL TUTORS

KEY AREA	FACILITATION TECHNIQUE	MEANING	SAMPLE QUESTIONS
Meta-cognition	Elicitation	Elicitation involves the tutor asking a question to the group or particular member of the group. The purpose of this technique is to evoke a verbal response from the students.	What do you mean by that? Tell us what you know. Would you explain that? What are other possible reasons for this? Is there a reason to question this information? Why? What are other possibilities? How does this information support or not support our original hypothesis?
	Re-elicitation	This technique is used when the previous response given was inadequate in some way. The tutor repeats the same elicitation question or rephrases it.	Why did you come to that conclusion? Could there be another alternative? Are there other possibilities that you may not have thought of? Turn to a student other than the one talking and ask "Do you agree with what she just said?" If what you say is true, then how would you explain . . . ? With this kind of problem, have you ever thought about . . .? What is the evidence to support that idea? Would you explain that a bit more? How do you know it is true? You seem to be assuming that . . . is due to . . . . Tell me more about your thinking. Please explain what you have just said so that I can understand your statement/opinion/conclusions.
	Prompting	Prompting is a technique used either to get students to expand upon a statement made or to gather more information.	Are there other possibilities that you may not have thought of? Let's stop and review our hypotheses again. Do you agree with that? What did that do for you? What does it mean in terms of your idea about the problem? So how are you going to decide what this is? What more do you need to know? What do you mean when you say . . . ? How might the client view this situation? Does anyone view this differently? If this occurs then what would you expect to happen next? Why? What are the consequences of each of these possible approaches? Are you satisfied with your explanations/hypotheses/alternatives or are there other issues you need to consider?

(continued)

■ TABLE 11-4 Techniques and Questions for PBL Tutors (continued)

KEY AREA	FACILITATION TECHNIQUE	MEANING	SAMPLE QUESTIONS
Procedural or inter-personal group dynamics	Refocusing	Refocusing is used when the students drifted off topic or dwelled on a minor point. This type of statement or question brings students back to the topic or the problem scenario.	How does the new information relate to our earlier discussion of . . . ? Let's stop and review what we know now about the issue. I'm not sure I'm clear about what you plan to explore further, it seems a bit broad to me. How will this information help in the management of the client situation?
	Directing	Directing refers to the tutor guiding the students in a certain direction, suggesting what to do next, or attending to group dynamics. This technique signaled an end to the students' discussion of a topic.	What is the situation about? What are the issues pertaining to this scenario? What further information do you require? What are your hypotheses for each issue? What are your group and individual goals? What resources are available? Let's revise our objectives and tackle those that are the most important to this scenario. Should we just tackle a piece of this problem? Maybe we ought to stop here and read some resources or go talk to an expert? Would it be better to get the big picture now and fill in the details later? What was identified as a learning need, but not explored? What does the group think we should do next? Perhaps there are better ways to examine this problem. Is there a resource that might be consulted? I'm not sure that you are right. Why don't you look that up and review it with us next time? (use sparingly)
	Evaluating	Formative and summative comments made to evaluate group process or individual student participation.	How do you feel about those facts you brought to the group today? Were you able to find all the resources you wanted? Are you comfortable with the way you have put that together? How well did we do today in working as a group? What were the major strengths of this session? What were the main areas in which we could improve? How much did the group learn by using this scenario?

(continued)

■ TABLE 11-4 Techniques and Questions for PBL Tutors (continued)

KEY AREA	FACILITATION TECHNIQUE	MEANING	SAMPLE QUESTIONS
Procedural or interpersonal group dynamics (continued)	Evaluating (continued)		What are some of the difficulties (if any) the group experienced with this scenario? What do you see yourself doing differently? What things did you not say that you might have? Actually, I thought you were unable to see beyond that one idea you had for the problem, and it limited your ability to see its real implications. The resources the group used seemed to be rather superficial and the group didn't bring the kind of information we needed to really understand. Do you agree?
	Summarizing	Before the group moves onto another topic, the tutor may ask questions or make summarizing comments about a particular area of discussion. Summarizing statements are usually made before moving onto another topic or part of the scenario.	What have we learned with this problem? What new facts or concepts? Do we have the entire explanation now? Do we have all the facts we need to move on? What have we learned from this problem? How might his new information be used in your clinical practice? In what way has working through this problem helped with understanding (e.g., how exercise affects heart disease)?
	Giving feedback	Giving feedback occurs when the tutor confirms what is heard or seen.	Are your sure of what you are saying? Do you feel you need to look that point up? You seem unsure. Could this be a learning issue that should be studied before we go further? There seems to be something going on here between us in this group. We seem to be going nowhere as a group. What do you suppose is going on? What shall we do about it? Depending on what work the group is doing, it may be appropriate to call a "time out" to discuss process. An effective way to start the discussion is to begin with phrases such as "I see . . .", "I hear . . .," or "I notice that . . ." and then the question, "Does anyone else share my experience." For example, I notice that people are coming late quite a lot and/or attendance is sporadic. I find this behavior disruptive to the learning process. Do others in the group notice this, and what does this behavior mean for the group?

(continued)

■ **TABLE 11-4 Techniques and Questions for PBL Tutors (continued)**

KEY AREA	FACILITATION TECHNIQUE	MEANING	SAMPLE QUESTIONS
Procedural or interpersonal group dynamics (continued)	Informing	Tutors providing facts, information, or ideas characterize this technique. In most instances no student response is required following informing.	

Adapted from: Alavi, C. (1995). *Problem-based learning in a health sciences curriculum*. London: Routledge; Barrows, H. S. (1988). *The tutorial process*. Springfield, IL: Southern Illinois University School of Medicine; Gilkison, A. (2003). Techniques used by "expert" and "non-expert" tutors to facilitate problem-based learning tutorials in an undergraduate medical curriculum. *Medical Education, 37*, 6–14; Wolff, A.C., & Rideout, E. (2001). The faculty role in problem-based learning. In E. Rideout, (Ed.), *Transforming nursing education through problem-based learning*. Sudbury, MA: Jones & Barlett.

The second corrective action used by tutors using a technique called time out. This technique involves the tutor stopping the process to check in with students regarding their individual opinion on a certain issue (Haith-Cooper, 2003). For example, the tutor might ask, "Should we stop here and discuss whether we should tackle a piece of this problem?" Time outs allow the tutor or students to clarify and redirect attention toward the essential features of the scenario. For example, to redirect the discussion back to the topic or the problem scenario the tutors could utilize refocusing techniques such as "Let's stop and review what we know about the issue" or "How will this information help us to manage the client situation?" Also, tutors commonly use directing techniques to check in with the students and guide their discussions. For example, "Would it be better to get the big picture now and fill in the details later?" Third, the tutor describes what he or she has heard or seen happening. This corrective action allows the tutor to validate his or her interpretation of the events and provides cues to prompt further student discussion. A common way for the tutor to seek validation is by redirecting the discussion using words such as "I see. . . ," "I hear . . . ," or "I notice that . . . ."

Fourth, the tutor utilizes refocusing, summarizing, feedback, and evaluating techniques in response to students going off topic or to maintain group dynamics (see Table 11.4). For example, the tutor may make summarizing comments about a particular area of the discussion or ask a question such as "In what way has working through this problem helped with understanding (e.g., how exercise affects heart disease)?" Throughout the PBL process tutors subtly provide feedback to individuals or the group making remarks such as "You seem unsure, could this be a learning issue that should be studied before we go further?" It is common for tutors to lead the group in the evaluation process; for example the tutor might say, "How do you feel about the facts you brought to the group today?" or "How well did we do today in working as a group?" The corrective actions of reminding and reflecting ensures that the group process flows well, and keeps the students on task and focused on their learning objectives (Haith-Cooper, 2003). The fifth, and perhaps most controversial intervention, is providing information to the students (Haith-Cooper, 2003). Some agree that the tutor can provide information only if it does not impede or short circuit the learning process (Katz, 1995). It is generally agreed that such teacher-directed actions should be used sparingly as it may inhibit further student discussion (Wolff & Rideout, 2001). Regardless of the type of tutor intervention, it is generally agreed upon that the level of intervention on the part of the tutor should decrease as the students gain experience with the PBL process.

While the faculty tutor's primary responsibility is that of facilitation, to function competently they must possess the requisite competencies in four areas: knowledge, skills, attitudes, and judgment. The attitudes and beliefs held by a tutor form the foundation upon which teaching practices and judgments are based. To develop these competencies a number of supports must be in place to adequately prepare faculty for this role.

COMPONENTS OF FACULTY DEVELOPMENT PROGRAMS

For many, adopting the faculty tutor role as described earlier is merely an application of their current role in a nonPBL curriculum. For others, the change requires a considerable shift in philosophy and beliefs about being a teacher as well as changes in behavior. Faculty members have reported decreased levels of self-confidence and feeling of uncertainty about when and how to intervene in a tutorial group (Bernstein, Tipping, Bercovitz, & Skinner, 1995; Creedy, Horsfall, & Hand, 1992). To ease the role transition and maximize their role, it is essential that faculty receive *orientation* and ongoing support. Because traditional didactic programs teach *what is known* and PBL programs focus on *what we know*, the challenge is to persuade faculty members to move from efficient teaching to effective learning. This section will provide an overview of the essential ingredients in an effective faculty development program and describe some strategies to successful implementation of these programs. While the list of issues to be considered in faculty development is long, the predominant challenges faced by faculty are:

- Reframing the theoretical basis of education.
- Developing an understanding of PBL.
- Acquiring and maintaining the qualities of effective tutors.
- Developing leadership for the future (Irby, 1996).

Reframing the Theoretical Basis of Education

The first step toward adopting the PBL approach is a redefinition of the word teacher. Whether consciously or not, most faculty members teach, "in ways that suggest we equate telling with learning and that we view teachers as the ultimate sources of knowledge" (Wilkerson & Hundert, 1991, p. 16). All faculty teaching in a PBL model need to redefine their relationship to the content to be learned and the students to be taught. Moreover, Barrows and Pickell (1991) suggest that faculty also need to make themselves vulnerable and admit they do not know all the answers. Reframing views of the educational process also requires faculty to develop increased levels of professional and personal awareness of self in relation to others (Creedy, et al., 1992; Wilkerson & Hundert, 1991). Such awareness can be achieved through reflection on one's current teaching ideologies, approaches, and practices. This fresh image of faculty as facilitators of learning is a major pedagogical shift for those new to PBL approaches. Before faculty members can move on to where they need to go, they need to have awareness of who they are as faculty and what beliefs they hold. Such reflection indirectly shapes one's future action (Olsen & Singer, 1994; Schön, 1987) and has been found to promote the development of competence (Wolff, 1998).

As faculty are rethinking assumptions about teaching and learning, they should also be introduced to the PBL model and to the theoretical underpinnings of the model (i.e., constructivism, social constructivism, and adult learning theory). The goal here is to assist faculty to question their old ways of knowing and become aware of PBL as an alternative approach to education. Both the theoretical basis for PBL and the research regarding PBL provide rationale. So this step in the faculty development process serves to explain why a new model of education is needed and provides rationale for one model that is both congruent with current educational theory and effective in practice.

Experiencing the process of PBL is a persuasive approach to increasing acceptance of the model. As Irby (1996) notes, "Reading and talking about PBL are not as powerful as experiencing the method. When they (faculty) experience the power of learning in this model at an emotional level, their assumptions about teaching and learning will be challenged" (p. 74). Participating in a PBL session should be an essential first step in any faculty development program.

Acquiring Effective PBL Skills

Next, faculty must achieve competence as skilled facilitators of the PBL process, which includes the complex and sometimes conflicting roles of consultant, learner, mediator, challenger, negotiator, director, evaluator, and listener. As Irby (1996) indicates, these are indirect forms of instruction that facilitate conversation, dialogue, and debate rather than the transmission of information. Identifying and practicing these roles is an essential feature of becoming an effective faculty tutor. Irby goes on to say that, "Faculty development programs (to help faculty acquire PBL skills) should be skill based with clearly articulated guidelines and rationale" (p. 75). Practicing the faculty tutor role in a small group, videotaping the practice sessions, and obtaining feedback based on rationale are powerful strategies for learning new skills. It is useful to incorporate examples and exercises that highlight situations that faculty new to PBL often describe as difficult to deal with, such as giving up control, not delivering a lecture if the topic is close to the faculty member's heart, providing feedback on student performance, and confronting group conflicts. Participation in such highly interactive sessions can be stressful, so it is essential that a safe environment be provided for faculty members as they take risks and practice these new skills.

Maintaining and Building on PBL Skills

The third component of faculty development for PBL has several aims. First, it is important to review and critique the experience of teaching in the PBL approach. Wilkerson and Maxwell (1988) suggest regular meetings of faculty teaching in a particular course. Such meetings provide the opportunity for faculty members to learn from and work with one another, dealing with both the content and process of tutoring. These meetings offer the benefits of ongoing collegial support and dialogue, and promote personal reflection.

A focus on developing advanced conceptual knowledge about PBL and advanced teaching skills should be incorporated in faculty development programs. Reviewing relevant literature and determining alternative strategies for dealing with new or recurring difficult situations in tutorials would be useful at this stage. According to Irby (1996), "this is less skill-oriented and more a process of reflection on experience and reconceptualization of ideas" (p. 75). A seminar format is appropriate here, where faculty share common problems and successes, experts can be called upon to provide their insights, and other mediums, such as the series of videotapes for tutor training prepared by Maastricht University, can be used to stimulate discussion (see Additional Resources).

Developing Effective Leadership Skills

The final component of a faculty development program should focus on the future, through inclusion of knowledge and skills in leadership and educational research for those faculty who have an aptitude and interest in leadership positions. Irby (1996) suggests activities such as workshops and fellowships aimed at leading groups, developing courses and curriculum, evaluating programs, and conducting research.

Success of any curriculum that incorporates the PBL philosophy is dependent on a cadre of faculty who have a commitment to the method, the self-awareness, and intellectual sensitivity to adopt and maintain the role, the ability to facilitate group learning, and sufficient expertise in the subject being explored by students to ensure rigor in learning. Faculty development is therefore crucial to prepare faculty for this new role. The most comprehensive faculty development programs extend over a substantial period of time thereby allowing for the learning and change process to occur. These programs incorporate all domains of learning while featuring experiential learning. Typically, these programs also provide ongoing support to new PBL tutors.

STRATEGIES FOR DEVELOPING SUCCESSFUL FACULTY DEVELOPMENT PROGRAMS

The aim of all faculty development programs should be to foster a positive attitude toward the PBL approach, promote confidence in the ability to serve as faculty tutors, and result in a change in focus from a teacher-centered to a student-centered educational philosophy. Comprehensive faculty development programs share several common threads, including provision of information on theory and practice; acquisition of facilitation skills, progressing from general to specific; multiple roles for faculty members who serve both as student and tutor in a small group; consideration of various tutor functions (e.g., questioning, facilitating, and evaluating); and provision of feedback to program participants (Kaufman, 1995). A number of resources can be accessed to learn more about the programs that embody these desired outcomes and incorporate all or most of the components discussed above (Alavi, 1995; Benor & Mahler, 1989; Branda & Sciarra, 1995; Creedy & Hand, 1994; Grand'Maison & Des-Marchais, 1991; Wilkerson & Irby, 1998). The following section offers eight strategies for incorporation into faculty development programs. Moreover, the aforementioned core competencies should also be used as a guiding framework for developing such programs (Box 11.3). Box 11.4 offers some survival tips for educators who make the transition to PBL.

BOX 11.4 SURVIVAL TIPS FOR TRANSITIONING TO THE PBL TUTOR ROLE

Often educators experience feelings of anxiety and uneasiness when implementing less familiar models of teaching. Stress, decreased levels of self-confidence, and fatigue when coping with workloads are important areas to monitor to prevent the hindrance of learning. If an individual experiences too much discomfort, change will not occur and he or she may maintain their current behaviors and beliefs instead of adapting the PBL philosophies.

SURVIVAL TIPS

1. Anticipate and manage anxiety by scheduling regular weekly (or biweekly) meetings with peers.
2. Implement changes based on tutorial experiences.
3. Integrate relevant suggestions that arise from the tutor–student evaluation process.
4. Conduct ongoing faculty development to orientate, reflect, and refresh.
5. Record thoughts; for example, many nurse educators find it helpful to keep a personal journal. It may also be used to analyze teaching beliefs and identify experiences that created difficulties when making the transition from traditional teaching methodologies to student-centered, problem-based approaches.

Adapted from Bernstein, P., Tipping, J., Bercovitz, K., et al. (1995). Shifting students and faculty to a PBL curriculum: Attitudes changed and lessons learned. *Academic Medicine, 70*(3), 245–247; Creedy, D., & Hand, B. (1994). The implementation of problem-based learning: Changing pedagogy in nurse education. *Journal of Advanced Nursing, 20*(4), 696–702; Holmes, D. B., & Kaufman, D. M. (1994). Tutoring in problem-based learning: A teacher development process. *Medical Education, 28*(4), 275–283.

First, successful adoption of the PBL model depends largely on the acceptance by the institution and participation by all those who teach (Wilkerson & Maxwell, 1988). Successful programs should be designed with faculty involvement and those responsible for instituting the PBL method should encourage an alteration of the organizational environment to ensure specific individuals are allocated to the faculty development task. This includes the appointment of an effective leader, as well as the designation of consult experts who have read the literature and who can determine faculty members' needs (Holmes & Kaufman, 1994; Wilkerson & Maxwell, 1988).

Second, faculty development programs should begin with educational sessions that focus on attitudinal competencies. Opportunities should be provided for educators to deal with current beliefs and assumptions about teaching and learning. Workshop topics should include philosophies of teaching, educational approaches, and identification of self as teacher (Creedy, et al., 1992). As eloquently stated by Wilkerson and Hundert (1991), "becoming a problem-based teacher requires both a desire to change, and an increased awareness of self and others" (p. 167). The learning activity in this chapter identifies useful questions for guiding the examination of one's teaching beliefs. After dealing with conceptual changes associated with the new pedagogy, entry-level educational sessions should address basic teaching skills and orient faculty members to the academic values, norms, and expectations of the PBL approach.

Third, faculty development programs for PBL must be experiential, so faculty walk the talk of participating in PBL, thereby learning about the principles of PBL (Barrows & Pickell, 1991). Programs that expect faculty to develop their own learning objectives and engage in the learning program are congruent with PBL. As such, faculty should be expected to determine specific and personal learning goals, and seek out the necessary resources. Group sessions should allow faculty to role play their approach to various representative issues confronted in PBL sessions. The group facilitator acts as a coach, observing and giving feedback.

Fourth, written materials should be developed to enhance participants' knowledge base. One such resource is an orientation guide developed for faculty adopting the PBL model (Wolff, 2000). This orientation guide includes a user-friendly, concise, thorough resource that provides a background on PBL and focuses on particular strategies faculty can use in specific situations. It is a useful complement to the interactive workshops that should be the centerpiece of any PBL faculty development program.

Fifth, to enhance tutors' professional understanding of PBL, effective faculty development programs should provide opportunities for tutor reflection about their instructional skill development and for opportunities for further refinement of their tutor skills. Creedy and Hand (1994) concluded that opportunities for reflection increases self-confidence and provides a sense of control and power to the teachers' learning process. Through a process of trial and error, accompanied by reflective thinking, teachers changed their beliefs about teaching and embraced the innovative PBL pedagogy.

Sixth, a process should be instituted for ensuring that collegial support is offered to all PBL faculties. Personal contacts and social support play major roles in influencing individuals to adopt an innovation. Such support can take a variety of approaches, including regular faculty tutor meetings held at the beginning, during, and at the end of a course; peer observations of tutorials and feedback; and dialogue through personal journals.

Seventh, developing a method of rewards and recognition for teaching will reinforce faculty commitment to a new approach to education. Incorporating methods of faculty evaluation, acknowledging excellence in teaching through faculty and university awards for teaching, and including contributions to education as an expectation for tenure and promotion are some of the methods used to encourage and reward PBL teaching and continual learning.

Finally, the outcomes of the faculty development program should be evaluated. Although the aforementioned programs include some degree of evaluation, it is often limited. When devising a new program, it is recommended that a method of evaluation be built into the program. The desired outcomes should be made clear and specific and a model of program evaluation selected. Economic evaluations have been underrepresented in the literature on PBL. Therefore, an approach to cost analysis should be considered an integral component of outcome research. Studies should be conducted that use rigorous and appropriate methods of design and analysis.

SUMMARY

Problem-based learning is an educational model that transforms the role of the teacher and alters the student–teacher relationship. Based on the tenets of constructivism, the eight-step PBL process is characterized by the use of a specially prepared problem as the context for a small group of students to learn clinical reasoning skills, to construct knowledge in the context of social environments, and to integrate and apply concepts of nursing to the context of a clinical situation. Within the PBL model, the faculty member's role as expert becomes secondary as the role of guide or facilitator taking precedence. As facilitator, the faculty tutor leads a task-oriented group of students to achieve the objectives of the nursing program. While this may sound relatively easy, it is clear that the role of the tutor involves a great deal of expertise. Moreover, in addition to the tutor's expertise there are various contextual and situational factors which impact on tutor behavior. Given the complex nature of the PBL tutor role, faculty development programs are crucial to prepare faculty for this role. Overall, successful programs foster unconditional acceptance among faculty, focus on the teaching attitudes and beliefs of faculty, offer support, acknowledge the feelings conjured by the change process, provide opportunities for reflection, and utilize the influence of crucial educational leaders. Over a significant period of time, the focus of such programs should promote professional, instructional, organizational, and leadership development. Finally, all programs for faculty development should include formal and rigorous evaluation of their outcomes and cost effectiveness.

LEARNING ACTIVITY

Becoming a Tutor: Increasing Self-Awareness

Adopting a new philosophical position for teaching and learning will require educators to reflect on their intentions, the values they espouse, and the objectives to be achieved. Critical reflection is a useful tool for analyzing personal beliefs about learning and the kinds of rewards that are important to a teacher.

Directions for Critical Reflection

The following questions can be used as a guide for critical reflection. Once the tutor has reflected on these questions, assumptions can be drawn regarding the nurse educator's underlying teaching philosophies.

1. Answer the following questions:
   a. How would you describe yourself as a teacher?
   b. How have you changed as a teacher since you began as a classroom teacher?
   c. What is the most important aspect of your teaching?
   d. If I observed your teaching, what would I see?
   e. Give me an example of a dilemma you faced as a classroom teacher and how you responded to it. Why was it a dilemma for you?
   f. How do you provide feedback to learners?
   g. How do you evaluate what students have learned?
   h. Describe a typical classroom session.
   i. How do you respond to questions from learners?
   j. How do you deal with questions you cannot answer?
   k. How do you select learning experiences for students?
   l. How do you react when you observe less than ideal performance by students? By other faculty and staff?
   m. What do you tell learners about your expectations of them in the classroom setting?
   n. How does the classroom setting affect the way you teach and learners learn?
   o. What are you trying to accomplish in your teaching? How do you know when you accomplish it?
   p. What would you like to do better in your teaching?
2. Review the answers searching for common themes.
3. Identify main concepts for each theme and describe the relationships among them.
4. Cognitive mapping techniques are useful for depicting your ideas of teaching. On a piece of paper draw a concept map or mind map. Refer to the following resources about cognitive mapping techniques: Buzan and Buzan (1998 or www.http://www.mind-map.com/EN/), All and Havens (1997), Daley (1996), and Chapter 2 of this textbook.
5. Analyze the map to examine the interrelatedness among concepts in the map and the implication of your perspectives in the context of the PBL tutor and the student.
6. Now that you have developed a clear idea of your beliefs, values, and attitudes about teaching and learning, you can now move on to identify your learning needs as you become a tutor and practice according to the principles and philosophies of PBL.

RESOURCES FOR EDUCATORS

PLANNING THE TEACHING/LEARNING EXPERIENCE

Questions to Support a Thoughtful Reading

1. Novice students require more intervention by the facilitator. Discuss how the tutor's role shifts in working with PBL groups composed of first year students as opposed to upper level students. Should more experienced PBL tutors facilitate novice PBL groups, and those with less experience facilitate proficient PBL groups?
2. Groups typically face a number of issues such as developing an approach to decision making; establishing group leadership; and learning how to deal with conflict. Consider how you would guide a group of students to deal with these issues.
3. Respect is a critical element of a successful PBL group. Think about why it would be important for individuals within the PBL group to respect each other. What happens when you or the students do not respect each other? How would you address the group members about their concerns that you were unfair in failing a student in the clinical area?
4. What would you say or do in the following situations:
   a. The group is discussing a topic in which you have expertise. You know the students are heading in the wrong direction.
   b. After reading the first part of the scenario, the students come up with what they believe to be a plausible answer and feel there is no point in continuing to work on the scenario.
   c. After reading the first part of a scenario and having a brief discussion, several members of the group say that they are unable to identify issues without more information.
   d. The students in the group listed several issues relevant to the scenario. No discussion took place. Assignments for research were identified and divided among the group members. Since they finished early, the group decided to go to the library to start researching the issues identified.
   e. The students have researched issues at a previous tutorial and after the discussion they are ready to move on to the next scenario; however, they have not related the issues discussed to the scenario at hand.
5. Determine how you would deal with the following situations. If required, what intervention techniques would you utilize?
   a. At the end of the tutorial, during the evaluation of the group's performance, a student remarks that the format, in which the students take turns presenting the learning issue, is boring. Another student agrees with this concern.
   b. Despite your efforts, the group is not functioning. There is silence, no one listens, the topics of discussion are disjointed, and there is no enthusiasm.
   c. For the last hour, there has been a great deal of confrontation and conflict between members of the tutorial group about a specific topic. This has disrupted the functioning of the group.
6. Inevitably you will be facilitating a group that will have the temptation to learn everything about a subject in the first case. Think about how you are going to help the

group resist this urge. How will you instill the confidence in them that other cases will give then an opportunity to learn more about the subject matter?

7. How do you balance the demands of content and process in programs such as PBL that feature teaching in small groups?

Instructions for Educators

Small group learning is affected by structural factors such as group size, physical environment, and course design. Group size influences member participation, group cohesiveness, relationship building, and group evaluation. It is generally agreed upon that the optimal size for PBL groups is five to ten members, with seven being the preferred. The physical layout of the classroom should be structured in a way that promotes nondominant, face-to-face interaction and opportunities for equal participation. Group dialogues can be influenced by a number of factors such as: bright glaring colors, inappropriate lighting, external noise, and inadequate room temperature and airflow. To ensure that students have time to adequately acquire the necessary knowledge and allow time for the PBL process to unfold, a number of factors must be considered with regards to designing PBL courses. These include the length of the term, group composition, frequency of sessions, duration of each session, and experience of the tutor (Benson, et al., 2001).

Tips for Developing a Student-Centered Learning Environment

The first clues that you are working in a PBL environment reside with the chairs in which you sit, and the rooms in which you gather. A flexible physical environment equipped with moveable furniture and writing equipment for brainstorming (e.g., flip chart and white boards) set the scene for approaching PBL learning. The educational environment should be transparent in that everything regarding the curriculum, learning objectives, evaluation tools, etc. are open and declared. A program handbook is a useful resource for providing faculty information, term and course objectives, a learning grid, timetables, program expectations, details pertaining to student evaluations, and required/suggested learning materials and equipment. The principles of PBL also shape the institutional environment, including policies, procedures, and guidelines. In PBL institutions students are often involved in many committees/task forces and curriculum evaluation.

During the initial PBL session the learning climate begins to be established. An attitude of acceptance and openness is essential to encourage group participation. Ground rules are established and expectations regarding attendance, promptness, completion of group tasks, and ongoing evaluation are some common topics for decision making. Faculty tutors assist in the creation of a safe and supportive learning environment that encourages: the expression of different opinions; embraces risk taking behaviors; and explores mistakes objectively as part of the learning process (Wolff & Rideout, 2001). The following activities may be useful in the first PBL session of a course with a new group:

1. List 25 things that you do not like about group work. Then brainstorm ways to overcome each. Use a mind map to display your results.
2. With your group, brainstorm the things that might make working together frustrating. Agree on policies to handle each.

EVALUATING THE TEACHING/LEARNING EXPERIENCE

Sample Evaluation Strategies and Tools

A SAMPLE TOOL TO EVALUATE YOUR CONTRIBUTION TO GROUP PRODUCTIVITY

Please complete a midterm and final self-evaluation providing examples of how you exhibited some of the following behaviors:

DESCRIPTION	SPECIFIC EXAMPLES OF. . .
1. Initiating and contributing ideas and information.	
2. Providing and inviting information, ideas, opinions, and feelings.	
3. Clarifying, synthesizing, and illustrating examples.	
4. Periodically paraphrasing or summarizing what has taken place and the major points being discussed.	
5. Encouraging and supporting the participation of each group member, for example: • giving others the opportunity to speak as much as self • waiting for others to finish speaking before beginning to speak • recognizing the right of others to express views without being put down • maintaining confidentiality of information and experiences.	
6. Actively listening to each group member and acknowledging the contribution of each group member.	
7. Observing and describing the process of group interaction during the discussion or at the end of the session.	
8. Giving direction to the discussion (e.g., asking open-ended questions, focusing, and clarifying assumptions/misunderstandings)	
9. Identifying when the group is off topic and redirecting the focus of the group.	
10. Initiating the discussion and speaking directly to group members.	
11. Participating in self-evaluation openly and honestly.	
12. Participating in peer evaluation by giving constructive criticism and feedback to individual members.	

On a scale of 0 to 10, 10 being the best you've ever done at promoting a productive group discussion and 0 being the opposite, how would you rate yourself?

Reflective Questions for Educators

1. How would you describe yourself as a teacher when working with students in a small group learning situation?
2. What is or would be the hardest part of the PBL tutor role for you to adopt?
3. How have you changed since you began as a PBL tutor?
4. What is the most important aspect of your role as a PBL tutor?
5. How do you respond to questions from students? How do you deal with questions you cannot answer?

References

Alavi, C. (1995). *Problem-based learning in a health sciences curriculum.* London: Routledge.

All, A. C., & Havens, R. L. (1997). Cognitive/concept mapping: A teaching strategy for nursing. *Journal of Advanced Nursing, 25,* 1210–1219.

Baker, C. M. (2000). Problem-based learning for nursing: Integrating lessons from other disciplines with nursing experiences. *Journal of Professional Nursing, 16,* 258–266.

Baptiste, S. E. (2003). *Problem-based learning: A self-directed journey.* Thorofare, NJ: Slack Incorporated.

Barrows, H. S. (1988). *The tutorial process.* Springfield, IL: Southern Illinois University School of Medicine.

Barrows, H. S., & Pickell, G. G. (1991). *Developing clinical problem-solving skills: A guide to more effective diagnosis and treatment.* New York: W.W. Norton.

Benor, D. E., & Mahler, S. (1989). Training medical faculty: Rationale and outcomes. In H. G. Schmidt, M. Lipkin, M. W. deVries, et al. (Eds.), *New directions for medical education: Problem-based learning and community-orientated medical education* (pp. 248–259). New York: Springer-Verlag.

Benson, G., Noesgaard, C., & Drummond-Young, M. (2001). Facilitating small group learning. In E. Rideout (Ed.), *Transforming nursing education through problem-based learning* (pp. 75–102). London: Jones & Bartlett.

Bernstein, P., Tipping, J., Bercovitz, K., et al. (1995). Shifting students and faculty to a PBL curriculum: Attitudes changed and lessons learned. *Academic Medicine, 70,* 245–247.

Branda, L. A., & Sciarra, A. F. (1995). Faculty development in problem-based learning. *Annals of Community-Oriented Education, 8,* 195–208.

Brooks, J. G., & Brooks, M. G. (1993). *In search of understanding: The case for constructivist classrooms.* Alexandria, VA: Association for Supervision and Curriculum.

Burrows, D. E. (1997). Facilitation: A concept analysis. *Journal of Advanced Nursing, 25,* 396–404.

Buzan, T., & Buzan, B. (1998). *The mind map book.* London: BBC Books.

Corey, M. S., & Corey, G. (1997). *Groups: Process and practice.* Pacific Grove, CA: Brooks/Cole.

Creedy, D., & Hand, B. (1994). The implementation of problem-based learning: Changing pedagogy in nurse education. *Journal of Advanced Nursing, 20,* 696–702.

Creedy, D., Horsfall, J., & Hand, B. (1992). Problem-based learning in nurse education: An Australian view. *Journal of Advanced Nursing, 17,* 727–733.

Cust, J. (1996). A relational view of learning: Implications for nurse educators. *Nurse Education Today, 16*(4), 256–266.

Daley, B. J. (1996). Concept maps: Linking nursing theory to clinical nursing practice. *Journal of Continuing Education in Nursing, 27,* 17–27.

David, T. J., & Patel, L. (1995). Adult learning theory, problem based learning, and paediatrics. *Archives of Disease in Childhood, 73,* 357–363.

Davis, W. K., Nairn, R., Paine, M. E., et al. (1992). Effects of expert and non-expert facilitators on the small-group process and on student performance. *Academic Medicine, 67,* 470–474.

De Grave, W. S., Dolmans, D. H. J., & van der Vleuten, C. P. M. (1999). Profiles of effective tutors in problem-based learning: Scaffolding student learning. *Medical Education, 33,* 901–906.

DesMarchais, J. E. (1991). From traditional to problem-based curriculum: How the switch was made at Sherbrooke, Canada. *Lancet, 338*(8761), 234–237.

Dolmans, D. H., Gijselaers, W. H., Moust, J. H., et al. (2002). Trends in research on the tutor in problem-based learning: Conclusions and implications for educational practice and research. *Medical Teacher, 24*, 173–180.

Eagle, C. J., Harasym, P. H., & Mandin, H. (1992). Effects of tutors with case expertise on problem-based learning issues. *Academic Medicine, 67*, 465–469.

Gijselaers, W. M. (1996). Connecting problem-based practices with educational theory. In L. Wilkerson & W. H. Gijselaers (Eds.), *Bringing problem-based learning to higher education*. San Francisco: Jossey-Bass.

Gilkison, A. (2003). Techniques used by "expert" and "non-expert" tutors to facilitate problem-based learning tutorials in an undergraduate medical curriculum. *Medical Education, 37*, 6–14.

Grand'Maison, P., & DesMarchais, J. E. (1991). Preparing faculty to teach in a problem-based learning curriculum: The Sherbrooke experience. *Canadian Medical Association Journal, 144*, 557–567.

Haith-Cooper, M. (2000). Problem-based learning within health professional education. What is the role of the lecturer? A review of the literature. *Nurse Education Today, 20*, 267–272.

Haith-Cooper, M. (2003). An exploration of tutors' experiences of facilitating problem-based learning. Part 2: Implications for the facilitation of problem based learning. *Nurse Education Today, 23*, 65–75.

Harvey, G., Loftus-Hills, A., Rycroft-Malone, J., et al. (2002). Getting evidence into practice: The role and function of facilitation. *Journal of Advanced Nursing, 37*, 577–588.

Holmes, D. B., & Kaufman, D. M. (1994). Tutoring in problem-based learning: A teacher development process. *Medical Education, 28*, 275–283.

Irby, D. M. (1996). Models of faculty development for problem-based learning. *Advances in Health Sciences, 1*, 69–81.

Katz, G. (1995). Facilitation. In C. Alavi (Ed.), *Problem-based learning in a health sciences curriculum* (pp. 52–70). London: Routledge.

Kaufman, D. M. (1995). Preparing faculty as tutors in problem-based learning. In W. A. Wright (Ed.), *Teaching improvement practices: Successful strategies for higher education* (pp. 101–126). Bolton, MA: Anker.

Kaufman, D. M., & Holmes, D. B. (1996). Tutoring in problem-based learning: Perceptions of teachers and students. *Medical Education, 30*, 371–377.

Knowles, M. (1975). *Self-directed Learning. A guide for learner and teachers*. New York: Association Press.

Mayo, W. P., Donnelly, M. B., & Schwartz, R. W. (1995). Characteristics of the ideal problem-based learning tutor in clinical medicine. *Evaluation and the Health Professions, 18*, 124–136.

Olsen, J. R., & Singer, M. (1994). Examining faculty beliefs, reflective change, and the teaching of reading. *Reading Research and Instruction, 34*, 97–110.

Pang, S. M. C., Wong, T. K. S., Dorcas, A., et al. (2002). Evaluating the use of developmental action inquiry in constructing a problem-based learning curriculum for pre-registration nursing education in Hong Kong: A student perspective. *Journal of Advanced Nursing, 40*, 230–241.

Reilly, D. E., & Oermann, M. H. (1999). *Clinical teaching in nursing education*. Sudbury, MA: Jones & Bartlett.

Rideout, E. (1999). Doing it: The roles, influences and behaviors of tutors. In J. Conway & A. Williams, (Eds.), *Themes and variations in PBL* (pp. 169–179). Callaghan, Australia: PROBLARC.

Rideout, E. (2001). *Transforming nursing education through problem-based learning*. Sudbury, MA: Jones & Bartlett.

Rideout, E., & Carpio, B. (2001). The problem-based learning model of nursing education. In E. Rideout (Ed.), *Transforming nursing education through problem-based learning* (pp. 21–45). London: Jones & Bartlett.

Savery, J. R., & Duffy, T. (1995). Problem-based learning: An instructional model and its constructivist framework. *Educational Technology, 33*(5), 31–38.

Schmidt, H. G., & Moust, J. H. (1995). What makes a tutor effective? A structural-equations modeling approach to learning in problem-based curricula. *Academic Medicine, 70*, 708–714.

Schmidt, H. G., van der Arend, A., Moust, J. H., et al. (1993). Influence of tutors' subject-matter expertise on student effort and achievement in problem-based learning. *Academic Medicine, 68*, 784–791.

Schön, D. A. (1987). *Educating the reflective practitioner*. San Francisco: Jossey-Bass.

Silver, M., & Wilkerson, L. A. (1991). Effects of tutors with subject expertise on the problem-based tutorial process. *Academic Medicine, 66*, 298–300.

Stinson, J. E., & Milter, R. G. (1996). Problem-based learning in business education. In L. Wilkerson & W. H. Gijselaers (Eds.), *Brining problem-based learning to higher education: Theory and practice*. San Francisco: Jossey-Bass.

Tiberius, R. G. (1990). *Small group teaching: A troubleshooting guide*. Toronto: OISE Press.

Wee, K. L., Kek, Y. C., & Sim, H. C. (2002). *Crafting effective problems for problem-based learning*. Retrieved May 16, 2004, from http://pbl.tp.edu.sg/CEP.htm.

Westberg, J., & Jason, H. (1996). *Fostering learning in small groups: A practical guide*. New York: Springer.

Wilkerson, L., & Hundert, E. M. (1991). Becoming a problem-based tutor: Increasing self-awareness thorough faculty development. In D. Boud & G. Feletti (Eds.), *The challenge of problem-based learning* (pp. 159–171). London: Kogan Page.

Wilkerson, L., & Irby, D. M. (1998). Strategies for improving teaching practices: A comprehensive approach to faculty development. *Academic Medicine, 73*, 387–396.

Wilkerson, L., & Maxwell, J. A. (1988). A qualitative study of initial faculty tutors in a problem-based curriculum. *Journal of Medical Education, 63*, 892–899.

Williams, B. (2004). Self direction in a problem based learning program. *Nurse Education Today, 24*, 277–285.

Wolff, A. C. (1998). *The process of maturing as a competent clinical teacher*. Unpublished Masters Thesis, University of British Columbia, Vancouver.

Wolff, A. C. (2000). *The role of the problem-based tutor: A resource guide for nursing faculty*. Unpublished manuscript (available a.wolff@shaw.ca).

Wolff, A. C., & Rideout, E. (2001). The faculty role in problem-based learning. In E. Rideout (Ed.), *Transforming nursing education through problem-based learning*. Sudbury, MA: Jones & Barlett.

Wong, J., & Wong, S. (1987). Towards effective clinical teaching in nursing. *Journal of Advanced Nursing, 12* (4), 505–513.

Additional Resources

Branda and Sciarra (1995) provides a series of tutorial situations illustrating problems commonly occurring in tutorial groups.

de Grave, W. (1998). *Improving tutoring: How to deal with critical incidents (Video No. V2901)*. Maastricht University. Available http://www.unimaas.nl/pbl/, accessed on August 5, 2004.

de Grave, W., Hommes, J., & Majoor, G. (1993). *Problem-based learning in the tutorial group (Video No. V2177)*. Maastricht University. Available http://www.unimaas.nl/pbl/, accessed on August 5, 2004.

de Grave, W., Huismans, E., Luth, M., et al. (2003). *Evaluation in the tutorial group: What now tutor?* Maastricht University. Available http://www.unimaas.nl/pbl/, accessed on August 5, 2004.

de Grave, W. & Majoor, G. (1993). *Task of the tutor in the report phase (Video No. V2281)*. Maastricht University. Available http://www.unimaas.nl/pbl/, accessed on August 5, 2004.

Jensen, E. (1997). *Completing the puzzle: The brain-compatible approach to learning* (2nd ed.). Del Mar, CA: The Brain Store, Inc.

Map Your Mind [Online]. Available: http://www.mapyourmind.com/, accessed on July 25, 2004.

Schwartz, P., Mennin, S., & Webb, G. (Eds.). (2001). *Problem-based learning: Case studies, experience, and practice*. London: Kogan Page Limited.

The Graphic Organizer [Online]. Available: http://www.graphic.org, accessed on October 25, 2005.

Wilkerson and Hundert (1991). Identify three case studies to use with new tutors in learning how to deal with the struggles encountered in teaching within the problem-based tutorial.

Woods, D. R. (1994). *Problem-based learning: How to gain the most from PBL*. Hamilton, ON: Donald R. Woods.

Chapter 12

Lectures for Active Learning in Nursing Education*

Marilyn H. Oermann

You are asked to teach a course with more than 200 students in it. Your own philosophy supports active learning and student participation, but you are faced with teaching this large group. The class meets in a large lecture hall on campus with immovable chairs. Your department chair confirms that there are no rooms available for break-out sessions or small group work. You are *stuck* in that lecture hall. How can you meet the realities of this teaching situation and still foster active learning among your nursing students?

INTENT

To promote active learning in nursing and other fields, many creative teaching strategies have been developed in recent years. These strategies foster development of problem solving, critical thinking, and communication skills, and they encourage students to work collaboratively with peers. However, in some nurse educators' rush to embrace active learning, they have viewed lecture negatively. Integrating active learning within lecture, rather than positioning active learning against lecture, emphasizes the benefits of both methods. An integrated approach also takes into consideration the situation of teaching large groups of students such as the one faced by the educator in the account that introduces this chapter.

This chapter examines benefits of an integrated approach to teaching rather than an either–or position. The purpose of the chapter is to describe how active learning can be incorporated into the lecture method of teaching in nursing and to present strategies for using active learning in the classroom. The chapter also discusses how to develop a lecture using an integrated approach. Sample strategies for active learning intended for use with lecture are also provided in the chapter.

* This chapter was expanded and revised with the permission of The Berkeley Electronic Press from an article that originally appeared by Marilyn H. Oermann (2004). Using active learning in lecture: Best of both worlds. *International Journal of Nursing Education Scholarship*, *1*(1), Article 1. Reprinted with permission of The Berkeley Electronic Press, 2004.

OVERVIEW

MOVE TOWARD ACTIVE LEARNING AND AWAY FROM LECTURE IN NURSING EDUCATION

The emphasis in nursing education on active learning and critical thinking has led to the development of many innovative instructional strategies for teaching in the classroom and clinical setting in recent years. Cooperative learning strategies, problem-based learning, group work, activities in which students discover knowledge themselves, and other creative teaching strategies have been developed as a means of promoting active learning in nursing courses. Many of these strategies foster problem solving and critical thinking, which are important outcomes of any nursing program. However, in nurse educators' rush to embrace active-learning methods, lecture has been criticized as an outdated teaching method. In some schools of nursing, educators have succumbed to "lecture bashing" (Woodring, 2001). Active learning and lecture need not be at opposite ends of a continuum; both have their place in teaching in nursing.

STUDENT-CENTERED LEARNING AND TEACHER-CENTERED INSTRUCTION

Active learning, or student-centered learning, is often contrasted to teacher-centered instruction. With active learning, students are engaged in the learning process; they are not merely listening to the teacher present information but instead are doing something with the content and then reflecting on the process of learning.

In **teacher-centered instruction**, in contrast, the teacher delivers content to students who listen to formal presentations but are in a passive role. In this approach, the teacher is central to the learning process—the teacher decides the content and how it will be presented and structures the learning for students. In most educational settings, teacher-centered instruction involves a traditional **lecture** in which the teacher presents information to a group of students who in turn listen, memorize, and recall the information.

ACTIVE LEARNING AND IMPORTANCE IN NURSING EDUCATION

There are many benefits of active learning for nursing students. Because students are engaged in the learning process, they are able to assess their own learning needs and take an active role in meeting them. Oermann (1998) suggested that active learning fosters critical thinking because students can explore alternate perspectives, examine different decisions that might be possible in a situation, analyze and weigh consequences of those decisions, and arrive at reasoned judgments.

Active learning in the form of problem-based learning improves problem-solving skills and use of knowledge in clinical practice (Richardson & Trudeau, 2003). Students explore how concepts and theories are used to solve patient and other problems and gain experience in analyzing clinical situations. Active learning also encourages them to reflect on their thinking and explore their ideas with peers and the teacher, fostering the development of critical thinking.

Many active-learning strategies are group oriented, and students benefit from group process. They develop communication skills, learn how to promote their ideas in a group, learn how to work with students who may have different backgrounds and approaches from their own, and realize the importance of being accountable individually and to the group (Baumberger-Henry, 2003). When students have extended experiences in the same groups, they also develop interdependence, learning to trust one another.

Active learning also encourages students to take responsibility for their own learning rather than relying on the teacher as the predominant source of information. In active learning, the student, not the teacher, is central to the process. There is collaboration between teacher and student with each sharing in the responsibility for learning. There also is collaboration among students. Given that students can pay attention in a lecture for only a short period of time (about 15 minutes) (Wankat & Oreovicz, 2003), active-learning strategies keep students involved and focused on the content, which is another advantage of using them in the classroom.

LECTURE METHOD AND IMPORTANCE IN NURSING EDUCATION

There are many advantages to using the lecture method in a nursing course. With lectures, teachers can synthesize information from varied sources extending the content presented in the student's textbook. Lecture also provides a way of delivering the most up-to-date information to students and sharing new research and ideas that may not be available yet in the literature.

Considering the growth of knowledge in nursing and related fields, teachers can select the most important content to present in lectures based on the learning outcomes, curriculum design, knowledge needed for clinical practice, and time constraints within the curriculum. Because of their lack of knowledge, students often have difficulty differentiating essential from nonessential content; but in the lecture method, the teacher can focus on critical information for learning both from a theoretical perspective and for clinical practice.

Lecture also provides a means of explaining difficult concepts and demonstrating their application in patient care. Teachers can review complex concepts in lectures until students understand them. Examples from clinical practice and case studies integrated with lectures demonstrate how new knowledge is used in patient care, which is important in students transferring their learning to the clinical setting and developing critical thinking skills (Oermann, 1998, 2000).

Lectures are particularly valuable for fostering problem solving. In a lecture the teacher can present concepts and information for solving clinical and other problems, demonstrate through examples how those concepts can be used in analyzing the problems, and explore with students as a group varied approaches to solving them. Presenting clinical examples that demonstrate the problems and related interventions assists students in applying the information in lecture to clinical practice. In this way, all students gain experience in thinking through clinical problems before they encounter them in practice.

Lecturing conserves time; faculty can present a substantial amount of information to a large group at one time (Bo-Linn, n.d.). Delivering information in the form of a lecture requires less time than using other active-learning strategies, particularly small-group work. The teacher has control over the content presented and discussed in lecture, can prepare ahead of time clinical examples that demonstrate how the concepts are used in clinical practice, and can develop carefully thought-out questions to ask the class. With good delivery and enthusiasm of the teacher, lectures also create interest in a subject.

RATIONALE FOR INTEGRATING ACTIVE LEARNING WITHIN LECTURES

Given the advantages of both approaches, the question is whether active learning and lecture need to be positioned at either pole of a continuum. Palmer (1997) suggested instead that teachers need a synthesis of these two views that embraces the best of both.

There are multiple reasons why an **integrated approach**, in which active-learning methods are interspersed within a lecture, is an effective strategy for teaching in nursing. The extensive knowledge to be gained in a nursing program, limited time for teaching, and an often large number of students in classes make lecturing a viable alternate. By interspersing active learning within the lecture, teachers can present essential content, synthesized from multiple sources, and also provide for involvement in the learning process. Many of the active-learning strategies are geared toward problem solving, critical thinking, and assisting students to apply concepts presented in lecture to clinical practice. These are important outcomes of any nursing course. With an integrated approach, students continue to receive essential information about nursing that they need to meet the objectives for the course and clinical practice and, at the same time, learn to think independently about that information.

STRATEGIES FOR IMPLEMENTATION OF INTEGRATED APPROACH

The first step is for the teacher to make a conscious decision to allow time within the class for active learning. Many of the strategies involve discussions among students and other small-group activities, which are more time consuming than presenting information. However, the strategies presented later in the chapter can be accomplished in 5 to 10 minutes. Given that students can pay attention for only a short period of time, by interspersing these methods throughout a class, teachers not only involve students in learning the content but also keep them focused on it. While many teachers are not willing to redesign their entire courses for active learning, they are able to integrate these methods within a more traditional lecture.

Decisions About Active-Learning Strategies Within Lecture

A shift toward using active learning within lecture requires preplanning, which involves preparing the lecture, developing the active learning methods, and deciding how to implement them as part of the class. Decisions about which methods to use and how to intersperse them within a lecture are made as the lecture is being prepared. One general plan is to lecture for 15 minutes and then provide an active-learning strategy (Wankat & Oreovicz, 2003). Alternatively, strategies might be integrated midway through the lecture and at the end, or for only the last 10 to 15 minutes of class time.

The active-learning strategies developed by the teacher depend on the outcomes to be achieved—what knowledge and skills will be learned from these activities? Other considerations are the size of the class, time available, and classroom setup (for example, if chairs are movable). Even with large groups and seats that are immovable, many strategies can be done individually, in pairs, or in groups of three, with selected students reporting to the entire class. Stringer (2002) compared small-group to individual case analysis and discussion as methods for incorporating active learning in a classroom. Student feedback about both methods was positive, and rooms for small-group and individual work were not needed.

Process for Developing and Presenting Lecture

In addition to these decisions about active-learning methods, there is a process to follow for developing and implementing an effective lecture in nursing courses. This process is described below.

KNOW STUDENTS' LEVEL OF UNDERSTANDING

The lecture should relate to the course objectives and should be at an appropriate level for the students. If guest lecturing or team teaching a course, it is incumbent on the educator, prior to developing the lecture, to assess the level of knowledge of the intended student group. Some of this information can be gained by reviewing prior course materials, but often it is best to ask course faculty carefully designed questions about the background knowledge of students relevant to the particular lecture content being planned. The teacher also should review the materials, readings, and learning activities of prior courses.

By beginning the lecture with open-ended questions, the teacher can assess background knowledge and review essential concepts. Preclass activities can be used to encourage students to review on their own prior to the lecture, which places the responsibility on students and allows the teacher to focus on new information. The teacher should make it clear how this new information relates to previous lectures.

PLAN LECTURE CONTENT AND ACTIVE-LEARNING STRATEGIES

The teacher can begin by listing the broad content areas to include in the lecture within the time frame for the class and considering the time required to carry out the active-learning strategies. It is critical in this planning phase to avoid listing content that can be read in the textbook or in an article. Instead, the lecture should synthesize literature from varied sources, which students could not read themselves; present examples to assist them in applying these new ideas to clinical practice; and encourage thinking about this new content and how it relates to prior learning. At this time the teacher also develops the active-learning strategies to be integrated within the class and makes other decisions about their implementation, such as when they will be used and if completed by small groups or with the entire group of learners.

DEVELOP OUTLINE

Lectures should never be written out in sentence form; instead, the teacher should develop an outline of the content or list topics to present in their order. On the outline, the teacher can list sample questions to ask students and make notes about clinical examples and short cases to share with them, demonstrating application of the content

BOX 12.1 GUIDELINES FOR DEVELOPING POWERPOINT FOR USE IN LECTURE

Develop PowerPoint presentations that highlight main concepts from lecture.
Ask questions about these concepts to actively involve students.
Select contrasting colors for text and background so they are easy to read; do not use red.
Make sure slides are not too busy—use a few key words or short phrases, not sentences.
Remember 6: 6 words/line and 6 lines/slide.
Use font size of 32.
Use uppercase and lowercase letters; IT IS HARD TO READ SLIDES THAT ARE ALL UPPERCASE LETTERS.
Avoid using animation and sounds unless relevant to students' understanding or discussion.
Do not vary fonts, font sizes, **bold,** and *italic*.
Use visuals when students need to "see" the concept.
Check your PowerPoint before class; also check its appearance if you are using it on the Web or for videoconferencing (its appearance may change).

to clinical practice. The teacher also can indicate on the outline the active-learning strategies selected for the class, their structure, when to implement, and time frame for completion. Highlighting with different colors the questions, clinical examples and cases, and where the active-learning methods will be introduced helps the teacher ensure adequate time for these and avoid presenting for the entire time period.

At this point in the process, the teacher also develops visuals such as PowerPoint and media clips to accompany the lecture to highlight and demonstrate the main concepts. Visuals can be overdone, so these should be planned carefully and used as basis for discussion in the class. Box 12.1 presents guidelines for developing PowerPoint for use in a lecture.

TIME LECTURE AND ACTIVE-LEARNING STRATEGIES

As a new teacher, it is sometimes difficult to gauge the time for a lecture and for implementing active learning methods in it; the same may be true for experienced teachers presenting new material or using new teaching methods. As such, it is a good idea to practice delivering the lecture, or a portion of it, and timing it. Even when the lecture and active-learning strategies appear to fit within the allotted time frame, it is prudent to plan additional learning activities in case the lecture is completed in less time than expected.

DELIVER THE LECTURE

Although planning the lecture content and developing active-learning strategies for it are critical, the delivery is just as important. Oermann (1999) suggested opening a lecture or speech with an interesting anecdote, a question, statistics that illustrate the importance of this content, a cartoon or photograph, a humorous story, or another statement that gets the students' interest in the topic. Being enthusiastic, speaking clearly and at an appropriate pace, highlighting important points, and maintaining eye contact with students throughout the lecture contribute to its overall effectiveness.

ACTIVE-LEARNING STRATEGIES FOR LECTURE

Questions

One of the predominant active learning methods is questioning students during a lecture. Questions can be answered by students individually or in small groups. Questions should assist students in clarifying their understanding of the information presented in the lecture, applying it to clinical practice, examining different perspectives and alternative approaches, and relating the readings and other activities to the lecture topic. In most instances, the intent is to ask thought-provoking questions that encourage students to think beyond the obvious rather than questions that ask for recall of facts and specific information. An advantage of using questions for active learning is that questions are an effective method for promoting critical thinking about the content (Oermann, 1997, 1998; Oermann, Truesdell, & Ziolkowski, 2000).

Questions range from low level, in which students answer by recalling relevant facts from the lecture, to higher level questions requiring application, analysis, synthesis of knowledge, and evaluation. Low-level questions such as "What does q.o.d. stand for?" generally have a single correct answer. Higher level questions, which often have more than one answer, ask students to apply information they have learned in class to a different situation or to a scenario, analyze a complex situation, synthesize concepts, or evaluate a series of alternates (Mertler, 2003; Oermann & Gaberson, 2006). These questions are useful for exploring other possibilities, important for critical thinking. An example of a higher level question is: Considering the evidence, what alternate interventions would be equally effective for a patient with chronic pain?

The teacher can begin by asking factual questions that review the content presented in lecture, the readings, and out-of-class assignments, then progress to higher level questions. Questions developed in this way use the cognitive taxonomy as the basis for sequencing. An example of a series of questions leveled using the taxonomy is in Table 12.1.

TABLE 12.1 QUESTIONS LEVELED USING COGNITIVE TAXONOMY

LEVEL OF TAXONOMY	SAMPLE QUESTION
Knowledge	What are physiological changes associated with the aging process?
Comprehension	Describe changes in metabolism that often accompany aging.
Application	Mrs. Smith is a 75-year-old with congestive heart failure (CHF). She comes to the clinic requesting help in losing weight. What data would you first collect from Mrs. Smith, and why is this information important?
Analysis	Mrs. Smith is covered only by Medicare. She tells you she is running out of money to buy her heart medicines. What questions would you ask her about her coverage and other resources? Provide two scenarios for her response. What would you suggest to her in both of these scenarios?
Synthesis	In the clinic where you work, you see many patients with CHF who were recently discharged from the hospital and have limited understanding of how to manage their CHF at home. What educational plan would you develop for these patients?
Evaluation	How would you evaluate the outcomes and cost effectiveness of your plan?

The questions should be planned ahead of the lecture to elicit the outcomes and cognitive skills intended. While open-ended questions are most appropriate, they need to be specific enough for students to know how to answer. For active learning to work effectively in the allotted time frame, it is best to write down the questions to be asked during the lecture, or at the end of it, in the intended order. Otherwise, teachers may be so focused on presenting the content that they neglect to ask the questions.

One-Minute Question and Answer

This active learning strategy is intended for use either with the class as a whole or in pairs of students. The intent is to clarify difficult concepts presented in the lecture and review major points. In this strategy the teacher poses a question about the lecture content. Each student has one minute to think about the answer, followed by students reporting on their answers and the teacher providing immediate feedback on their accuracy. As a small group activity, students have one minute to explain their answer to the person sitting next to them or to a small group, with peers confirming accuracy or raising new questions about the content.

Students also can do a one-minute paper in which they answer a question about the lecture in writing. For example, the question might ask students to identify unclear points from the lecture, similarities and differences between the lecture and their readings, and how the lecture concepts could be used in clinical practice. Another activity is to announce at the beginning of class that the lecture will be stopped midway for students to write a one-minute paper on a topic presented earlier in the lecture, thus encouraging students to listen attentively during the class (University of Pittsburgh Faculty Development Services, 2004).

Discussion

Another active-learning method that can be integrated within a lecture is a structured discussion about the content. Discussions promote problem solving, decision making, and critical thinking, and in small groups encourage cooperative learning and group-process skills (Crabtree, Royeen, & Mu, 2001; Gaberson & Oermann, 1999). Small-group discussions at the end of lecture are particularly appropriate for assisting students to apply the content presented in the lecture to patient care. In planning a discussion, the teacher should be clear about its intended goals: for example, to review the concepts presented in class, examine how those concepts are used in clinical practice, compare the lecture with students' readings and own experiences with patients, and examine approaches not presented in the lecture that might be equally effective.

The questions for discussion are important because they need to elicit the intended outcomes. For example, if the goal of the discussion is critical thinking about concepts presented in class, "what if" type of questions and ones that address alternate perspectives are needed (Gaberson & Oermann, 1999). If the goal instead is to review the content and identify areas needing more explanation, different questions would be used to structure the discussion.

Short-Case Analysis

Short cases within a lecture are valuable for applying concepts from lecture to clinical practice and developing the ability to problem solve and think critically. Cases provide an opportunity for students to integrate and apply clinical and basic science knowledge to simulated situations (DeMarco, Hayward, & Lynch, 2002). In this way, cases help bridge the gap between theory and practice.

Students can identify problems in cases, develop multiple approaches to solving them, discuss different points of view and assumptions they made about the situation that influenced their thinking, and propose alternate decisions that might be possible, weighing the consequences of each. Tomey (2003) reviewed the literature on the use of cases in nursing education and found that case methods led to the development of problem solving and critical thinking skills. When cases are analyzed in small groups, students become more comfortable in face-to-face communication, learn how to promote their ideas in groups and give feedback to others, and learn about individual and group accountability (Baumberger-Henry, 2003).

Cases have two components: a short case for analysis by students and questions to discuss about the case or as a result of the analysis. The case should apply concepts from lecture to simulated situations or clinical scenarios and should be short to avoid directing the students' thinking and discussions in a particular way. Questions should be open-ended and ask for alternatives rather than one possible answer. Cases analyzed in small groups allow for sharing of responses so students can learn from each other. Box 12.2 provides examples of short cases for active learning.

Jarrott and Blieszner (2001) developed a series of cases for active learning that required application of course material. In this strategy, students role-played family scenarios, which engaged them in active learning and gave them a better understanding of real-life issues related to the course content on family.

Bookend Approach

Yuretich, Khan, Leckie, and Clement (2001) developed an active-learning method termed the "bookend approach" for use in large classes. With this method, the teacher carefully organizes the topics to be presented in the class, then delivers a 10 to 12 minute lecture. Following the lecture, students work in groups of three on a specific problem or question related to the lecture content. They are allotted approximately 5 minutes for group work, followed by the teacher leading a discussion with all of the students in the class and then summarizing the discussions of the various groups. This method promotes active and collaborative learning and can be used with both small and large classes.

Writing as Active Learning

Active-learning strategies not only encourage critical thinking but also can be used to help students develop writing skills (Oermann, 1997; Richardson & Trudeau, 2003). Students can work in pairs or small groups to complete short and focused writing

BOX 12.2 SAMPLE SHORT CASES FOR USE WITH LECTURE

You have a follow-up visit with Ms. S in her home. She tells you that she has a terrible headache, is nauseated, and has been vomiting all morning. She also says that sometimes she has trouble seeing.

- Analyze this case in terms of content presented today in class.
- What data are most important in this case and why? What questions would you ask Ms. S?
- How do Ms. S's symptoms compare with what you read in Chapter 7 in your book?

You learned about the diagnosis of bronchitis today and interventions for it. Describe one other diagnosis that is similar. How will you differentiate these two in your practice?

From the lectures this week and your readings, develop a short case study about a school-aged child with one of the problems we discussed. Describe signs and symptoms you would expect to find in an assessment of children with this problem. Write only the signs and symptoms on a sheet of paper and pass the paper to the group next to you. The second group's task is to identify the problem from those signs and symptoms. Then share analyses. Was the other group correct? Why or why not? What other problems fit those signs and symptoms?

You are working night shift, and the resident orders a drug you are unfamiliar with for one of your patients complaining of pain. In reading about the drug, you find that the amount ordered is higher than the usual dose. You tell the resident, who says to give it as ordered because the patient is in so much pain. In small groups identify different options for the nurse. What are the consequences of each of these options? Decide as a group what you would do and develop a rationale for that decision using one of the theories we discussed in class.

Your clinical experience is in an assisted living facility. When you meet your client, you find her tied to her wheelchair. What would you do? Why? What did you learn today in class to guide your actions?

Mr. D, 61 years old, is seen in the clinic with increasing shortness of breath. He has had three chest colds this month. You hear crackles in the lower bases of his lungs and expiratory wheezes.

- What additional data would you collect in the initial assessment? Why?
- What are Mr. D's priority problems?
- How will the data you plan on collecting help you confirm the priority problems?
- Mr. D returns to the clinic 3 days later, with fatigue and a high temperature. His white blood cell count is elevated, and he is coughing constantly. He says he is spitting up green mucus. Mr. D is diagnosed with pneumonia.
- Describe nursing interventions for Mr. D and provide a rationale for them.
- What outcomes will you measure to determine if Mr. D is progressing?
- Share your plan of care with the group next to you. What are other interventions that might be used? Why would these also be effective?

Divide into groups of three and select one of the diagnoses presented in lecture. Develop a case that is consistent with that diagnosis and plan interventions.

assignments about the content presented in the lecture. With many of these assignments, only one to two paragraphs are necessary. Keeping the writing activity short assists students in focusing their writing and avoids their summarizing from other sources without thinking critically about the information. Richardson and Trudeau (2003) used problem-based and collaborative learning in the classroom to develop undergraduate students' writing skills. Focused writing assignments encouraged students to think critically and independently and to improve their writing skills. Students also learned to work collaboratively with peers and communicate their ideas effectively to an audience.

With in-class writing activities, students can pass what they wrote to another group for critique and feedback on content and clarity. Some of the assignments can then be continued as out-of-class work and submitted for feedback from the teacher or for grading purposes. The examples that follow, however, are intended for use in class as active-learning strategies. Teachers often complain about the extensive number of papers to grade. Many of those assignments, though, are nothing more than summarizations of what others have written with no original thinking by the student. In-class writing, in contrast, fosters critical thinking and avoids students reporting only from the literature. Although it is unlikely that peers can critique writing style, they can review for accuracy of content and clarity in how the ideas are presented.

Examples of in-class writing activities are:

- Compare a diagnosis discussed in the lecture with one learned in an earlier class.
- Compare two interventions and the strength of evidence.
- Develop a clinical scenario that matches the content presented in class.
- Identify information from the lecture that is still unclear, write questions about that information, and pass the questions to another student or a small group of students to answer in writing.
- Respond in writing to teacher-prepared questions (that review the content presented in lecture and readings).
- List interventions you used for one of your patients, identify alternate interventions for that patient, and provide a rationale for why they would be as effective.
- Write a narrative about these data (data set provided by the teacher) including the meaning of the lab results.

Concept Map

A concept map is a graphic or pictorial arrangement of main concepts or ideas that help students visually connect information (Gaberson & Oermann, 1999). An example of a concept map is provided in Figure 12.1. While often used in clinical teaching, students may develop concept maps from their readings to assist them in linking new facts and concepts to information already learned. Then, as part of the lecture, students can work in small groups to review and compare their **concept maps** and discuss new links between the lecture and their map. In this way, concept maps are useful in encouraging students to prepare for class and complete their readings and other out-of-class assignments. As an alternate at the end of a lecture, students can work in small groups to develop a concept map about that lecture, drawing on their readings for its development. Activities such as these enhance critical thinking and group process, and encourage students to learn from one another. If students present the results of their discussion to the class, teachers can provide immediate feedback.

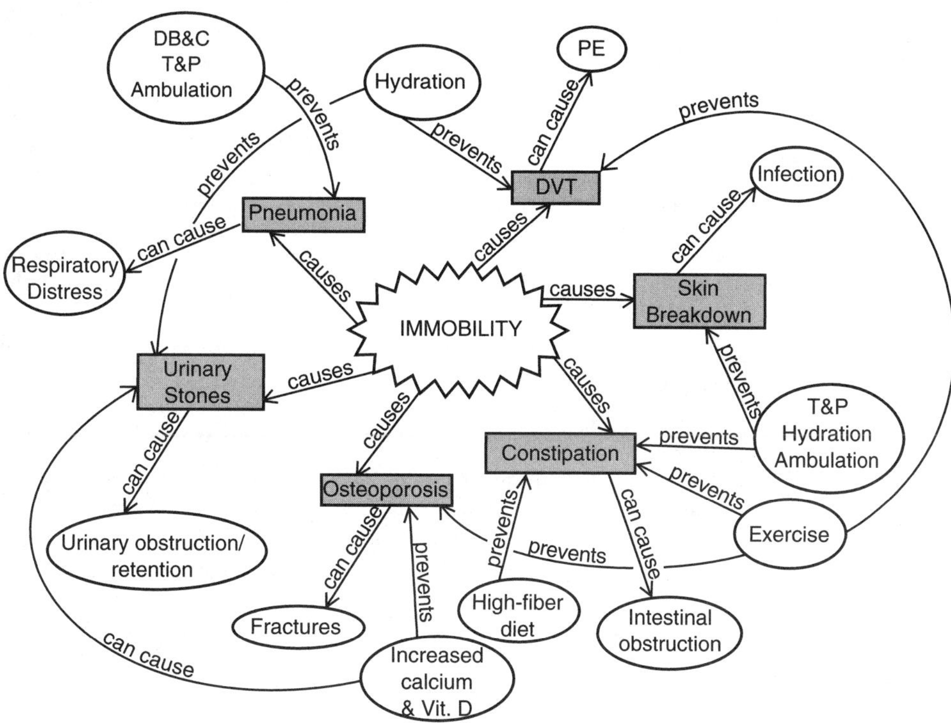

■ **FIGURE 12.1** Concept map. Adapted from Ignatavicius, D. D. (2004). From traditional care plans to innovative concept maps. In M. H. Oermann & K. Heinrich (Eds.), *Annual review of nursing education* (Vol. 2, p. 210). New York: Springer Publishing Company. Reprinted by permission of Springer Publishing Company.

SUMMARY

There are numerous benefits of active learning for students, but there also are benefits of lecture as a method for teaching. Both have their place in nursing education. Even with the growth of online nursing courses, many courses are still taught with traditional methods. Active-learning strategies incorporated within lecture provide for involvement of students and at the same time build on the strengths of lecture as a teaching method—reflecting the best of both worlds.

LEARNING ACTIVITY

You are teaching a maternity nursing course in a prelicensure program. One of the topics in an upcoming class is family assessment. Your goal is to integrate active-learning methods in that class. You have 30 students in the course, and the class meets for 2 hours. Use the Instructions for Educators section to plan your lecture and active-learning methods for this class.

RESOURCES FOR EDUCATORS

PLANNING THE TEACHING/LEARNING EXPERIENCE

Questions to Support a Thoughtful Reading

1. What is active learning, and how does it compare to teacher-centered instruction?
2. Why are both active learning and lecture important teaching methods in nursing education?
3. What are the outcomes, advantages, and disadvantages of active-learning and lecture methods?
4. Develop a rationale for integrating active-learning strategies within lectures. Would you use an integrated approach in your teaching? Why or why not?
5. Make a list of the active-learning strategies you read about in this chapter. Briefly describe each strategy. Which ones might you use in your own classes and for post clinical conferences? How do these fit within your philosophy of teaching in nursing?
6. What levels of questions can be asked during class and in other interactions with learners?
7. What are examples of in-class writing activities that foster active learning?

Instructions for Educators

First, you need to make a conscious decision to allow time within the class for active-learning strategies. Second, plan the lecture content and then ask yourself what types of strategies would help students understand the basic concepts to be presented in that lecture, apply them to clinical practice, and develop their problem-solving and critical thinking skills as related to that content. Third, develop the active-learning methods and decide how and when to implement them in the class. Will you intersperse them throughout the lecture? Stop at midpoint for an active-learning strategy? Or use them at the end of the class when students are often less attentive? Consider, too, the size of the student group, time available, and classroom setup, for example, if chairs are movable or not. Keep in mind that with large groups and seats that are immovable, students can complete the strategies individually or in pairs, with selected students reporting to the entire class.

Next, develop an outline of the content for your lecture. On the outline, list sample questions to ask students, clinical examples and short cases to share with them, the active-learning strategies you have planned, and where you will start and finish those strategies. Even though you have a plan for class, you need to be flexible with these strategies, gauging their time based on student needs. Use different colors to highlight on your outline the questions, clinical examples and cases, and where the active learning methods will be introduced.

Finally, implement your strategies as part of your lecture and again be flexible with your time. Evaluate their effectiveness in terms of student achievement, ability to apply the concepts to clinical practice, and satisfaction with the teaching methods.

EVALUATING THE TEACHING/LEARNING EXPERIENCE

Questions to Elicit Feedback from Students on Their Learning

1. Plan a lecture that you might give. Develop an outline for that lecture and list all possible active-learning strategies that you could use. Provide a rationale of why those strategies would be appropriate including the outcomes they would achieve.
2. Of the active-learning strategies presented in this chapter, select three and develop those strategies for in-class use.
3. Write examples of questions you could ask students during a lecture or in other interactions with them that are leveled using the cognitive taxonomy.
4. Develop one short case for use in a lecture to foster active learning and promote critical thinking.

Reflective Questions for Educators

1. Are students learning from your lectures or are they only taking notes?
2. How effective are your teaching strategies in motivating students to learn and take an active role in their learning?
3. How important is active learning in your philosophy of teaching in nursing? If important, what are strategies you can use to foster active learning within your classes?

References

Baumberger-Henry, M. (2003). Practicing the art of nursing through student-designed continuing case study and cooperative learning. *Nurse Educator, 28*, 191–195.

Bo-Linn, C. (n.d.). Advantages and Disadvantages of the Lecture Method. Division of Instructional Development, University of Illinois. Accessed September 3, 2003, from http://www.oir.uiuc.edu/Did/docs/LECTURE/Lecture1.htm.

Crabtree, J. L., Royeen, C. B., & Mu, K. (2001). The effects of learning through discussion in a course in occupational therapy: A search for deep learning. *Journal of Allied Health, 30*, 243–247.

DeMarco, D. R., Hayward, L., & Lynch, M. (2002). Nursing students' experiences with and strategic approaches to case-based instruction: A replication and comparison study between two disciplines. *Journal of Nursing Education, 41*, 165–174.

Gaberson, K., & Oermann, M. H. (1999). *Clinical teaching strategies in nursing education*. New York: Springer.

Jarrott, S. E., & Blieszner, R. (2001). Creating families in the classroom: An active learning approach. *Gerontology & Geriatrics Education, 22*, 15–27.

Mertler, C. A. (2003). *Classroom assessment*. Los Angeles: Pyrczak Publishing.

Oermann, M. H. (1997). Evaluating critical thinking in clinical practice. *Nurse Educator, 22*, 25–28.

Oermann, M. H. (1998). How to assess critical thinking in clinical practice. *Dimensions of Critical Care Nursing, 17*, 322–327.

Oermann, M. H. (1999). Public speaking: Tips for flying solo. *Home Health Focus, 5*, 61–62.

Oermann, M. H. (2000). Clinical scenarios for critical thinking. *Academic Exchange Quarterly, 4*, 85–91.

Oermann, M. H., & Gaberson, K. (2006). *Evaluation and testing in nursing education* (2nd ed). New York: Springer.

Oermann, M. H., Truesdell, S., & Ziolkowski, L. (2000). Strategy to assess, develop, and evaluate critical thinking. *Journal of Continuing Education in Nursing, 31*, 155–160.

Palmer, P. J. (1997). The courage to teach: Exploring the inner landscape of a teacher's life. San Francisco: Jossey-Bass.

Richardson, K., & Trudeau, K. J. (2003). A case for problem-based collaborative learning in the nursing classroom. *Nurse Educator, 26*, 83–88.

Stringer, J. L. (2002). Incorporation of active learning strategies into the classroom: What one person can do. *Perspective on Physician Assistant Education, 13*, 98–102.

Tomey, A.M. (2003). Learning with cases. *Journal of Continuing Education in Nursing, 34*, 34–38.

University of Pittsburgh Faculty Development Services. (2004). The lecture method. Accessed July 1, 2004, from http://www.pitt.edu/;ciddeweb/FACULTY-DEVELOPMENT/FDS/lectmeth.html.

Wankat, W. P., & Oreovicz, F. (2003). Breaking the 15-minute barrier. *ASEE Prism, 12*(8), 40.

Woodring, B. C. (2001). Lecture is not a four-letter word! In A. J. Lowenstein, & M. J. Bradshaw (Eds.), *Fuszard's innovative teaching strategies in nursing* (3rd ed., pp. 65–82). Gaithersburg, MD: Aspen.

Yuretich, R. F., Khan, S. A., Leckie, R. M., & Clement J. J. (2001). Active-learning methods to improve student performance and scientific interest in a large introductory oceanography course. *Journal of Geoscience Education, 49*, 111–119.

Additional Resources

Gaberson, K., & Oermann, M. H. (1999). *Clinical teaching strategies in nursing education.* New York: Springer Publishing Company.

Ignatavicius, D. D. (2004). From traditional care plans to innovative concept maps. In M. H. Oermann & K. Heinrich (Eds.), *Annual review of nursing education* (Vol. 2, pp. 205–216). New York: Springer Publishing Company.

Sedlak, C. A., & Doheny, M. O. (2004). Critical thinking: What's new and how to foster thinking among nursing students. In M. H. Oermann, & K. Heinrich (Eds.), *Annual review of nursing education* (Vol. 2, pp. 185–204). New York: Springer Publishing Company.

Shellenbarger, T., Palmer, E. A., Labant, A. L., & Kuzneski, J. L. (2005). Use of faculty reflection to improve teaching. In M. H. Oermann, & K. Heinrich (Eds.), *Annual review of nursing education* (Vol. 3, pp. 343–357). New York: Springer Publishing Company.

Zygmont, D. M., & Schaefer, K. M. (2005). Journey taken by two educators transitioning from teacher-centered to student-centered instruction. In M. H. Oermann, & K. Heinrich (Eds.), *Annual review of nursing education* (Vol. 3, pp. 125–142). New York: Springer Publishing Company.

Models and Strategies for Teaching by Distance Education Using Student-Centered Approaches

Chapter 13

Cynthia K. Russell, Victoria S. Murrell, Margaret T. Hartig, W. Dean Care, Susan Jacob, Carol Lockhart, Sarah Mynatt, James Pruett, Cheryl Stegbauer, and Carol Thompson

Barbara T. is a first-year PhD student majoring in nursing education. She has a particular interest in student-centered approaches to distance learning. Barbara has just completed a history of nursing education course and was amazed to discover that distance education started in the late 19th century. Barbara examined the roles and responsibilities of universities and colleges as they responded to the learning needs of widely dispersed, nontraditional, off-campus students. She discovered there have been several generations of distance education. This first-generation method of delivery was print based, highly structured, and teacher centered. Beginning in the Industrial Revolution era, the distance education movement focused on efficiency, bureaucracy, control, and mass production of printed materials. Moving forward in time, the introduction of the telephone allowed for two-way interaction between the teacher and students. Radio and television technology brought with it the ability to transmit audio and visual images to the student. As the digital age and fifth generation technologies emerged, there was greater capacity for expedient and simultaneous interaction among students and between teacher and students. Today, distance education has evolved to a predominantly Web-based delivery model, one that is highly flexible, allows for maximum interaction, and focuses on the learner. Barbara was interested and pleased to see that the emergence of student-centered distance education has mirrored the evolution of instructional technology. This course raised several questions in her mind: Will new generations of instructional technology affect student learning experiences?; Will faculty continue the move away from traditional institution-based approaches and migrate to interactive distance education strategies?; What technical supports will faculty need to design and implement student-centered courses?; and, How can pedagogical practices be adapted to address the new, emerging instructional technologies? Barbara wonders if one of these questions will form the basis for her doctoral dissertation.

Early in her doctoral program, Barbara has discovered that, throughout history, advances in instructional technology have influenced and powered paradigmatic shifts in education. She is beginning to understand that distance education, and students studying by distance, have benefited from these advancements.

INTENT This chapter provides a description of five generations of distance learning models. The impact of advancing technology on teaching, learning, and student-centered education is addressed. Teaching and instructional design strategies that foster student centeredness are suggested and supported by the literature. The chapter concludes with a look at several issues facing faculty as they pursue student-centered distance education.

OVERVIEW

MODELS OF DISTANCE EDUCATION

Several models have been advanced to depict the variety of distance-education delivery used in contemporary institutions (Pennsylvania State University, 1998; Taylor, 1995, 2001a, 2001b; University of Maryland, 1997). Of these models, the most sophisticated is Taylor's five generations of distance education models. Taylor's conceptual framework focuses on the associated delivery technologies, the characteristics of those delivery technologies, and institutional variable costs for each generation. The models are not mutually exclusive and, in reality, institutions employ more than one model. See Table 13.1 for a conceptual framework of Taylor's five models.

First Generation: Correspondence Model

Print is the delivery technology for the correspondence model of distance education. Print has the **flexibility of time**, **flexibility of place**, and **flexibility of pace**, in that students and faculty are not required to be in the same place at the same time nor must all students progress through the content together as a cohort. **Interactivity**, in any advanced way, is limited with print technologies and the **institutional variable costs** for production and delivery are high. Students, however, appreciate and benefit from well-designed print materials. Most students are familiar with correspondence models of education, even though not all students do well in this model of learning. Typically there is no interaction among students or between faculty and students. There is also limited immediate feedback because the correspondence model is asynchronous and often relies on postal mail for communication.

Second Generation: Multimedia Model

The multimedia model supplements print materials with audiotapes or videotapes, computer-based learning, and interactive video. Each of these additional technologies has the flexibility associated with print, but audiotape and videotape suffer from the same limited interactivity as print materials. Depending on their design, computer-based learning and interactive video can provide students with opportunities to interact with materials. However, the institutional variable costs do not decrease, given the costs associated with producing materials for each student.

TABLE 13.1 TAYLOR'S MODELS OF DISTANCE EDUCATION: A CONCEPTUAL FRAMEWORK

MODELS OF DISTANCE EDUCATION AND ASSOCIATED DELIVERY TECHNOLOGIES	CHARACTERISTICS OF DELIVERY TECHNOLOGIES					
	FLEXIBILITY			HIGHLY REFINED MATERIALS	ADVANCED INTERACTIVE DELIVERY	INSTITUTIONAL VARIABLE COSTS APPROACHING ZERO
	TIME	PLACE	PACE			
FIRST GENERATION: THE CORRESPONDENCE MODEL						
Print	√	√	√	√	—	—
SECOND GENERATION: THE MULTIMEDIA MODEL						
Print, audiotape, videotape	√	√	√	√	—	—
Computer-based learning	√	√	√	√	√	—
Interactive video	√	√	√	√	√	—
THIRD GENERATION: THE TELELEARNING MODEL						
Audioconferencing and videoconferencing	—	—	—	—	√	—
Audiographic communication	—	—	—	√	√	—
Broadcast TV/Radio	—	—	—	√	√	—
Audioteleconferencing	—	—	—	√	√	—
FOURTH GENERATION: THE FLEXIBLE LEARNING MODEL						
Online interactive multimedia	√	√	√	√	√	√
Access to Internet resources	√	√	√	√	√	√
Computer-mediated communication	√	√	√	√	√	—
FIFTH GENERATION: THE INTELLIGENT FLEXIBLE LEARNING MODEL						
Online interactive multimedia	√	√	√	√	√	√
Access to Internet resources	√	√	√	√	√	√
Computer-mediated communication, using automated response systems	√	√	√	√	√	√
Campus portal access to institutional processes and resources	√	√	√	√	√	√

√, yes; —, no.

Third Generation: Telelearning Model

In the telelearning model, real-time two-way conferencing takes precedence, whether via telephone, video, or any form of broadcast. While these methods of interaction offer increased opportunities for **advanced interactive delivery**, they are not as flexible as the other models. As with the prior models, the institutional variable costs do not decrease.

Additionally, **audioconferencing** and **videoconferencing** are the two delivery technologies that are not **highly refined materials**. The sophistication of content delivered via audioconferencing or videoconferencing is highly dependent on the faculty, the specific mix of students, and the subject matter. Reliance on spontaneously generated conversation in real-time conferencing replicates the traditional face-to-face classroom model while taking limited advantage of the potential of new delivery technologies.

Fourth Generation: Flexible Learning Model

The flexible learning model is also referred to as technology mediated flexible learning, because of its move to incorporate interactive multimedia, Internet-based resources, and computer-mediated communication via e-mail and other modalities. This model makes use of the benefits of flexibility, allows highly refined instructional materials, and advanced interactive delivery. Institutional variable costs for the flexible learning model begin decreasing with the development of sophisticated instructional materials that can be easily and quickly set up at limited or no additional costs even given increasing enrollment. The initial costs in developing interactive multimedia resources tend to be substantial, given the broad range of people and products required to produce materials that will stand the test of time in facilitating learning.

Fifth Generation: Intelligent Flexible Learning Model

The final model, intelligent flexible learning, incorporates the use of all the technologies in the previous model, with the addition of automated response systems for computer-mediated communication and campus portal access to institutional processes and resources. This model is flexible in terms of time, place, and pace. It incorporates highly refined materials and advanced interactive delivery. The institutional variable costs approach zero for each delivery technology in this model, given the potential of automation to provide on-demand access and decrease person-to-person requests for those matters that involve personal contact.

In summary, the models of distance education for contemporary educational institutions take into account location, timing, pacing, interactivity, and costs. Institutional adoption of delivery methods is influenced by constraints at the levels of the (a) institution (i.e., costs and available resources), (b) faculty (i.e., time, motivation, and resources), and (c) student (i.e., available and accessible technologies and time). In addition, several other factors such as outcomes of the learning experience, content and experience to be conveyed, students' backgrounds, and dimensions of instructional design influence the selection of appropriate strategies for student-centered distance education.

FACTORS IN SELECTING STRATEGIES FOR STUDENT-CENTERED DISTANCE EDUCATION

Each distance education model allows for the use of several strategies that foster student-centered distance education. The sheer number of options may be overwhelming for faculty, causing them to continue to use familiar strategies. Faculty may also be reticent to explore and adapt the strategy that is optimal in a given situation. However, the decision-making process can be facilitated when approached in a logical fashion. Several factors are foundational to selecting appropriate methodologies that best support specific teaching–learning experiences.

Outcomes of the Learning Experience

One of the most important issues to be resolved early in the planning for an educational experience is identifying **outcomes**, or what students should take away from the experience. The purpose of some learning experiences is active learning, in which students engage with the content to learn something new. **Community building** is another goal for learning experiences. In this sort of experience, students engage with relevant content with a goal of reinforcing the sense of community in distance education. A third purpose of some learning experiences is assessment or evaluation, wherein students demonstrate their comprehension/competency or mastery/proficiency of the content.

Determining expected student learning outcomes and how they will be assessed provides the faculty with structure to produce outlines at the class, chapter/module, and course levels. If applied across a curriculum, outcomes provide scope and sequence in planning a course of study. Determining appropriate outcomes is an important process that facilitates the expert's provision of relevant course content to students.

The construction of outcomes often adheres to the following format:

> *At the end of the [lesson/chapter/course], the student will be able to [verb] [object of the verb].*

For example, at the completion of a class session on heart sounds, one of the outcomes might state "the student will be able to discriminate between a normal and abnormal adult heart rhythm." More specific outcomes can use the "ABCD" method proposed by Heinrich, Molenda, Russell, and Smaldino (1996). Using this framework, the **a**udience, **b**ehavior, **c**ondition, and **d**egree are all defined within the outcome. Further development of the previous outcome using the ABCD method might read:

> *Using a stethoscope (condition), the student (audience) will be able to discriminate between a normal and abnormal adult heart rhythm (behavior) with no errors (degree).*

There should be several outcomes for each class that support the outcomes for the chapter/module, as well as those for the course. The outcomes should be measurable so that each student's level of competency can be assessed. Using the outcomes, appropriate and adequate assessments can be used to determine if the student has reached the desired level of competency.

In keeping with student-centered learning, faculty may offer students a variety of options for demonstrating that they have achieved the outcomes of a course. For example, in a qualitative research course options for a culminating project may be to (a) prepare a proposal for a qualitative study or (b) conduct a qualitative study. While both options result in different end products, students have the option of selecting the manner by which they will fulfill the course requirements and may choose whichever option best meets their needs.

Content and Experience to Be Conveyed

A clear view of desired outcomes and consideration of multiple formats and delivery processes available in distance education can assist experienced faculty. Complex information and processes can be broken down into digestible components for novice students to grasp and integrate into their knowledge base. Often it is difficult for those with understanding of complex concepts or skills to step through the processes necessary to develop that understanding. For the student, these steps compose crucial information that must be acquired in the educational process. Therefore, a major factor in course planning consists of determining what specific content and experiences will be incorporated and in what format.

Outcomes focused on attainment of mechanical and/or technical skills generally require concrete content and opportunities for application. Online resources allow supplementary step-by-step instructions in text format with drawings, photos, and/or streaming video to demonstrate steps in the process. Audio programs add another dimension. Students may be as successful in mastering techniques taught online that were previously taught in clinical laboratory situations. For example, blood pressure measurement can be taught with detailed listing of the steps for applying and using the equipment, accompanied by photos or video descriptions of the process. Learners can experience Korotkoff sounds through audio enhancement. Practice in determining the difference of amplitude can help students learn the skill of blood pressure measurement. When students are then in their clinical and laboratory sessions, they have the foundation to apply their psychomotor skills related to cuff placement and deflation.

Abstract content, such as a nursing theories course, can use different experiences to promote understanding. Reading assignments and questions about content can be followed by asynchronous discussion board postings or synchronous chat sessions. In these activities, students are provided with opportunities to defend, challenge, and potentially change or strengthen their personal perceptions.

Students' Backgrounds

The Net Generation, Digital Natives, the Millenials, Generation Y, the Digital Generation—these are the incoming students, born from 1980 through 2000 (Raines, 2002), and they have changed radically from the people our institutions were designed to educate (Prensky, 2001a). As **digital natives**, these students are "native speakers of the digital language of computers, video games, and the Internet" (Prensky, 2001a, p. 1), whereas faculty are **digital immigrants** who speak in a predigital language.

The diverse backgrounds of students and faculty present several challenges for enacting student-centered distance education. No longer will the traditional, established methods of conducting class be sufficient for promoting student learning. Compare the characteristics of digital native students and digital immigrant faculty in Table 13.2.

TABLE 13.2 CHARACTERISTICS OF DIGITAL NATIVES AND DIGITAL IMMIGRANTS

DIGITAL NATIVES	DIGITAL IMMIGRANTS
Prefer receiving information quickly and from multiple multimedia sources.	Prefer slow and controlled release of information from limited sources.
Prefer parallel processing and multitasking.	Prefer singular processing and single/limited-tasking.
Prefer processing pictures, sounds, and video before text.	Prefer to provide text before pictures, sounds, and video.
Prefer random access to hyperlinked multimedia information.	Prefer to provide information linearly, logically, and sequentially.
Prefer to interact/network simultaneously with many others.	Prefer students to work independently rather than network and interact.
Prefer to learn just in time.	Prefer to teach just in case.
Prefer instant gratification and instant rewards.	Prefer deferred gratification and deferred rewards.
Prefer learning that is relevant, instantly useful, and fun.	Prefer to teach to the curriculum guide and standardized tests.

Adapted from Jukes, I. (2005). Understanding Digital Kids (DKs): Teaching & learning in the new digital landscape. Retrieved October 28, 2005, from http://thecommittedsardine.net/infosavvy/education/handouts/ndl.pdf.

Creating truly engaging learning for this group of students requires that faculty change their instructional styles. Jukes (2005), Prensky (2001a, 2001b, 2002), and EDUCAUSE (Oblinger & Oblinger, 2005) are excellent starting references to learn more about the backgrounds of incoming students and the changes that faculty must make if they are to avoid merely **e-Teaching** and meaningfully engage students in e-Learning. Some suggestions for redesigning instruction include (Jukes, 2005):

- Make learning fun and relevant to students.
- Use mechanisms to deliver learning faster.
- Use less step-by-step instruction and more random access, just-in-time learning.
- Use less text and more pictures, sounds, and video.
- Provide more opportunities for multitasking, networking, and interactivity.
- Understand that there are two kinds of content: (a) traditional—reading, writing, history, sciences, and (b) 21st century content—critical thinking, problem solving, process as well as personal skills.

It is also important to account for students' previous experiences in the classroom or in the workplace in determining the foundation for developing new knowledge. While this foundation may be included in a review process to "ramp up" for the core course material, it should not be necessary to provide instruction in any prerequisite knowledge. Communicating expectations of previous knowledge is, however, a requirement. Providing resources for individual remediation, including Web sites and/or articles, can be helpful.

Dimensions of Instructional Design

Once the outcomes, type of content and experiences to be provided, and students' backgrounds have been considered, the next step is to determine what approaches will aid students in achieving mastery of that content. Figure 13.1 diagrams some of the various dimensions involved in considering the design and development of instructional materials. In planning for student-centered distance learning, a combination of approaches is possible in view of the continuum of possibilities.

PERSON FOCUS

This dimension ranges from a focus on the individual to focus on a group. The permutations between those poles are endless as one considers large groups, small groups, and the various ways to facilitate and mentor groups, as well as individuals. The course must be designed with teaching methodologies that facilitate appropriate student engagement, interactions, and responses. For example, in a one-on-one online setting, the instructor and student can have a much more intimate discourse. The ability to engage in Socratic questioning decreases proportionally to the size of the group. However, possibilities for collaboration, teamwork, and discursive interactions in larger online classes provide a different dynamic. For example, larger groups of online students result in a broader set of perspectives that may be helpful in challenging individual students' assumptions. **Course management systems** (CMS), such as Blackboard, Moodle, and WebCT, provide instructors with an easy structure for setting up small-group collaboration environments that include functions for e-mail, discussion boards, and chats among group members.

ENGAGEMENT

Prensky's (2005) provocative article, entitled "Engage me or Enrage me: What today's learners demand," describes three types of students: those who are self-motivated, those who go through the motions, and those who tune out faculty. Prensky (2005) claims that while our educational system handles the first two groups fairly well, educators are

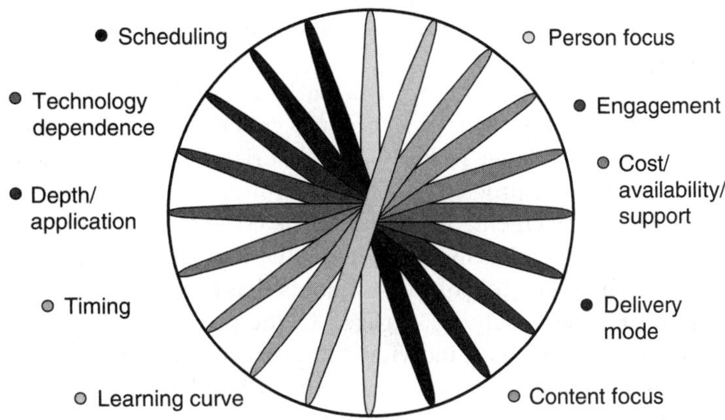

■ **FIGURE 13.1** The instructional design sphere.

not effectively reaching the third group of students, those who resent the fact that their time in school is being wasted. While students of prior generations were not always particularly engaged in educational settings, today's students expect to be engaged by what they do. The formative years of these digital natives have been filled with video games, the Internet, instant messaging, and computers except, as Prensky rightly points out, when they are in school. While higher education faculty may believe this phenomenon is isolated to elementary and secondary schools, these students are aging and arriving in institutions of higher education. The challenge for educators is to take advantage of new technologies and methods for offering students multiple and simultaneous interaction with content so that students engage with the curriculum and avoid becoming enraged.

As this chapter is written, researchers from institutions such as Harvard, Princeton, and George Mason University, among others, are exploring new mechanisms for student engagement and learning that take advantage of students' multitasking and learning styles. Fascinating research is being conducted in the use of **Multiuser Virtual Environments** (MUVEs) for designing and delivering classroom-based situated learning and the ways in which virtual environments may aid transfer of learning from the classroom to real world situations. MUVEs have their basis in the Internet and games such as "Dungeons and Dragons." MUVEs support socialization and problem solving and are highly constructivist environments. Consider this example:

> *A virtual hospital is constructed, wherein multiple users who are health professions' students and practitioners interact in real time. The virtual institution offers opportunities for interprofessional interaction among different professions as well as the different disciplines within those professions. All components of a typical care environment are included. Students interact not only with an individual patient scenario, but also other professions and in various roles, such as direct care provider, nurse manager, administrator, and so on.*

For an example of one such environment, see the Penfield Virtual Hospital at http://www.hud.ac.uk/hhs/departments/nursing/penfield_site/default.htm. This resource, developed by faculty and staff at the University of Huddersfield in the United Kingdom, is a notable step forward to develop stimulating and challenging educational resources. Educators must become involved in creating more of these environments that will engage students.

Engagement, therefore, is a particularly important consideration in the student-centered distance course. In order to gain the most from any learning situation—and to generate knowledge rather than memorize facts—the student should be interested and invested in the process. Different techniques can be used to promote varying levels of student engagement. The poles of the engagement continuum are anchored by passivity and activity. **Passive learning** is the type of learning commonly encountered in the lecture hall. The role of the student is that of a recipient of information provided by the teacher, who is actively engaged in the process. This passivity can also take place in small groups or with individual students if the instructor does not center the learning on the student. Faculty lectures that are videotaped and delivered on CD/DVD or in streaming video foster the same type of passive observation experience among students as the large lecture hall experience.

Active learning, on the other hand, provides more of an engaging learning environment for the students in that they can participate more in the discovery and creation of their own knowledge. Focusing on student engagement encourages a different perspective about presentation, processing, and assessment of learning materials. In distance education, active learning may be supported by the use of discussion boards. Students become actively engaged in answering questions about course material that require application in specific contexts. Discussion boards also support active learning when students synthesize course content to answer questions about situations or cases.

COST AND AVAILABILITY OF SUPPORT

Financial costs, time investment, and technology support are important considerations for faculty and institutions that are developing student-centered education materials, as well as the students who access these materials. Many of the more sophisticated software programs useful for developing content and interactive materials are expensive. Sophisticated software programs also require a significant investment of time on the part of faculty or staff who must learn how to use them in preparing materials. Although newer technologies, such as audioconferencing and videoconferencing and streaming video, are relatively easy to use, their costs for hardware, high speed Internet access, and ongoing staff support for faculty and students are high.

Technology support is a final consideration that should not be overlooked. It is inappropriate to assume that all faculty could, would, or should learn the finer details about the software or hardware they use to engage in student-centered distance education. The costs are sometimes overwhelming for an institution, particularly if a solid information technology infrastructure is lacking. Students also require technology support. In recognition of this, some of the most highly regarded institutions provide around-the-clock, 365 days per year, e-mail and/or telephone support. Chapter 22 discusses these challenges to student-centered distance education more fully.

DELIVERY MODE

Student-centered distance education can be delivered in print format or with audiotapes or videotapes. The introduction of multimedia into the course content, as distributed on CD/DVD, provides opportunities for delivery of more advanced and interactive content. Still, the learning process remains a solitary one with the prior content delivery modes. The speed of communication via the Internet introduced a new world of potential to that of distance education, and new ways of delivering course content are available to both students and teachers. In addition, what had been an isolated experience for the student has evergrowing capacity for interactivity between and among participants. While some distance education is still conducted via mail, there is a growing supply of learning tools that include text, video, audio, interactive television, Internet-based chat rooms and discussion boards, e-mail, interactive programs, computer-based instruction, Web-based instruction, **Internet telephony**, and document sharing technologies, to name a few.

CONTENT FOCUS

There are really four points on this scale of considerations, and this touches somewhat on the topic of learning preferences. One dichotomous pair that represents the type of information that is introduced, concrete and abstract, is positioned at the opposite ends of the continuum. However, superimposed is how that information is processed—by application (doing) or by reflection (thinking). Concrete and abstract content often require different kinds of presentation as well as various opportunities for processing. Applied content begs for an approach different from reflective content.

Concrete learners focus on detail and stress being correct or accurate. They want step-by-step directions. Practical information with real life examples provides the connection to the real world that a concrete learner desires. Structured course content with precise and measurable expectations or outcomes will increase student comfort. Opportunities to practice skills are important. A computer program demonstrating ear examinations with examples of tympanic membrane appearance would be appreciated. Once the concrete knowledge is attained, students could apply their knowledge of appearance in determining how to discriminate between a normal ear drum and an ear canal or ear drum that shows evidence of infection.

Learning often occurs in a progression from concrete to abstract, though some students are likely to initiate their learning from an abstract perspective. Abstract learners are able to conceptualize and understand the overall process of what is going on. They make connections between topics and see the patterns in bits of information. They are deductive, imaginative, and enjoy questions of "What if. . . ?" Conversely, they may ignore important details in a process, unlike concrete learners who often cannot grasp the big picture because of the attention to minute detail.

Most students are able to combine aspects of both learning styles and process information differently when necessary. Some students, however, identify more strongly with one dimension over another. Concrete learners are often afraid to be wrong and take risks. They also have difficulty accepting their work as "good enough." Abstract learners can be innovative in their approaches, but may ignore facts. Providing experiences for both types of learning can expand student abilities. The variety is likely to create anxiety when students have to adapt to a different style, but coping with that anxiety is a learning experience in itself.

The previously mentioned examination of an ear provides a good example for understanding the differences between how a concrete and an abstract learner approach and process content. Once students become comfortable with the basic knowledge of tympanic membrane appearance, they progress to activities that require more abstract abilities and reflection. Concrete learners are likely to study tympanic membrane appearance in multiple situations while abstract learners will look quickly and want to apply the knowledge. Concrete learners will prefer to write a care plan for a case study with clear-cut symptoms, while abstract learners will eagerly accept the challenge of a vague case study with multiple possible diagnoses and treatments. Resulting care plans will be easy to distinguish between the many pages of precise and minute details identified by students who tend to take a concrete approach and the few pages outlining broad categories of care needs without any such detail provided by the more abstract student.

LEARNING CURVE

This term can apply to many aspects of the teaching and learning experience: use of technologies and/or the content itself. For students, **learning curve** refers to the degree of difficulty with which the student grasps something before he or she is able to truly comprehend and apply it. For example, for someone learning to play the piano, it is imperative to learn the notes of the scale before learning to read music. For some, this learning curve may be steeper than for others. Those in charge of developing instructional materials should ask themselves what the learning curve for specific information is likely to be for the students. This curve should be taken into consideration when introducing materials or other learning activities.

A similar learning curve exists for faculty who are using distance education technologies. Institutions may provide faculty development workshops to introduce faculty to new technologies. Faculty success in using new technologies, however, is not assured by workshop participation. In addition to workshops, faculty require continued hands-on experience and expert guidance by other faculty or support staff. A well-designed faculty development program will decrease faculty's learning curves and assist them in becoming proficient with the technology.

TIMING

The terms "synchronous" and "asynchronous" have become part of the distance education vocabulary. Synchronous defines activities that occur in the same time space—for example, online chats, audioconferencing and videoconferencing, interactive Web casts or other broadcasts that may or may not be archived for later access. These kinds of activities do not require that participants be together physically, but they require that participants use a communication tool such as a computer or telephone at the same time. Asynchronous activities are those activities that do not require participation at the same time. A common example of an asynchronous activity is homework, something with which most people in a learning situation are familiar. More electronic examples include e-mail, discussion boards, archived broadcasts or conference presentations, and recordings on CD or DVD. Consideration of the appropriate timing for activities in the development phase for course materials can provide students with greater flexibility.

DEPTH/APPLICATION

Bloom (1956) provides one set of guidelines for the progression of learning (Figure 13.2). Starting with the most basic level of learning, Bloom (1956) theorized that students can achieve various levels of learning that include (in order of cognitive challenge) knowledge, comprehension, application, analysis, synthesis, and evaluation. The last three—analysis, synthesis, and evaluation—comprise the higher level critical thinking skills required of nurses in the workplace. Another set of terminologies include surface and deep learning. Surface learning comprises the lower three levels of Bloom's taxonomy: knowledge, comprehension, and application. These require memorization of facts or details. Deep learning requires the ability to take knowledge and relate new ideas and information. The complexity of the tasks and strategies (especially assessment) should correlate with the necessary level of learning required of the student.

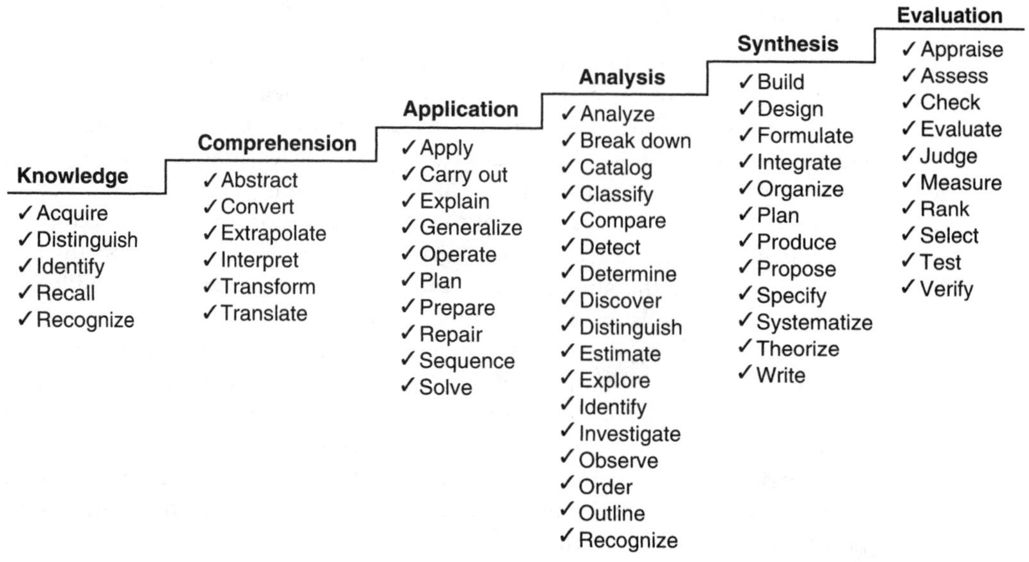

■ **FIGURE 13.2** Bloom's Taxonomy.

TECHNOLOGY DEPENDENCE

Student-centered learning does not require electronically-mediated technologies such as computers and the Internet. However, when teaching and learning at a distance, the technologies that have and continue to be developed can facilitate communication and collaboration that challenges the traditional face-to-face resources. The explosion of the Internet in the last decade of the 20th century, coupled with the everdropping prices of personal computers, have made relatively low tech resources like e-mail and listservs widely available to both faculty and students. The ability to burn data onto CDs, providing a relatively inexpensive way to exchange data, has also made learning at a distance more reasonable, especially for those students who may not have consistent Internet access. However, with the growth of the Internet and its potential for the use of multimedia have come sophisticated programs and delivery systems that can require a significant outlay of resources for the teaching institution, the faculty, and the students. Examples of these include streaming audio and video, videoconferencing, and content authoring programs. Faculty and student resources of time, money, equipment, and access must be considered as the learning materials are planned.

SCHEDULING

Online and distance learning can be organized so that the completion of course requirements has flexibility. As the course is being structured, the faculty will want to consider whether or not students can progress at their own pace or if the students should follow through the curriculum together as a cohort. Another consideration is whether the materials are presented and are accessible in a linear fashion or if they may be accessed in a **nonlinear learning** fashion so that students have the materials they need or want to access at their disposal. Is the course content to be organized in modules? Chapters? By a time span (e.g., "for the week of. . .")? The options are numerous.

Available Methodologies

Numerous methodologies exist that can be tailored to the outcomes of the learning experience, the content and experience that needs to be conveyed, students' backgrounds, and the dimensions of the instructional design sphere. Figure 13.3 depicts the multiple spheres of consideration that should guide the choice of appropriate methodologies.

An additional area of interest when determining the appropriate methodologies for any given situation is the size of the class and the level of faculty involvement. Methodologies and activities that work well in a smaller course or in a course where the faculty desire to be in the middle differ from those appropriate for large enrollment courses or those courses where faculty elect to move out of the middle (MOOM) with respect to the focus of course activities and communications.

Taylor's (1995, 2001a, 2001b) five generations of distance education models assist faculty in selecting the most appropriate methods for delivery, given the spheres of consideration for each course. Within the five generations of models for distance education, essentially there are three types of media/methods that can be used (Benjamin, 2003):

- Static
- Broadcast
- Interactive

STATIC MEDIA

Static media, including print text and images, are typically delivered via paper, CD/DVD, or Internet, from faculty to students (one-way directionality). Examples of static media include traditional quizzes or examinations, scholarly papers, visuals

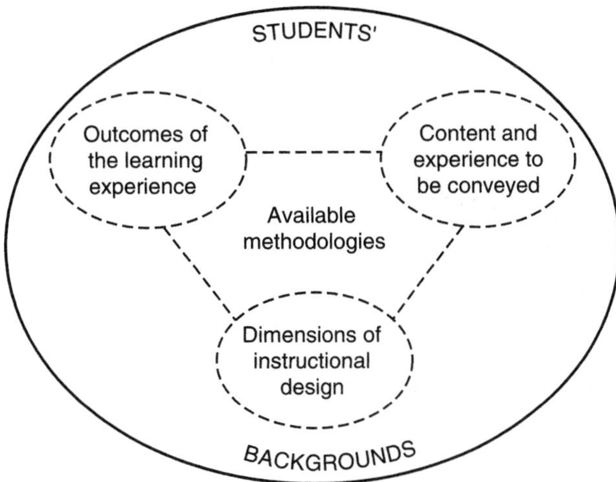

■ **FIGURE 13.3** Multiple spheres in choosing appropriate distance education methodologies.

for courses, and journal articles. The benefits of static media include their familiarity to faculty and students, low cost, easy indexing and retrieving, and their potential for graphic richness. Issues associated with static media include the intensiveness of viewing/reading, ineffective communication of action and emotion, limited spontaneity, and delayed feedback, either from faculty in response to a student paper or from students in regard to their understanding of the material.

When delivered via the Internet, using a CMS such as Blackboard, Moodle, or WebCT, static media can be quickly and economically delivered to small or large groups of students, archived for use in subsequent courses, and provide a foundation for common discussion and reflection. Use of a CMS for testing purposes offers faculty options such as (a) allowing students to retake tests until they achieve a predetermined level of mastery, (b) selecting test questions from a large bank of test items to provide individual tests for each student, (c) setting a time limit for test completion that mimics a nurse registration or certification examination, and (d) providing preprogrammed rationales for correct and incorrect responses.

BROADCAST MEDIA

Broadcast media add audio and video components to the text base of static media. Typically delivered from faculty to students (one-way directionality), broadcast media are most often found in television, radio, CD/DVD, streaming video, or sophisticated content management programs. Broadcast media are dynamic, immediate and familiar, and approximate the traditional classroom in their use of video and audio. Limitations of broadcast media include their one-way communication, ineffective tailoring of materials to individuals, lack of learner–learner interaction, and the special hardware, software, or other equipment required to develop, deliver, or access sophisticated materials.

Examples of situations where broadcast material may be particularly helpful include content areas that are repetitive for faculty to review, particularly problematic for students, or demonstrate physical examination techniques. For example, a faculty member who conducts an epidemiology course may be videotaped presenting a complicated epidemiological principle. The faculty member may also develop PowerPoint slides to accompany the presentation and identify relevant Web sites for students. Using programs such as eTeach or Macromedia's Breeze, this content can be packaged into a learning module and delivered via the Internet or a streaming video server, thereby serving as a repository for students in that course or future courses to review and re-review to enhance their understanding of the course material. Faculty at the University of Tennessee Health Science Center have used Macromedia's Flash to prepare materials on the oxygen–hemoglobin dissociation curve for nurse anesthesia students, as well as arterial blood gas interpretation for acute and critical care students. Faculty may find the resources listed in Box 13.1 to be helpful.

Broadcast media are often expensive to produce and deliver, given the special hardware, software, and equipment needed for production and delivery of a quality product. A significant amount of time also is required for the development of broadcast media, if they are to stand the test of time within courses. Other individuals, such as instructional designers and video producers, often need to be involved with the design and production of these materials, which adds to the time and cost of any project. Once produced,

BOX 13.1 RESOURCES FOR DISTANCE EDUCATION

Low Threshold Applications
- http://www.tltgroup.org/ltas/home.htm

MERLOT (Multimedia Educational Resource for Learning and Online Teaching)
- http://www.merlot.org/Home.po

Harvey Project
- http://harveyproject.org/index.htm

broadcast media can be delivered to small or large groups of students, even though the expense of delivery may involve a significant cost outlay for a streaming video server. Student connectivity to the Internet must be considered with the use of broadcast media, with alternative delivery modes provided for students with dial-up connections. Most broadcast media may be delivered on CD/DVD and videotape in addition to the Internet.

INTERACTIVE MEDIA

Interactive media includes audio, video, and text, in two-way communication between or among faculty and students. Delivered via audioconference, telephone conference, text or voice chat, discussion boards, listservs, simulations, interactive television, and journals or blogs, interactive media have the potential for enhancing interactive dialogue among participants. In addition, interactive media often help to establish a more personal relationship and connectedness among students and faculty. Examples of use for interactive media are class sessions, virtual office hours, guest lectures, interactive games, and virtual clinics. Some of the modalities of interactive media (conferencing, interactive television, simulations) are expensive in terms of the equipment and bandwidth that their delivery requires. The technology training and support required of faculty and students to ensure seamless application of these media provide yet another associated cost.

Some uses of interactive media place restrictions for time, place, and pace among students. For example, videoconferencing, audioconferencing, and interactive television require students and faculty to convene at the same time, in possibly different places, for synchronous sessions. Without sufficient planning, however, these sessions may replicate the classroom's "talking head" and not offer added value to the interactivity. Other forms of interactive media, including interactive games, offer students opportunities to interact with content while affording them asynchronous flexibility in terms of time, place, and pace.

Experience-based learning is a particular type of active learning that is well suited for delivery by interactive distance education media. Related learning types include situational learning, case-based learning, contextual learning, service-based learning, and problem-based learning. Preparing experience-based learning content requires the use of software applications that enable merging desired learning outcomes with real world situations that students encounter. The resulting multimedia instructional presentations coordinate verbal and visual messages to deliver engaging, adult learner-focused, interactive, and modular content (Mayer, 2001; Wittrock, 1989). Virtual patients and virtual clinics are examples of experience-based learning.

One example of experience-based learning is the Virtual Primary Care Clinic (VPCC) prepared at the College of Nursing, University of Tennessee Health Science Center (http://www.utmem.edu/nursing/DHEP/index.htm). The VPCC offers students in a core primary care family nurse practitioner course opportunities to apply didactic course content to the assessment of a virtual patient. As students progress through each VPCC case they may refer to other materials, thereby increasing their learning opportunities. Once they complete each case, students enter a Blackboard course discussion board where they dialogue about treatment aspects and how the progression or outcome of the case may have changed given alterations in the patient's demographics, health conditions, and family situation.

In summary, selecting the content and delivery mechanisms for student-centered distance education demands a type and level of sophistication on the part of faculty that has not historically been required. Many factors must be considered in order to ensure that the teaching/learning experiences will meet the needs of both faculty and students. Table 13.3 summarizes the preceding discussion through offering questions for faculty to take into account as they plan for the best student-centered learning experiences for specific content areas.

TABLE 13.3 QUESTIONS FOR SELECTING STRATEGIES FOR STUDENT-CENTERED DISTANCE EDUCATION

QUESTIONS	DIMENSIONS
1. What are the desired outcomes of the learning experience?	• Active learning • Community building • Assessment/Evaluation ○ Comprehension/Competency ○ Mastery/Proficiency
2. What type of content or experience needs conveyed?	• Concrete • Applied • Abstract
3. What background do students bring to the educational experience?	• Experience with higher education • Experience with the content • Experience with technology
4. What dimensions of the Instructional Design Sphere are appropriate to consider?	• Person-focus • Engagement • Cost/Availability/Support • Delivery mode • Content focus • Learning curve • Timing • Depth/Application • Technology dependence • Scheduling
5. Given the answers to the prior four questions, what specific methodologies best support the teaching–learning experience?	• Static • Broadcast • Interactive

EVOLVING CONSIDERATIONS IN PROVIDING STUDENT-CENTERED DISTANCE EDUCATION

Distance education is rapidly evolving in its research base, theoretical background, and practice. The issues that face faculty electing to provide student-centered distance education, likewise, are a rapidly changing target. Some of the current issues that occupy many listserv discussions and publication pages are verification of student effort, student-centered academic support services, quality standards and benchmarking, technology changes, and lifelong learning and knowledge management.

Verification of Student Effort

Verification that a specific student performs the work that results in a grade for an assignment and a course is a faculty concern, whether courses are face-to-face or delivered online. While some faculty, administrators, and accrediting agencies are concerned about the increased potential for cheating in online courses, in reality the potential for cheating is about the same in online and face-to-face courses (Carnevale, 1999; Roach, 2001). The institutional commitment to honesty and the design of online courses, however, can help to ensure students operate with honesty, trust, fairness, respect, and responsibility, five fundamental values that support academic integrity (Center for Academic Integrity, 1999).

Hinman (2000) offers three possible approaches that institutions may implement, singly or in combination, to prevent cheating and plagiarism. The first, the virtues approach, is concerned with developing students who do not want or seek to cheat. University honor codes are an example of a virtues approach, wherein the institution seeks to mold students who desire to be honorable and virtuous in their student academic life. In the second approach, prevention, faculty and administrators strive to eliminate or reduce the opportunities as well as the pressure to cheat. Examples of prevention approaches include individualized assignments and proctoring of examinations. The final approach, the police approach, has as its goal to catch and punish students who cheat. Plagiarism resource sites are an example of the police approach which is, by its nature, an after-the-fact strategy. Box 13.2 discusses strategies that facilitate student-centered learning and minimize the likelihood of student cheating or plagiarism.

Student-Centered Academic Support Services

Academic support services include such areas as tutoring, individualized instruction, peer-to-peer support, and teaching assistants. The best practices literature (CHEA, 2002; Dirr, 1999) clearly notes that, in addition to these services that support students' academic work, students who study at a distance require access to all the traditional student services such as the library, bookstore, and support for using instructional technologies.

An important aspect of student-centered academic support services provided to students who are studying at a distance is that students should not be required to be present on campus to access these services. All services that on-campus students can access should be accessible at a distance. This aspect may create challenges for these campus services that are often understaffed when trying to provide services in traditional face-to-face environments.

BOX 13.2 STRATEGIES THAT FACILITATE STUDENT-CENTERED LEARNING AND MINIMIZE THE LIKELIHOOD OF STUDENT CHEATING OR PLAGIARISM

1. ACKNOWLEDGE THAT CHEATING AND PLAGIARISM MAY OCCUR AND TAKE STEPS TO ADDRESS IT

Virtues approach

Adopt a prevention focus:

- Inform students about academic integrity and, if applicable, the institution's honor code.
- Provide information about plagiarism and its meaning in the online environment.
- Explain proper citations and fair use guidelines.

Prevention approach

To ascertain who is taking an assessment:

- Use a log-in system.
- Use several short assessments throughout the course to provide multiple checkpoints.
- Include assignments that require some degree of cooperation and/or collaboration among students.
- Build on a high level of faculty–student interactivity via e-mail and synchronous chats.
- Have proctored examinations.

To control student use of unauthorized resources in completing assessments:

- Make all assessments open-book.
- Use tests or quizzes more as self-assessments.

To prevent students from collaborating with each other in taking assessments:

- Set time limits.
- Control number of permissible accesses to assessments.
- Create large question pools for generating randomized assessments.

2. DESIGN EFFECTIVE ONLINE ASSESSMENTS

- Ask mastery-type questions, as well as other questions that require students to demonstrate higher-order thinking.
- Ask students to relate topics to their own personal and/or professional experience.
- Design process-oriented assessments with pieces of work submitted throughout the duration of the course.

3. EMPLOY MECHANISMS TO CATCH AND PUNISH THOSE WHO CHEAT

Police approach

- Keep a log of discussion group participation by students and review writing styles.
- Ask students to provide a writing sample at the beginning of the course for comparison with future written work.
- Know what is available online before assigning a paper.
- Have assignments submitted electronically and archive copies.
- Subscribe to a plagiarism detection service.

Adapted from Cercone, K. (2002). Tips, tricks, and how to prevent cheating in distance education. Retrieved October 19, 2005, from http://web-pt.net/wyoming/index.htm; McVay Lynch, M. (2004). *Learning online: A guide to success in the virtual classroom.* New York: Routledge Falmer; Olt, M.R. (2002). Ethics and distance education: Strategies for minimizing academic dishonesty in online assessment. *Online Journal of Distance Learning Administration, 5*(3). Retrieved October 19, 2005, from http://www.westga.edu/~distance/ojdla/fall53/olt53.html.

Some institutions have found the provision of academic support services is best handled through contracts with outside agencies. Particularly in terms of technology support services that should be provided around the clock, 365 days per year, institutions often find that the cost to contract these services to other agencies is less than staffing an in-house center.

Quality Standards and Benchmarking

Educators, administrators, and accreditors agree on the need for quality standards and benchmarking in distance education programs. Numerous documents have been published to help guide institutions in ensuring that their programs reflect best practices in the provision of online programs (see Table 13.4). The Council for Higher Education Accreditation (CHEA), a private, nonprofit national organization that coordinates accreditation activity in the U.S., lists three major challenges that assuring quality in distance education presents for accreditation (2002):

1. Alternative design of instruction that differs from traditional classroom-based learning environments.
2. Alternative providers of higher education that are new online degree granting institutions as well as online consortia of institutions and corporate universities.
3. Expanded focus on training that is especially relevant for professional fields, but is often independent of the longer term and more structured offerings of degree programs.

Regional accrediting organizations in the U.S., such as the Southern Regional Education Board (SREB), have developed standards, policies, and/or processes for evaluating distance learning. These standards focus on seven features deemed fundamental to assuring quality in distance learning, including (a) institutional mission, (b) institutional organizational structure, (c) institutional resources, (d) curriculum and instruction, (e) faculty support, (f) student support, and (g) student learning outcomes (CHEA, 2002). Just as institutions are well advised to develop or adopt a set of benchmarks and quality guidelines for their distance programs, it is advisable for prospective students to ask to review such documents to ensure that the institution is well equipped to provide quality distance programs.

Another initiative that holds promise for fostering quality student-centered distance courses in nursing programs is the Flashlight/TLT Evaluating Educational Uses of the Web In Nursing (EEUWIN, n.d.) benchmarking project. Developed by the TLTGroup in collaboration with the Indiana University School of Nursing, University of Colorado Health Sciences Center, and the University of Kansas School of Nursing, the EEUWIN project allows participating programs to administer a standardized, online benchmarking survey to students across their programs, or a series of courses. Data are pooled, with programs receiving individualized reports for their programs by course, raw data for their program, and a benchmarking report by course comparing each course against a multi-institution pool. Participating programs compare themselves across 11 indices measuring success in three major areas: technology use, educational practices, and outcomes.

Having accessible, transparent, and up-to-date standards and practices is becoming increasingly important in an environment of savvy students who are critically evaluating distance education programs. For example, EDUCAUSE (2004), a nonprofit association

TABLE 13.4 STANDARDS AND BENCHMARKS FOR DISTANCE EDUCATION PROGRAMS

TITLE	ORGANIZATION	URL	IMPORTANT ASPECTS
Best practices for electronically offered degree and certificate programs	Western Cooperative for Educational Telecommunications	http://www.wcet.info/resources/accreditation/Accrediting%20-%20Best%20Practices.pdf	Five components: 1. Institutional context and commitment 2. Curriculum and instruction 3. Faculty support 4. Student support 5. Evaluation and assessment
Quality on the line: Benchmarks for success in Internet-based distance education	National Education Association and Blackboard, Inc.	http://www.nea.org/he/abouthe/Quality.pdf	Seven categories: 1. Institutional support 2. Course development 3. Teaching/learning 4. Course structure 5. Student support 6. Faculty support 7. Evaluation and assessment
Five pillars of quality online education	The Sloan Consortium	http://sloan-c.org/effective/pillarreport1.pdf	Five pillars: 1. Learning effectiveness 2. Student satisfaction 3. Faculty satisfaction 4. Cost effectiveness 5. Access
Putting principles into practice: Promoting effective support services for students in distance learning programs	Western Cooperative for Educational Telecommunications	http://www.wcet.info/projects/studentservices/Survey%20Report.pdf	Six areas: 1. Pre-enrollment services 2. Academic advising 3. Learning resources 4. Course advising, counseling, social support 5. Technical support for distance students 6. Financial aid

whose mission is to advance higher education by promoting the intelligent use of information technology, developed a publication entitled, *Student Guide to Evaluating Information Technology on Campus*, that offers prospective students and their parents specific questions to assess an institution's computing and information technology environment.

Technology Changes

Whether they are called third-generation devices, next-generation technologies, or cutting edge technology, **handheld electronic devices** are becoming more ubiquitous in everyday life and in distance education environments. These devices combine many of the functions of today's computers into a small package that is easily held in users' hands.

McVay Lynch (2004) notes "the future of technology in online education is toward diversification, increasing functionality, and overlapping modes of learning" (p. 188).

Handheld electronic devices, such as cell phones and personal digital assistants (PDAs), have the potential to enhance student-centered distance education through their "download and go" interface for educational games, just-in-time training, streaming video, electronic books or **e-books**, and reference books for clinical areas, and drug databases for clinicians. These devices also create new challenges for faculty in terms of content design issues, such as preparing and distributing class materials, and compatibility/interoperability issues, such as interfaces among various devices. Handheld devices make it possible for students to communicate with each other via wireless, infrared, or Internet technologies, which may be an issue in testing situations. Additionally, user satisfaction may be affected by the lack of a keyboard for text generation, as well as the need to read material on a small screen.

In contrast to the usefulness of cell phones and PDAs for students, **pen-based computing** using **Tablet PCs** is a technology that holds great promise for faculty. Tablet PCs enable the development of innovative presentations that integrate text with diagrams (Anderson, et al., n.d.). A particularly useful feature of tablet PCs is the ability for faculty to download student papers, use their handwriting to make digital annotations, and then return them to students in tablet PC Journal or Acrobat PDF format. Students who have received such documents comment on the personalization that they felt from receiving documents with faculty handwriting as compared to using something as impersonal as Microsoft Word's track changes feature.

Lifelong Learning and Knowledge Management

If the half-life of general knowledge is 3 to 4 years (McVay Lynch, 2004) it is not a far stretch to assume that the half-life of health care-related knowledge is as little as half that. Before graduating from their nursing programs some of what students have learned is already out of date and in need of revision. Combined with the rapid turnover in knowledge is the awesome increase in the amount of information in the world, and within health care specifically. Dawes (2001) illustrated this rapidly increasing health care knowledge by using hypertension as an exemplar. In his research, he found 27 kilobytes of guidelines for treating hypertension, 3,000 new papers per day, 1,000 new articles per day indexed on Medline, and 46 randomized controlled trials. Health care providers, Dawes noted, have too many patients with too many problems, and too many journals to read with a lack of time to read them, which contributes to information overload and an overall tendency for clinicians to read what they are familiar with and avoid difficult or new issues. A final factor to consider is the trend in the frequency with which workers change jobs. By some U.S. Department of Labor estimates, 40% of the workforce change jobs yearly and, on average, every 10 years workers change careers (Cetron & Davies, 2003). All these matters raise issues for retraining, retooling, and accelerated learning programs that are geared to adult students.

Fennema (2003) notes that the Information Age is requiring educational environments to provide students with lifelong learning, interactive and collaborative learning, and asynchronous learning. Learning must go beyond the traditional boundaries of academia to become part of the culture of graduates' lives, where they must have opportunities to actively engage with others in the learning process. Learning must become more relevant to students' immediate needs through just-in-time learning opportunities.

SUMMARY

Student-centered distance education has come a long way yet, in many ways, there is a great distance to go to ensure that the styles and attitudes of today's students are not forced to fit yesterday's course design. The evolution of technology for the creation and delivery of distance education materials seems to occur at lightening speeds. Without a firm grounding in the pedagogy of the teaching–learning experience, faculty may find themselves wrongly embracing the technology over the pedagogy. This would be a terrible mistake. When designing student-centered learning, it is important to recall that the technology is not the thing—whether or not students learn is what counts. Without student learning, all the distance education technologies are for naught.

LEARNING ACTIVITY

1. For at least one topic in a subject area, create at least three learning objectives utilizing verbs that reflect analysis, synthesis, and evaluation as defined by Bloom's (1956) *Taxonomy*. Keep in mind the objectives must be measurable, so verbs like "understand" will not suffice.
2. Utilize the Sphere of Instructional Design to create and complete a matrix for teaching one topic in your course which results in a focus on the student's experience rather than the teacher's objectives. Once you have thought through one topic, it should be much easier to contemplate subsequent ones.
3. Think about your digital native students. Consider at least one of your current teaching approaches that may not be as effective as you would like. How can you re-engineer your teaching to encompass their instant messaging way of life while encouraging contemplative and reflective thinking skills?

RESOURCES FOR EDUCATORS

PLANNING THE TEACHING/LEARNING EXPERIENCE

Instructions for Educators

1. If you had to learn the content of a class, how would you go about it? Thinking about this question helps reframe the approach to one of guide from the side. The teaching work is then to set up the experience so the students can go through those steps.
2. Reframe your teaching work as grocery shopping rather than growing the food yourself. Often your work is selecting the best of the materials already available in books or online, and so on. When lecturing, the approach was like growing the food yourself. You were providing good food, but probably not the variety that can come from

shopping. More importantly, you have deprived the students of learning how to shop. Knowledge changes so quickly that learning to shop is just as important as preparing the food for today's meal.

3. Clearly set forth expectations for an assignment. In planning an assignment that will be graded, the first thing that needs to be done is to think through the outcomes of the assignment and design it to meet those outcomes. Providing students with clear instructions and weights of expected outcomes helps them to meet faculty's expectations.
4. Plan the necessary time to develop an online course or segments of online instruction. Placing courses online requires the faculty member to master the system that is used and to carefully plan the semester's schedule. Time also includes the training, support, and consultation from technology experts and instructional designers to convert existing face-to-face and new content to the required format of each department and university.

Tips for Developing a Student-Centered Environment

- The toughest part is making the time and effort to complete the task reasonable. Generally there will need to be multiple sources to achieve the desired outcomes, so carefully evaluate the optimal mix for the student, as well as resources available and their costs. For example, in one week of a graduate critical care class, students were to learn five pulmonary areas, one being chest tubes. Initially the faculty member identified seven sources for this content that would have meant 450 pages of reading and three interactive tasks. The final chest tube assignment was one reading and an interactive exercise that covered four of the five content areas for the week.
- Redundance of material through different learning styles will maximize the group's learning. For example, give visual material along with auditory, inductive, and deductive approaches.
- Develop a template for how the course is delivered. Tweak the template as needed to achieve specific outcomes. Standardization will help you keep the learning focused on the content rather than the process.
- Set expectations with a comprehensive syllabus that includes policies such as e-mail expectations, honor code, grading requirements, and so on.

Questions to Support a Thoughtful Reading

1. What methods and media are already familiar to you? Consider one new one at a time, since your learning curve may require all the extra preparation time available.
2. What experiences do the students have to build upon?
3. Has there been a recent public event that would help the adult learner better see the immediate utility of the content to be learned? For example, when the President of the U.S. choked on food while watching the weekend game, the Monday morning exercise on obstructive airway was placed in the scenario of the president choking.
4. What content is really just memorization and what is really synthesis? Plan the learning accordingly.
5. Explain how distance education engages students.

6. Explain three factors to consider to prepare faculty for teaching in distance education.
7. What two or three standards would you suggest for your college or university to adopt for distance education?

EVALUATING THE TEACHING/LEARNING EXPERIENCE

Questions to Elicit Feedback from Students on Their Learning

1. Write at least three outcomes that are measurable and require more than memorization.
2. Explain two kinds of support that an institution needs to put in place for a quality student-centered distance education program.

Sample Evaluation Strategies and Tools

1. Ask students for feedback on what they would change in the specific unit.
2. Use a checklist with criteria for distance education courses developed by faculty with expertise in distance education.
3. Ask other, more experienced, faculty to review the course and make suggestions.

Reflective Questions for Educators

1. Was the process of learning fun?
2. Have you used a variety of methods that engage the students, foster interaction, appeal to different learning styles, and develop higher levels of learning?

References

Anderson, R., Anderson, R., Hoyer, C., et al. *Lecture presentation from the tablet pc*. Retrieved October 19, 2005, from http://www.conferencexp.net/community/Library/Papers/WACE.doc.

Benjamin, J. (2003). Interactive online educational experiences: E-volution of graded projects. In S. Reisman, J. G. Flores, & D. Edge (Eds.), *Electronic learning communities: Current issues and best practices* (pp. 1–26). Greenwich, CT: Information Age Publishing.

Bloom, B. S. (Ed.). (1956). *Taxonomy of educational objectives*. New York: Longman, Green & Co.

Broadbent, B. (2002). *ABCs of e-Learning: Reaping the benefits and avoiding the pitfalls*. San Francisco: Jossey-Bass/Pfeiffer.

Carnevale, D. (1999, November 12). How to proctor from a distance: Experts say professors need savvy to prevent cheating in online courses. *The Chronicle of Higher Education*. Retrieved October 19, 2005, from http://chronicle.com/free/v46/i12/12a04701.htm.

Center for Academic Integrity. (1999). *Fundamental values project*. Retrieved October 19, 2005, from http://www.academicintegrity.org/fundamental.asp.

Cercone, K. (2002). Tips, tricks, and how to prevent cheating in distance education. Retrieved March 19, 2005, from http://web-pt.net/wyoming/index.htm.

Cetron, M. J., & Davies, O. (2003). *50 trends shaping the future*. Special Report published by the World Future Society.

Council for Higher Education Accreditation. (2002). *Accreditation and assuring quality in distance learning*. CHEA Monograph Series 2002, Number 1. Washington, DC: CHEA Institute for Research and Study of Accreditation and Quality Assurance.

Dawes, M. (2001, April 9). *Practice of evidence-based medicine*. Prepared for the Centre for Evidence-Based Medicine. Retrieved October 20, 2005, from http://www.cebm.net/downloads/april_01/ebm_intro.ppt.

Dirr, P. J. (1999). *Putting principles into practice: Promoting effective support services for students in distance learning programs: A report on the findings of a survey*. Western Cooperative for Educational Telecommunications. Retrieved October 19, 2005, from http://www.wcet.info/projects/studentservices/Survey%20Report.pdf.

EDUCAUSE. (2004). *Student guide to evaluating information technology on campus.* Publication No. 2301. Washington, DC: EDUCAUSE, American Association of Collegiate Registrars and Admissions Officers, and the National Association for College Admission Counseling. Retrieved October 20, 2005, from http://www.educause.edu/studentguide.

EEUWIN. (n.d.). *Evaluating the educational uses of the web in nursing: A Flashlight benchmarking project.* Retrieved October 19, 2005, from http://www.tltgroup.org/services/EEUWIN/Home.htm.

Fennema, B. (2003). Preparing faculty to teach in the e-Learning environment. In S. Reisman, J. G. Flores, & D. Edge (Eds.), *Electronic learning communities: Current issues and best practices* (pp. 239–269). Greenwich, CT: Information Age Publishing.

Heinrich, R., Molenda, M., Russell, J. D., et al. (1996). *Instructional media and technologies for learning.* Englewood Cliffs, NJ: Merrill.

Hinman, L. M. (2000, November 2). *Academic integrity and the World Wide Web.* Presented at the 10th Annual meeting of the Center for Academic Integrity. Retrieved October 19, 2005, from http://ethics.acusd.edu/presentations/cai2000/index_files/frame.htm.

Jukes, I. (2005). Understanding Digital Kids (DKs): Teaching and learning in the new digital landscape. Retrieved October 28, 2005, from http://thecommittedsardine.net/infosavvy/education/handouts/ndl.pdf.

Mayer, R. E. (2001). *Multimedia learning.* New York: Cambridge University Press.

McVay Lynch, M. (2004). *Learning online: A guide to success in the virtual classroom.* New York: Routledge Falmer.

Moodle. (2005). Retrieved October 2, 2005, from http://moodle.org

Oblinger, D. G., & Oblinger, J. L. (2005). *Educating the net generation.* Retrieved October 30, 2005, from http://www.educause.edu/educatingthenetgen.

Olt, M. R. (2002). Ethics and distance education: Strategies for minimizing academic dishonesty in online assessment. *Online Journal of Distance Learning Administration, 5*(3). Retrieved October 19, 2005, from http://www.westga.edu/~distance/ojdla/fall53/olt53.html.

Pennsylvania State University. (1998). *An emerging set of guiding principles and practices for the design and development of distance education.* Retrieved October 12, 2005, from http://www.outreach.psu.edu/de/ide/.

Prensky, M. (2001a). Digital natives, digital immigrants. *On the Horizon, 9*(5). Retrieved October 27, 2005, from http://www.marcprensky.com/writing/Prensky%20-%20Digital%20Natives,%20Digital%20Immigrants%20-%20Part1.pdf.

Prensky, M. (2001b). Digital natives, digital immigrants, Part II: Do they really *think* differently? *On the Horizon, 9.* Retrieved October 27, 2005, from http://www.marcprensky.com/writing/Prensky%20-%20Digital%20Natives,%20Digital%20Immigrants%20-%20Part2.pdf.

Prensky, M. (2002). e-Nough! *On the Horizon, 11*(1). Retrieved October 27, 2005, from http://www.marcprensky.com/writing/Prensky%20-%20e-Nough%20-%20OTH%2011-1%20March%202003.pdf.

Prensky, M. (2005). "Engage me or enrage me": What today's learners demand. Retrieved October 19, 2005, from http://www.marcprensky.com/writing/Prensky-Engage_Me_or_Enrage_Me.pdf.

Raines, C. (2002). Managing millenials. Retrieved October 30, 2005, from http://www.generationsatwork.-com/articles/millenials.htm.

Reinert, B. R., & Fryback, P. B. (1997). Distance learning and nursing education. *Journal of Nursing Education, 36*, 421–427.

Roach, R. (2001). Safeguarging against online cheating: Distance education standards and plagiarism. *Black Issues in Higher Education.* Retrieved October 19, 2005, from http://www.findarticles.com/p/articles/mi_m0DXK/is_8_18/ai_76651873.

Taylor, J. C. (1995). Distance education technologies: The fourth generation. *Australian Journal of Educational Technology*, 11, 2, 1–7. Retrieved October 23, 2005, from http://www.ascilite.org.au/ajet/ajet11/taylor.html.

Taylor, J. C. (2001a). *Fifth generation distance education.* Retrieved October 8, 2005, from http://www.dest.gov.au/archive/highered/hes/hes40/hes40.pdf.

Taylor, J. C. (2001b). *Fifth generation distance education.* Retrieved October 23, 2005, from http://www.usq.edu.au/electpub/e-jist/docs/old/vol4no1/2001docs/pdf/Taylor.html.

University of Maryland. (1997). *Models of distance education: A conceptual planning tool.* Retrieved October 19, 2005, from http://www.umuc.edu/ide/modlmenu.html.

Usability First. (2005). *Usability glossary.* Retrieved October 29, 2005, from http://www.usabilityfirst.com/glossary/main.cgi.

Webopedia. (2005). *Terms*. Retrieved October 21, 2005, from http://www.webopedia.com.

Wikipedia. (2005). *Wikipedia: The free encyclopedia*. Retrieved October 22, 2005, from http://www.en.wikipedia.org/wiki/Main_Page.

Wittrock, M. C. (1989). Generative processes of comprehension. *Educational Psychology, 24*, 345–376.

Additional Resources

1. http://ide.ed.psu.edu/iDDE/
   Integrating Instructional Design in Distance Education
   A tool that allows faculty to search for and match appropriate instructional strategies to types of distance education delivery. The site demonstrates the integration of instructional strategies into distance education through including information about, and demonstration of, instructional classes, strategies, tactics, and examples. The example delivery systems include Web-based courses, audioconferencing and videoconferencing, and so on. The site also has a complementary section of three instructional theories (Robert Gagne's *Nine Events of Instruction*, John Keller's *Attention, Relevance, Confidence, and Satisfaction (ARCS) Motivation Theory*, and Charles Reigeluth's *Elaboration Theory*) that permits searching for instructional strategies that support each of these theories.
2. http://www.academicintegrity.org
   The Center for Academic Integrity
   The Center for Academic Integrity operates out of the Kenan Institute for Ethics at Duke University. The Center offers a forum for members and nonmembers to review and promote the academic integrity of various campus constitutents, including students, faculty, and administrators. A particularly useful section of their site includes the honor codes, modified honor codes, and academic integrity policies of a large set of academic institutions. Bill Taylor, a Professor of Political Science, wrote a six-page letter to his students, detailing the importance of integrity and identifying what integrity means for the faculty and student roles within a course. This letter can be freely adapted to other organizations and is located at http://www.academicintegrity.org/pdf/Letter_To_My_Students.pdf.
3. http://www.esac.org/fdi/
   Eastern Association of Colleges
   The Faculty Development Institute of the Eastern Association of Colleges, a collaboration among five colleges and universities on Maryland's Eastern Shore, has some excellent resources to encourage and enable faculty's innovation with technology. In particular, they offer a peer course review rubric entitled, Quality Matters: Inter-Institutional Quality Assessment in Online Learning, that enables peer review of online courses through specific questions in eight sections: (a) course overview and introduction, (b) learning objectives (competencies), (c) assessment and measurement, (d) resources and materials, (e) student interaction, (f) course technology, (g) student support, and (h) ADA compliance. Access this document at http://www.esac.org/fdi/rubric/finalsurvey/demorubric.asp.

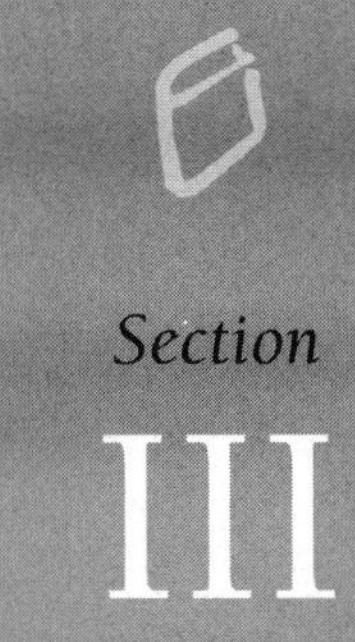

Section

III

CONSTRUCTING NURSING CURRICULA: CHALLENGES AND ISSUES

Chapter 14

Historical Influences of Nursing Curriculum

JoEllen Dattilo
M. Kathleen Brewer

The Nurse

The world grows better, year by year,
Because some nurse in her little sphere,
Puts on her apron and grins and sings.
Keeps on doing the same old things
The temperatures, giving the pills
To remedy mankind's numberless ills;
Feeding the baby, answering the bells
Being polite with a heart that rebels
Longing for home and all the while
Wearing the same old professional smile;
Blessing the new born babe's first breath,
Closing the eyes that are still in death.
Taking the blame for
The doctor's Mistakes,
Oh Dear, what a lot of patience it takes,
Going off duty at seven o'clock
Tired, discouraged, and ready to drop.
When we lay down our caps
And cross the bar
Oh Lord, will you give us just
One little star,
To wear in our crowns with
Our uniforms, new
In that city above, where the
Head Nurse is you.

—AUTHOR UNKNOWN

As one reads the poem, "*The Nurse,*" images of starched, white uniforms and caps, glass thermometers, and a Madonna-like presence easily come to mind. The saintly nurse seems to carry out her duties with routine efficiency. The doctor's reputation is safeguarded because the dutiful nurse accepts the responsibility for his errors. Fast-forward to the 21st century's perception of a nurse and the contrast is dramatic. This quaint poem reflects the educational preparation and mindset that were characteristic of hospital training schools. However, on closer observation, some of the abilities described are still relevant today. The notion that nurses "answer the bells" parallels the role of contemporary nurses who respond to their clients' needs. The depiction of caring and concern and professional demeanor is still relevant in today's world. Thoughtfully analyzing the history of nursing education curricula may create a connection to our professional past and a guideline for the future.

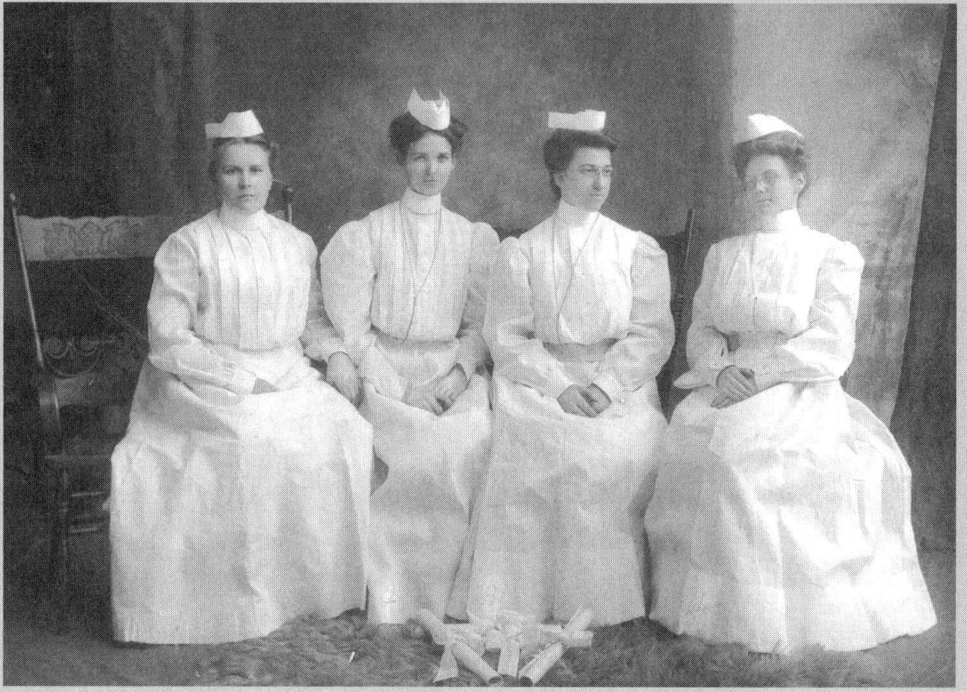

First graduating class (1904) of Tabernacle Training School for Nurses. Used with permission of Georgia Baptist College of Nursing of Mercer University.

INTENT

This chapter traces the evolution of nursing education from the early training schools to contemporary programs within institutions of higher learning. Placed in a chronological context reflective of societal needs and educational objectives of the time, the primary aim of hospital diploma schools, associate degrees, and baccalaureate nursing programs becomes evident. Various conceptual and organizational frameworks and curriculum designs are described. The reader will gain an appreciation and understanding of the historical influences and trends that have shaped nursing education today.

For nurse educators to be better prepared to meet curricula challenges, an understanding of the history of nursing education is essential. It *is* the curriculum plan that primarily supports the philosophy and purposes of the educational institution. As philosophies and purposes about nursing and nursing education change, so do nursing curricula. After a historic review, it becomes evident that current beliefs about the role of the nurse shaped the curriculum blueprint. As you will see, some curricula notions have become part of nursing education history while other notions are surprisingly visible in today's nursing programs.

The purpose of studying any history is to gain a perspective and an appreciation of how a phenomenon develops over time. Historical analysis is essential to acquiring insights into why changes occurred. Studying history supports planning a preferred future because historical analysis surfaces the merits and mistakes of the past, allowing planners to be discerning in their work. Nursing curricula is a phenomenon that can be addressed using a historical analysis; thoughtful reflection on how nursing curricula contributed to the progression of nursing education can support nurse educators in working creatively and effectively in designing new programs of study.

The chapter concludes with a section that addresses why the evolution to student-centered teaching has occurred and the historical influences that threaten the practice of student-centered teaching and teachers' and students' willingness to embrace it.

OVERVIEW

Overview of the Evolution of Nursing Programs
- The Early Hospital Training Schools
  Analysis of Early Hospital Programs
  Committee Recommendations
  The Bellevue Study
  Ginzberg Committee
- Beginnings of Baccalaureate Education
- Associate Degree Programs

Evolution of Nursing Curricula
- Entry-Level Curriculum Plans
- Curriculum Design
- Conceptual and Organizational Frameworks
- Curriculum Patterns

Future Implications
Preparation for the Future
Summary
Learning Activity
Resources for Educators
- Planning the Teaching/Learning Experience
  Instructions for Educators
  Tips for Developing a Student-Centered Learning Environment
  Questions to Support a Thoughtful Reading

OVERVIEW OF THE EVOLUTION OF NURSING PROGRAMS

The Early Hospital Training Schools

The history of modern nursing education began with Florence Nightingale. Her theoretical model for nursing practice emphasized discipline, good character, a nursing service hierarchy, and a strong ability to follow protocol and physicians' orders. Independent thinking and intellect were not perceived as desirable attributes of a nurse, or criteria for admission into **hospital training schools** (Hood & Leddy, 2003).

These training schools were first established in the northeastern United States and Canada in the early 1870s (Bramadat & Chalmers, 1989; Ross-Kerr, 2002). The pri-

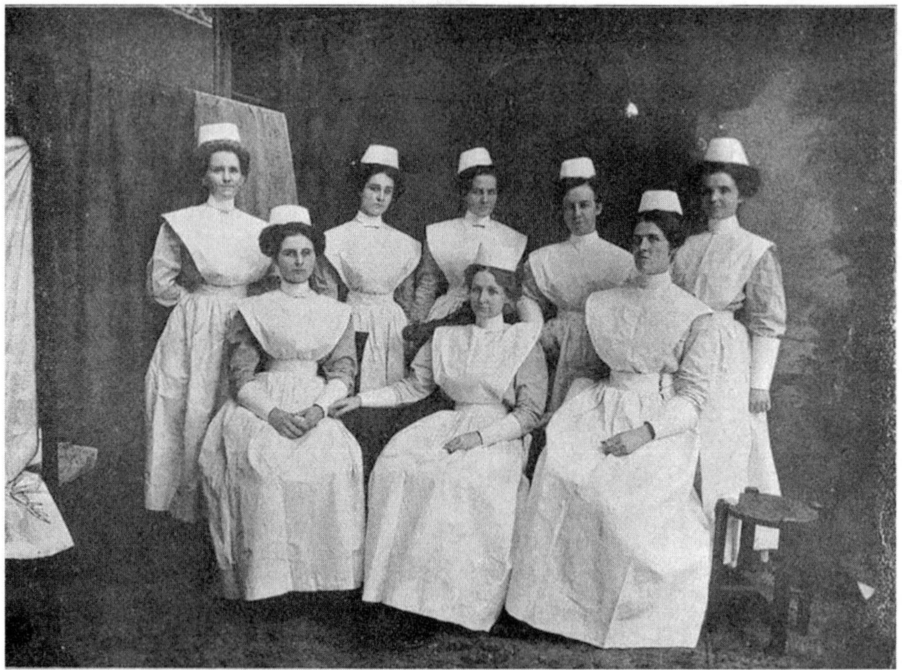

Ninth graduating class (1911) of Tabernacle Training School for Nurses. Used with permission of Georgia Baptist College of Nursing of Mercer University.

mary purpose of the hospital school was to train young women to provide care within the parent institution. Students were viewed as apprentices and given on-the-job training, providing a source of cheap labor for the hospital. Because there were no accreditation standards for programs of nursing education, each hospital school decided on the length of its program and curriculum. Clinical experiences were determined by the number of patients admitted to the hospital, and the types of diagnoses. Hospital staffing, not the education of nurses, was the purpose of the hospital schools. As the benefits of student staffing became known, the number of hospitals opening schools increased rapidly. By 1890, 15 schools were established in the United States, and those multiplied to 432 schools by 1900 (Bullough & Bullough, 1994). Prior to the Great Depression in 1929, 2,300 hospital schools of nursing were in operation (Fitzpatrick, 1983).

ANALYSIS OF EARLY HOSPITAL PROGRAMS

The Committee on the Grading of Nursing Schools was formed in the mid-1920s to conduct a review of hospital training schools in the United States. Early studies of hospital schools conducted by the National League of Nursing Education and a committee supported by the Rockefeller Foundation:

> *made it clear that there was one fundamental condition which was handicapping progress, a condition which must be removed if satisfactory results were to be achieved. This basic weakness lay in the fact that nursing schools were operated for the most part as adjuncts to the management of hospitals and not primarily as educational institutions. (The Committee on the Grading of Nursing Schools, 1934, p. 12)*

The report ended with the opinion that a proliferation of hospital training schools resulted in a "great overproduction of nurses inadequately selected and imperfectly educated. . . . We believe that studies of this Committee have made the evils of overproduction and undereducation so clear that the need for radical reform is obvious to the most conservative" (The Committee on the Grading of Nursing Schools, 1934, p. 12). After 8 years of study, the Committee published its findings and proposed recommendations to improve nursing education. The notion of grading schools was the committee's attempt to raise educational standards. One of the first observations was that there was a high unemployment rate among graduate nurses, which was unrelated to the national economic condition. As more and more young women were recruited into training schools, students provided most of the nursing care. The student would receive room and board, and a nominal allowance, in return for her service to the hospital. This staffing strategy greatly reduced the number of positions available for graduate nurses who demanded a higher fee. Interestingly, the committee included students when calculating the number of trained nurses. By 1930 there was one nurse for every 416 people or one trained nurse for every 100 families (The Committee on the Grading of Nursing Schools).

Concerned about the poor quality of nurses and nursing education, the Committee on the Grading of Nursing Schools' initial action was to establish what a professional nurse should "know and be able to do" (The Committee on the Grading of Nursing Schools, 1934, p. 61). The objectives and competencies proposed to reform nursing education were published in 1934 in *Nursing Schools—Today and Tomorrow*, and may well be the historical origin of curriculum standards. Before competencies were formulated, the committee solicited the opinions of patients, physician, hospital administrators, and nurses about the role of the nurse. Patients expected nurses to keep them comfortable during illness and get along amiably with their families and friends. Physicians demanded "a personal loyalty to himself" (The Committee on the Grading of Nursing Schools, p. 63). It was required that the nurse "build up the confidence of the patient and family in his (the doctor's) competence and skill" (The Committee on the Grading of Nursing Schools, p. 63). The doctor also expected the nurse to possess knowledge, judgment, and skill (The Committee on the Grading of Nursing Schools). Hospital administrators expected nursing staff to meet the needs of the patient and physician. The community perceived the nurse as someone who should be prepared to deal effectively with catastrophic events, promote health, and prevent illness. Finally, the nurse was expected to recognize her duty to all others. Yet, the nurse was to be aware of her abilities and work in areas that best suited her "personal traits and temperamental character" (The Committee on the Grading of Nursing Schools, p. 66).

COMMITTEE RECOMMENDATIONS

Based on the expectations of the profession at the time, several conclusions or educational mandates were proposed in the report that addressed the questions about what nurses should know and be prepared to do. According to the committee, nursing training schools should prepare the graduate to:

- Be able to render expert bedside care; this expertise was seen as the cornerstone of learning in nursing education, including a familiarity with 43 varieties of beds and bedmaking; the making and adjustment of beds for various types of patients are difficult and complicated nursing activities.
- Possess the special knowledge and skills which are required in dealing effectively with situations peculiar to certain types of illnesses; especially diseases or conditions which are prevalent in the community.
- Be able to observe the patient; to interpret physical manifestations; develop a sixth sense; not only detect instantly but interpret correctly the significance of obscure symptoms.
- Apply principles of mental hygiene; better understand psychological factors in illness and recovery.
- Take part in promotion of health and disease prevention.
- Personally attain some degree of economic security; to live a balanced life through spiritual and cultural activities. (The Committee on the Grading of Nursing Schools, 1934, pp. 66–78)

Many of the notions described in the committee's conclusions are evident in the program outcomes of today's nursing schools and colleges. Seeking educational reform, the Committee on Grading addressed what it perceived as the essential conditions for a basic professional school. Components included an independent: board of trustees;

nances; head of the school; faculty; students; curriculum; relation of schools to each other; and the relationship to the community and other professions (The Committee on the Grading of Nursing Schools, 1934). The curriculum component, in the context of this chapter, requires more discussion.

Emphasizing the schools' responsibility to educate students about what they needed to know to meet the needs of the community for professional care, clinical "types" were identified (The Committee on the Grading of Nursing Schools, 1934, p. 133). It was proposed that:

- Students have experience in medical; surgical; maternity; pediatrics; tuberculosis; mental; communicable disease; outpatient; and home care nursing.
- College credit be given for nursing school course work.
- Traditions of the profession be respected and understood, but not sanctified.
- Schools agree what courses are basic to the study of nursing.
- Assignments based on types of patients requiring care, not number of months spent on a service. (The Committee on the Grading of Nursing Schools, 1934, p. 133)

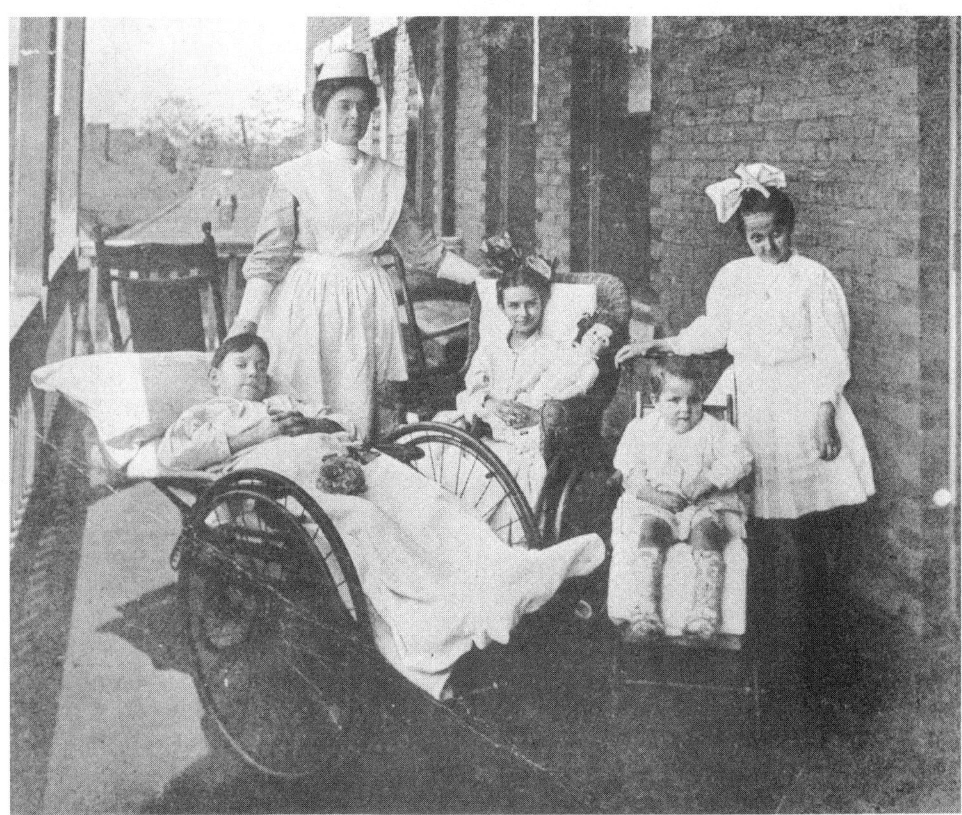

Children's Charity Ward of Tabernacle Infirmary, which later became known as Georgia Baptist Hospital. Used with permission of Georgia Baptist College of Nursing of Mercer University.

The Committee on Grading cited the National League of Nursing Education (NLNE) recommendations for educational programs in the 1934 report. The NLNE advocated a 3-year course of study that included 6,252 hours of practice, and 885 hours of theory. The committee advised that the 885 theory hours should be regarded as the minimum number. The committee members encouraged faculty to increase the number of theory hours and require less, but better, clinical experiences. A strong suggestion was made that schools not only offer more theory but also provide experiences where the theory can be applied. To this end, the NLNE proposed the length of time which students should spend on each of the major services as follows:

- Surgical and operating room—6 months.
- Medical—4 months.
- Obstetric and delivery room—3 months.
- Communicable and tuberculosis—3 months.
- Psychiatric and neurological—2 months.
- Eye, ear, nose, throat, skin, metabolism, other specialties—1 month.
- Diet kitchen—1 month.

In the report, the committee endorsed that the "32 subjects recommended by the League should be taught" (The Committee on the Grading of Nursing Schools, 1934, p. 167); however, the exact courses were not listed in the report. It was only implied that courses focused on sciences, ethics, and nursing history be included. Conditions not tolerated were also described. These conditions addressed the accreditation of the hospitals, staffing ratios of graduate nurses, and student eligibility to sit for the state exam. Even "refresher courses" (The Committee on the Grading of Nursing Schools, p. 217) offered by hospitals to graduate nurses were suggested to improve the quality of nursing care.

In the final chapter of the report, the committee recommended the closing of training schools that did not meet educational standards. Other schools were encouraged to raise their standards to a professional level with the leadership of the NLNE.

Although the Committee on Grading of Nursing Schools document, *The Final Report, Nursing Schools—Today and Tomorrow* (1934), has been described in lengthy detail, many of the proposed mandates for educational reform are evident in contemporary nursing education. Understanding the historical influences of hospital training schools curricula on today's programs of nursing education provides an appreciation and insight on how we began and where we are going.

THE BELLEVUE STUDY

Another assessment of nursing education, **The Bellevue Study**, was published in *Clinical Education in Nursing* (Pfefferkorn & Rottman, 1936). The intent of the study was to "again point the way for constructive development in a field of activity so universally accepted as of fundamental importance but the growth in which has been too rapid, too undirected for the most effective results" (Pfefferkorn & Rottman, 1936, p. xii). To this end, several educational principles were proposed as curricula mandates:

- Assignments considered more fundamental should precede more complex activities; beginning students should be assigned to convalescent or chronic patients "as they give good practice experience to the young student" (Pfefferkorn & Rottman, 1936, p. 100).

- Students should rotate in a systematic way.
- Students should have a comparable theory and practice experience.
- Bedside care performed by students must be supervised.

Before a student began her clinical practice, she took 16 weeks of preparatory courses. Sciences, "basic to nursing," (Pfefferkorn & Rottman, 1936, p. 107) were required. The courses included anatomy and physiology, chemistry, bacteriology, nutrition and cookery, personal hygiene, principles and practices of elementary nursing, ethics, history of nursing, and drugs and solutions (Pfefferkorn & Rottman).

The report further describes the blocks or recommended rotational patterns for clinical teaching. For example, in a 3-year course of study, 48 weeks covered the medical and surgical specialties. A mathematically planned schedule was devised which rotated students to all identified clinical areas after the preparatory courses were completed. To begin, students were assigned to medical or surgical rotations. The teaching program correlated with the clinical practice. At Bellevue Hospital, students rotated blocks every 4 weeks. Each block consisted of four lectures, usually given by physicians, four nursing classes and four clinics. Exams were given at the end of each block section. The average exam scores for the four blocks constituted the theory grade in that area of study. Students then progressed into medical or surgical specialties depending on what the initial rotation was. For example, neurology and psychiatry were part of the medical rota-

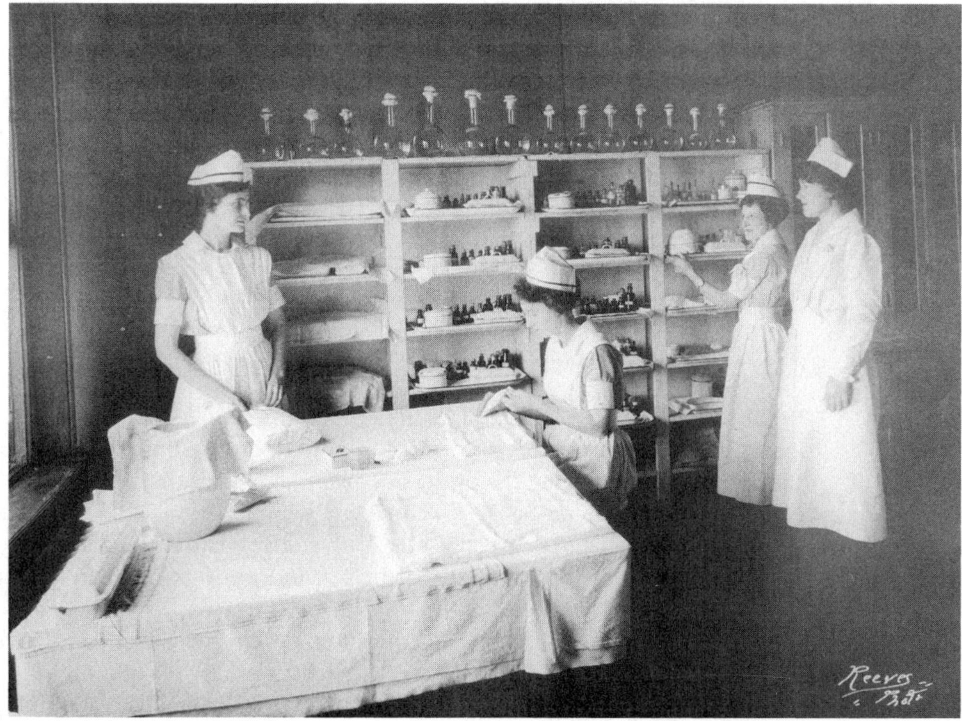

Georgia Baptist Hospital School of Nursing students working in central supply. Used with permission of Georgia Baptist College of Nursing of Mercer University.

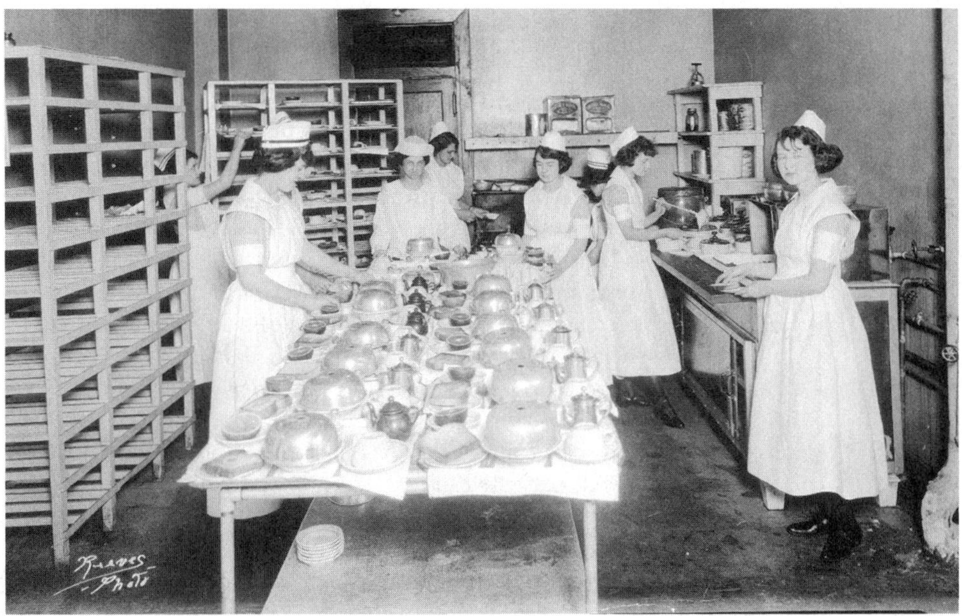

Georgia Baptist Hospital School of Nursing students working in diet kitchen. Used with permission of Georgia Baptist College of Nursing of Mercer University.

tation. The operating room, diseases of the eye, ear, nose, and throat, and gynecological conditions followed the surgical route. All students eventually rotated to communicable disease units, outpatient departments, pediatrics, and obstetrical nursing areas. The students were required to scrub for ten deliveries and observe a minimum of 30 other births. Senior students were assigned to night duty. Students had periodic vacations that complemented the rotation schedule. Additionally, each student was permitted 4 weeks of "health allowance" (Pfefferkorn & Rottman, 1936, p. 133) in case of illness during the 3-year program. Any unused time was given back to the students as a bonus.

GINZBERG COMMITTEE

In the fall of 1947, the Director of the Division of Nursing Education at Teachers College, Columbia University, formed a **Committee on the Function of Nursing** to study the problems confronting the profession, especially the nursing shortage, and offer curriculum revision strategies. Dr. Eli Ginzberg, who was Associate Professor of Economics in the School of Business at Columbia University, chaired the committee. The twelve-member group composed of three nurses and various medical and social science experts, met only six times.

The movement to place nursing education within the colleges and universities began in 1909, but by 1948 only about 10,000 students were enrolled in higher education institutions with approximately 92,000 students still enrolled in hospital training schools. The hospitals dictated the length of study and the curriculum. The committee decided to critique the hospital schools. It noted that the amount of theory taught was minimal and was usually placed at the beginning of the program. There was poor correlation between the didactic component and the students' clinical experience. "The content and the fragmentation of the curriculum are also subject to criticism. Biology, physiology, and other sciences are presented in such condensed form that they contribute little to illuminating clinical experience" (The Committee on the Function of Nursing, 1948, p. 50). The committee went on to report that "The clinical program is repetitive, and is frequently of poor quality" (The Committee on the Function of Nursing, p. 51). It was even observed that those nurses in positions of authority suffered from an "exaggerated sense of responsibility for the private lives of their charges" (The Committee on the Function of Nursing, p. 51).

Beginnings of Baccalaureate Education

The Committee on the Function of Nursing recommended that nursing education should be similar to that of teachers and engineers; that is, it recommended a 4-year program that led to a baccalaureate degree as the requirement for professional nursing education. These nurses, they suggested, would be the leaders of the profession who would direct the care given by the less-educated practical nurse. It was envisioned that the professional nurse and the practical nurse would function as a unit. The notion of practical nursing was new and had not yet been widely implemented.

Around the same time as the committee issued its report, A Program for the Nursing Profession (1948), Dr. Esther Lucille Brown published a report for the National Nursing Council. In ***Nursing for the Future***, Brown (1948) observed that "there was something not only drastically but chronically wrong with a system of education which could not meet the demand either for qualitative or quantitative service" (p. 10). The nursing education conditions in 1948 were largely apprenticeship training in nature. Brown (1948) argued that nursing education belongs within institutions of higher learning.

> *The kind of preparation for the professional nurse that nurse educators have now come to advocate is strikingly like that provided by schools of engineering. Students are to be admitted directly from high school to a basic curriculum that is the product of attempts to integrate general and technical training. (p. 143)*

This idea of an integrated curriculum was heralded as the curriculum of the future and was being tested both in the United States and Canada. The integrated approach was the development of a 4-year or 5-year program of study. General education courses and nursing courses were placed throughout the curriculum plan. A Bachelor of Science in Nursing (BSN) was awarded at program completion.

Written for directors of nursing education programs, *Administration of Schools of Nursing* (Williams & Stewart, 1950), was meant to be a guide about managing schools of nursing. The authors claimed that one vital aspect of operations was curriculum development and implementation. Williams and Stewart (1950) described two patterns of curriculum plans, segregated or integrated curricula (p. 160). In segregated curricula, the academic and professional courses were pursued in separate units and even at separate institutions. The responsibility for implementation was divided between an academic institution, which oversaw the general education courses, and the hospital school that taught the nursing courses. In an integrated curricula, academic and professional courses were part of a continuous program of study entirely under the control of the college or university which secured hospital placements for clinical experience.

By the 1970s, hospital schools were still prevalent. However, momentum was building for the establishment of nursing education programs within institutions of higher learning. The American Nurses' Association (ANA) published a position paper in 1965 that created controversy and separation among nurses and nurse educators. The paper, titled **Educational Preparation for Nurse Practitioners and Assistants to Nurses**, endorsed baccalaureate education as the entry-level preparation into professional nursing practice. The associate degree was for **technical nurse** preparation. Diploma school education was not even mentioned in the report. In 1979, the ANA furthered its position by advocating that the BSN be required for professional nursing practice by 1985. The National League for Nursing (NLN) published their support of the BSN as the entry-level credential in the *Position Statement on Nursing Roles: Scope and Preparation* (National League for Nursing, 1982).

Although there was increasing advocacy for baccalaureate programs, the development was initially slow. "The growth in the numbers of these programs was slow both because of the reluctance of universities to accept nursing as an academic discipline and because of the power of the hospital-based diploma programs" (Chitty, 2001, p. 39). Historically, the first collegiate program in the United States was established at the University of Minnesota in 1909. In 1919, the University of British Columbia School of Nursing was approved and located within the Faculty of Applied Science (i.e., Engineering) (University of British Columbia, School of Nursing History, Health Care Information Resources, 2004). Zerwekh and Claborn (2003) noted that there were 695 baccalaureate programs in the U.S. according to a 2001 NLN report. In Canada, there are currently 36 generic and 21 post R.N. baccalaureate programs in nursing (UBC, 2004).

Early baccalaureate curriculums were usually 5 years in length. Students typically studied liberal arts during the first 2 years, followed by 3 years of nursing courses. The curriculum emphasized theoretical concepts and scientific principles. Clinical experience was limited in number of practice hours and complexity of patient assignments. In contrast, the diploma school curriculums continued to teach nursing using the medical model. Diseases and treatment of diseases, grouped according to body systems, was the framework of learning. Notably, diploma students continued to have more clinical practice than classroom hours. Although no longer the apprenticeship of earlier times, diploma students were given a multiple of complex patient assignments. This resulted in a wide discrepancy between the hands-on clinical skills of diploma-prepared school students and students enrolled in baccalaureate programs. This discrepancy fueled the controversy about the optimal educational preparation for nurses.

Associate Degree Programs

In response to the nursing shortage, a 2-year associate degree program was developed. The aim of the associate degree, according to Mildred Montag's 1951 doctoral dissertation *The Education of Nurse Technicians*, was to produce a technical nurse. Montag envisioned the technical nurse as a semiprofessional "prepared for hospital or nursing home employment" (Hood & Leddy, 2003, p. 28). The associate degree nurse (ADN), who was to provide direct patient care, was to be supervised by the professional nurse. Montag (1951) developed a curriculum that included first-year general education courses and second-year nursing courses. The ADN was intended to be a terminal degree with a separate licensure exam. Intended as the terminal degree, there were no articulation options for completion of a baccalaureate degree. The ANA noted the distinction between the technical and professional nurse in 1965. A particularly candid summation of the educational controversy about the type of program (hospital, baccalaureate, or associate degree) declared:

> *For close to five decades, we've been arguing about the best way to prepare a nurse . . . Perhaps the most concrete measure of our progress is that we are now divided into three factions instead of two. No longer is hostility concentrated between the collegiate and hospital-based programs . . . it's now split three ways. (Lysaught, 1981, p. 90)*

Endorsing baccalaureate preparation for professional nursing, The National Commission for the Study of Nursing and Nursing Education (1970) developed a conceptual scheme for educational mobility for the 2-year technical nurse (Lysaught, 1981). The plan allowed access to baccalaureate programs for the associate degree graduate. One variation, the two-plus-two design, offered an associate degree curriculum for the first 2 years and then enrollment into the upper division BSN program. Shortly after the commission's mandates were announced, the Council of Diploma Programs of the National League for Nursing voted not to support the recommendations. The Assembly of Hospital Schools of Nursing of the American Hospital Association had an even stronger response. It was resolved to "repudiate any individuals or groups who alluded to the phasing out of diploma programs for nursing education" (Lysaught, 1981, p. 98). The commission fired back that

> *so long as these institutions remain open it will be a long-lasting reminder that nursing alone, of all the emergent professions, maintains a divided and divisive system of education that militates against its own and should have been abandoned in the early decades of the 20th century. (Lysaught, 1981, p. 101)*

From 1950s on, associate degree programs proliferated and diploma schools significantly decreased. Baccalaureate education experienced a steady growth. By 2001 the National League for Nursing reported that only 86 diploma schools remained opened. The same source counted 885 associate degree programs and 695 baccalaureate programs (Zerwekh & Claborn, 2003).

EVOLUTION OF NURSING CURRICULA

Entry-Level Curriculum Plans

Curriculum plans are the reflection of the parent institutions' purpose or mission. These documents define why the entity exists and identify the primary institutional goals or objectives. The curriculum plan provides the foundation for the purposes and goals. For example, hospital schools were created to provide nursing service to its institution;

students rotated to all areas of the hospital. Content was organized according to the **medical model** of education. Body systems and specialty areas of care provided the organizing framework of the 3-year curriculum plan. Emphasis was placed more on clinical practice and less on didactic learning. No college credit was awarded for any diploma nursing courses.

Today's associate degree programs in the United States, generally 2 academic years in length, about 60 semester hours, require introductory general education courses in the sciences and liberal arts. The second-year nursing courses usually are organized according to specialty areas. Although most of the practice takes place in acute care settings, ADN students do have some community and leadership experience. Community and leadership practicums, once thought to be only included in the BSN programs, were often cited as a major distinction between the technical and professional nurse.

More varied in length and curricula design is the baccalaureate program. Time spent in generic programs can range from an accelerated 16-month curriculum to a 5-year course of study. Usually, a requirement for admission into an accelerated program is an earned degree, or completion of all prerequisite courses. Also, some **accelerated programs** require that the prospective student complete a certified nursing assistant course prior to matriculation. The course of study is extremely intense with an expectedly steep learning curve. Some prelicensure programs begin nursing courses during the first year. Commonly, this is limited to an introductory course that focuses on the evolution of the nursing profession. The **diagonal curriculum plan** introduces nursing courses at the start of the second year. Upon entry to this level, the student begins the clinical practicum experience. This curriculum plan requires 3 years of nursing practice. Although clinical competency is a major aim of this type of plan, it may be a barrier to the nontraditional student who has previous college credit or another degree. Enrolling in a diagonal curriculum as a nontraditional student would add to the total number of years one spends in undergraduate education.

A more common length of program is what is known as an **upper two**. Students complete most of the core requirements during the first 2 years. Nursing courses begin at the start of the third year of the program. The advantage of this plan is the easy access for transfer students. Students can complete the core courses anywhere, usually at an accredited college or university, and then transfer into the program of choice. Often this is the less expensive option in terms of tuition costs. The upper two programs also allow the student to enjoy the experience of a general education course of study before the major is declared. A disadvantage of the upper two program is limited clinical experience. A student in this type of curriculum plan has only four semesters of clinical compared to the student in a diagonal plan who will have six semesters of practice. Additionally, there is a recruitment risk that the student may lose interest in nursing while in the general studies component and select another major.

Curriculum Design

Although length of program establishes program timelines, it is the **curriculum development**, or **curriculum design**, that defines the composition and outcomes of the educational experience. A major influence during the 1950s through the 1970s was the

Tylerian behaviorist curriculum development paradigm. Grounded on the work of curriculum theorist, Ralph Tyler, the framework for nursing education was transformed. According to the Tyler model, curriculum design was organized around four essential questions:

1. What educational purposes should the school seek to attain?
2. What educational experiences can be provided that are likely to attain these purposes?
3. How can these educational experiences be effectively organized?
4. How can we determine whether these purposes are being attained? (Murdock, 1986, p. 27)

Tyler recommended that learning objectives, learning experiences, and evaluation measures could be developed from the responses to these inquiries. This Tylerian paradigm guided curriculum design for many years.

Em Bevis and Jean Watson (1989) took exception to the Tylerian model. In their book, *Toward a Caring Curriculum: A New Pedagogy for Nursing,* they criticized the Tylerian behaviorist model. Specifically, they noted three problematic assumptions:

1. There is one type of learning and one coherent group of compatible theories sufficient to support and explain learning.
2. Educated, mature learners can be graduated using behaviorist theory and the teaching methods that are consistent with it.
3. The schooling system based on behaviorism is capable of liberating, educating, and helping people to be integrated. (Bevis & Watson, 1989, p. 3).

Bevis and Watson (1989) defended their criticisms based on what they believed to be the limitations of behaviorist doctrine in nursing curriculum design, namely: (a) the widespread acceptance, without questioning, of the behaviorist theory approach to nursing curriculum development; (b) that learning could only be achieved if empirically validated; (c) behaviorism is a masculine theory which supports deductive logic and procedural knowledge; (d) nursing is a feminine field based on human sciences, intuitive and constructed knowledge, and multiple realities; and (e) nursing philosophies and research were shifting from a quantitative, objective reductionistic perspective focusing on diagnoses and treatments to a qualitative, holistic, experiential, phenomenological, and human experience orientation (pp. 4–5).

Bevis and Watson (1989) questioned how nursing education philosophies speak to holism, caring, and the human experience, but plan curriculums based on behavioral objectives. The central themes of their reflections revolve around the notion that "curriculum is the interactions and transactions that occur between and among students and teachers with the intent that learning occur" (Bevis & Watson, p. 5). Learning is considered an active process in which teachers facilitate the learning, and students are responsible for their own learning agendas. This new paradigm of curriculum development embraces a transformative perspective where the teaching–learning process is seen as a uniquely human activity. Knowledge is considered to be something that is constructed, contextual, and emotional. Within this framework, an ethic of caring as a moral imperative is integrated throughout the curriculum. Bevis & Watson (1989) proposed that four "mini-models" (p. 77) compose the theoretical position of the proposed paradigm: the learner maturity continuum, the typology of learning, criteria for teacher–student interactions, and criteria for selecting and devising learning activities. The student is no longer trained but guided to become a self-directed, self-motivated, lifelong learner with a passion for inquiry. Subject matter is considered secondary to the actual teaching–learning process.

Conceptual and Organizational Frameworks

Another defining aspect of the curriculum design is the **conceptual** or **organizational framework**. Beginning in the early 1970s, an NLN accreditation criterion required that a conceptual framework provide the foundation for baccalaureate curriculum design. The framework should reflect the mission, philosophy, program outcomes, and level objectives of the educational unit. It was held that a conceptual framework should direct or structure a cohesive and logical program of study. Bevis and Watson (1989) envisioned a conceptual framework as an:

> *Interrelated system of premises that provide guidelines or ground rules for making all curricular decisions—objectives, content, implementation, and evaluation. The conceptual framework . . . is the conceptualization and articulation of concepts, facts, propositions, theories, phenomena, and variables relevant to a specific nursing educational system. (p. 26)*

Early examples of conceptual frameworks based on the work of theorists from other disciplines included Maslow's hierarchy of human needs, Erickson's developmental stages, and Seyle's physiological stress and adaptation theory (Webber, 2002). Although these nonnursing theories had merit and applicability to the nursing profession, there was a need for nursing-based conceptual frameworks. The nursing process was the start of such frameworks. By the 1970s, the nursing process had evolved into a five-step decision-making model. Although frequently used as the main element in curriculum design, it proved insufficient as a framework for nursing and nursing education. It was concluded that the nursing process was too limited, functional, and linear to encompass the depth and scope of nursing. Dissatisfaction with the nursing process as a conceptual framework encouraged the generation of nursing theory. The theoretical works of Hildegard Peplau, Virginia Henderson, Myra Levine, Martha Rogers, Dorthea Orem, Sister Callista Roy, Imogene King, and Dorothy Johnson began to emerge (McEwen & Brown, 2002). These nursing scholars developed their own unique theories and models of nursing and many programs selected one of these theorists on which to base their curriculum. What educators discovered rather quickly was that no one theory could encompass all of nursing. Nurse educators struggled with the single theory approach and eventually gave up the effort (Webber). Programs then began using multiple nursing and nonnursing theories to create their conceptual frameworks. These eclectic models were individualized according to faculty preferences. By 1999 the National League for Nursing Accreditation Commission (NLNAC) announced that programs would no longer be expected to base a curriculum on a specific conceptual framework. However, NLNAC continues to require that an organizational framework guide the development of curriculum, objectives, competencies, and leaning activities (NLNAC, 1999).

McEwen and Brown (2002) conducted a national survey to determine:

- Conceptual frameworks in current use.
- How conceptual frameworks are used in curriculum design.
- What tools, concepts, and processes are emphasized.
- What differences in the application of a conceptual framework between diploma, ADN, and BSN are evident.

In this study, 300 schools were sampled with 160 surveys returned. The percentage of returned questionnaires proportionally represented the percentage of surveys sent to diploma, ADN, and BSN programs. The findings suggest that there are more similarities than differences in the components and application of conceptual frameworks across the three program types. Most conceptual frameworks are eclectic, with the nursing process as the most common component. There appeared to be a decline in the nursing theory-based curriculum. Critical thinking was stressed more in baccalaureate programs, while diploma schools tended to still use the medical model with a content orientation. Associate degree programs focused on the development of problem-solving skills. The majority of participants reported a balance between content and the process of learning.

Curriculum Patterns

Another feature of contemporary baccalaureate curriculums is the curriculum pattern. The two most commonly used are the integrated curriculum pattern and block curriculum pattern (Billings & Halstead, 1998, p. 124). Popular during the late 1970s and early 1980s the integrated curriculum pattern was the antithesis to the medical model. Conceptual in approach, the integrated pattern identified selected themes as the organizing element. For example, if the renal system were to be taught, discussing the regulatory function of the system would be the starting point. Next, the consequences of altered function would be addressed, followed by a discussion of common nursing interventions. This approach eliminated time spent on multiple etiologies. However, the integrated approach became somewhat less manageable when concepts were carried to an extreme. It became difficult for the generic student to grasp the concept of cellular proliferation when everything from fetal development to cancer was included in this category. It also was difficult at times to apply the concept in the clinical setting. For instance, if students happened to have their practicum on the maternity unit, concepts of immobility would be more difficult to apply. Another consequence of considerable concern was an increased failure rate on the licensure exams taken by students who matriculated in an integrated curriculum.

To be fair, there are some positive aspects of an integrated curriculum. Some concepts such as principles of nutrition, health assessment, pharmacology, and research are easily integrated across the curriculum. And by integrating some content, space is created in the curriculum plan for other courses.

Conversely, blocking the curriculum results in a rigid and inflexible pattern. A common blocking pattern is positioning courses in the curriculum plan according to areas of practice (adult health, pediatrics, etc.) or body systems (gastrointestinal, endocrine, etc.). These are probably the most common blocking approaches. This pattern is usually sequential because it is believed, for example, that students must have maternity nursing before they are eligible to take pediatric nursing. Using a blocking pattern makes evaluation somewhat easier because the area of learning is precisely defined. The clinical experience directly correlates with the didactic content of the course. However, the components of this pattern are taught in isolation. Faculty members teaching in their area of expertise may have little awareness of what is included in other courses. This may lead to repetition and student disinterest.

FUTURE IMPLICATIONS

What becomes evident from an historical review of nursing curriculum development is that the process of change is never ending. Yet, some issues seem to persist or re-emerge such as the notion to integrate nutritional and pharmacological principles into clinical courses, or to offer them separately. The American Association of Colleges of Nursing (AACN) 2002 publication, *Nursing Education's Agenda for the 21st Century,* states:

> *Preparation for the entry-level professional nurse now requires a greater orientation to community-based primary health care, and an emphasis on health promotion, maintenance, and cost-effective coordinated care that responds to the needs of culturally diverse groups and underserved and other populations in all settings. (p. 1)*

To this end, the AACN has made curriculum recommendations that address the need for processes and outcomes as well as content in the preparation of baccalaureate nurses. The teaching–learning relationship should facilitate role modeling, collaborative problem solving, and professional socialization (AACN, 2002, p. 7). Essential cognitive and interpersonal behaviors such as critical thinking, ethical decision making, and information seeking, sorting, and selection, among other abilities are identified. Not only should high acuity content be included, but also health promotion. It is within a baccalaureate program of study that the AACN believes this entry-level generalist should be prepared.

PREPARATION FOR THE FUTURE

There is still work to be done. Cognizant of the evolution of curriculum development makes the nurse educator better informed to create the curriculums of the future. However, questions remain. What is the best preparation for professional nursing? What curriculum design would best prepare a professional nurse? What should be included in the curriculum? How long should the program be? Should nursing education teaching be student centered? Many educators believe that it should be student centered. One major factor that has affected this change is the profile of today's student. Many of today's students enter colleges and universities as adult learners with life experiences and responsibilities. They have not only multiple career path choices but also numerous institutions offering the nursing major. Their expectations of the program and the faculty can be discriminating. The teaching–learning relationship is seen as a reciprocal partnership between faculty and student. Furthermore, the notion of student-as-customer has forced many institutions to reassess how the academic program is delivered. A student-centered approach also requires faculty to give up traditional ways of instruction and places the responsibility for learning squarely on the student. But, is this not what we desire the professional nurse to be, a self-directed, responsible, active learner? Simply, the student-centered approach challenges the faculty to continuously stay current and be flexible. Their primary role is that of a resource person and a facilitator. Concurrently, students are challenged to be active participants in their learning. An argument can easily be made that to participate in a student-centered curriculum requires more effort on both parties.

The student-centered approach may be jeopardized if the traditional opinion is held that students are not capable of making decisions about their learning. Also, if the faculty is reluctant to shift the balance of power in the learning setting, by giving up the position of absolute authority, then student-centered teaching will not thrive. Ultimately, student-centered learning necessitates change from both teacher and student, and challenges what has been historically practiced. However, there exists a contingent which actually prefers the antiquated methods of teaching; possibly it is preferred because it is familiar; possibly it is easier to be a passive learner than an active participant in one's learning. Embracing the old methodology may be more cost-effective, particularly during periods of a nursing shortage. Lecturing 100 students in an auditorium who passively listen and take notes is more efficient than forming multiple small student learning groups with a faculty facilitator. The question remains: What approach best prepares the nurses of the future? As future nurse educators, this becomes your decision to make.

SUMMARY

The chapter described the historical evolution of nursing education curricula. Three types of nursing preparation programs were discussed: hospital training schools, baccalaureate programs housed in institutions of higher learning, and the associate degree programs. The missions of each of these entities were explained, and how the curriculums were developed to support these tenets. Curriculum plans, curriculum designs, and the purposes of conceptual and organizational frameworks were discussed. Connections were proposed which suggest that some early nursing education constructs are evident in contemporary programs.

LEARNING ACTIVITY

After thoughtful reflection upon the historical influences of nursing curriculum, debate the notion that a professional nurse needs a baccalaureate degree for career mobility. Consider the ANA Standards of Professional Performance as the measurement criteria in the American Nurses Association's (2004), *Nursing: Scope and Standards of Practice*.

RESOURCES FOR EDUCATORS

PLANNING THE TEACHING/LEARNING EXPERIENCE

Instructions for Educators

- Consider offering as a **hybrid** online course.
- Consider peer grading of seminar leadership and participation.

Tips for Developing a Student-Centered Learning Environment

- Present topics in historical order to enhance understanding about nursing education evolution.
- Utilize the seminar format rotating student facilitators.
- Student leaders should distribute seminar objectives and participant assignments one week prior to class.

Questions to Support a Thoughtful Reading

1. Synthesize information about the historical influences from early training schools and distinguish if some are evident in contemporary nursing education.
2. Examine some of the curricula commonalties among diploma, associate degree, and baccalaureate nursing programs. Ascertain the differences.
3. Articulate the primary purpose of a conceptual framework or organizational framework. Compare and contrast the similarities and differences.
4. Analyze the advantages and disadvantages of the block and integrated curriculum design.
5. Resolve if there should be separate licensure exams for the diploma, associate degree, and baccalaureate prepared graduate.
6. Determine if the BSN should be the entry-level credential into professional nursing practice.

EVALUATING THE TEACHING/LEARNING EXPERIENCE

Questions to Elicit Feedback from Students on Their Learning

1. Synthesize the historical information about nursing education and the influence on curriculum development today.
2. Determine what critical components should be included in a baccalaureate curriculum plan for the 21st century.

Sample Evaluation Strategies

- Have students search the Internet for several nursing program catalogs and critique the curriculum plan.

- Have students debate the question "Are BSN graduates better prepared as professional nurses?"
- Develop a curriculum plan.
  - Have students divide into small groups.
  - Give class time for group work.
  - After thoughtful discussion, have the group write a philosophy of nursing and nursing education; develop program and level outcomes; select or develop a conceptual or organizational framework; develop a curriculum plan; and identify the accreditation criteria that would be used in assessment.
- Invite members of the college community to attend the presentation.

Reflective Questions for Educators

1. Do students articulate an appreciation for the historical influences on curriculum?
2. Are students able to appraise the positive and negative factors inherent in each type of nursing program?
3. What strategies used in the class were most effective in shifting the center of learning to the students? Least effective?
4. What teaching/learning strategies were most effective in providing students with opportunities to judge educational practices, rooted in a historical context, that operate in their everyday lives as nursing students?
5. In class, how did I develop students' expertise to critique historical elements of nursing curricula presented in this chapter?

References

American Association of Colleges of Nursing. (August, 2002). *Nursing education's agenda for the 21st century*. Retrieved on October 22, 2005 from http://www.aacn.nche.edu/publications/positions/nrsgedag.htm.

American Nurses Association. (1965). *Educational preparation for nurse practitioners and assistants to nurses: A position paper*. Kansas City, MO: American Nurses Association.

Bevis, E., & Watson, J. (1989). *Toward a caring curriculum: A new pedagogy for nursing*. New York: National League for Nursing.

Billings, M., & Halstead, J. (1998). *Teaching nursing: A guide for faculty*. Philadelphia: Saunders.

Bramadat, I., & Chalmers, K. (1989). Nursing education in Canada: Historical "Progress"—Contemporary issues. *Journal of Advanced Nursing, 14*(9), 719–726.

Brown, E. (1948). *Nursing for the future: A report prepared for the National Nursing Council*. New York: Russell Sage Foundation.

Bullough, B., & Bullough, V. (1994). *Nursing times for the nineties and beyond*. New York: Springer.

Chitty, K. (2001). *Professional nursing concepts and challenges* (3rd ed.). Philadelphia: Saunders.

Committee on the Grading of Nursing Schools. (1934). *The final report, nursing schools today and tomorrow*. New York City.

Fitzpatrick, M. (1983). *Prologue to professionalism: A history of nursing*. Bowie, MD: Robert J. Brady.

Hood, L., & Leddy, S. (2003). *Leddy & Pepper's conceptual bases of professional nursing* (5th ed.). Philadelphia: Lippincott Williams & Wilkins.

Lysaught, P. (1981). *Action in affirmation: Toward an unambiguous profession of nursing*. New York: McGraw-Hill.

McEwen, M., & Brown, S. (2002). Conceptual frameworks in undergraduate nursing curricula: Report of a national survey. *Journal of Nursing Education, 41*(1), 5–14.

Montag, M. L. (1951). *The education of nurse technicians.* New York: G.P. Putnam's Sons.
Murdock, J. (1986). Evolution of the nursing curriculum. *Journal of Nursing History, 2*(1), 16–35.
National Commission for the Study of Nursing and Nursing Education. (1970). *An abstract for action.* New York: McGraw-Hill.
National League for Nursing. (1982). *Position statement on nursing roles: Scope and preparation.* New York: National League for Nursing.
National League for Nursing Accrediting Commission (1999). *Directory of accredited nursing programs.* Retrieved October 22, 2005 from http://www.nlnac.org/DirectoryMainp1.htm.
Pfefferkorn, A., & Rottman, M. (1936). *Clinical education in nursing.* New York: Macmillan.
Ross-Kerr, J. D. (2002). Nursing in Canada from 1760 to the present. In J. D. Ross-Kerr & M. J. Woods (Eds.), *Canadian nursing: Issues and perspectives* (4th ed., pp. 34–53). Toronto: Mosby.
The Committee on the Function of Nursing. (1948). *A program for the nursing profession.* New York: Macmillan.
University of British Columbia, School of Nursing History, Health Care Information Resources (2004). Retrieved April 24, 2004, from http://www.nursing.ubc.ca/about/history.html.
Webber, P. (2002). A curriculum framework of nursing. *Journal of Nursing Education, 41*(1), 15–24.
Williams, D., & Stewart, I. M. (1950). *Administration of schools of nursing.* New York: Macmillan.
Zerwekh, J., & Claborn, J. (2003). *Nursing today: Transition and trends* (4th ed.). St. Louis: Saunders.

Additional Resources

American Association of Colleges of Nursing. (January 2004). *Faculty shortages in baccalaureate and graduate nursing programs: Scope of the problem and strategies for expanding the supply.* Retrieved October 22, 2005 from http://www.aacn.nche.edu/publications/whitepapers/facultyshortages.htm.
American Association of Colleges of Nursing Web site. Available at: http://www.aacn.nche.edu.
American Association for the History of Nursing Web site. Available at: http://www.aahn.org.
Center for Nursing Historical Inquiry Web site. Available at: http://www.nursing.virginia.edu/centers/history.html.
Center for the Study of the History of Nursing Web site. Available at: http://www.nursing.upenn.edu/history.
Csokasy, J. (2002). A congruent curriculum: Philosophy integrity from philosophy outcomes. *Journal of Nursing Education, 41*(1), 32–33.
Kalish, P., & Kalish, B. (2004). *American nursing: A history* (4th ed.). Philadelphia: Lippincott Williams & Wilkins.
Mawn, B., & Reece, S. (2000). Reconfiguring a curriculum for the new millennium: The process of change. *Journal of Nursing Education, 39*(3), 101–108.
National League for Nursing Web site. Available at: http://www.nln.org.
Wineburg, S. (1991). Historical problem solving: A study of cognitive processes used in the evaluation of documentary and pictorial evidence. *Journal of Educational Psychology 83*(1), 73–87.

Conceptualizing the Purpose of Nursing: Philosophical Challenges in Creating Meaningful Theoretical Learning Experiences

Chapter 15

Sally Thorne

As a returning RN entering a postbasic nursing program in the mid-1970s, I was horrified to be told I had to learn nursing all over again; this time from the perspective of a conceptual model. In that era, it seemed an embedded wisdom within the baccalaureate nursing education community that those of us who originally trained in hospital programs were beyond hope for conceptual thinking. And that the only way for us to unlearn our medical model habit pattern was to engage us in repetitive meticulous data gathering, followed by compulsive sorting and organizing according to whatever nursing model we were meant to apply. Those nursing assessment documents, often ranging to 70 or 80 pages of handwritten notes (well before the days of computers), represented compilations of the theoretical totality of what nursing considered potentially relevant to decisions about and on behalf of a client. Experientially, however, this process seemed the direct opposite of learning. Although the scope and complexity demanded of the models may have broadened our horizons in some ways, it also led to some amusing debates over whether hair color constituted a coping behavior or a force, and what symbolic meanings human excretions might have for their owners.

Over the years, I surprised myself by coming to value systematic thinking as a core element in excellent clinical reasoning, and subsequently to include it prominently in my undergraduate and graduate teaching. Later, I was fortunate enough to engage in doctoral study at a time when the philosophy of nursing science was gaining prominence as a priority in our discipline. Watching the progression of thinking within our discipline over these decades has been a source of deep satisfaction. I now stand in awe of the intelligence that has characterized nursing's theorizing over the course of its historical development. When I think of the challenge facing educators in making the conceptual structure of nursing relevant within a student-centered context, I reflect back to that skeptical learner in my own post-RN program. Given the choice, I would never have selected nursing theory as a relevant focus of study, and I think it is safe to say that remains the case for our students today. However, what our students do expect of us is not to impart information, but to inspire curiosity and to facilitate engagement in the beginning phases of a lifelong learning process. Recognizing that many educators of today are likely to approach nursing theory with a significant degree of cynicism at the outset, student-centered educational strategies may actually compound the challenge of articulating what possible relevance all of this theorizing might possibly play. I write this chapter in the hopes of engaging student-centered educators in reflection about the inherent dialectic between conceptual structures and conceptual capacities, with the intent of sparking some excitement for what nursing theory might offer to the nursing educational imagination.

INTENT

In this chapter, I invite the reader to consider the possibility that engaging students in a study of nursing theory—something that seems antithetical to the real world of practice—might actually have a powerful role to play in the professional practice of nursing. Nursing's relationship to the social mandate requires a dynamic reframing of its nature, scope, and definition as conditions change over time. The profession must respond to repeated challenges related to what nurses do and how they do it. Something about nursing seems so fundamentally straightforward because caring for the sick is a basic function of any society, but articulating what constitutes nursing is an exceptionally complex challenge. This becomes immediately apparent to those who attempt to defend why nurses require comprehensive education; or who argue for suitable working conditions for nurses; or who engage with policy makers in planning for health service delivery; or who engage in the challenging process of designing forward-thinking nursing curricula. In their time, the scholars we now refer to as nursing theorists took up the challenge of trying to define the conceptual structure of this complex discipline—to really understand how it is that nurses handle so much complex information, interpret it systematically, consider its implications within the wider context, and apply it to the unique complexities of each individual case. Their attempts to theorize nursing were sometimes awkward, and the profession's efforts to apply theory were often literal and rigid. However, if we allow this next generation of nurses to discard the relevance of nursing theory, a worry that has been expressed by recent observers (Edwards & Liaschenko, 2003; Flaming, 2004), we may place the profession at considerable risk for losing its center and its core purpose. By critically recounting aspects of the history and context of nursing theory, and by trying to create some enthusiasm for the complexity and relevance of its intellectual project, I encourage curriculum builders and the nursing educators who implement those curricula back into the debate and invite them to take up the challenge.

OVERVIEW

Introduction
Background to the Challenge
- Changing Health Care Systems
- Changing Role Definitions

A History of the Model Movement
- Florence Nightingale
- Postwar Science
- An Era of Model Building
- Metaparadigm Thinking

INTRODUCTION

The history of curriculum building for the explicit purpose of educating nurses is inextricably tied to the emergence of nursing theories and conceptual frameworks. Although such conceptual devices formed the core of thought about the discipline during many of its evolutionary phases, they have been more recently overlooked within some quarters as outdated or misguided attempts to build the science of our discipline in a social and political context that is no longer relevant. In this chapter, I reconsider the foundational knowledge that was developed during a generation of model building, theorizing, and philosophizing in the context of our current educational and theoretical challenges. As will be evident in my discussion, I take the nursing theory movement not as a flawed and outdated conceptual process, but rather as an early and brave attempt at theorizing what we now understand to be highly complex systems and processes associated with conceptualizing the purpose and intent of nursing. From that perspective, I explore and analyze the insights that emerged from that aspect of our discipline's **philosophical** thinking.

In the late 1960s and early 1970s, nursing scholars began what would eventually become a project within our discipline to try to make explicit that which was self-evident about shaping students into nurses. For a generation or more, **nursing models** and frameworks dominated the conceptual structure of what was understood to be our disciplinary knowledge, and the business of formal **theorizing** became something of a fetish within the discipline. After two decades of consistent advocacy for **conceptualizing** and **systematic thinking**, nursing educational theory took another dramatic turn in the late 1980s. In many quarters, nursing theory was abandoned as a misguided and outdated form of scholarship (Hardy, 1986; Holden, 1990; Timpson, 1996). In its place, such intellectual stances as postmodernism, **complexity science**, holism, and human science were posited as more advanced and sophisticated forms of thinking and philosophizing within the discipline (Huntington, Gilmour, & O'Connell, 1996; Lister, 1991).

In an era of multiple coexisting realities and **relativism**, however, it becomes increasingly important that we continue to examine the core of systematic thinking as a foundation of nursing excellence so that it can once again be rendered relevant to our modern curricular projects in nursing education.

BACKGROUND TO THE CHALLENGE

From the time of Florence Nightingale's early attempts to elevate nursing from the lowest form of service to a trained vocation, the challenge of articulating what it is that nursing is, does, and can be has been a prominent focus of concern. In the early stages, the definition of nursing created a means by which drudgery and physical labor were distinguished from the capacity to reason, problem solve, and apply knowledge (Nightingale, 1946/1859). Throughout our history, nursing leaders have wrestled with questions of what nursing is and what it is not, attempting to pinpoint those essential elements that define it and distinguish it from other professions, acts, and social roles. This struggle to conceptualize the discipline has taken place within the context of various sociopolitical challenges. These have included the shift from home to hospital care, the transition within nursing education from hospital schools into the academy, and the change from earlier grounding of nursing educational curricula within medical science toward a conceptual structure that represented nursing's own professional identity and interpretive logic.

Changing Health Care Systems

In the current context, our sociopolitical challenges may have changed somewhat, but the core difficulty remains quite similar. For example, as we face increasing pressure from governments and health authorities to rationalize the need for nurses in diverse clinical contexts, we are challenged to articulate distinctions within the "family" of nursing, a phrase which reflects the wide range of professional and technical activities and roles that are developed to address practical problems in delivering health services to populations. Beyond the identity that most of us would recognize as registered nurse or professional nurse, many of our health care systems utilize more economical workers in the form of practical nurses, care aides, or others who perform limited nursing acts often under the guidance and supervision of a nurse. In such a context, our challenge becomes one of being able to conceptualize what it is that distinguishes these more economical laborers from the professional practice of nursing. At the other end of the spectrum, we also recognize an increasing number of advanced practice nursing roles, such as those of advanced specialty practice or the nurse practitioner primary care provider. In those contexts, our conceptual challenge is to distinguish the contributions they might make to the health care system from those of the medical specialist resident or the family practice physician.

Thus, the dynamic social contexts within which nursing is enacted force the profession to continually grapple with what it is that distinguishes nursing from that which is not nursing. As the health care system diversifies, and the everyday practices of nurses become increasingly distinctive (compare, for example, the community-based street nurse from the nurse whose primary practice is scrubbing up in the operating theater), it becomes critically important to articulate this core of understanding within our discipline in a manner that is sufficiently broad to encompass a wide range of nursing practices without jeopardizing the coherence that represents our collective orientation to knowledge and action.

Changing Role Definitions

While many attempts have been made over time to create a conceptual definition of this discipline of ours, the effort has been likened to "nailing down jelly" because of its intellectual and theoretical slipperiness and complexity. Our leaders have consistently recognized that the essence of nursing constitutes something about the knowledge that is brought to bear on and enacted within caring practices, but have not found it useful or even possible to distinguish substantive knowledges that are nursing's unique domain and those that are shared with other disciplines. What used to be called "borrowed knowledge," because it was originally developed in relation to some other discipline's academic project, has increasingly been considered part of the vast domain of knowledge developed by (theoretically) all disciplines with which nursing is privileged to engage. These can include not only the applied disciplines such as health sciences, education, and the law, but also the basic sciences, social sciences, and even the humanities. Further, the substantive knowledge that nursing creates through its own research and scholarship is generally considered to be relevant to a broader audience, including other health professions, policy makers, and the public at large. Thus the knowledge that is unique to nursing cannot be the substantive, factual, particular knowledge that is constantly under development and from which all disciplines might draw. Rather it is a form of "how to" knowledge that represents nursing's unique angle of vision on a problem, with all of the inherent assumptions, beliefs, and values that nursing brings to its distinctive understanding. What theorists have consistently recognized is that it is a particular set of reasoning processes, intellectual linkages, emphases, and ways of working out problems that distinguishes nursing thinking from the thinking of other disciplines and differentiates the conditions for nursing acts from the acts performed by nonnurses.

The challenge to nurses charged with designing educational curricula, then, has remained one of conceptually distinguishing nursing as a particular disciplinary orientation and as a unique role within society under changing circumstances. In the context of this challenge over the course of our history, individual theorists have set out a wide range of claims about how nursing ought to decide which of the possible knowledge sources to privilege in any given situation, how to deconstruct and rationalize certain clinical problems, and how to best articulate that which is core to the beliefs, values, and assumptions of our discipline. In so doing, they have created a climate of lively discourse and, at times, heated disputation.

A HISTORY OF THE MODEL MOVEMENT

In attempting to make sense of the current intellectual challenges faced by our discipline, it is useful to remind ourselves that, although caring for the sick is a cultural universal across temporal and spacial contexts (Yura & Walsh, 1983), that which we consider modern nursing is deeply rooted within 19th century England, and has borne the legacy of the defining features of that particular society.

Florence Nightingale

A visionary leader within that complex era, Nightingale violated the roles traditionally associated with her gender and class by taking principles developed during field nursing in the Crimean War into a proposal to revolutionize care of the sick and injured within the English hospital care system. An accomplished epidemiologist and a passionately committed nursing advocate, she was able to accomplish demonstrable improvements in clinical and public health systems through her various reforms (de Graaf, Mossman, & Slebodnick, 1986). Despite constant opposition, she was able to spark the common uptake of a vision that encompassed not only care of the sick but also the health of the public, and was able to articulate an essential role for knowledgeable nursing in enacting that vision (Gill, 2004). Although Nightingale's contributions to the profession are well recognized, it is important to note that early nursing was also blessed by the presence of similarly courageous, inspirational, and creative thinkers such as Catherine McAuley in Ireland (Meehan, 2003) and Lavinia Dock and Adelaide Nutting in the United States (Williamson, 2000). Although these early scholars recognized nursing as "intimate, dirty and hard work in the service of others at their lowest ebb", they fully recognized its capacity, done well, to provide "solace for the human condition" (source unknown).

Postwar Science

The post–World War II era in North America has been identified as another significant juncture in Western social history that stimulated another wave of advances within the conceptualization and definition of nursing (Thorne & Perry, 2001). Wartime investments in a range of scientific and technological developments had a profound effect on the way in which health care was delivered and created a climate within which nursing began to formally acknowledge and exploit its scientific nature. In attempting to establish science as the legitimate basis for nursing, the leaders of our discipline began to recognize nursing knowledge as something beyond mere application of the knowledge produced by other disciplines, but a form of scholarship that had a character and nature all its own (Chinn & Kramer, 1999). Building on the foundation for nursing research that had been established in the 1950s, which was an era of massive scientific development within many disciplines, including the health sciences, the 1960s marked a turn toward the challenge of thinking through how nurses ought to use and apply all of the various knowledge forms that were increasingly available to them (Henderson, 1966). Leaders within our discipline of this era began to recognize that in order to use knowledge within a complex practice discipline, nursing required explicit mechanisms to guide the systematic organization of facts and theories relevant to their practice as well as to foster critical interpretation of the implications of applying those facts and theories in the context of actual practice contexts (Meleis, 1997). The work toward making explicit these intellectual processes became the grand project that we have now come to refer to as nursing theory (Beckstrand, 1978).

An Era of Model Building

Much of the theorizing found within the nursing literature of the late 1960s and early 1970s was motivated by the pressure nurse educators felt for clarity within the discipline. The traditional curricula (such as medical science) and pedagogical strategies (such as apprenticeship) characteristic of most nursing schools were quickly becoming outdated (Orem & Parker, 1964; Torres, 1974). Within this context, the idea of a theoretical structure that could define and distinguish nursing and nursing science was highly valued as a mechanism by which to generate curricula that would optimally serve the practice of nursing (Dean, 1995). In this spirit, a cadre of nursing scholars began to wrestle with the fundamental questions underlying the discipline, such as: "What is the focus and scope of nursing? How is nursing unique and different from other health care professions? What should be the proper knowledge base for professional practice in nursing?" (Thorne & Perry, 2001, p. 88). Their embryonic answers to these profound questions took the form of conceptual frameworks capable of organizing the concepts central to nursing and explicating relationships between these concepts. In this manner, they were intended to serve as "mental maps" for the fundamental informational and decisional processes inherent within nursing practice (Ellis, 1968; Johnson, 1974; McKay, 1969; Wald & Leonard, 1964).

While it can be argued that the model-building enterprise was distinctly philosophical in nature, its origins within that particular moment in history led to its processes being framed using the syntax of nursing science, such that nursing's conceptualization was understood as theory building. This quirk of historical chance has left us the heritage of a terminological morass that has produced considerable confusion and misunderstanding over the subsequent years. Although terminology such as nursing theory to refer to a conceptual framework may have conferred some needed scientific legitimacy at a time when such external credibility seemed scarce within the discipline (Cull-Wilby & Peppin, 1987; Jones, 1997), it also created a significant division between nursing education and mainstream nursing practice, for whom the role and scope of nursing theories was never well understood or accepted (Levine, 1995).

Metaparadigm Thinking

In contrast to the formal theories of "normal" science, with their laws, propositions, and predictive potential, nursing theories emerging from that era represented conceptual structures intended to inform and organize the line of reasoning that a nurse would use in order to apply a diverse range of general forms of knowledge within the practice context of an infinite number of unique clinical cases. Each of the conceptual models represented a distinct attempt to work out these relationships in a manner that consistently produced excellent clinical reasoning across the diverse contexts that nurses confront on a daily basis. Common to all of these models were conceptualizations of four basic elements of nursing reasoning: ideas about the *person* as client of nursing, claims about *nursing* as a set of actions and activities, definitions of *health* as the intended outcome of nursing, and explanations of the *environment* as the context within which all of this takes place. These elements came to be known as the metaparadigm concepts of nursing (Fawcett, 1984). While the term **metaparadigm concepts** may have represented another misnomer, it represented an attempt to locate the models that governed the clinical reasoning inherent in nursing squarely within the scientific advances that were so strongly influencing all of health care while, at the same time, setting nursing apart from its cousins in medicine and the other health disciplines. All of the conceptual models further organized ideas about these four common elements in such a manner that they would be applied through a sequential reasoning process known as the nursing process, essentially a problem-solving process that required assessment and planning before intervention, and then evaluated the effects of intervention before the cycle began again.

While many of these core features represented considerable commonality among and between all of the models, the history of the times was characterized by diversity and divisiveness. As a peculiarity of the evolution of nursing's theoretical project, the earliest manifestations of these conceptual models were almost exclusively known by the name of the theorist (such as Orem, Roy, Newman, Rogers, Parse). Later, writings about these theories began to associate them with their unique central conceptualizations or core identifying features (such as *Self-Care, Adaptive System, Expanding Consciousness, Unitary Human Beings, Human Becoming*). For a time, these model builders stood in direct competition with one another for conceptual control of the discipline, and it was assumed by many that, in this preparadigmatic science, one or another of them would win out and become the new **normal science** of the discipline. In the context of this competitive scholarly climate, it was perhaps understandable that the early nursing theorists and their adherents furthered the divide by endorsing a culture of rigidity surrounding the use and application of these models.

BACKLASH TO CONCEPTUAL FRAMEWORK THEORIZING

Much as the syntax of a language must be understood as a complete system, and may not be applicable across languages, the model builders tended to press for a complete allegiance to their system of thinking within educational curricula, in nursing service delivery contexts, and within the conceptual foundations of nursing research (Kikuchi, 1997). In this environment, in a manner reminiscent of its Victorian military and convent roots (Marshall & Wall, 1999), nursing began to apply what it understood as the rule structure of its conceptual models with an unparalleled literalism and rigidity through the 1970s and 1980s.

The Challenge of Application

In nursing education, the prescriptive and formulaic approach to applying models did provide a guiding structure for developing nursing curricula based on the profession's self-definition rather than the beliefs held by medicine about what nurses ought to know. However, much as an overly rigid adherence to the tenets of behaviorism dominated much of nursing educational evaluation at the time (Gronlund [1985] was a particularly popular authority of the day), this codified form of model application became increasingly problematic for those attempting to implement it. Since the models tended to focus their attention on ideal reasoning processes rather than tangible outcomes, they provided little guidance with regard to the larger concerns associated with safe and effective standards for professional practice. As many educators discovered, if you fail to attend to objective measures of enacted competencies in a professional practice discipline such as nursing, you create the space within which it becomes difficult to claim that a particular student is or is not safe to practice. Thus, although the model movement's contribution to obtaining control of the discipline's own curricula was highly valued within the community of nursing educational scholars, there was also an emphatic resistance among many nurse educators to the overly enthusiastic application of a conceptual model as a primary educative tool.

In the nursing practice community, there was a similarly strong upsurge of resistance to this rigid method of model application. In the clinical context, the rigidity arose because of the problematic assumption that practice excellence would be optimally achieved by prescriptive theorizing taking direction from one particular conceptual structure alone. Thus, nurses applying models in practice focused on generating detailed lists of the variables highlighted within the particular model to which their workplace ascribed, working out in a probabilistic manner how the bits of assessment data might relate to one another under the unique circumstances of a particular patient, and thereby directing their clinical reasoning process. Nurses working in clinical settings using different models found it increasingly difficult to consult across practice languages and to articulate disciplinary rather than model perspectives. Unfortunately, much of the model implementation activity of the era reflected unsophisticated interpretations of the possibilities to which the original model builders had originally aspired. Instead, practice leaders of the day typically advocated a somewhat formulaic approach to nursing practice that failed to reflect the creativity, inspiration, and passion apparent in the original theoretical works (Holden, 1990). As an outcome of these misguided model implementation initiatives, many expert nurses felt constrained by practice environments in which overt adherence to a particular model was expected and thinking beyond the scope of the model was discouraged.

Over this period of time, the nursing scholarship community became similarly disenchanted with conceptual models as the panacea for nursing's scientific advancement. Afaf Meleis (1987) spoke for many when she advocated a turn from internal reflection upon nursing's intellectual processes and toward theorizing the fundamental substance of the discipline. Although many researchers made valiant efforts to locate their scholarly projects within the theoretical underpinnings of nursing as explicated by these conceptual frameworks, many began to understand that such grounding all too often led to research questions whose primary focus was to advance the theory rather than to deal with the substantive matters that the theory was intended to frame. Thus, it became increasingly common for nursing research to be grounded within theoretical frameworks distinct from those that were understood to represent the unique disciplinary knowledge of nursing. As curriculum builders at both undergraduate and graduate levels came to dissociate that which was research methodology training from that which was nursing theory, the relationship between nursing theory and other forms of nursing scholarship became severely strained.

Through the 1990s, the reactions of nursing's education, practice, and research communities to the rigidly applied tenets of nursing's conceptual frameworks created the context for a widespread backlash against the theoretical model project overall. From an earlier stance of uncritical acceptance of nursing theory, on the assumption that adherence to it would inherently advantage the profession, many scholars, educators, and leaders responded with harsh criticism of the model movement, even to the point of emphatic rejection of its relevance (Holden, 1990). During this era, it became the fashion within some nursing scholarship communities to actively disparage those who continued to see any value in the models, who included the study of them in their graduate curricula, or who made reference to them in the development of their clinical practice guidelines (Engebretson, 1997; Varcoe, 1996).

Rethinking Nursing Knowledge

Fueling the model bashing of this era was the sweeping uptake of Benner's (1984) seminal work *From Novice to Expert,* which was often cited as proof that experiential knowledge, obtained through reflection on paradigm case exemplars, was more influential in developing expertise than was adherence to a conceptual framework. A more careful read of Benner's original might have contextualized her claims as being based on expert nurses who were building experiential knowledge upon a base of highly developed mechanisms for systematic thinking. However, in the mood of the day, this critical distinction seemed relatively unimportant and the idea was widely taken up, even in basic undergraduate education. The subsequent trend toward experiential nursing curricula based on reflection-in-action rather than systematic thinking (Bevis & Watson, 1989) can be traced to this interpretation of Benner's original work. Defining curriculum as the context within which learning may take place rather than that which ought to be learned reoriented curriculum builders in many nursing programs toward the theoretical foundations of adult education and community development rather than the theoretical underpinnings and conceptual structures underlying their own discipline.

The backlash against the conceptual models was also fueled by a number of converging events in nursing's scholarly context, including the paradigm debates within nursing and the popular emergence of alternatives to conventional scientific thinking. Although many of the original conceptual models were formulated during an era in which logical positivism was the dominant scientific form, nurses had been aware since the influential work of Carper (1978) that their discipline heavily relied upon multiple knowledge sources or ways of knowing. However, taking up Kuhn's (1962) claim that scientific change occurred by revolution, not evolution, some theorists began to argue for a conceptualization that distinguished conventional nursing models as being part of the outmoded science rather than the more enlightened forms of thinking (Newman, 1992; Parse, 1987). By conceptualizing the models as belonging to one of two fundamentally mutually exclusive paradigms, which they labeled *totality* (the inherently reductionistic outmoded version) and *simultaneity* (the enlightened version) (Cody, 1995; Nagle & Mitchell, 1991), these scholars created a fierce tension within the conceptual model scholarship community. Thus, while much of the scholarly nursing world was looking elsewhere, ignoring the overall relevance of the nursing theoretical world in favor of more substantive foci, those still involved in the theoretical project got caught up in heated ideological and positional debates (Cody, 2000; Pilkington & Mitchell, 2003; Rodgers, 1991; Thorne, et al., 1998). Although most nursing scholars comfortably sidestepped the debates by discounting the relevance of the theoretical project in the first place, those attending to the unfolding saga found it a curious episode in our discipline's intellectual history—one in which passionate adherence to what they understood as revolutionary new ways of thinking led some scholars to uncompromising rejection of the insight and wisdom contained within the conceptual foundations of our discipline's scholarly history.

Finally, these disciplinary trends and debates were played out within a context of increasing popular discourse in the philosophy of science itself. Although Kuhn's challenge of the logical order of scientific advancement was first published in 1962, it came gradually to the attention of theorists and scholars across all scientific disciplines over the next 30 years. Within the health sciences, Kuhn's scientific revolution as a reference point created a sense of permission to extend scholarly thought well beyond the traditional confines of scientific thinking and to embrace a wide range of social and philosophical theories. The release from a linear causation mode of science was particularly important, and nurses quickly explored such ideas as chaos theory and complexity science, theoretical positions that might help their inherently messy practice discipline engage more effectively within the world of science and link it to the wider sphere of philosophy. Until that time, while there had always been a certain subtext of excellent philosophizing within the discipline, such as is apparent in the work of Nightingale, Orlando, Peplau, Travelbee, and many others, science and philosophy had been generally understood as essentially separate enterprises, with the philosophical enterprise largely irrelevant to nursing science (Kikuchi, 1997).

In the wake of this deconstruction of conventional science's hold on the discipline, nursing scholars have increasingly taken up a wide range of social and philosophical stances from which to generate their scientific inquiry, including critical, feminist, postcolonial social theory, poststructuralist, postmodern, constructivist methodologies, theoretical relativism, and pragmatism. While these expanded options have certainly enlivened the scholarship of the discipline, and produced a wealth of new knowledge, it might also be argued that a good portion of the work that is currently undertaken within these contexts seems to have lost the core of its fundamental disciplinary purpose. Outside of the context of a strong theoretical grounding relative to the nature of nursing, it could become increasingly problematic for nursing to sustain a strong and meaningful professional and disciplinary identity. Thus, we once again seem to be at a crossroads in which there is some urgency to embark again on the quest for philosophical understanding as to the nature, scope, and purpose of this discipline we call nursing.

A CHALLENGE TO EDUCATORS

In articulating this rather extended (and opinionated) review of recent events in our discipline's theoretical history, I attempt to lay the foundation for what I hope will be a convincing argument toward renewed enthusiasm for conceptualizing the purpose of nursing and for explicitly including that agenda within our nursing education curricula. Because it is nurse educators who hold within their grasp the potential to inspire the thinking of the next generation, that audience seems a pivotal partner for generating ideas that are central to the discipline's future. If we in the nursing education community can find our way toward rediscovering the excitement inherent in considering these matters of fundamental importance to our discipline, we will make progress toward solidifying our role and function in a manner that securely grounds our science. In so doing, we might, as Edwards and Liaschenko (2003) have suggested "salvage the very idea of a theory of nursing" (p. 3).

Reclaiming Our Intellectual History

From my perspective, academic nursing must find a way to reclaim this aspect of its intellectual history if it is to truly educate nurses toward the full scope and complexity of this complicated human endeavor we call nursing. Toward this end, we in the nursing education sector can do much to ensure that the next generation of nurses learns to appreciate the impressiveness of those early attempts to wrestle with complexity, made outside of the context of the ideas and understandings to which we now have ready access. Our matriarchs (for the early model builders were all women) struggled with matters of holism, context, and complexity as fundamentally important to the practice of nursing long before they had the words and the concepts with which to render these ideas into scientific language. They really were the intellectual giants upon whose platform our current grasp of what constitutes excellence has been built. As such, we owe them, ourselves, and our students a prominent place within our nursing curricula.

Similarly, I believe that it behooves the nursing education community to reflect critically on the implications of the trends and fancies it takes up in revising and reforming basic nursing curricula, so that perhaps we can resist our characteristic tendency to throw the proverbial baby out with the bathwater. While the early rigid adherence to what educators thought conceptual models represented within our nursing educational programs was clearly problematic, the problem seems more appropriately located within the limited understanding and unimaginative thinking of those engaged in the application efforts rather than in the fundamental aspirations and intentions of the original theorists. Thus, it seems timely to revisit some of these frameworks and theories, to mine them for guidance and direction, as we ground the socialization of our next generation of nurses within the scholarship that has been associated with conceptualizing its purpose. We can do this as a co-learning project, educators in partnership with nursing students.

Rethinking Our Curricular Approaches

It seems self-evident that our curricular approach should not be one of attempting to inculcate each new nurse with one or another perspective such that he or she can never work effectively within a context outside of that paradigm. Neither should our students be forced to learn in intricate detail the workings of a dozen or so conceptual frameworks. These approaches to applying conceptual models within nursing education were clearly counterproductive, missed opportunities for mining the richness of students' thinking, and have been discarded. On the contrary, we can be equally counterproductive if we abandon our efforts to engage in the processes of systematic reasoning in our efforts to become more student centered in our curricula and pedagogical approaches.

Knowing as we do that students tend to be drawn to the practical realities of clinical nursing and have difficulty appreciating the relevance of conceptual and theoretical thinking in relation to that practice imperative, it seems apparent that it is the educators who must inspire/model a commitment to a grounding within the critical scholarship of our discipline, including its conceptual history, by inviting students into this fascinating space as colearners. When educators and students together engage in this enterprise with sufficient intellectual curiosity to discover how fascinating the traditions of our discipline really are, and how relevant are the struggles of the early theorists for our modern disciplinary projects, we can create learning environments in which the history comes alive and the next generation takes up the challenge of interpreting the unique role of nursing within its own particular set of social and political challenges.

Reorienting Our Pedagogical Practices

Learning the complexity of systematic, contextually driven, and defensible clinical reasoning within nursing requires a thoughtful strategy, engaging both learners and educators in a dynamic interaction characterized by critical reflection and a clearly articulated understanding of excellence. Rather than asking our students to memorize and regurgitate the names of theorists and the main elements of their frameworks, which remains the primary mechanism by which nursing theory seems to be addressed in many of our disciplinary texts and curricula, our educational efforts would be most well placed if they orient our attention toward engaging students in an appreciation of the underlying intentionality inherent in all of these theoretical enterprises. These intentions symbolize core values such as:

- Comprehensive assessment.
- Critical reflection on the contexts in which nurses and persons interact.
- Recognition of the implications of taking action in relation to any aspect of the human person.
- Accountability for an auditable reasoning process by which one reaches sound and defensible clinical judgements.

Each of these values underscores the reasons that conventional science, as it was known to our discipline in those early days, was insufficient to answer nursing's pressing questions and therefore inappropriate as a primary source for guiding its clinical reasoning processes.

Over time, as their colleagues in other health care disciplines come to realize the inherent limits of conventional Western science for resolving matters of human health and illness experience, the nursing students of today will be ideally placed for showing leadership in their capacity to work with complex knowledge forms in a dynamic and evolving practice context. By wrestling with the questions that attracted the attention of our model builders, by suspending the search for easy answers, by helping them discover how exciting it is to think deeply about this social act, this profession, this thing we call nursing, and by designing curricula within which this history of our thought tradition can be brought to life, we will engage educators and nursing students of this era as co-learners in an appreciation for the marvelous philosophical grounding and complexity science that constitute our disciplinary heritage.

SUMMARY

As nursing scholars continue to explore an increasing array of scientific methodologies and philosophic approaches to resolving the core questions of our discipline, nursing educators and students will continue to be challenged with questions of relevance and applicability to the everyday practice of nursing. In the current idiom, we might more comfortably consider this the philosophy rather than the theory or science of nursing. If we fully appreciate the continuing complexity inherent in the nature of our discipline's social mandate, we will be inspired to create learning environments in which we can effectively nurture a new generation of nurses to accept our invitation to enjoy the creative and profoundly inspirational theorizing of the conceptual model builders. As has been the tradition of each generation of nursing scholars throughout our intellectual history, the nursing students of today will take up the challenge and offer us new ways of thinking about the nature of nursing. From one generation to the next, we are inspired by how beautifully simple and yet incredibly complex is this discipline that has drawn us so passionately into its grasp.

LEARNING ACTIVITY

Group Projects: The theoretical history of nursing is amenable to visual and graphic depiction in the form of posters and displays. These projects can become a secondary reflective mechanism to engage students in thinking about their own differences in approaching an intellectual challenge and imagining how it was that the theorists engaged with other scholars to develop the kinds of models that emerged to describe the profession.

Short Essays: The key to understanding the theoretical work of the discipline is to dig below the surface of terms and relationships and enter the world of conceptualizing and philosophizing. Students can uncover some of the complexity inherent in the concepts that make up any of the nursing theories if they are encouraged to reflect not on what is said, but what it might mean, reframing ideas in language that makes sense within the current context and setting them against current practice challenges. The kinds of questions that make excellent assignments are "what if?" questions, challenging students beyond that which a theorist has defined and into the domain of what else might have been implied or intended, such as:

- A number of the nursing theorists used the notion of basic human needs as their organizing framework for understanding how the human person operated. What does

it mean about human nature and experience to understand people as being comprised of basic human needs?
- Some nursing theorists considered the human person as a behavioral system, in which all parts interacted in an open and dynamic manner. What does it mean to understand all parts in relation to one another? Does that mean it is never appropriate to study parts in isolation?
- Nursing theorists vary in their interpretations of what the proper object of nursing ought to be. What does it matter if nursing considers health to be an achievable outcome as compared to an unachievable theoretical ideal?

RESOURCES FOR EDUCATORS

PLANNING THE TEACHING/LEARNING EXPERIENCE

Instructions for Educators

The history of nursing theorizing is a fascinating one, but can be made more fascinating by encouraging an understanding of the individual nurses who have contributed to it over the course of the last century and a half. Rather than having students dissect a theory, you might find it far more productive for them to get to know a theorist—the character and motivation of a particular nurse scholar and the unique species of theorizing in which he or she engaged. Using a simple electronic search engine, students can discover a great deal about nursing theorists and their works. Our colorful intellectual history can be brought to life by having them try to discover what they can of the personality quirks that remain a part of their historical legacy and the linguistic gymnastics in which many of them attempted to overcome the limitations of mere words. Each of the nurse theorists emerged out of a particular professional and academic context, drew from a distinct set of popular theoretical trends of their time, and engaged with each other in some rather heated and lively debates. Encouraging students to discover what was driving these differences of opinion can bring the topic of nursing theory alive. Although some of our history is amusing and some of the ideas have become outdated, what underscores the field is the creative imaginations of these scholars and their passionate concern for creating the intellectual conditions under which excellent nursing could be developed and practiced.

Questions to Support a Thoughtful Reading

1. What historical traditions created the urgency for defining and conceptualizing the nature of nursing?
2. How have the social contexts of nursing contributed to the need for a shared understanding of its scope and nature?
3. What trends in the advancement of knowledge have led to the dramatic shifts in how nursing has responded to its theoretical scholarship?
4. What do we understand now about knowledge—scientific and otherwise—that the original model builders could not have understood?

EVALUATING THE TEACHING/LEARNING EXPERIENCE

Questions to Elicit Feedback from Students on Their Learning

1. What is it about nursing that makes it so difficult to clearly and succinctly define?
2. What is happening within the current context of nursing work life in your community that makes it important for nurses to be able to define their scope of practice?
3. What can we learn from the era of model bashing?

Reflective Questions for Educators

Consider your own initial experiences in learning about nursing theory. What "vintage" do you represent, and how was nursing theory conveyed and studied during your own socialization into the profession. What biases have characterized your own relationship to theory—either for or against it as a useful aspect of nursing scholarship?

References

Beckstrand, J. (1978). The notion of a practice theory and the relationship of scientific and ethical knowledge to practice. *Research in Nursing & Health, 1*(3), 131–136.

Benner, P. (1984). *From novice to expert: Promoting excellence and power in clinical nursing practice.* Menlo Park, CA: Addison-Wesley.

Bevis, E., & Watson, J. (1989). *Toward a caring curriculum: A new pedagogy for nursing.* New York: National League for Nursing.

Carper, B. (1978). Fundamental patterns of knowing in nursing. *Advances in Nursing Science, 1*(1) 13–23.

Chinn, P. L., & Kramer, M. K. (1999). *Theory and nursing: Integrated knowledge development* (5th ed). St. Louis: Mosby.

Cody, W. K. (1995). About all those paradigms: Many in the universe, two in nursing. *Nursing Science Quarterly, 8*(2), 144–147.

Cody, W. K. (2000). Paradigm shift or paradigm drift? A meditation on commitment and transcendence. *Nursing Science Quarterly, 13*(2), 93–102.

Cull-Wilby, B. L., & Peppin, J. C. (1987). Towards a coexistence of paradigms in nursing knowledge development. *Journal of Advanced Nursing, 12*(4), 515–521.

Dean, H. (1995). Science and practice: The nature of knowledge. In A. Omery, C. E. Kasper, & G. G. Page (Eds.), *In search of nursing science* (pp. 275–290). Thousand Oaks, CA: Sage.

de Graaf, K .R., Mossman, C. L., & Slebodnick, M. (1986). Florence Nightingale: Modern nursing. In A. Marriner (Ed.), *Nursing theorists and their work* (pp. 65–79). St. Louis: Mosby.

Edwards, S., & Liaschenko, J. (2003). Editorial: On the quest for a theory of nursing. *Nursing Philosophy, 4*(1), 1–3.

Ellis, R. (1968). Characteristics of significant theories. *Nursing Research, 17*(3), 217–222.

Engebretson, J. (1997). A multiparadigm approach to nursing. *Advances in Nursing Science, 20*(1), 21–33.

Fawcett J. (1984). The metaparadigm of nursing: Present status and future refinements. *Image, 16*(3), 84–87.

Flaming, D. (2004). Nursing theories as nursing ontologies. *Nursing Philosophy, 5*(3), 224–229.

Gill, G. (2004). *Nightingales.* New York: Ballantine.

Gronlund, N. E. (1985). *Stating behavioral objectives for classroom instruction* (3rd ed.). New York: Macmillan.

Hardy, L. K. (1986). Identifying the place of theoretical frameworks in an evolving discipline . . . the nursing profession. *Journal of Advanced Nursing, 11*(1), 103–107.

Henderson, V. (1966). *The nature of nursing.* New York: Macmillan.

Holden, R. J. (1990). Models, muddles and medicine. *International Journal of Nursing Studies, 27*(3), 223–234.

Huntington, A., Gilmour, J., & O'Connell, A. (1996). Reforming the practice of nurses: Decolonization or getting out from under. *Journal of Advanced Nursing, 24*(2), 364–367.

Johnson, D. E. (1974). Development of theory: A requisite for nursing as a primary health profession. *Nursing Research, 23*(5), 372–377.

Jones, M. (1997). Thinking nursing. In S. E. Thorne & V. E. Hayes (Eds.), *Nursing praxis: Knowledge and action* (pp. 125–139). Thousand Oaks, CA: Sage.

Kikuchi, J. F. (1997). Clarifying the nature of conceptualizations about nursing. *Canadian Journal of Nursing Research, 29*(1), 97–110.

Kuhn, T. S. (1962). *The structure of scientific revolutions*. Chicago: University of Chicago Press.

Levine, M. E. (1995). The rhetoric of nursing theory. *Image: Journal of Nursing Scholarship, 27*(1), 11–14.

Lister, P. (1991). Approaching models of nursing from a postmodernist perspective. *Journal of Advanced Nursing, 16*(2), 206–212.

Marshall, E. S., & Wall, B. M. (1999). Religion, gender, and autonomy: A comparison of two religious women's groups in nursing and hospitals in the late nineteenth and early twentieth centuries. *Advances in Nursing Science, 22*(1), 1–22.

McKay, R. (1969). Theories, models, and systems for nursing. *Nursing Research, 18*(5), 393–399.

Meehan, T. C. (2003). Careful nursing: A model for contemporary nursing practice. *Journal of Advanced Nursing, 44*(1), 99–107.

Meleis, A. I. (1987). Revisions in knowledge development: A passion for substance. *Scholarly Inquiry for Nursing Practice, 1*(1), 5–19.

Meleis, A. I. (1997). *Theoretical nursing: Development and progress* (3rd ed.). Philadelphia: Lippincott-Raven.

Nagle, L. M., & Mitchell, G. J. (1991). Theoretic diversity: Evolving paradigmatic issues in research and practice. *Advances in Nursing Science, 14*(1), 17–25.

Newman, M. A. (1992). Prevailing paradigms in nursing. *Nursing Outlook, 40*(1), 10–13, 32.

Nightingale, F. (1946/1859). *Notes on nursing: What it is and what it is not*. Philadelphia: Lippincott.

Orem, D. E., & Parker, K. S. (1964). *Nursing content in preservice nursing curriculums*. Washington, DC: Catholic University of America Press.

Parse, R. R. (1987). *Nursing science: Major paradigms, theories, and critiques*. Philadelphia: Saunders.

Pilkington, F. B., & Mitchell, G. J. (2003). Mis-takes across paradigms. *Nursing Science Quarterly, 16*(2), 102–108.

Rodgers, B. L. (1991). Deconstructing the dogma in nursing knowledge and practice. *Image: Journal of Nursing Scholarship, 23*(3), 177–181.

Thorne, S., Canam, C., Dahinten, S., et al. (1998). Nursing's metaparadigm concepts: Disimpacting the debates. *Journal of Advanced Nursing, 27*(6), 1257–1268.

Thorne, S. E., & Perry, J. A. (2001).Theoretical foundations of nursing. In P. A. Potter, A. J. Perry, J. C. Ross-Kerr, et al., (Eds.), *Canadian fundamentals of nursing* (2nd ed., pp. 86–100).Toronto: Mosby.

Timpson, J. (1996). Nursing theory: Everything the artist spits is art? *Journal of Advanced Nursing, 23*(5), 1030–1036.

Torres, G. (1974). Curriculum process and the integrated curriculum. In National League for Nursing (Ed.), *Unifying the curriculum: The integrated approach*. New York: National League for Nursing.

Varcoe, C. (1996). Disparagement of the nursing process: The new dogma? *Journal of Advanced Nursing, 23*(1), 120–125.

Wald, F. S., & Leonard, R. C. (1964). Toward development of nursing practice theory. *Nursing Research, 13*(4), 309–313.

Williamson, L. (2000). History of nursing. Retrieved September 15, 2004, from http://www.thoemmes.com/social/nursing_intro.htm.

Yura, H., & Walsh, M. B. (1983). *The nursing process: Assessing, planning, implementing, evaluating*. Norwalk, CN: Appleton-Century-Crofts.

Chapter

16 Aftermath of the Curriculum Revolution: What Did We Overthrow?

Mary Ellen Purkis

I graduated from a four-year degree program in Nursing in 1981. At that time, we were experiencing a shortage of nurses in Canada. As a new graduate, the shortage was a good thing for me because it meant that I had my pick of jobs. I chose to work in the emergency room (ER) of a busy downtown hospital. I spent my final preceptorship in that area and had been pleased that finally, at the end of my long program of educational studies, I found a practice setting that really drew me in. I loved the unpredictable pace of work and the unending variety of issues that brought people to the ER.

About a year and half later, I left that job, which I still look back on with great fondness. I decided that I needed some additional challenges and excitement in my life. Taking advantage of the flexibility afforded me by my education, I decided that a move to a different country would satisfy my curiosity. What might I learn about nursing in a different health care system? With relatives to support me in England, I moved there where I stayed with family while searching for a nursing position. Eventually, I ended up in Scotland having negotiated a complex regulatory process enabling me to obtain employment there as a registered nurse.

My first job was in a small rural hospital approximately 50 miles south of Edinburgh, Scotland. Talk about culture shock. Nursing took place in long Nightingale wards with about 12 patients down each side of the room. Patients requiring constant observation were placed at the top of the ward, and those nearing discharge were at the bottom. Most shocking to me was that, as a new staff nurse, I was required to get to work as soon as I arrived in the morning while the ward Sister and senior staff nurses went into the Sister's office to receive report from the night Sister. The idea of providing care for patients I had not been introduced to previously through the mechanism of report was unknown to me. Initially, I was worried about giving breakfast to someone who would be going to the OR that morning or juice to someone who, for other reasons, might be NPO. Gradually I began to rely on my own capacities (talking with patients and trusting that they would tell me that they were not to eat, reading signals at the patient's bedside, checking with my nurse colleagues) to gain a sense of how to provide appropriate care for the patients in the ward. I was not assigned to specific patients but rather helped out generally with early morning care, meals, and mobilization of patients needing such assistance. This too was foreign to me. I felt somewhat at a loss because I did not have patients who "belonged" to me and for whom I was responsible.

The final challenge was in providing a report of my activities to my colleagues. Because there was a fairly hierarchical system in place, only the Sister was responsible for reporting what she determined each category of professional needed to know. She would ask for information when she needed it. There was no place for me to record my observations and interpretations of how patients were responding to the medical treatment plan. More significantly, there did not seem to be any acknowledgement of a nursing treatment plan that would complement that medical treatment plan. There were treatments, understood clearly as being directed by physicians, and then there was care. There was no way of making a nursing presence known other than through the absence of care issues (i.e., patients were not hungry, patients did not have bed sores, patients did not develop infections, and so on). Indeed, it was quickly my observation that the level of physical care and attention received by patients was of a high quality. It was difficult for me, however, to resolve this outcome with the utter lack of an intellectual presence of nursing—which would have been signaled to me, based on my own education and early practice experience as the writing up of my nursing care in nurses' notes, and the sharing of my actions and the results of those actions with my colleagues during shift report.

INTENT

The opening scenario above offers a context for reflection. As a new graduate from a 4-year, North American degree program, I took a particular form of nursing practice for granted. There was a practical component to the work, the provision of care and there was an intellectual component, writing up the care provided, including the responses of patients to that care. My move to a different health care delivery system, that of the National Health Service in the early 1980s, forced me to reconsider much of what I had taken for granted in relation to my nursing practice.

Since entering into the formal work of nursing education in the later half of the 1980s, I have held this example close in my reflections on what it means to educate nurses. Is nursing inherently a scholarly practice demanding that intellectual skills be taught to students in order to support their professional practice? Or, is nursing inherently a practical activity that seeks legitimacy with other health care sciences and so dabbles in the academy to satisfy this interest?

In asking these questions, I am in good company. As one sets about writing about the development of nursing education, it is impossible to miss a particularly turbulent time in that history: the time of the so-called curriculum revolution. The revolution gained momentum through the later half of the 1980s and resulted in a compilation of papers published at the end of the 1980s, (Chinn, 1989) as well as several individual papers published by the revolutionaries (Allen, 1990; Moccia, 1990; Thompson, 1987).

In this chapter, I want to locate my own individual experience of nursing in two different health care systems, one Canadian and the other British, look forward into the effects of the revolution on the educational system, and then consider the impact of the revolution on nursing education and nursing practice. Having offered an interpretation of the effects of the curriculum revolution, I will move on to argue that systemic separation of education from practice has undermined the effects that possibly may have arisen out of a successful revolution. Contemporary efforts to establish processes of accountability between education and practice offer opportunities to achieve some of what the revolutionaries wanted to see happen. These processes of accountability also hold significant challenges for educators. These challenges will be explicated in an effort to set out an agenda for seeing the revolution through.

OVERVIEW

IDEOLOGY AND REVOLUTION

The language of revolution has specific historical references. We can think of the American Revolution and the Russian Revolution, so how can a curriculum revolution be understood within such historical contexts? As consumers of this literature, should we imagine that the language of revolution was drawn on in an attempt to dramatize the efforts of the authors of these curriculum plans? Or should we consider the use of the metaphor of revolution as a deliberate linguistic device?

The sociopolitical references to revolution are, I believe, deliberate. Those involved in the curriculum revolution sought to model that revolution on historical precursors through a signaling of a desire to overthrow dominant views and practices.

Dominance and Conformity

Forms of dominance rest close to the surface for most nurses; we are taught early in our professional identity formation to think of ourselves in contrast to medicine. The focus of medical practice, we are told, is cure; the focus of nursing practice is care. Few people would likely choose care over cure. Most wish to be cared for while being cured. But on such a distinction of cure versus care, cure is typically understood to dominate over care.

This division is so widely held that many nurses could be excused for thinking that this was what the revolution aimed at from the start: the overthrow of medical domination over nursing practice. But indeed that revolution had begun a good 20 years earlier with the move of nursing education into the academy and the development and expansion of the nursing theory movement (Dickoff & James, 1968; Donaldson & Crowley, 1978; Flaskerud & Halloran, 1980). While commentators have since criticized the capacity of those early theoretical attempts to create a unique basis within the discipline for nursing practice, that was clearly the aim at the time (Cody, 1999; Daly, et al., 1997; Mitchell & Cody, 2002; Paley, 1996, 2001).

By the time of the curriculum revolution in the late 1980s, nearly two decades of academic (i.e., university-based) curriculum development was behind us. In the late 1980s it was the dominance of our own language that the revolutionaries were primarily focused on. Allen's (1990) descriptions of the practices of nursing education he encountered in the decade preceding the revolution were clearly influential on his future revolutionary writings.

> *My very first class in nursing, like many, was an "introduction to nursing." The first day of that first class, the faculty spent an entire 2 hours of my life patiently explaining that, and I quote, "man is influenced by his environment." Startling examples included wearing more clothes when it is cold than when it is hot. . . . In all honesty, I waited quietly for the first half hour actually thinking this was a joke—surely the instructors would soon switch gears dramatically and make some meta-analysis point. At least discuss the archaic semantic choice of generic "man." Alas, it never happened. (p. 312)*

Allen (1990) initially thought that his teachers were joking; after all, everyone knows that when it is hot outside, we tend to wear less clothing, lighter weight materials—cotton rather than wool. He waited 30 minutes for the punch line, but it never came. After 30 minutes, he began to realize that these teachers had so seriously aligned themselves with the theoretical position they were sharing with students that they had lost touch with the reality of what everyone knows. They were in a theoretical space, and students were required to enter that space to participate in the construction of a form of nursing within that space. The students would demonstrate that they understood by not treating what was being told to them as a joke.

Such a demand to conform in particular ways to specific theoretical models of nursing perhaps represents an amalgam of the old with the new; nurse training schools are often caricatured as operating under the firm rod of the Matron who regulated students' social as well as work lives. To the extent that educators of the time were shaped by such apprenticeship systems, it should not be too surprising that they took academic language up within the context of an apprenticeship training. As Allen's (1990) example illustrates, systems theory was taken to the extreme, used to make the most mundane of points and then turned into a direct and general application for nursing practice:

> *Systems tend towards homeostasis—when the external temperature increases, human bodies require more exposed surface area in which to dissipate heat—when it is hot outside good nurses will ensure patients wear lightweight cotton clothing.*

The way in which systems theory (as well as other general theoretical positions) was introduced into nursing education encouraged this value for direct application of ideas. It is important to note that von Bertalanffy (1968) developed systems theory as a reaction against reductionism (Heylighen, Rosseel, & Demeyere, 1990), and yet this is precisely what we see in nursing's employment of this theoretical position. The function of nurse education through the 1960s and 1970s was largely about drawing on understandings of science in particular sorts of ways (i.e., reductionistic) in an effort to construct a disciplined, regularized type of professional identity (for a critical appraisal of this movement, see D'Antonio, 2004; Karseth, 2004; Nelson, 1997).

Constructing a Professional Identity

What stands out so clearly in the example provided in the opening scenario is that for me at least, the notion of a professional identity had clearly taken shape through my educational and early experience as a registered nurse. This identity was linked closely to the intellectual practices associated with nursing: writing up nursing practice episodes and relaying these verbally through the event of shift reports. Parker (1996) has written eloquently about these effects of reporting on practice within the Australian context.

> *The days of a separate nursing structure, separate reporting mechanisms, separate documentation and separate enclaves are fast disappearing. The question then arises of how nurses can remain open to change and at the same time hold on fast to those aspects of nursing they believe need to be preserved. The study of the handover gives some clues. In the best handovers observed there was an authoritative nursing voice transmitting authentic nursing knowledge. In the best handovers, the nurse responsible for direct nursing care handed over at the bedside to the nurse responsible for direct nursing care over the following shift. This is a model for hospital nursing in the future. (p. 25)*

In contrast, the nurses I worked with in Scotland had a strong sense of identity, but it was not articulated through the practices of shift report. Instead, it was signaled primarily through adornment, and the privileges associated with rank. Sister wore a navy blue belt with an elaborate buckle. Staff nurses work pale blue belts, usually with much more modest buckles. Enrolled nurses, with similar educational preparation to licensed practical nurses within the Canadian context, wore dark green belts. As a newcomer to this practice world, I quickly caught on to the sorts of activities one could observe enrolled nurses engaging in (morning care), when and how they would work more collaboratively with staff nurses (staff nurses would prepare meals from the trolley, enrolled nurses would distribute the meals), the sorts of activities only staff nurses did (distributing medications around the ward) and how Sister interacted with all of this (accompanying the medical consultant on his rounds of the ward, speaking quietly with a staff nurse between visits to patient's bedsides; at which point the staff nurse would mobilize equipment and people to carry out the orders of the physician). I do not recall any conflict between the ranks. Everyone seemed to understand their place in the order of the ward and they conducted themselves accordingly. Relying perhaps more on implicit models or theories of hierarchy and military training to which the British system of nurse education has been compared (Moore, 1988), these nurses had learned how to conform to a way of practicing nursing where there were clear divisions of labor and little explicit questioning of the value of those divisions. Nursing practice was guided by these divisions and not by theoretical understandings of bodies as described by Allen (1990). While the disciplining of mind and body (i.e., how a student thinks about the practice of nursing and then puts such thinking into action) was quite different (i.e., an application of general systems theory versus an enactment of a militaristic division of labor), the outcome of conformity to an accepted norm was quite similar between these two systems of nursing education.

This was the case even up to the point of the night staff standing in concert when the night supervisor entered the ward. This was perhaps my most vivid memory of conformity within that foreign experience. Having been raised in the apparently more democratic context of the Canadian health care system, I always made sure I was busy with a patient at the time when the night supervisor would enter the ward. Unwilling to risk a more public form of resistance by remaining seated when all of my colleagues stood to acknowledge a senior nurse's presence on the ward, I resisted more quietly by relying on what I hoped was a deeper value that patient need should take priority over professional protocol.

Challenging Conformity

The contrast between nursing practice in rural Scotland in 1983 and nursing practice in Canada and throughout North America in the early 1980s stands in some uneasy tension. The Scottish context that I describe can be ridiculed for its apparent unquestioning authoritarianism. It is important to note however, that the nursing care that arose out of that organizational context seemed to be extremely good. Patients did not languish without efforts to keep them mobilized and ready to return home or to supportive living arrangements. There were no bedsores anywhere in evidence and in the unusual circumstance of a patient having fluid replacement, no instances of phlebitis. By contrast, debate about the best treatment protocols for decubitus ulcers was common on the Canadian hospital units I had worked on as a student; there was never any debate about why patients were developing ulcers. It was almost as though we took for granted that ulcers and phlebitis were common side effects of advanced treatment.

It is true that one elderly woman with significant visual impairment was admitted to the Scottish rural hospital with general malaise and she experienced rather rapid cognitive deterioration. In my view, her deteriorating condition was largely because of a complete lack of regard for how the constant noise of a Nightingale ward would impact the cognitive abilities of an elderly person with a significant visual impairment. I observed that no systematic efforts were made to accommodate her visual disability; for example, ensuring that she had access to her white cane, that regular events occurring in the ward were explained to her so she could begin to recognize them as daily events, and that she could link these to the time of day by having access to the clock located on her bedside table. Further, no one appeared to acknowledge or question the impact of lack of attention to her visual limitations on her rapid deterioration. Excellent, routine physical care proceeded for this woman and for all others on the ward. And so, while she was ultimately moved to a long term care facility, now with a significant cognitive impairment along with her visual impairment, she went there in a physically robust state.

While the Scottish example demonstrates *professional* authoritarianism, it could be argued that my memory of Canadian nursing reflects a form of variation on *academic* authoritarianism. Authority in the Scottish case was housed in the person of the Sister. All information and direction for patient care emanated from her. By contrast, I was experiencing the culture shock of the British system having been inculcated within a different system of authorities. Roy's (1976) adaptation model organized and guided my practice as a student and followed me into practice as a new graduate. So, while I felt the necessity of resisting the personal authority embedded in the body of the night supervisor as she made her rounds (checking to be sure every *thing* was in order), I did not at that time recognize or acknowledge the extent to which the intellectual authority of my own educational experience stood against that personal authority, how it fueled my resistance to some aspects of professional practice in the Scottish context but was incapable of helping me articulate an alternate form of professional practice that would have addressed the cognitive deterioration of my elderly patient. Indeed, I conformed to the practices that organized nursing care in that place. And it is this powerful effect of place that I believe stands behind the efforts of the revolutionaries.

Discourses of Relevance

It can be argued that those advocating for change in educational programs for nursing exploited the flexibility in the language of revolution. Calls for revolution supported demands as diverse as democratization in the classroom (Allen, 1990) and more holistic nursing practice (Bevis & Watson, 1989), as well as the expansion of nursing into the political arena. Those advocating revolution never pinned down precisely where the action was going to take place, where the frontline of this revolution was going to be. Was all the action going to take place in the classroom? In the hospital? At the patient's bedside? In the community? Where should we look for the positive outcome of this revolution?

At the time of the curriculum revolution, most nurses assumed that nursing's legitimate concerns could be fulfilled in their entirety within hospital contexts (Moccia, 1990). Seeking to broaden the intellectual and political horizons for nurses, the revolutionaries proposed new teaching methods and new topics as necessary to achieve a change in practice that would create a context within which nurses could be less constrained in their contributions to health care.

Driving the demand for revolution was—and is still to a great extent—an assumption that nursing's traditional curricular efforts have focused on issues irrelevant to the wider social and political good. The revolutionaries were keen to open people's eyes to the fact that "political and economic reforms have changed the underlying philosophies and structures of health care and of education. This has created a level of social, political and cultural upheaval in recent years which has affected the lives and health status of all people" (Clare, 1993, p. 1033). The revolutionaries encouraged nurses and educators alike to consider the nursing curriculum not merely as a device for organizing biomedical knowledge but as a mechanism that could support social change. Specifically, the interests of patients would receive greater emphasis—and nursing's place in the health care hierarchy would also be the subject of debate within this new curriculum.

Debates that raise questions about the relevance of any given nursing curriculum create tension within nursing, focused as we are on the practicalities of situations. Indeed, it could be that organizing the revolution in these terms, seeking to shift the nursing gaze away from the natural sciences (biology, pathophysiology, pharmacology) over to the social and political sciences, may well have had negative implications for its effectiveness. As nurses in traditional locations of practice have experienced increases in the intensity and acuity of the patient care workload, it is educators who are so easily targeted as being irrelevant. As those advocating curriculum revolution aimed at producing a workforce that would challenge the status quo, those debates did not diminish. For example, when a curriculum embeds a value for questioning the good of all students doing head-to-toe assessments in a standardized way, such questioning is heard as frivolous at best and encouraging poor practice at worst by nurses who experience the intensification in their workload common to restructured health care systems of the early 21st century. Here is a frontline; educators on one side, experienced practitioners on the other, and often students and their patients in between trying to negotiate the tricky terrain of appearing to be responsive to satisfying the demands of the workplace against the demands of living up to a revolutionary curriculum.

While this example may seem extreme, and divisive, it is, I argue, an outcome of the revolution that demands serious consideration. This outcome is counter to the claims of what the revolutionaries hoped to accomplish. In classrooms in our program and others that have taken up the ideas inherent to the curriculum revolution we see courses on "Change Processes in Health Care" and "Ethics and Nursing Practice"—but the health care workplace is experienced by the same teachers who teach in those classrooms as being remarkably effective in resisting the translation of this knowledge into practice settings. In the end, all we seem to have accomplished is a more serious (and complete) separation between education and practice.

EDUCATION AND PLACE

At work in such processes of separation is an archaic worry of nurses—a worry that reaches far back into historical memories of what brought us to nursing, a memory that draws out ambivalent feelings of being called into this service of caring for the sick and the vulnerable. At those times when we give ourselves over to that archaic worry, we might ask ourselves questions such as, "To what extent is nursing practice an inherent, intuitive, artistic performance—something we're born to engage in, versus an intellectual endeavor, based in some form of scientific reasoning and the result of deliberative, rational thought?" Tapping into these worries, Benner (1984) had a role to play in the revolution by offering both of these stories—the intuitive and the rational—to nurses (Padgett, 2000). Benner's work, offering nursing a staged description of how nurses evolve from novice to expert practitioners, draws on language of both of these competing views of practice. Nurses are attributed with having more knowledge of patients and their experiences of health and illness than is typically acknowledged by more powerful players in the health care delivery system, namely, physicians. At the same time, Benner's descriptions of practice frequently portray nurses as happening upon patients in the midst of dire events and then struggling to have their intuitive judgment taken seriously by physicians. It was perhaps never Benner's intention to resolve the inherent tensions in her descriptive work. Those who have extended her initial study have focused on valorizing nursing's privileged use of intuition as a central mechanism underpinning knowledgeable practice (Hams, 1998; Nash, 1999; Woodall, 2000). The resulting tension created by such stories, or fictions as the philosopher of history, Michel de Certeau (1974/1984) describes them, might be usefully examined to further explicate not so much the *content* of nursing practice as the *effects* of our fictions on the construction of our identities as particular kinds of health professionals.

Our history binds us into holding open the possibilities of entering the patient's room just at that moment he goes into cardiac failure, that somehow we knew this was going to happen and we were brought to that threshold by some invisible hand. The power of that image of intuitive presence displaces the significance of disciplinary knowledge and specifically how, in practice, we draw on particular, structured knowledge from particular and structured environments and locations in order to enact our caring practices; that our knowledge is relevant and contextual. The careful cultivation of these forms of knowledge, their articulation within circumstances of caring, and how those circumstances produce certain effects are often glossed over in nursing's persuasive fictions. But in seeking an answer to the question of just what it is that was overthrown in the revolution, we must look to *all* of our practices of organizing knowledge in order to determine if anything happened at all.

The Significance of Practice in Nursing Education

One way in which educators seek to address troubling questions of relevance is to develop curricula that expose students to the full range of possible practice contexts. This response to contemporary nursing brings with it a number of associated challenges such as determining how much time to spend in what sort of practice contexts; how much time to spend in the community in contrast to the hospital; how to determine whether in-patient pediatric experiences should now be relegated to the category of specialty education and so on. Here again we see a tension between attending to questions of relevance inside nursing (can you call yourself a generalist nurse if you haven't spent 6 weeks on an in-patient pediatrics unit?), all the while being determined by processes of rationalization outside (as the CEO of the Health Authority decides that the pediatric unit is no longer sustainable and all acutely ill children must be transported out to the designated tertiary care center). While we seek to address one question of relevance, others are being determined for us. When we get caught out on these processes, we become acutely aware of attending to breadth while not considering depth. The question that intrigues me is this: Does nursing represent a multitude of quite historically unique depth experiences?

Michel de Certeau in *The Practices of Everyday Life* argues that

> *the modern age, which first arose out of a methodic effort of observation and accuracy that struggled against credulity and based itself on a contract between the seen and the real, now transforms this relation and offers to sight precisely what must be believed. Fiction defines the field, the status, and the objects of vision. The media, advertising, and political representation all function in this way. (1974/1984, pp. 186–187)*

The fictions that nursing students and their teachers see each day in mediated versions of contemporary health care are shaped by discourses of nursing shortages, wait lists for surgical and diagnostic procedures, and by the politically motivated nursing curriculum. As products of a revolution, we aim for relevance and against conformity. In so doing, we get caught in our own deep desire to produce rational, professional caregivers. These caregivers are the recipients of all our calculated rationality, a rationality that is exemplified in our efforts to create just the right mix of practice placements within which students can *complete* themselves and graduate as registered nurses.

Of course almost any period of time in practice itself can be used to undermine this fiction of the completed nurse. Good care all too often fails to rely on the knowledge of nurses or physicians. Instead, as teachers often hear from students at the end of a set of exhausting shifts, it often relies on the cultivation of friendships in places like Radiology (where you can squeeze in an extra patient if you can talk to someone you know there) or ICU where, when you are absolutely desperate, you can send a patient away who otherwise is going to expire right in front of your eyes.

A student I worked with once during a hospital-based practice experience was making full use of the language and actions of her preceptor to engage in a performance of doing nursing. She described for me the regularity of the observations she had made of her patient's failing body over the course of the 12-hour shift. She and her preceptor both clearly hoped that recitation of these facts for the troupe of physicians who, one after another, attended this man, would be taken up by them as a sufficient reality and evidence of his illness. Their hope was that someone would take responsibility for instituting a medical plan that would save the patient from what seemed like an inevitable movement toward death. The physician's responsibility would be relayed to the nurses through the enunciation of a plan of care that would entail more things for them to "do and to say" (de Certeau, 1974/1984) about the man as someone who had a legitimate place on their nursing unit. Despite their repeated attempts, such an outcome did not occur. The only thing left for them to do was to call on a nurse colleague who worked in the ICU and have their patient transferred to a place where a greater range of things to say and do might be available.

de Certeau (1974/1984) comments on this practice of recitation that the nurses hoped would create possibilities for action with this patient:

> *Our society has become a recited society, in three senses: it is defined by stories, by citations of stories, and by the interminable recitation of stories . . . the spectator-observer knows that they (the fictions) are merely "semblances," the results of manipulations—"I know perfectly well that it's so much hogwash"—but all the same he assumes that these simulations have the status of the real: a belief survives the refutation that everything we know about their fabrication makes available to him . . . citation thus appears to be the ultimate weapon for making people believe. Because it plays on what the other is assumed to believe, it is the means by which the "real" is instituted. (pp. 186–188)*

In her story of desperation to bring medical expertise to bear in the prevention of death, the student performed the ultimate fiction of the acute care hospital; that it is a place of expertise where efficient and effective treatment of illness is found, delivered, and, on the basis of which, people's health returns and they are discharged home, whole and well. She knows "perfectly well that it's so much hogwash—but all the same" must engage in the performance of the belief in this fictive reality.

So, what is this student nurse practicing in practice? She is practicing overlooking the fractures in the fictions. Her work as a student and soon-to-be graduate nurse will have to focus on finding examples of expert interventions, her own as well as the interventions of others, others that will serve to "offer to *sight* precisely what must be *believed*" (de Certeau, 1974/1984, pp. 186–187). And this is why agreement—conformity—in practice as to what is to be held by all as relevant work, relevant knowledge, relevant outcomes is so important. It is only through such conformity that the identity work can be accomplished.

As much as practice is a place for students to accrue experience, it is also a place to perform one's identity as a nurse. Of course the revolutionaries knew this. They hoped to give a new shape to nursing through revolutionized students. Having contemplated the problems of conformity however, they traded one ideology for another—and then they did not follow their ideology through to practice in recognition of those depth experiences of place. In not following through, they may well have left education and practice more seriously divided than ever before. It is to this possibility that the chapter now turns in an effort to suggest an alternative approach to practice education that does not seek to resolve the division between practice and education but to hold both in tension for the purposes of learning.

The Functions of Place

The revolutionaries clearly acknowledged the powerful effect that the practice setting had on students, new graduates, and experienced staff. However, it is unclear whether such acknowledgement extended to an explicit recognition that education extends beyond the classroom and into those complex practice settings. Whether this was recognized or not, the revolutionaries failed to implement mechanisms that would *take the revolution into the practice*, to take the ideology to the frontline to explicate the myriad processes of conformity and their operations from *that* place.

In contrast to those who work tirelessly at determining the right mix of placements to produce a complete nurse at the end of a 4-year program of studies, I do not believe that it ultimately matters *where* students are placed in practice nor what configuration of placements they move through. There is an established range of skilled practices that students learn and practice in some isolation from the wider field as first-year and second-year students. Once they have handled the instruments and artifacts through which nursing is made explicit (catheters, syringes, stethoscopes, etc.) it is then a matter of students manipulating these extensions of themselves to enact the visible fiction of nursing that must be believed by them and their instructors, preceptors, and potential employers. That is, there are conformities that they must perform in order to be accepted as members of the profession. We disregard the significance of these performances only at our own peril. The fiction of the skilled, competent nurse is a serious fiction indeed. And it is certainly the case that our reliance on traditions in nursing that the opportunities for rendering oneself visible as a skilled and competent nurse are much greater within a hospital. This is perhaps what underlies teachers' anxieties about ensuring students have sufficient opportunities to engage in practice in that setting. This may be as strong for teachers as it is for students.

However, there is so much operating in our wider desire to unify and to totalize, that one nursing unit within a hospital can be treated much like the next. There are differences of juxtaposition that show up when you turn left hoping to enter the nurse's station, only to find yourself standing in front of the elevators. But de Certeau (1974/1984) argues that this is not the order of difference that defines a place. Rather, he writes of imbricated and stratified places: those "opaque and stubborn places" (p. 201) that remain even after a rationalist process of system restructuring has written a new purpose for this particular nursing practice unit, changing it from one concerned with care before and after abdominal surgery to that demanded around the accomplishment of ENT and plastic surgery.

These stubborn places reside "beneath the fabricating and universal writing of technology," including those technologies that seek to obtain the ultimate efficiency from the human and material resources deployed into this activity of patient care. "The revolutions of history, economic mutations, demographic mixtures lie in layers within it, and remain there, *hidden in customs, rites and spatial practices*" (de Certeau, 1974/1984, p. 201, italics added).

I would like to propose, for consideration, that these stratified places await those who are practicing performances of nursing—students and the nurses they seek to distinguish themselves from and those they seek to emulate. These places produce opportunities for the consumption of *hidden customs* (of celebrating after a successful transfer of a problem patient), *rites* (of creating opportunities for a student to recite her part in this heroic adventure), and *spatial practices* (of excluding the dying from a unit focused solely on the living) by people seeking to render themselves visible as nurses. It is within these customs, rites, and spatial practices that conformity binds. And so, it is in *these places* that ideologies of discipline, of relevance, and of revolution must be made explicit.

REVOLUTIONIZING ACCOUNTABILITY

Following de Certeau (1974/1984), I would argue that these places "cannot be reduced to their unregulatable and constructable surface" (p. 200). That is, their power cannot be diminished through illumination. We cannot banish them by merely shining a light on them. They continue to be available—in their richness and their weakness, in all their irregularities—to students who seek to practice the fictions of professional nursing practice. Rather than looking for the regularities of a nursing performance, one that may lend temporary security that a student is taking up the lessons of the classroom in this foreign and separate place of practice, we could instead be looking at students' practices of consumption—what out of those stratified places do these new young professionals find and take up in order to make us believe they are nurses? Here is the beginning of a new set of questions that could fuel a different conversation around the curriculum table and one that could take us out of our exhausting efforts to fulfill our duty to provide for the complete nurse.

Explicating Contemporary Ideologies

What I am suggesting here is a process of accountability that runs both ways in the student–teacher relationship. All curricula are ideological, just as all places of practice too are ideological, even where the ideology is one of practicalities devoid of theoretical mumbo-jumbo. Rendering the curricula's ideology visible—to the extent that is possible—becomes the responsibility of the teacher in the classroom *as well as in the practice setting*. It is important to recall de Certeau's (1974/1984) caution here that we are not simply seeking to raise some aspects of ideological practice to the surface. He does not see benefit in rendering visible the structured (and ideological) routines of daily practices in this way. Rather than being able to draw back the ideological curtain to show dominant structures in need of revolutionary overthrow, de Certeau instead insists that we must look at practice.

And so, how conformity plays out *in practice* becomes a joint responsibility of student and educator. Ideological clashes can become the subject of dialogue and debate and should form the basis of accountability in practice. We explore this a little more closely through reference to an example already presented.

Ideological Knowledge in Practice

Earlier I described briefly the circumstances of decline I witnessed in an elderly female patient admitted to the medical ward I worked on for a time in the rural Scottish hospital. While that ward was accustomed to having elderly patients admitted, this woman's visual impairment was an associated factor that nurses on the ward seemed unable or uninterested in incorporating into their daily nursing activities. I was working the day this woman was admitted to the ward and I worked with the senior staff nurse who did the formal work of admission. The woman attempted to explain to the staff nurse the various supports she had brought with her into the hospital, supports the woman knew would assist her in remaining oriented while outside of her usual living circumstances. The nurse seemed to disregard this information, focusing instead on the physical symptoms the woman had been experiencing—the real reason for her admission. The nurse treated the visual impairment as something the woman herself would need to deal with. It would be up to the nurses to deal with her physical concerns.

The next day, I recall assisting this elderly woman with her morning care. She seemed so much more frail to me that morning than she had been when she had quite confidently walked onto the ward the day previously. Now she was in a hospital gown, her white cane was not visible anywhere. The clock with extra-large and bright numbers was on her bedside table but she was having difficulty locating it there.

I was away for 2 or 3 days and by the time I returned to the ward, the woman had deteriorated even further. She mumbled quietly and her fingers were constantly in motion twisting the sheets of her bedding, calling out when she heard loud noises. Her clock was now also gone from the bedside table—I assumed because there was not room for it given the need for nurses to use that space for their own tools and implements.

I was greatly saddened to see how quickly this woman's condition had deteriorated. I tried talking with some of the other staff about it but was unable to frame my concerns in ways that they could help me help the patient. Over the following weeks, the woman became understood increasingly as a problem patient as her calling out behaviors increased. At that time I did not know of the significant literature in nursing that addressed environmentally induced delirium. Clearly this information would have been vitally important for us as a nursing team to create a different plan of care for this woman. She was eventually transferred to a long-term care facility after several weeks on the ward. Physically she was robust. The breathing difficulties she had been admitted with had resolved with adjustments in medication. She was however, incapable of conversation where she had been completely intellectually engaged upon admission. She was functionally immobile because her visual impairment necessitated additional efforts on the part of the nursing staff in assisting her to walk.

Critique

Excellent physical care was a source of great pride on this medical ward. That was accomplished in this case. However, because the conceptualization of the work relied upon an assumption that the cognitive capacities of the patient are unrelated to the environment in which they live, there seemed to be no recognition on the part of the nursing staff that they could influence the course of this woman's evident decline. This was what I found so frustrating. Having been educated to understand something of the relationship between persons, health, environment, and nursing (the four metaparadigm concepts), I had a conceptualization of how nursing care could be planned and implemented that would have changed the outcome to some extent. Given the environmental constraints of an open, Nightingale ward, it would have been challenging to the extreme to create quiet time for this woman. However, I am confident that had it been understood as essential to the practice of nursing on this ward that not only physical outcomes were important but also cognitive outcomes, that this creative and committed group of nurses would have implemented that plan extremely well.

The fictions that kept order in that ward meant that if the medical consultant and ward Sister noticed the woman's cognitive decline, they certainly did not think to ask me for my views on the rapidity of that decline. Being an outsider—in more ways than one—I was at a loss to know how to make my observations visible and important to those who might have helped me create an effective plan of care. It is entirely possible that everyone reading the chart saw that the woman was 93 years of age and her confusion and delirium were treated as typically associated with that age. Ageist attitudes such as these are endemic in acute care institutions. This is important, because while my description of the patient's decline sounds as though the care delivered was poor indeed, it was entirely within the bounds of normal practice for that ward. All the staff were conforming to usual modes of practicing nursing there. Perhaps it was only because I was so struck by the confidence and intellectual acuity of this 93-year old woman at admission that the contrasting decline was so vivid to me. Why that difference was so invisible to others is still a mystery to me. Eventually, the patient conformed to the expectations of the staff; she became the cognitively impaired elderly woman they believed she was. And their practices in providing excellent physical care to her body continued to conform to the norm for the ward.

Accountability for Practice

How could a revolutionized educational curriculum respond in this sort of circumstance? Critical attentiveness to how an increasingly business-oriented health care system might encourage nurses to be aware of how their focus narrows to physical treatment of presenting concerns, disregarding wider emotional and social considerations. But such critical attentiveness will not, on its own, disrupt the same process of decline that I have described above. Such a curricular approach offers to students theoretical (some would say, ideological) framings with which to make sense of what they see in practice. As such, they represent what de Certeau (1974/1984) describes as "artifacts for consumption," practical exemplars that might be taken up by practitioners—students and staff—to help them make sense of the work they are doing. *How* such artifacts are consumed—what consuming them does for students and staff, how it positions them to ensure ongoing processes of conformity—could be a site for revolutionary education.

In order to engage in this sort of revolutionary education, educators must be engaged. By this I mean an educator who observes in detail the decisions made by staff and students in these sorts of circumstances and works to track the linkages between practices of theoretical or ideological consumption and the nursing practices that emanate. Particularly important would be rendering visible how discourses understood within the discipline as being implemented for the benefit of patients may, in fact, limit opportunities for the patient to participate in the decision making regarding his or her care. For example, when I asked the student who described her preceptor's heroic efforts to have their patient transfer to ICU whether anyone had asked the man what he wished for himself, she told me that no, everyone assumed that active treatment of the cascading physical deterioration was the only option to pursue. We talked for a while about what nursing care through this deterioration toward death might have looked like. We decided that on such an active treatment unit, many nurses would have viewed this as giving up. We agreed, however, that practice might also have been designed in such a way as to provide excellent end-of-life nursing care.

There would be tensions to negotiate here. The debates about relevance would certainly be raised. Who is better positioned to comment on the right decisions to base practice on? Educators? Frontline staff? Patients? Family members? But if education proceeded, not toward the right answer (therefore buying into a particular form of the discourse of relevance), but rather toward a critical dialogue about the fictive possibilities inherent in any "occasion for nursing" (Latimer, 2000), about the choices that we may engage in performing ourselves as professional practitioners, we can maintain vigilance that such choices shape us as nurses. We need to be present in practice, less I believe to oversee and regulate the practice of our students, and more to act as critical observers of the multiple and continuous practices of conformity that limit creative possibilities for patient care, limit the diversity of perspectives that could offer nurses and their patients choices in how quality of life is lived (Northrup, 2002).

Embedded here are also assumptions that we are all guided by particular perspectives—some of them acknowledged and claimed by nursing's intellectual heritage, others representative of perspectives yet to be articulated, and others still representative of perspectives from other disciplines. de Certeau's (1974/1984) insights on place invite critical dialogue and debate on the practices of unique individuals as they engage in structured and structuring spaces. The resulting conformities stand in testament to the powerful influence of these structures. But individuals who reach out and into those structured and structuring spaces to accomplish their nursing practice enact these. Understanding how these processes occur, what they result in and how they might be different stands as a new frontier for developing critical accountability in our practice.

de Certeau's (1974/1984) writing on practices of consumption offers a theory of action whereby social actors are understood as active creators of the forms of reality they inhabit and move about in. As such, his writings stand in some welcome contrast to the all-too-frequent constructions of people as passive followers of rules.

For those interested in studying the social organization of nursing practice, such writings offer interesting possibilities for investigating the effects of nurses' practices of consumption on patients and the construction of professional knowledge. This theoretical formulation also represents an interesting way to propose questions of central concern to educators who are, at the same time, subject to those same totalizing discourses of accountability surrounding the preparation of nurses who can be counted on to act for the public good.

Within that discursive space of accountability to the public, to say that it just does not matter where students learn how to practice may sound cavalier. But to suggest that it does matter is to perpetuate a belief that will always fail. And in the effort to avoid such inevitable failure, it will require effort that could be spent in so many more interesting and ultimately fruitful pursuits; those of exploring the diversities of nursing practices and all the myriad ways in which that diversity is governed, modified, and shaped to enable us to believe in its unified wholeness.

SUMMARY

The curricular purpose for students and teachers being in practice together, particularly in the latter stages of a program, could be reinvented as occasions for critical exploration of the consumption of nursing's historical location in space and time. The argument presented in this chapter is that those who attempted the original curriculum revolution did not perhaps go far enough. Having noticed the constraining effects of the hierarchical education system within the context of an equally hierarchical health care system, they assumed that making changes in education would effect the necessary changes in practice.

The intellectual efforts that have been put into exploring the causes and effects of curriculum change have not been matched by an appreciation and critical exploration of the influence and effects of institutional spaces but rather place it, as has been described here, on the development of professional nurses. In this chapter, I have offered one theoretical entrée into this underexamined aspect of educational practice. I have argued that educators have an important role to play in that place: that being as critical interpreter of how place is actively consumed in the performance of professional practice fictions. The use of the metaphor of fiction, I argue, ensures openness to diverse explanations for practice. It is a serious metaphor—one that can make all the difference in the world to the person's experience of being nursed.

LEARNING ACTIVITY

Think back to your initial education as a nurse. In your first or second year of your program, do you recall a situation where your learning in the classroom came in conflict with what you were experiencing in a related practice experience? Take 10 minutes to write about this experience. Be as explicit as you can about the classroom learning that you had been guided in. Be explicit also about the situation you encountered in the practice setting that you experienced as being in conflict with what you learned in the classroom. Now write about your response to this conflict. Did you discuss it with fellow students? Did you discuss it with your teacher? How was the conflict dealt with?

RESOURCES FOR EDUCATORS

PLANNING THE TEACHING/LEARNING EXPERIENCE

Instructions for Educators

Teaching/learning experiences drawing on the ideas found in this chapter need to treat curriculum as a form of ideology. Students could be asked to recall experiences where their plans for care were challenged, either by clinical teachers or by nursing staff, during their prelicensure educational experience. These challenges can be named as points of tension that may have arisen between what students were taught in classroom situations and how they were learning institutional practices of nursing. Students should be able to recall what the explicit curriculum goals of their nursing program were and how these were experienced by them as irrelevant within the context of institutionalized nursing practice.

Questions to Support a Thoughtful Reading

1. What do you recall experiencing as a point of tension in your early education as a nurse?
2. What was the curriculum goal embedded in this point of tension?
3. How did this curriculum goal come to be in conflict with values expressed by practitioners?
4. Was this conflict explicitly discussed as part of your nursing program?
5. If you were the educator in this situation, how would you deal with this point of tension or conflict now? What are the practices of conformity inherent in this tension or conflict? How might an educator demonstrate engagement and accountability for patients, students, and the nursing curriculum in this situation?

EVALUATING THE TEACHING/LEARNING EXPERIENCE

Sample Evaluation Strategies or Tools

1. Educators and students could evaluate the effectiveness of the learning by reflecting on the extent to which conflicts are not resolved but rather become the focus of the learning. Conflicting positions should remain visible. Engagement involves explicitly moving between the conflicting positions in an effort to render the complexity of quality patient care by nurses transparent.
2. It is likely that within a 3-hour class, teachers might only be able to address one or two examples brought forward by students. It is challenging to remain in the conflict and to keep conflicting positions open for discussion. The teacher will likely wish to discuss this experience with a knowledgeable peer. In this case, a coteaching arrangement might be organized to foster discussion among peers later.

References

Allen, D. (1990). The curriculum revolution: Radical re-visioning of nursing education. *Journal of Nursing Education, 29*, 312–316.

Benner, P. (1984). *From novice to expert: Excellence and power in clinical nursing practice.* Menlo Park, CA: Addison-Wesley.

Bevis, E. O., & Watson, J. (1989). *Toward a caring curriculum: A new pedagogy for nursing.* New York: National League for Nursing.

Chinn, P. (Ed.). (1989). *Curriculum revolution: Reconceptualizing nursing education.* New York: National League for Nursing.

Clare, J. (1993). A challenge to the rhetoric of emancipation: Recreating a professional culture. *Journal of Advanced Nursing, 18*, 1033–1038.

Cody, W. K. (1999). Middle-range theories: Do they foster the development of nursing science? *Nursing Science Quarterly, 12*, 9–14.

Daly, J., Mitchell, G. J., Toikkanen, T., et al. (1997). What is nursing science? An international dialogue. *Nursing Science Quarterly, 10*, 10–13.

D'Antonio, P. (2004). Women, nursing and Baccalaureate education in 20th century America. *Journal of Nursing Scholarship, 36*, 379–384.

de Certeau, M. (1974/1984). *The practice of everyday life* (Rendell, P. Trans.). Berkeley, CA: University of California Press.

Dickoff, J., & James, P. (1968). Symposium on theory development in nursing: Researching research's role in theory development. *Nursing Research, 17*, 204–206.

Donaldson, S. K., & Crowley, D. M. (1978). The discipline of nursing. *Nursing Outlook, 26*, 113–120.

Flaskerud, J. H., & Halloran, E. J. (1980). Areas of agreement in nursing theory development. *Advances in Nursing Science, 3*, 1–7.

Hams, S. (1998). Intuition and the coronary care nurse. *Nursing in Critical Care, 3*, 130–133.

Heylighen, F., Rosseel, E., & Demeyere, F. (Eds.). (1990). *Self-steering and cognition in complex systems: Towards a new cybernetics*. New York: Gordon and Breach Science Publishers.

Karseth, B. (2004). Curriculum changes and moral issues in nursing education. *Nurse Education Today, 24*, 638–643.

Latimer, J. (2000). *The conduct of care: Understanding nursing practice*. Abingdon, UK: Blackwell Science.

Mitchell, G., & Cody, W. K. (2002). Ambiguous opportunity: Toiling for truth of nursing art and science. *Nursing Science Quarterly, 15*, 71–79.

Moccia, P. (1990). No sire, it's a revolution. *Journal of Nursing Education, 29*, 307–311.

Moore, J. (1988). *Zeal for responsibility: The struggle for professional nursing in Victorian England, 1868–1883*. Athens, GA: Georgia University Press.

Nash, C. (1999). Applying reflective practice. *Emergency Nurse, 6*, 14–18.

Nelson, S. (1997). Reading nursing history. *Nursing Inquiry, 4*, 229–236.

Northrup, D. T. (2002). Time passing: a Parse research method study. *Nursing Science Quarterly, 15*, 318–326.

Padgett, S. M. (2000). Benner and the critics: Promoting scholarly dialogue. *Scholarly Inquiry for Nursing Practice, 14*, 249–271.

Paley, J. (1996). How not to clarify concepts in nursing. *Journal of Advanced Nursing, 24*, 572–578.

Paley, J. (2001). An archeology of caring knowledge. *Journal of Advanced Nursing, 36*, 188–198.

Parker, J. (1996). Handovers in a changing health care climate. *Australian Nursing Journal, 4*(5), 22–26.

Roy, C. (Ed.). (1976). *Introduction to nursing: An adaptation model*. Englewood Cliffs, NJ: Prentice-Hall.

Thompson, J. L. (1987). Critical scholarship: The critique of domination in nursing. *Advances in Nursing Science, 10*, 27–38.

von Bertalanffy, L. (1968). *General system theory*. New York: George Braziller.

Woodall, T. (2000). Clinical expertise: A realistic entity or a phenomenological fantasy? *Journal of Neonatal Nursing, 6*, 21–25.

Knowledge and Knowing Made Manifest: Curriculum Process in Student-Centered Learning

Carol Jillings
Kathy O'Flynn-Magee

Chapter 17

Faculty in a school of nursing have just completed a meeting at which the curriculum was a hot topic. At this meeting, there was disagreement among faculty members about the extent to which stakeholder input should be taken into account when making curricular decisions. The student representative voiced students' concerns about the relevance of some content for current clinical practice. They believe that many theoretical aspects of courses do not seem to relate to their everyday clinical experiences. Although the students appreciate the inclusion of core concepts and theories, their learning priority is acquiring the nursing skills necessary for survival in the practice world of nursing. Faculty agreed to engage in a debate about whose voice should be heard in curriculum.

INTENT Nursing education has the challenging mandate of preparing a generation of practitioners who are knowledgeable and equipped with values and critical thinking abilities required in an emerging and ever changing health care system. Nurse educators endeavor to develop curricula that reflect not only the complexities of the practice world (and the requisite knowledge, attitudes, and competencies), but the various forms of knowledge influencing and influenced by practice. The process of curriculum development requires both logic and a comprehensive view of the many contexts of nursing. There is a need for both vision and leadership in constructing the blueprint for learning that will serve present and future needs. A concomitant challenge is for nursing education to become and remain more student centered. Curriculum implementation is not a dictatorial process; curriculum and instruction do not constitute dogma. Learners are catalysts of the curriculum, bringing knowledge, experiences, and perspectives that ultimately shape their learning and acquisition of practice competencies. In this chapter, it is our intent to explore the intricacies of curriculum development by first discussing the nature of the knowledge at its core. Since curriculum development is a form of knowledge exchange, we will then move to an overview of curriculum process, its historical roots and configurations, the common elements that have remained after debate and critique, and the phases of curriculum development that are relevant in the current educational and practice climates. We will conclude by examining issues surrounding the curriculum and its implementation in a climate of change.

OVERVIEW

INTRODUCTION

The nature of nursing knowledge, and the processes of knowing in nursing, have been discussed in the literature of the discipline for over 25 years. Beginning with Carper's (1978) analysis and discussion of patterns of knowing in nursing, later extended by White's (1995) introduction of an additional dimension, the profession has embraced the cornerstones of empiric, aesthetic, personal, ethical, and sociopolitical knowing as fundamental to understanding the forms of knowledge embodied in nursing practice. The realm of nursing education is concerned with structuring and conveying knowledge so that learners can master the core competencies required for practice. The nursing curriculum provides the infrastructure for organizing and delivering content and learning experiences, building toward cognitive, affective, and psychomotor outcomes. The crucial interplay between forms of knowledge, ways of knowing, and the process of curriculum development cannot be understated; if the curriculum is to provide experiences that extend beyond mere content delivery and skill acquisition, it must reflect all dimensions of nursing and in addition, achieve a profound connection with the learner who must ultimately understand and enact the core concepts, theories, and competencies. The ensuing discussion will explore knowledge and knowing in nursing education and, building from this examination, describe the process of curriculum development in its historical and contemporary contexts. Challenges and issues, particularly as they relate to student-centered learning, will be addressed in order to provide food for thought and a basis for critique and debate.

FORMS OF KNOWLEDGE

> *It [the knowledge of nursing] is recognized as the knowledge which everyone ought to have—distinct from medical knowledge, which only a profession can have.*
>
> *(Nightingale, 1860)*

There are several approaches to conceptualizing forms of knowledge that serve us well in creating a backdrop for a discussion of knowledge in the nursing educational context, and we highlight a selection that is by no means all inclusive. These conceptualizations have arisen because scholars recognize that a singular category of knowledge does not exist and that educators, in particular, benefit from considering a variety of knowledge forms. Burnard (1987) puts forth an epistemological theory that encompasses three domains of knowledge: propositional, practical, and experiential, as foundational to a theory of experiential learning. While propositional knowledge equates with textbook and theoretical knowledge, practical knowledge relates to development of functional skills, including, but not exclusive to, psychomotor abilities. Burnard likens experiential knowledge to Polanyi's (1958) personal knowledge, and describes it as subjective, affective, and embedded in personal encounters. Eraut (1994) expands our understanding of professional knowledge by describing six categories of knowledge: people, situational, educational practice, conceptual, process (or know-how), and control (knowledge about self). In particular, his inclusion of educational knowledge is an important one for nurse educators to consider. While some forms of knowledge can be grasped intellectually, Eraut reminds us that others such as aspects of know-how knowledge can only be learned through practice. A hugely important role of the clinical educator is to help students make sense of theoretical knowledge as they apply what they know to the context of clinical practice (Keating, 2006).

Of considerable interest to nursing is the somewhat elusive tacit knowledge that was first described by Polanyi (1958). This form of knowledge is well recognized in practice professions and is often expressed as intuition, another somewhat elusive term that Dickenson-Hazard (2004) defines as an "active expression of tacit knowing" (p. 4). Understanding tacit knowledge as beyond one's rational awareness (Carlsson, Drew, Dahlberg, & Lutzen, 2002), thus rendering it as somewhat invisible and inaccessible, serves to hinder nursing students' knowledge acquisition (Edmond, 2001). Therefore, we need to consider how we teach and help students learn that knowledge which is intuitive or tacitly embedded in experienced and knowledgeable nursing practice. As they begin to acquire such knowledge in their everyday practice encounters, students should be given ample opportunity and guidance to reflect on this newly acquired knowledge so that it can move to a conscious level (Herbig, Bussing & Ewert, 2001). Although intuitive knowledge may be respected in practice, Ruth-Sahd (2003) claims that it is seldom incorporated into nursing curricula. In an effort to do so, she recommends that teachers share their intuitive experiences with students and encourage them to develop and value their own intuitive knowledge.

VALUING VARYING KNOWLEDGE FORMS

An exploration of varying conceptualizations of knowledge encourages us to think about how these forms of knowledge are addressed, valued, and legitimized in nursing education. While a variety of knowledge forms and patterns of knowing may be evident in the literature, our exploration begs the question as to whether this diversity is being addressed in curricula and in everyday teaching practice. If not, is it because particular forms are valued more than others? If so, it is crucial to understand why this occurs. Ceci (2000) acknowledges the importance of exploring who and what makes nursing knowledge legitimate and cautions us to consider how issues of power and marginalization may relate to legitimizing knowledge. Tabak, Adi, and Eherenfeld (2003) agree that "a critical approach to education requires that teachers acknowledge the relationship between power and knowledge and come to terms with the fact that both can be used for multiple ends" (p. 252). Therefore, curricula designers need to be conscious of who decides the legitimacy of knowledge within a curriculum, thoughtfully critique those choices, and perhaps even more importantly, reflect on what and why some knowledge forms may be missing altogether.

Some authors claim that the focus of nursing education has been on propositional and practical knowledge with a spotlight on the former by academia, (Burnard, 1987; Freshwater & Stickley, 2004), thus resulting in a devaluing of other forms of knowledge (Beach, 2002; Dickenson-Hazard, 2004; Edmond, 2001; Eraut, 1994; Freshwater & Stickley, 2004; Ruth-Sahd, 2003). On the other hand, from a practice perspective, theoretical knowledge may not be regarded as highly as practice and intuitive knowledge. Yet, just as it is important to recognize the limitations of theoretical forms of knowledge, it is equally important to do so for various other forms (Johnson & Ratner, 1997; Kaeding & Rambur, 2004). Viewing knowledge solely through the academic versus the practice lens and vice versa does not always allow a broad appreciation of the inherent worth of all knowledge forms and may contribute to the theory/practice and practice/theory gaps that continue to exist today in nursing education.

It is up to us, as educators, to help students experience and value all forms of nursing knowledge as legitimate and to encourage them to critique, question, and challenge inappropriate, unclear, or unfair legitimizing practices. At times however, in an effort to survive the daunting challenge of clinical practice experiences, students, particularly as they begin their nursing careers, often want the survival guide version of what they need to know. As a result, they may believe that some of the knowledge embedded in the curriculum is superfluous. Being student centered in this situation means that teachers respect students' voice in the context of what Pratt (1998) refers to as "legitimate, though incomplete, ways of knowing" (p. 47). Thus, a student-centered approach does not ignore the reality of the teacher's knowledge; while such knowledge may result in an inequality of function between student and teacher, a respect for the equality of identity or students as persons allows an equitable and student-centered partnership to exist (Paterson, 1998).

Tabak et al. (2003) maintain that "in the workplace, nurses' knowledge is likely to be discounted through the social organization of health care, a hierarchical and patriarchal organization that privileges scientific knowledge and physicians who control it" (p. 250). Kaeding and Rambur (2004) agree that society continues to believe that the nursing profession has few intellectual components and they insist that "there are serious risks to underemphasizing knowledge" (p. 137). Within the nursing profession, relentless debate and a lack of consensus about the nature of nursing knowledge result in considerable ambiguity in designing nursing curricula (Thorne, 2003; Trnobranski, 1997). If we, as a profession, cannot articulate the value of our knowledge such that governmental decisions override professional beliefs and values about educational preparation for entry to practice, how can we expect society to understand the value of knowledge that is unique to nursing? As nurse educators, we need to explore the divisiveness that accounts for the ways in which knowledge is valued within the profession and move toward agreement about the importance of knowledge in all its forms. It is important to remember that the purpose of nursing knowledge and theory resides in its relevance for practice (Beach, 2002). The tension that exists as a result of differing values is crucial to resolve so that when future nurses (today's students) take on the profession's values, they include all forms of nursing knowledge.

KNOWING

Patterns of knowing as theoretical, empirical, critical, ethical, technological, personal, interpersonal, and aesthetics are discussed in Chapter 2. The classic presentation of patterns of knowing in nursing was done by Carper in 1978, who proposed four distinct orientations: empirics, aesthetics, personal knowledge, and ethics. Empirics encompass the science of nursing and aesthetics, the art of nursing, the two most obvious orientations of a practice profession. Personal knowing is the nurse's own awareness of self, critical to engagement in a caring relationship with the recipient of nursing care. Lastly, ethics comprise the moral component of nursing. White's (1995) expansion of Carper's work proposes sociopolitical knowing, that larger context of the nurse–client relationship or, as she puts it, the "wherein" (p. 9). Chapter 2 presents a model of decision making that includes eight elements of a knowledge base that, as in earlier conceptualizations, mirrors different patterns of knowing. Each of the foregoing views contributes to a broad view of nursing knowledge and knowing; there is not one exclusive perspective or lens, and nursing, but by its nature, is multidimensional and complex.

A number of other perspectives on knowing have been advanced by scholars in nursing and other disciplines, and these perspectives are often articulated in ways resembling the forms of knowledge described earlier in this chapter. Belenky, Clinchy, Goldberger, and Tarule (1986), feminist educators whose landmark presentation of women's ways of knowing has shaped discourse in education and diversity, describe five categories for the organization of knowledge: silence, received knowledge, subjective knowledge, procedural knowledge, and constructed knowledge. Rancourt, Guimond-Papai, and Prud'homme-Brisson (2000) present three ways of knowledge acquisition: noetic, involving intuition and insight; rational, involving reason and thought; and empirical, involving perception and the senses. Rancourt et al. posit that these reasoning processes constitute epistemic styles, noting that they "have been in part responsible over the centuries for the development as well as the subsequent fracturing of knowledge into various classification systems known as disciplines" (p. 4). Although the work by Rancourt et al. focuses on knowledge acquisition, it is still relevant for any consideration of ways of knowing. Within nursing, Chinn and Kramer (2004) have continued Carper's (1978) legacy by building on empirics, ethics, aesthetics, and personal knowing as foundations for the discussion of integrated knowledge development. Each conceptualization identifies categories, dimensions, or epistemologies with the goal of describing the multifaceted nature of knowing and knowledge in ways that reflect rationality, perception and insight, objectivity and subjectivity, the received and the internal, the tacit and the explicit. Familiarity with these perspectives has served nursing well, capturing elements of knowledge and practice that resonate with its core values of caring and evidence-based practice.

In the context of nursing education, the forms of knowledge and patterns of knowing lead us to examine the ways in which we operationalize such diversity within the curriculum and its component parts. If we as educators value multiple forms of knowledge and ways of knowing, how does this play out in the design and construction of curriculum and instruction? Furthermore, are there parallel (or, at least, concomitant) considerations with respect to knowledge in teaching and learning that should be accounted for in the structures and processes of nursing education?

CONVEYING WHAT WE KNOW: THE ENTERPRISE OF NURSING EDUCATION

The forms of nursing knowledge and ways of knowing are foundational to nursing education: the educational process should reflect all perspectives on knowledge in a balanced manner. The nursing curriculum, as the "formal plan of study" (Keating, 2006, p. 2), comprises the structures and processes whereby knowledge is conceptualized, organized, and operationalized. Beyond knowledge, the curriculum also embodies core values concerning nursing practice and weaves knowledge and values together in ways that lead students to the achievement of outcomes reflecting competencies required for professional practice.

Nursing educators have, throughout history, endeavored to articulate curricular structures and instructional strategies in ways that reflect the science of nursing—the essential values, beliefs, assumptions, concepts, theories, and critical thinking processes that form the basis for the provision of care to clients. Educational programs have embraced the multiple client contexts and breadth of knowledge necessary for the attainment of standards of professional practice. The complexity of nursing education has led educators to discover and remediate many challenges: making explicit the nature of the recipients of nursing care (individuals, families, groups, communities, populations); describing the dynamics of client behaviors in and responses to issues of health and illness; developing statements of beliefs about nursing generally and teaching and learning processes specifically; attending to the processes of knowledge generation and dissemination as they contribute to evidence-based practice; promoting educational practices which contribute to the development of learners' professional values, ethical practice and critical thinking abilities; maintaining a focus on caring as a core value of the profession; and ensuring that outcomes reflect the necessary competencies required of beginning practitioners. Teaching and learning in nursing have evolved from an era when the educational mandate focused on distinguishing nursing knowledge from the purely biomedical to the current age of health promotion, population health, and global thinking. The design of curriculum and instruction, then, resembles a novel perspective on a complex algebraic equation: multifactorial, with the need for the expression of many interrelated ideas and accompanied by a detailed explanatory narrative.

The curriculum provides the structure or blueprint for achieving the desired outcomes of the nursing educational experience. It has its basis in core values, beliefs, and assumptions about the nature of nursing and the processes of teaching and learning. As noted earlier, it comprises the arrangement of core content and learning experiences and the sequencing, continuity, and integration of fundamental concepts. The curriculum, however, does not stand as a monolith of content. It encompasses pedagogy—he art and science of teaching. Lather (1991) discusses pedagogy as the "transformation of consciousness that takes place in the intersection of three agencies—the teacher, the learner, and the knowledge they together produce" (Lusted, cited in Lather, p. 15). Lather further notes that pedagogy "focuses attention on the conditions and means through which knowledge is produced" (p. 15). When Lather's points are considered in light of what has been discussed earlier in this chapter with respect to forms of knowledge and ways of knowing, the concept of pedagogy is magnified. With its mandate for structuring and communicating all forms of knowledge, the nursing curriculum can be complex and daunting to the educator; furthermore, the curriculum can be built on a solid foundation that may then be forgotten (or from which teaching/learning practices deviate) in the midst of ever changing and demanding clinical practice and classroom milieu. An additional possibility in the nursing education scenario is that the curriculum and its components may have evolved out of past practices and traditions without clear articulation or embracing of foundational values and beliefs, including those values which focus on, and set the tone for, student-centered learning. In any case, the forms of knowledge at the core of nursing must be visible, and the ways of knowing acknowledged and fostered in the myriad approaches to content and learning experiences, teaching and learning, and formative and summative evaluation.

Structuring Nursing Knowledge Within the Curriculum

Nursing knowledge gives rise to the core elements of clinical nursing practice: the recipient of nursing care; issues of health and illness; patterns of clinical decision making; and therapeutic approaches in the design and delivery of nursing interventions.

Outcomes in the areas of cognitive, affective, and psychomotor learning reflect learners' mastery of core content and competencies across the curriculum. Historically, nursing curricula have articulated levels of learning and achievement at various benchmarks and have included conceptual frameworks or maps indicating concepts central to the program of study. Knowledge has been structured to reflect the numerous clients and contexts of nursing practice wherein learners gain exposure and valuable clinical experience as they progress from term to term, or year to year. In the 1970s, the notion of the integrated curriculum (National League for Nursing, 1974) provided the guideposts for framing nursing knowledge and promoting student learning in a cumulative manner. In the late 1980s, up until the present day, theoretical knowledge (hence, knowing) has been presented in concert with processes such as partnership and caring, which were felt to be less evident in the elaborate frameworks and meticulously crafted statements of outcomes of the preceding era in education (Bevis & Watson, 1989). In addition, elements of practice (skills and competencies, for example) have been linked to their theoretical foundations—often concepts and principles—in order to facilitate students' application of knowledge to practice. Herein lies a great challenge: linking the abstract to the concrete, the theoretical to the practical. These linkages should be manifest in the design and structure of courses, laboratory sessions, seminars, and clinical experiences; they should reflect the various forms of knowledge and ways of knowing. Yet, it is interesting that, in the design of nursing curricula, educators have often continued to perpetuate the theory/practice dichotomy by designating certain course elements as theory and others as clinical. This tendency seems to fly in the face of a balanced approach to the consideration and inclusion of nursing knowledge (and knowledge from outside of nursing that we apply regularly in practice).

The Process of Curriculum Design

What, then, are the elements of and processes involved in the curriculum, and how do they become part of a construction that contributes to student centeredness? In architecture and design, the maxim "form follows function" refers to the need for careful and deliberate consideration of the purposes and intents of an undertaking before, and concurrently with, making decisions about its structural components. In the history of curriculum building in nursing, teachers have drawn on theories and principles from the discipline of education, while at the same time being mindful of the need to prepare graduates for the realities of clinical nursing practice.

Early curriculum work in nursing was greatly influenced by the work of Tyler (1949) and Taba (1962), whose presentations of curriculum theory and practice afforded a logical and systematic approach to curriculum development that was well suited to university nursing education. Both theorists were proponents of a model of curriculum that laid out objectives to be achieved, explicated core curricular experiences, and identified centers of organization (subjects or topics) (Taba, p. 438). The notions of scope of learning, and of sequence and continuity, were vital to the selection of content and learning activities (Taba, 1962; Tyler, 1949, p. 84). These characteristics formed the integrated curricular approach advocated by the National League for Nursing in the seventies

(NLN, 1974). Torres (1974, p. 2) defined the integrated approach as "blending the nursing content in such a way that the parts of specialties are no longer distinguishable." The goal of this approach was to move the nursing curriculum away from the medical model or body systems approach. The integrated curriculum comprised the program philosophy, terminal behavioral objectives, a conceptual framework (drawing on main concepts from the beliefs statements, the outcomes, and the nursing theory or model used as the basis for the program), horizontal and vertical strands (threads), and the total curriculum design including level objectives and nursing and support courses and the related content and learning experiences. This approach allowed academic nursing to configure programs that were tightly woven, with clear benchmarks for assessing learning outcomes. The attention to behavioral objectives at various levels ranging from the temporal (semester or year) to the minute (specific subobjectives illustrative of the behaviors stated in general objectives) allowed nurse educators to focus on cognitive, affective, and psychomotor learning and to devise detailed evaluation plans. The devices known as threads or strands promoted sequencing and breadth, ideas promulgated by McNeil (1981); in this schema, sequential presentation of content and learning experiences (such as simple to complex, familiar to unfamiliar, concrete to abstract) was considered vertical organization, with horizontal organization attending to features such as concentration and correlation of concepts and experiences (McNeil, pp. 183–193). In addition, the centrality of the nursing model or theory was intended to ensure that core concepts were nursing oriented as opposed to being driven by the biomedical model that was so evident in diploma education. Finally, the detailed curriculum framework allowed educators to make explicit the core concepts of the program and track their emphasis in both nursing and support courses; this, of course, underscored the importance of a breadth of learning in courses within nursing and from other disciplines. Interestingly, Beauchamp (1975), another educational theorist who advocated an integrated approach to curriculum development, noted that a curriculum "contains a body of culture content that tentatively has the potential for the realization of the goals" (p. 128). The culture to be learned in this era of nursing education embodied the values of professionalism, leadership for change, and collaboration—all hallmarks of baccalaureate preparation for practice.

Curricular perspectives of the 1970s and early 1980s also included attention to contextual factors influencing nursing education: societal trends, characteristics of the health care system, and political issues. Conley (1973), in her classic text on curriculum development, wove numerous environmental factors into the backdrop for her description of curriculum process; in her description of sources of curriculum decisions, she included focal points such as cultural values, social and scientific forces, psychological and learning theories, the nature of nursing and nursing education, and the student. Her approach added depth to the complex matrix of levels and concepts created by the integrated model and was revolutionary in its attention to the critical role of the student in shaping the curriculum. A similar argument was introduced by Bevis (1978), who proposed that the student of nursing was an equally important component of the curriculum, not just the vagabond on the learning journey. Bevis' conception on the curriculum framework differed from earlier iterations by proposing a tripartite notion of the curriculum framework: subject/knowledge, setting, and student. This is not to say that students were not important focal points in the approaches to curriculum described earlier, for program philosophies were replete with statements about learner participation, learning needs, and styles; the spin, as we would say today, was just somewhat different.

The latter 1980s heralded the infamous curriculum revolution and the arrival of the caring curriculum, a movement which encouraged educators to return to valuing caring as a core component of the discipline and to more closely attend to matters of teaching and learning process in nursing education (Bevis & Watson, 1989). The hegemony of behaviorist approaches was challenged and, as discussed in Chapter 15, the literal interpretation and overreliance on nursing models and theories was criticized. Curricular literature of this era focused on teaching and learning to a much greater extent than on the actual structure or process of curriculum building (although it is interesting to note that accreditation and program approval standards and criteria were still steeped in the rigid design formulae of the preceding decade). Having carved out its educational identity in the academy, nursing education turned more to function than to form. Education theory in the 1980s and early 1990s was focused on orientations to the curriculum (Miller & Seller, 1990), positions that reflected underlying values and beliefs concerning educational aims, the learner, the learning process, the learning environment, the teacher's role, and the ways in which learning should be evaluated (Miller & Seller, p. 5). The transmission, transaction, and transformation positions articulated by Miller and Seller (pp. 5–9) depicted the relationship and engagement (or lack thereof) of student and curriculum, with the latter transformative position being most linked to humanistic and social change orientations. This theoretical viewpoint seemed to echo the curriculum revolution (and indeed, devolution) in nursing, wherein there was a renewed focus on the learner and the teaching/learning process.

In the curriculum evolution in nursing education, we seem to be returning to a balance wherein attention is focused on the structural integrity of the curriculum, as well as on the processes of teaching and learning. Additionally, the larger contexts—and the characteristics of the health care system in particular—are shaping the construction of courses and their associated learning experiences. Nursing practice concepts have evolved to include health and illness as social constructions, collaboration and partnership with clients, respect for lived experience, and globalization. The diversity of the student population has led nurse educators to become more student centered, recognizing the heterogeneity of contemporary learners; for example, not only are students more culturally diverse, but they often enter nursing programs after having pursued a previous career, or build on an undergraduate degree or other postsecondary education in a different field. They enter nursing with a variety of life experiences that influence their learning needs and approaches to learning. It is not surprising, then, that our present efforts at curriculum development are multifaceted and ever changing. Dillard and Leidig (1998) provide an overview of curriculum components which include: foundations (consisting of sociological and political forces, historical perspectives, and theories of teaching and learning); philosophy/mission; design; organizing frameworks; outcomes/competencies/objectives; educational activities; and evaluation. These components are not unlike those described in the nursing curriculum literature 20 years earlier, but they are presented with additional depth, incorporating variables such as student needs and abilities, workforce expectations and technological advances (Dillard & Leidig, pp.73–78). In a similar vein, Iwasiw, Goldenberg, and Andrusyszyn (2005) discuss numerous facets of curriculum development in the current climate, detailing a model that not only describes steps in the curricular process but integrates faculty development needs and accounts for the human and organizational complexities of the change process. They infuse the development process with deliberation, organization, and decision strategies and emphasize the significance of contextual data. Finally, Keating (2006) proposes crucial components of the curriculum echoing the foregoing elements, but includes emphasis on critical thinking, cultural competence, and nursing workforce diversity. She further discusses the need for curricular approaches that apply across various types and levels of postsecondary institutions, accounting for the increasing trends in collaborative education. Clearly, as the nursing curriculum development process has taken root, grown, undergone modification and been reborn, core elements have been embraced and maintained and the values promoting and permitting attention to multiple forms of knowledge have persisted; in addition, trends toward increasing student centeredness have led to greater attention being paid to learner needs and approaches to learning and to diverse perspectives on the core components of the curriculum.

Instructional Design and Implementation

If the curriculum, as the blueprint for learning, provides the framework for conveying nursing knowledge and ways of knowing, then the design of instruction (and its enactment in multiple settings for learning) is the means by which knowledge comes to life and is applied to actual nursing situations. Instructional design comprises the selection and organization of core content and experiences in a logical and sequential form that acknowledges and reflects faculty beliefs about the flow of learning, the contexts of nursing practice, and the cumulative building of nursing competency. Typically, this process involves the construction of discrete courses and the linkage to clinical nursing practice in a variety of settings and with different clients as the focus of practice. The enterprise of course development involves many decisions, some made and communicated by a departmental curriculum committee or coordinating group, and others determined by faculty directly involved with teaching specific courses. Attention is given to the content and experiences necessary for learners to achieve program outcomes and meet requirements for professional practice.

Instructional design is often the locus for the tensions characterized as the theory/practice gap: he potential disconnect between nursing knowledge as embodied in core concepts and processes, and the realities of the clinical practice context. The essence of this gap has been foreshadowed earlier in this chapter; certain forms of knowledge or ways of knowing may be deemed to be more accurate reflections of what is often alluded to as the reality of nursing practice. For example, it might be argued by some educators (and by practitioners) that empirical knowledge/knowing constitutes the reality of nursing and encompasses the tangible, visible, and often emergent issues that nurses face daily in the delivery of patient care. Personal, aesthetic, or ethical knowing/knowledge may present as value added but may not constitute the priority issues to be managed by the nurse. This perspective might be seen to echo the practical/theoretical split. Again, it may be less important at this juncture to elucidate and defend positions on knowledge/knowing in nursing education; an awareness of the various perspectives, though, is critical if educators are to design and implement strategies of teaching and learning that reflect both the complexities of the discipline and the realities of the work of nursing.

The design of instruction is incomplete, however, without attention to the processes involved in facilitating student learning. This focus entails reflection on and validation of faculty beliefs about teaching and learning, and the application of theories, concepts, and principles of adult learning. We have alluded earlier in this chapter to teaching and learning knowledge, something that goes beyond the conceptualizations presented to this point. The implementation of teaching is more than a simple internalization of the intended outcomes and proposed learning activities for a unit of instruction. It must include consideration of relevant theories, concepts, and principles of education and the selection of approaches that promote content delivery, learner engagement, and mastery of desired outcomes. "The traditional didactic transference of knowledge is now, more than ever, being challenged, with the use of art, poetry, dance, drama, and music in the classroom slowly being encouraged in nursing curricula. These expressive modalities can penetrate in an instant the heart of the learning" (Freshwater & Stickley, 2004, p. 95). Thus it seems that nurse educators, in addition to valuing multiple forms of knowledge and perspectives on knowing in the broad realm of nursing, also embrace a body of pedagogical knowledge that may also possess empiric, aesthetic, personal, ethical, and sociopolitical forms. This observation is not dissimilar to Grundy's (1987) notion of curriculum as praxis, rather than product; curriculum is not a static document or prescription, but is a gestalt of educational practice and structure.

A Synthesis of Phases of Curriculum Development and Instructional Design

Given the overview of the past 30 plus years of curriculum history, what vital elements remain in the process of curriculum development? The critical phases are presented next; note that they are named phases, rather than steps, out of the belief that each denotes a process of engagement among faculty, students, and external stakeholders and none stands alone without critical linkages to the others.

CONTEXTUAL ELEMENTS

This foundational phase of curriculum development involves gathering data and determining the actual and potential impact of a number of factors: health care trends, educational trends, sociopolitical forces, institutional philosophy and structures, professional association requirements and standards of practice, and stakeholder views and expectations. The notion of students as stakeholders values and reinforces the idea of student-centered teaching and learning. The environmental scan that examines contextual elements is broad and inclusive.

PHILOSOPHY AND MISSION

This encompasses faculty discussion and articulation of beliefs about nursing and about teaching and learning in the academic and clinical practice environments. It includes the vision of the academic unit's contribution to the educational enterprise and to the growth of the profession. It reflects the mission, vision, and purpose of the educational institution. It might also indicate a valuing of the various forms of nursing knowledge and ways of knowing.

PROGRAM OUTCOMES OR GOALS

These statements capture the knowledge, values, and competencies to be demonstrated upon completion of the program of study. Ideally, they should reflect the diverse forms of knowledge, as well as the multiple contexts of nursing practice. They will also clearly link to the competencies and standards of practice articulated by the professional nursing body.

CURRICULUM FRAMEWORK

This phase of development entails the delineation of core concepts in the curriculum. Concepts will arise from main aspects of nursing: the client, the environment, health and illness, aspects of the practice of nursing (assessment; decision making; domains of practice, such as prevention, health promotion, support, teaching; and characteristics of professional practice, such as leadership, critical thinking, evidence-based practice). These nursing concepts may arise from a nursing model or conceptual framework, and from the philosophy/mission and outcome statements; using these elements as sources of major concepts ensures that main ideas about nursing roles and competencies, and concerning the recipient of nursing care, are included. Concepts may be configured as a map, diagram, or matrix—the arrangement should indicate interrelationships and linkages, and the concepts selected should reflect the program belief statements and outcomes. Threads or strands may be used to convey sequence, continuity and integration of core concepts, and learning experiences.

CURRICULUM DESIGN

This blueprint includes the various levels or benchmarks within the program and the delineation of courses. Courses include those in nursing and those designated as support coming from other disciplines; courses also reflect program requirements and areas where electives may be chosen. For example, in an accelerated or upper division curriculum, all support courses may be structured as foundational for immersion in nursing courses occurring later in the program; this approach differs from that of traditional designs where both nursing and support/elective courses are combined across the entire 4 years of the program. The model or pattern chosen for course delivery will reflect linkages with other departments and disciplines in the institution as well as the realities of timetabling and clinical resources; hopefully, a degree of student choice will be built in to allow for pursuit of individual interests and learning needs. The configuration of courses will attend to sequencing and interfacing of discrete courses and reflect the teaching/learning philosophy of the academic unit.

INSTRUCTIONAL DESIGN

This phase involves the explication of the details of individual courses: outcomes/competencies, core content and concepts, learning experiences, settings for learning (classroom, clinical, laboratory), teacher-directed and independent activities, and strategies for teaching, learning, and evaluation. The design of instruction should logically flow from the other major elements of the curriculum. Furthermore, curriculum and instructional design should not be viewed as mutually exclusive. *This is a crucial phase wherein attention to student centeredness may be either enacted or ignored.* It is often tempting for this phase to be delegated to a few individuals, creating the huge potential for a disconnect from the overall curriculum process. The success of this phase is highly dependent on good communication among faculty and students and on shared decision making with respect to content and learning experiences, their interrelationships and synergies. In addition, if committed to student-centered approaches, faculty should ensure student input, feedback, and participation as courses are developed, evaluated, and refined.

ISSUES IN THE CURRICULUM PROCESS

It is not surprising that, given the complexity of the process of curriculum development, and the multifaceted entity that results, there are numerous challenges and issues to be addressed by nurse educators. These include, but are certainly not limited to, the following:

- Maintaining a balance of focus and attention to the various forms of knowledge and ways of knowing that are at the core of nursing.
- Addressing potential tensions between theory and practice, content and process, and curricular rigidity versus flexibility.
- Attending to the internal dynamics of the nursing faculty/school/department, including the process of curricular development, evaluation, and change.
- Acknowledging faculty needs in relation to expanding knowledge and skills of teaching and learning theories, concepts and principles, and current nursing practice.
- Fostering critical perspectives on emerging trends and technological developments that have an impact on nursing education.

Each phase of the curriculum process can be influenced by the impact of these issues, and each issue has the potential to disrupt or derail the systematic approach to design and implementation that is desirable. Student centeredness can also be obscured in the face of these issues. The ensuing discussion is not intended to be an in-depth exploration of each; we will, however, attempt to capture the essence of the issue and the critical considerations to be addressed by faculty.

Forms of Knowledge/Ways of Knowing

The multiple forms of knowledge and ways of knowing discussed at the beginning of this chapter present a challenge to nurse educators as they attempt to address not only the diverse learning needs and styles of students but the multiple ways in which nurses look at the world. Reflecting empirical, personal, aesthetic, ethical, and sociopolitical knowing in the curriculum goes beyond giving lip service to these dimensions in stating the philosophy and outcomes; faculty must ensure a balanced approach in the design and delivery of content and learning experiences. In an effort to do this, faculty must value different ways of knowing and knowledge forms and make these explicit in their everyday teaching practices with students. Although curricular and instructional design are inextricably linked (and, some might argue, really elements of one comprehensive process), they have been designated as two foci here in order to draw attention to the core considerations for each. If nurse educators adopt student-centered approaches to teaching and learning, it is necessary to consider the ways in which student centeredness promotes consideration of all forms of knowledge/knowing in the nursing curriculum and all it encompasses. Curricular structures (outcomes, levels, benchmarks, core concepts, and elements of content) should reflect all forms of knowledge, and curricular processes (the design, delivery, and evaluation of courses and learning experiences) should be geared to student diversity. Faculty should engage in continual reflection on and validation of approaches to teaching and learning, examining the extent to which teaching strategies are geared to types of knowledge and ways of knowing. Attention to knowledge and knowing in nursing education, while an abstract and often perplexing notion, is an important challenge to be addressed in order to ensure that students graduate with a balanced approach to professional practice.

The interface of knowledge and practice in teaching and learning determines how the cornerstone patterns of knowing are actually accounted for in the planning, implementation, and evaluation of the nursing curriculum. It is quite straightforward to acknowledge that educators need to expose students to multiple forms of knowledge and to different ways of looking at the world. It is even logical to take the view that students of nursing must gain insight, not only into the complex clinical situations they will face daily, but into their own values, beliefs, and assumptions. The challenge, however, is to create an educational environment that permits the achievement of these ends and provides a breadth of experiences, rather than simply paying token attention to the ways of knowing or providing recipelike experiences that do not promote critical thinking. Nursing education has a tradition of promoting prescriptive thinking, including the application of rules and principles to clinical situations. Attention to patterns of knowing is perhaps the vehicle for expanding practice into an evolving praxis in the promotion of student learning; and nowhere is educational praxis more evident than in the logic, cohesiveness, and scope of the curriculum development process.

Potential Tensions

The intricacy of the nursing curriculum gives rise to several challenges that are both structural and functional. One example of this is the theory/practice tension. Historically, nursing curricular and instructional design have designated specific courses or their elements as theory or practice, the former term denoting classroom-based learning, and the latter clinical learning. This dichotomy has served a somewhat administrative function, enabling educators to plan, implement, and evaluate the learning of core content separately from its application to clinical nursing practice. The split, however, has unintentionally perpetuated a schism between theory and practice, giving the illusion that they can be neatly separated when, in fact, they are intertwined. Educators must continually remind themselves that, although there may be value in separating out discrete elements of content and learning experiences, practice and theory are so intimately linked that they cannot always be neatly dissected when allocating credit values or grades, or when determining grading systems.

The flexibility (or lack thereof) of the curriculum is a second consideration as a potential tension. Curriculum development is a time-consuming and often tedious process. Once the final product has achieved departmental, institutional, and professional approval, faculty face the temptation to leave everything exactly as planned lest another revision process be deemed necessary. While this is an admirable goal—and while curricular changes should not be made capriciously or in isolation—it is nearly impossible in the current health care and educational environment to interpret the curriculum rigidly. It is important, therefore, that nursing faculty have strong mechanisms for monitoring curriculum implementation, identifying issues that arise (such as duplication and overlap of content, the need for introduction of new skills and technologies, or the need to adapt to changes in the clinical setting), and refining course content and learning experiences. Typically, a school or faculty curriculum committee would be responsible for these processes (and for parallel formative and summative evaluation of the curriculum). Student centeredness is particularly critical when considering curriculum flexibility, for student input may often give rise to the need for change, particularly at the level of instructional design.

Internal Dynamics

The structure and inner workings of the faculty or school of nursing have a tremendous impact on curriculum process. Implicit in the preceding discussion of tensions is the role that faculty engagement or disengagement with the curriculum may play. Faculty may be keen participants in all aspects of the development and evolution of the curriculum, or they may watch from afar and later deviate from the processes. Faculty involved in clinical teaching roles may not have the baseline knowledge of the curriculum structure and feel disconnected from core components of the courses in which they teach; on the other hand, faculty who are removed from clinical teaching and practice may not recognize when the curriculum is not grounded in current practice. Established processes of curriculum monitoring, review, and refinement may not include student voices as directly as they could. Communication seems to be the vital element in facilitating curriculum implementation and evolution, and faculty/school governance and administrative structures need to ensure openness, dialogue, and participation of all stakeholders.

Faculty Development

Just as forms of nursing knowledge and knowing underpin the curriculum, knowledge of perspectives, theories, and processes of teaching and learning play a critical role in curricular design and implementation. Faculty should be knowledgeable and competent practitioners of nursing, but what of their knowledge base in educational theory and practice? Teachers need to be able to ensure that their teaching practice is grounded in concepts and principles of adult learning and, in particular, student-centered approaches to education. Often faculty may be exposed to prevailing trends in education, or to current buzzwords and popular theories; they may lack the opportunity, however, to achieve a depth of knowledge in teaching/learning theory or to critically debate the merits and shortcomings of particular teaching strategies. The needs of faculty for ongoing development as teachers should be factored into departmental priorities in the same way that grant-writing skills and clinical practice development are accounted for in the school's strategic planning processes.

Critical Perspectives on Trends

Nurse educators have the dual challenge of responding to both clinical practice and educational trends. In the postsecondary environment, they are often bombarded by emerging research evidence, technological innovation, and new approaches to teaching. Educators may feel compelled to adopt every new trend in order to appear to be on the cutting edge, yet trends must be assessed and evaluated for their fit and synergy with the program philosophy and mission and with the curriculum itself. Opportunities to discuss and debate new ideas, the hallmark of the university, should be constructed and supported in order for faculty to respond to best practices while at the same time ensuring their own unique perspective on trends.

SUMMARY

Contemporary definitions of the curriculum account for the interplay of curricular elements and the teaching and learning approaches through which they are given life. They also acknowledge the characteristics of the world in which we live, where change is the norm and where the global context has primacy. Pinar, Reynolds, Slattery, and Taubman (1996) note that educators need to move from a mindset of "curriculum development" to one of "curriculum understanding" in order to embrace change and address interrelationships between discrete subjects and the larger sociopolitical context (Taubman, p. 6). Dillard and Laidig (1998) reinforce this argument and present an inclusive definition of curriculum that incorporates the following: foundations (historical, social, and political contexts), philosophy/mission, design, organizing framework(s), outcomes/competencies/objectives, educational activities, and evaluation (Dillard and Laidig, pp. 73–78). In a similar vein, McAllister (2001) interweaves curricular elements such as course design and content with student and teacher "input factors" (p. 305), environmental factors, assessment and evaluation approaches, and the learning climate. It seems that we have entered an era of nursing education where the boundaries between the blueprint and the construction of learning are less rigidly defined, providing the impetus for greater attention to diverse forms of knowledge and knowing. The current context challenges us to remain committed to an openness in curriculum and instruction, drawing on traditions that can now be refined to honor a student-centered approach.

LEARNING ACTIVITY

1. In an in-class writing exercise, students will reflect individually on their educational experiences that have and have not been student centered.
2. As a group project, examine a course outline from a nursing curriculum, compare it with the broader curricular documents, and identify the presence of various forms of knowledge and ways of knowing.
3. Students will participate in a debate considering one of the following statements:
   - Teachers should decide what knowledge students need.
   - Practice knowledge is more valuable than theoretical knowledge.
   - All faculty are responsible for the design, implementation, and evaluation of the curriculum.
   - Student centeredness is a nice-to-do rather than a need-to-do approach in nursing education.

RESOURCES FOR EDUCATORS

PLANNING THE TEACHING/LEARNING EXPERIENCE

Questions to Support a Thoughtful Reading

1. In a school/faculty of nursing, who designs curriculum? How is this decided? What does the ideal curriculum committee look like?
2. Who are the main internal and external stakeholders in the curriculum process?
3. Are we valuing and drawing on students' knowledge in the most constructive way?
4. In considering new knowledge, how do we move beyond Smythe's (2004, p. 327) question "could it be that we are merely asking nurses to unwrap prepackaged thoughts?"
5. In what ways do nurse educators use knowledge about teaching and learning processes in their everyday practice?
6. How do students learn to value all knowledge forms and ways of knowing? How does the notion of power influence this process?
7. Diversity is a term often used in referring to today's nursing student. How are curricula attending to this diversity?
8. How can quality environments be assured in the current hectic climate of nursing education?
9. Who is responsible for ensuring that educational environments are positive?
10. How is critical dialogue, a hallmark of the university, fostered in the world of nursing education today?
11. If institutions and educators value student-centered curricula, how do they build in the element of student choice (i.e., elective courses, preferred ways of learning, flexibility in full-time or part-time study)?
12. How can processes of curricular and instructional design perpetuate or resolve issues related to the theory/practice gap?

EVALUATING THE TEACHING/LEARNING EXPERIENCE

Sample Evaluation Strategies

1. Students will write a critical analysis of a course outline in the context of various knowledge forms and ways of knowing.
2. Students will engage in self and peer evaluation of the debate process outlined under the Learning Activity.

References

Beach, D. (2002). Professional knowledge and its impact on nursing practice. *Nurse Education in Practice, 2*(2), 80–86.

Beauchamp, G. A. (1975). *Curriculum theory.* (3rd ed.). Wilmette, IL: The Kagg Press.

Belenky, M. F., Clinchy, B. M., Goldberger, N. R., et al. (1986). *Women's ways of knowing.* New York: Basic Books.

Bevis, E. O. (1978). *Curriculum building in nursing: A process.* (2nd ed.). St. Louis: Mosby.

Bevis, E. O., & Watson, J. (1989). *Toward a new curriculum: A new pedagogy for nursing.* New York: National League for Nursing.

Burnard, P. (1987). Towards an epistemological basis for experiential learning in nurse education. *Journal of Advanced Nursing, 12,* 189–193.

Carlsson, G., Drew, N., Dahlberg, K., et al. (2002). Uncovering tacit knowledge. *Nursing Philosophy, 3,* 144–151.

Carper, B. A. (1978). Fundamental patterns of knowing in nursing. *Advances in Nursing Science, 1,* 13–23.

Ceci, C. (2000). Not innocent: Relationship between knowers and knowledge. *Canadian Journal of Nursing Research, 32,* 57–73.

Chinn, P. L., & Kramer, M. K. (2004). *Integrated knowledge development in nursing.* (6th ed.). New York: Mosby.

Conley, V. C. (1973). *Curriculum and instruction in nursing.* Boston: Little Brown.

Dickenson-Hazard, N. (2004). Notes from the chief executive officer: I have experienced this before. *Reflections on Nursing Leadership,* second quarter, *30*(2), 4.

Dillard, N., & Laidig, J. (1998). Curriculum development: An overview. In D. M. Billings & J. A. Halstead. *Teaching in nursing: A guide for faculty,* (pp. 69–83). Philadelphia: Saunders.

Edmond, C. (2001). A new paradigm for practice education. *Nurse Education Today, 21,* 251–259.

Eraut, M. (1994). *Developing professional knowledge and competence.* London: Falmer Press.

Freshwater, D., & Stickley, T. (2004). The heart of the art: Emotional intelligence in nurse education. *Nursing Inquiry, 11,* 91–98.

Grundy, S. (1987). *Curriculum: Product or praxis?* New York: Falmer Press.

Herbig, B., Bussing, A., & Ewert, T. (2001). The role of tacit knowledge in the work context of nursing. *Journal of Advanced Nursing, 34,* 687–695.

Iwasiw, C., Goldenberg, D., & Andrusyszyn, M. (2005). *Curriculum development in nursing education.* Toronto: Jones & Bartlett.

Johnson, J. L., & Ratner, P. A. (1997). The nature of the knowledge used in nursing practice. In S. E. Thorne & V. E. Hayes, (Eds.). *Nursing praxis: Knowledge and action,* (pp. 3–22). Thousand Oaks, CA: Sage.

Kaeding, T., & Rambur, B. (2004). Recruiting knowledge, not just nurses. *Journal of Professional Nursing, 20,* 137–138.

Keating, S. B. (2006). *Curriculum development and evaluation in nursing.* Philadelphia: Lippincott Williams & Wilkins.

Lather, P. (1991). *Getting smart.* London: Routledge.

McAllister, M. (2001). Principles for curriculum development in Australian nursing: An examination of the literature. *Nurse Education Today, 21,* 304–314.

McNeil, J. D. (1981). *Curriculum: A comprehensive introduction.* (2nd ed.). Boston: Little Brown.

Miller, J. P., & Seller, W. (1990). *Curriculum: Perspectives and practice.* Toronto: Copp Clark Pitman.

National League for Nursing. (1974). *Unifying the curriculum: The integrated approach.* New York: NLN.

Nightingale, F. (1860). *Notes on nursing: What it is, and what it is not.* New York: D. Appleton and Company. [First American Edition] Retrieved January 2005, from htttp://digital.library.upenn.edu/women/nightingale/nursing/nursing.html.

Paterson, B. (1998). Partnership in nursing education: A vision or a fantasy? *Nursing Outlook, 46*, 284–289.

Pinar, W. F., Reynolds, W. M., Slattery, P., et al. (1996). *Understanding curriculum.* New York: Peter Lang.

Polanyi, M. (1958).*Personal knowledge: Towards a post-critical philosophy*. Chicago: University of Chicago Press.

Pratt, D. D. (1998). Alternative frames of understanding: Introduction to five perspectives. In D. D. Pratt and Associates, (Eds.). *Five perspectives on teaching in adult and higher education* (pp. 33–53). Malabar, FL: Kreiger.

Rancourt, R., Guimond-Papai, P. & Prud'homme-Brisson, D. (2000). Faculty ways of knowing: The crux of nursing curricula. *Nurse Educator, 25*, 117–120.

Ruth-Sahd, L. (2003). Intuition: A critical way of knowing in a multicultural curriculum. *Nursing Education Perspectives, 24*, 129–135.

Smythe, E. (2004). Thinking. *Nurse Education Today, 24*(4), 326–332.

Taba, H. (1962). *Curriculum development: Theory and practice.* New York: Harcourt, Brace & World.

Tabak, N., Adi, L., & Eherenfeld, M. (2003). A philosophy underlying excellence in teaching. *Nursing Philosophy, 4*, 249–254.

Thorne, S. (2003). Theoretical issues in nursing. In J. R. Kerr and M. J. Wood (Eds.). Canadian nursing: Issues and perspectives (p. 116–134) 4th edition. Toronto: Mosby.

Torres, G. (1974). Educational trends and the integrated curriculum approach in nursing. In National League for Nursing, *Unifying the curriculum—The integrated approach,* (p. 1–6). New York: NLN.

Trnobranski, P. H. (1997). Power and vested interests—tacit influences on the construction of nursing curricula? *Journal of Advanced Nursing, 25*, 1084–1088.

Tyler, R. (1949). *Basic principles of curriculum and instruction.* Chicago: University of Chicago Press.

White, J. (1995). Patterns of knowing: Review, critique, and update. *Advances in Nursing Science, 17*, 73–86.

Chapter 18

Preceptorship Pathways for the Senior Undergraduate Nursing Student

Olive J. Yonge
Florence Myrick

Mary had worked for 5 years on an acute care psychiatric mental health nursing unit. She enjoyed her work, particularly the teamwork with the other health care professionals. She believed her nursing education had prepared her to begin working in this area but that her actual work experience had given her another perspective that could not be easily documented in books or articles. One day in the autumn, she was approached by her unit manager, Jolleen, who asked her if she would agree to act as a preceptor for a baccalaureate nursing student enrolled in the final year of the program. By way of background information, Jolleen told Mary that, if she agreed, the student would be scheduled to spend 10 weeks with her, working the same shifts inclusive of both night and weekend shifts. Mary's first reaction was: "No, what could I possibly teach a student?" Jolleen then gently reminded Mary that she was known as a nurse with considerable clinical expertise. Jolleen also indicated to Mary that it was not just nurses who valued her clinical competence, but other members of the health care team who validated this perception of her work weekly during multidisciplinary team meetings. Jolleen proceeded to convince Mary to assume this preceptor role by assuring her that she would not be expected to assume a management role on the unit without support. Rather, resources would be made available to support her throughout the practicum by a specifically designated faculty member, Jolleen herself, and the unit staff. Jolleen closed the discussion by cautioning Mary that being a preceptor might be stressful given the demands of teaching and the unknown abilities of the student. Mary reluctantly agreed to act as preceptor.

Prior to the commencement of the preceptorship practicum, the faculty member and later Anne, the student, contacted Mary and arranged for a coffee meeting. Following the meetings, Mary's anxieties were significantly decreased. Listening to Anne's goals for the practicum, Mary believed they could be achieved and furthermore she was looking forward to assisting Anne in becoming a beginning psychiatric mental health nurse. Anne thus began the practicum in February and by March, Mary was amazed at Anne's progress. Indeed, at the termination of the practicum, Mary was quite keen to recruit Anne as a staff member to the unit. During the practicum, Mary provided Anne with continuous feedback. Mary believed that Anne's final evaluation was merely a formality. During the documentation of the evaluation, however, Mary became aware that there were areas for further development that could be identified that would foster Anne in her development as a professional nurse. Anne appreciated

Mary's comments and the constructive manner in which the evaluation was delivered. On the final day of the practicum, Anne purchased and presented Mary with a corsage as a token of her appreciation and to recognize the work she had done and to formally display that recognition to the staff and patients. Mary agreed to serve as a reference for Anne as she embarked upon the process of job applications. The following autumn, Mary approached Jolleen, and this time Mary requested the pleasure of precepting another student. Both of them smiled at each other, remembering Mary's early reluctance.

INTENT The purpose of this chapter is to describe the pathways through which the preceptorship experience evolves. Specifically, the authors focus on the pathways related to the senior undergraduate students while recognizing the numerous other pathways that are applicable to different levels of students, other practice-oriented professionals and nursing staff who begin work in new clinical areas, and to registered nurses commencing their careers. Senior undergraduate nursing students provide a unique population because they are concerned not only with the acquisition of new skills and competencies but are also faced with the transition from the student to the professional nurse role. In this chapter, the authors address student, preceptor, and faculty preparedness; establishment of the preceptorship program in the clinical·area; facilitation of the preceptorship program; and the advantages, evaluation, and closure process involved in the preceptorship experience.

OVERVIEW

INTRODUCTION

In Canadian faculties and schools of nursing, **preceptorship** has become the leading method of choice for teaching and learning in almost all final years of the undergraduate curricula and is also increasingly becoming prevalent in graduate curricula as well (Goldenberg, Iwasiw, & MacMaster, 1997). Preceptorship is an arrangement in which a registered nurse or other health professional designated as **preceptor** is paired with an undergraduate in the final year of their educational program, or a graduate nursing student, called a **preceptee**, in the practice area for the purpose of role socialization and teaching. An alternative model, one that has been traditionally used in nursing education at all levels of teaching/instruction, is designed to assign a small group of students to a **faculty member** who assumes full responsibility for their clinical supervision. The size of these clinical groups can vary from 8 to 12 students. The preceptorship model was developed to address some of the perceived weaknesses of the traditional model of clinical supervision. Nurse educators came to recognize that students would benefit immeasurably from one-to-one teaching by a registered nurse in the practice environment. This particular kind of arrangement not only would allow students to be exposed to nurses with specific clinical expertise, but would also provide them with the opportunity to work the exact shifts of the nurses (preceptors) with whom they were paired, an arrangement that has not been previously an option in the faculty supervision model. From an organizational perspective then, the preceptorship model had the advantage of providing access to clinical and community settings that could only accommodate one or two students, or those that were located at a distance from the educational institution. Students, too, believed they could gain more competencies and skills in a preceptorship experience than in a traditional kind of clinical experience (Myrick, 1988). Because of the nature of the preceptorship experience—a one-to-one student/preceptor relationship, there was the assumption that students would not be competing for the attention of their preceptor with other students. In the more traditional clinical teaching model, 8 to 12 students would inevitably be required to rely on one instructor to assist them in developing their competencies and facilitate them through the teaching learning process. The faculty to student ratios allowed "little time for in-depth teaching– with each student individually, whereas preceptors are able to guide the student in the context of the one-to-one relationship" (Byrd, Hood, & Youtsey, 1997, p. 344). In the preceptorship model then, the one-to-one relationship came to be seen as offering the best possible arrangement in that it afforded students the preceptor's undivided and individualized attention. In turn that relationship could allow the students to capitalize on and maximize both the quantity and the quality of the experiences to which they would encounter.

STUDENT PREPAREDNESS

Throughout their nursing program students are systematically prepared for the preceptorship experience through clinical, laboratory, and classroom teaching. Typically, preceptorship is viewed as a capping project or practicum whereby the knowledge that the students have acquired throughout their program is integrated through practice and related scholarly work. By completion of the practicum, students are expected to perform for a sustained period of time at the level of a registered nurse. In fact, during the last third of their practicum, students may often function as staff members (Myrick & Yonge, 2004). This occurrence is rarely addressed overtly, but the authors would suggest it is a practice that, while discouraged, continues to transpire more frequently than is desired.

Not surprisingly, all students are not psychologically or even cognitively prepared for a preceptorship practicum. Recognizing the challenges of preceptorship, educators therefore assess student knowledge levels and preparation for the experience prior to its commencement. Typically, it is the responsibility of faculty members to assume a leadership role in organizing clinical skills' training. Faculty members must ensure that the curriculum is designed to adequately prepare students for their preceptee role. McGregor (1999) describes one instance in which students are required to register in courses such as pathophysiology, introductory nursing science, advanced technological skills, and managerial processes in nursing prior to beginning a preceptorship experience. Ensuring that students have mastered the course material provides them with the essential skills to be preceptored. The technical skills that may be mastered in support of assuming a preceptee role include: knowing advanced wound care, performing venipuncture, monitoring and interpreting electrocardiograms, and conducting cardiopulmonary resuscitation (CPR). After recognizing that her students were inadequately prepared to be preceptees, Souers (2002) developed a comprehensive performance review composed of a test situation of scenarios. Each scenario incorporated various teaching strategies such as interaction, computer programming, or case studies. Students were required to complete each scenario with their work subsequently evaluated as either a pass or redo. If students were required to redo a scenario, they were asked to work on a similar, but not identical, scenario. Prior to the preceptorship experience, each student was then required to complete ten scenarios over 2 days.

Students may be preceptored in any agency and even in international settings. Each setting reflects unique challenges for the student and faculty member alike. For example, if the setting for the preceptorship experience is home health care, the unstructured nature must be addressed by the student and preceptor (Neal, 1999). Thus prior to a placement in the practice setting, students can be prepared by role playing, engaging in critical thinking exercises, and working through practice scenarios.

While not frequently alluded to, there are also legal risks inherent in the preceptorship experience (Phillips, 2002). Both students and preceptors are held accountable for competent care. Such care requires knowledge and awareness of the ethical, legal, and professional responsibilities related to nursing practice. One of the first responsibilities that preceptees must assume is to become familiar with the agency's policy and procedure manual, with a particular focus on those policies that apply to their specific area of practice. If, however, the agency does not provide such policies, then decisions out of the ordinary must be made in consultation with the preceptor, agency administrator, and faculty supervisor.

One specific example related to the legal complexities of the preceptorship experience occurred during a student's northern nursing preceptorship placement. In this particular instance, the agency in which the placement occurred routinely used a small airplane when flying staff to conduct a weekly clinic in a remote settlement. The small aircraft accommodated four people: the pilot, physician, nurse, and in this case, the nursing student. At the time, it was determined that while this experience was not essential to the student/preceptee's learning, it would inevitably add to the richness of the student's knowledge about nursing in the north. The risk was judged to be minimal because the plane that would be transporting the student was perceived to be a typical mode of transportation even though the landing strip to which it had access was not a regular landing strip but rather a pasture. The pilot noted unequivocally that this particular unusual landing space was not an obstacle to landing. There were, however, no policies or procedures for nursing students in this agency pertaining to flying in an aircraft, nor would there likely be such documents developed in the future. The sponsoring agency was a mission hospital with scarce resources for developing such policies. Finally, the preceptor was informed that, should the student accompany him, he would be responsible for her nursing actions in that she would be seen to be practicing within the parameters of his license. Following an in-depth discussion with regard to these legal matters, the preceptor decided that he would support the student's learning experience. The student thus flew north with her preceptor and became a participant in an experience specific to rural and remote nursing. This nursing experience proved to be invaluable for the student. Through this exposure, she acquired a deeper understanding of the connection between access to health care and geography. As well, the student learned that some community members "saved up" their health care concerns for the "airplane professionals." Being witness to the effects of such relational patterns in this remote setting, she gained a greater appreciation for the importance of responding to and treating symptoms prior to a progression of symptoms leading to a severe illness. Students need to be prepared especially for the preceptorship approach to clinical teaching (Yonge, 1997). They need to be provided with specific content such as how to be a preceptee, how to contend with conflict effectively, and how to manage stress and even loneliness. Trevitt, Grealish, and Reaby (2001) developed a self-paced student module and an accompanying video to prepare students for the preceptorship experience. Consequently, one of the outcomes for the students was that the module was found to assist them in becoming aware of best approaches to preceptors as well as best strategies for eliciting constructive feedback from them. The evaluation of the module itself, however, indicated that the time required to review the materials contributed to student workload.

PRECEPTOR PREPAREDNESS

In an ideal world, all registered nurses with a particular number of years of experience would be eligible to assume the preceptor role. Regardless of that experience, however, some nurses are better prepared and better suited to be a preceptor owing to their own clinical and educational experiences such as having had a positive preceptorship experience when they were a student or a new nurse in an health care agency; enjoyed the patient teaching role; or worked in a clinical area that promoted education such as a school nurse. Some nurses have self-developed goals that include teaching and mentoring of others, while others believe preceptoring to be an intrinsic part of their professional responsibility.

The actual selection and recruitment of the nurse for the preceptor role is frequently based on the leadership style of the unit manager or administrator of the agency. While some negotiate with nurses, others assign preceptorship experiences. Depending on the method of selection used, a preceptor may or may not welcome the opportunity to precept. Freidburger (2001) described a program in which nurses must meet specific requirements such as participating in meetings, providing student feedback, and contacting faculty prior to assuming the preceptor role.

Preceptorship cannot be founded on the "warm body" syndrome, in which any nurse who is available will be sufficient as preceptor. Indeed, Andrews and Chilton (2000) found that, although preceptors felt inadequate in their role, they were often unwillingly assigned to the role by their superiors. Birx and Baldwin (2002) revealed that the majority of preceptors learn on the job, thus rendering preparation for the role highly variable. Preceptorship is a powerful relationship that directly impacts the student, preceptor, agency, and patient (Myrick & Yonge, 2003). In other words, it cannot nor should it be left to chance.

FACULTY PREPAREDNESS

While faculty prepare students and preceptors for their role, faculty themselves require preparation. Typically, faculty lecture, facilitate seminars, and teach in the clinical areas. They are, however, not often afforded the opportunity to precept a student in a formalized preceptorship relationship. Yonge, Myrick, Ferguson, and Haase (2003) using telephone semistructured interviews, questioned eight faculty members as to their preparation for the faculty role in a preceptorship course. The faculty participants taught in a fourth-year baccalaureate preceptorship course and were assigned up to 24 students each. Through a content analysis of the transcribed data, the researchers found that, if faculty stated they were prepared, it was usually because of their own development through reading, researching, attending presentations, past preceptor experience, faculty consultation, and as a result of their familiarity with the preceptorship teaching structures. Faculty who perceived they lacked preparation indicated that they had not been provided with background information about the preceptor or agency in a timely manner, were unaware of student expectations, and received no course orientation or directions as to how to evaluate the students. The findings of this study were limited owing to the small sample size and the collection of data from one institution. Ferguson (1996), in a qualitative study of 30 preceptors working in five clinical agencies, not surprisingly found that faculty are vital to the preparation of preceptors for their role. Faculty members are instrumental in providing information to preceptors about the principles of teaching and learning, offering ongoing support, and managing conflicts as they arise. In addition to being accessible, faculty need to provide relevant information to preceptors about program goals and objectives, serve as a resource regarding the teaching/learning process, assist the preceptor in evaluating the student, and actually mentor the preceptor throughout the experience (Ferguson, 1996). Beeman (2001), describing how she organized a preceptorship program for seven junior nursing students, echoes Ferguson's observations and advocates the need for faculty to be easily available to the preceptor. For Beeman, this availability included lunch meetings with the student and preceptor. Having lunch away from the clinical area allows for uninterrupted time to discuss relevant issues related to the preceptorship experience.

INSTITUTION OF THE PRECEPTORSHIP EXPERIENCE ON SITE

Prior to commencement of the preceptorship experience, students must acquaint themselves with their preceptor, agency, and location. Within that context, they are expected to develop personal learning objectives congruent with course objectives. By way of introduction, students may forward their photograph to the preceptor, together with a letter of intention and introduction, resume, and/or curriculum vitae. As previously alluded to, a student in a preceptorship practicum must abide by the legal and ethical requirements of professional practice of the jurisdiction as well as the policies and procedures of the agency to which they are assigned. Some agencies require that students devote a full day or multiple days to orientation prior to their beginning in the clinical area. During this time, students can not only become familiar with the physical setup and resources available in the agency, but also review its policies and usual practices.

Faculty typically begin the orientation process by contacting the preceptor and providing written material such as a course outline, a preceptor manual, and an itemized list of skills the student has either mastered or has yet to master. In some cases, students may provide the preceptor with the list of skills that they generate as they progress through the program. This list is called the practice portfolio. As well, the faculty may also provide the preceptor with student-generated learning objectives and expectations. Ideally, the faculty member meets one on one with preceptors to provide them with relevant information and to address any questions they may have with regard to the preceptorship experience. Because students may be preceptored in any location in the world, however, the meeting between the faculty member and the preceptor may take the form of a telephone call or a videoconference. The prudent faculty member also involves the unit manager or administrator in the orientation process. Subsequently, the preceptorship experience does not occur in isolation but is part of a web of relations among students, faculty at their home institution, and designated agency personnel. The more agency personnel who are informed about the expectations of the preceptor and student, the more likely the preceptor will receive the support required for a successful experience (Myrick & Yonge, 2003).

Students drive the preceptorship experience. Prior to arriving in the clinical area usually they have carefully assessed the quality, type, and kind of experience in which they would like to engage. To that end, they have thus selected a preceptorship experience in a particular clinical site, in consultation with faculty, and one that is derived from their self-identified areas for developing nursing competencies congruent with their career plans and personal interests. While there are course objectives to meet, students formulate, and reformulate in an ongoing manner, personal objectives as they progress through the practicum. Since the clinical area is dynamic and everchanging, they must continuously seek out different learning experiences, identify teaching resources, and manage the tension of being the only learner assigned to one teacher. In our experience, students often indicate they miss the support of a clinical group.

The preceptorship experience is not, however, only student driven but it is also student centered. This factor is especially evident in international placements. While students may be viewed frequently as strangers because of their appearance and manner of dress, they are generally treated with respect and regarded with intense interest. For example, preceptors welcome students into their agencies and even into their homes. It is also, however, a student-centered experience even if the student does not leave the country. Regardless of the location, students must assume responsibility for daily evaluations and assessments. While faculty may visit an agency to determine how the experience is progressing (unless they are there every day), they cannot fully assess either the student's progress or at time regress. Students may keep logs. Some will cojournal with their preceptors. Yet others may journal solely for the instructor, all as a means by which to assess their learning. Students may request daily or weekly meetings with their preceptor to review the attainment of objectives and to seek input to guide their development of new objectives. Within the context of student centeredness, a question often posed is related to student readiness or more specifically, "When is the student ready to fully capitalize on a preceptored practicum?" It is not sufficient that faculty recognize student capability, readiness or lack thereof. Students must be able to identify exactly what it is they need to achieve to become beginning competent practitioners since preceptorship experiences are often offered at the end of a nursing program when students begin to view themselves in the role of the registered nurse. This, too, is the time they still carry the student label and are able to ask questions as a student–learner. Preceptorship is used primarily in the final clinical practicum as a bridge between the completion of the nursing program and the commencement of professional nursing practice. Thus, if a student is unable to assume the role of preceptee then it becomes questionable as to their readiness for professional practice at that particular point in time. Journaling, focused preceptor-student meetings, and self-evaluations serve to contribute to the notion of student centeredness in that they afford students the opportunity to critically reflect on their performance and encourage them to question their own assumptions and readiness for professional nursing practice. Intrinsic to that critical reflection is their foundation of nursing knowledge which fosters in them the ability to be able to know what they do know and equally importantly generates a desire to know what they do not know.

Faculty also need to orient themselves to this method of teaching. They need to develop tools and resources to monitor student and preceptor nursing shifts, activities, and expectations regarding the roles and responsibilities of student, preceptor, and faculty. Potentially it is not uncommon for faculty in one course to be assigned to up to 24 students, and more preceptors since students may be paired with more than one preceptor. The actual teaching assignment could thus consist of over 48 students and preceptors at any given time. Owing to the fact that student and preceptor dyads work different schedules, it becomes a significant organizational challenge for faculty to keep abreast of these numbers and to contact the dyads in a timely manner. The use of technology in the form of e-mail, although not always reliable, has made it somewhat easier to contact preceptors and students. If students are assigned international placements, they are asked to obtain free e-mail addresses in public servers, which are accessible anywhere in the world. Worthy of note here is the recognition that it is not uncommon for faculty to experience teacher withdrawal as they observe the student now directly being taught by a preceptor. In other words, relinquishing their primary teaching responsibility to a preceptor can engender anxiety in some faculty as their role as teacher becomes increasingly more peripheral to the teaching/learning experience. Faculty thus need to be clear as to their newly designated role with the acknowledgement that while the teaching/learning experience is a shared responsibility among the student, preceptor, and faculty, the first line of teaching and learning is now situated within the context of the preceptor/preceptee relationship.

FACILITATION OF THE PRECEPTORSHIP PROGRAM

Once the preceptor, student, and faculty are prepared and oriented for their particular roles within the preceptorship experience, the actual preceptoring begins. The advantages of preceptorship include recruitment of students to the agency; acceptance of students as a valued member of the health care team; development of critical thinking (as students ask questions and offer new perspectives); and the evolution of some preceptorships into long-term mentoring relationships. Patients, too, benefit from being the recipients of care by the preceptor and student. In fact, during the last third of the preceptorship program, it is not unusual for preceptors to discover that they have extra time. Such time allows them to work on creative projects, review and revise policies and/or teaching tools, a development related to the ability of their students to assume part of the preceptor's patient assignment.

Occasionally, however, the preceptor can be confronted with issues or challenges pertaining to the experience. One particular challenge that can arise is an inadequately prepared or unmotivated student. Lack of motivation can emanate from illness, fatigue, cognitive dissonance about nursing as a career choice, dislike of the preceptor and/or clinical area, student arrogance about their nursing knowledge, or a struggle with disillusionment. To illustrate the latter, in one particular instance a student was noted to bitterly complain because her placement was not what she expected or requested, and her subsequent placement in the clinical area made her bored and listless.

While the preceptorship practicum typically occurs at the completion of the fourth year of a nursing program, the assumption cannot be made that the student is necessarily ready to be preceptored. Some students may be assigned to locations that are geographically distant from family or friends and are surprised and dismayed at the loneliness they experience. Sometimes, such a situation can become more stressful for the student than anticipated. Equally, prior to the practicum, the faculty and student may judge that the student is ready for practice in such a location but when confronted with the actual demands of the situation both realize that such an assignment was a misjudgment. There are also situations that arise in which students may not be equipped to perform in a manner conducive to the preceptorship experience. Throughout their program such students may have had poor grades, high absentee rates, and attitude issues. Despite the fact that these students may have been perceived to have met the minimum requirements for successful passing in each course, in the preceptorship, our experience would suggest that such students can quickly reveal a lack of commitment that cannot sustain them through the rigors of clinical practice. This particular situation can become untenable for the student, preceptor, faculty, and even the staff on the unit in which the preceptorship is taking place.

The preceptorship experience and the teaching/learning process entailed therein may be accurately perceived as additional responsibility for the preceptor. In other words, teaching students is not their primary role. It would be accurate to say that a student who lacks motivation presents a complex challenge even for a gifted clinical instructor much less for a preceptor. Of particular concern are those students who can be arrogant or overly self-confident. These students too quickly reveal their values in the practice environment. They can be difficult to trust and prove to be irritating in the work situation. As with the student who lacks motivation, the overly confident student requires complex interventions.

A major issue that can often occur as well is the nurses, on the other hand, who may not wish to assume the preceptor role (Myrick & Barrett, 1992). Such nurses may be distracted by personal issues or feel coerced into the preceptor role. They may be experiencing burnout or feel inadequate to assume the role. Some preceptors present as overbearing and intimidated by the responsibility of teaching a student. Others may perceive that because the student is practicing under their professional license, they must constantly monitor the student's behaviors. Such perceptions can result in a strained relationship between the student and preceptor and in turn, adversely affect other members of the health team. If, however, a student is found to actually engage in unethical or illegal behavior it may be difficult for the preceptor to confront the student despite the fact that the situation warrants immediate intervention. Occasionally, faculty may be perceived to be remote, inaccessible, disorganized, or even disconnected from the preceptee/preceptor relationship. Some preceptor/preceptee dyads may perceive that a faculty member induces stress when visiting the dyad. Faculty, on the other hand, can sometimes offer critique of the nursing care provided by the preceptor and the student that is perceived as being less than constructive (Corlett, 2000).

The preceptor/preceptee relationship most frequently necessitates a shadowing of the preceptor by the student particularly in the initial phases of the experience. There are, however, those preceptors who view this dimension as an intrusion by the student into their space. Consequently, to create a greater comfort level for themselves, preceptors may resort to assigning students in such a manner that can leave them feeling neglected and abandoned.

Of concern for students also is the realization that there exists on the unit in which their preceptorship experience is occurring a subculture that frequently involves the rumor mill and occasional negative interactions among the staff. Typically students in traditional practica are not privy to the social interactions among staff. Students thus may find such dynamics distressing, particularly as they are becoming socialized to the nursing profession. It is not unusual, therefore, for students to report to faculty that they have been exposed to gossip among staff and question, "If there is gossip about others, is there then gossip about us as well?"

ADVANTAGES OF PRECEPTORSHIP

For the most part, the majority of students and preceptors experience their preceptorship as a privilege that is often life changing. As a result of the experience, preceptors are frequently afforded workload relief, the opportunity to develop new skills in the area of teaching and learning, rewards for their efforts, and the good fortune to develop a mentorship relationship with the student. Many nurses feel privileged to be able to participate in a mutually beneficial professional relationship such as preceptorship. The preceptors' contributions are valued not only by management but also by other nurses and health professionals. Indeed, it is not uncommon for preceptors to report that they learn more from the students than the students learn from them; such a statement reflects the high regard preceptors hold for students.

Students view their preceptorships as extremely positive experiences and many remark it as the highlight of their nursing program. Through it they acquire independence, come to understand the rhythms of shift work, learn how to interact and thrive as members of a health care team, and begin to imagine a future as a registered nurse. Subsequently, it is not unusual for students to give gifts of chocolates or flowers to the agency staff and a special, individual-oriented gift to their preceptor. These gifts are reflective of the students' gratitude to the preceptor and to the agency for enhancing and promoting their development as a nurse.

One of the most long lasting and significant advantages of the preceptorship experience with regard to preceptors is their development in the teaching role. Specifically, preceptors use various teaching/learning behaviors on a routine basis. Depending on their teaching style and the learning style of the student, they may quickly explain how they would carry out a procedure and then carefully illustrate it for students who may be a visual learner. They may then require the student to repeat the procedure while observing; expecting the student to then complete the procedure. Other students may be more comfortable with verbal descriptions. These students are auditory learners and thus may require more time in this phase. Yet others, kinesthetic learners, may prefer the preceptor to be succinct in their description allowing them instead to carry out the procedure as opposed to observing or reading about it (Myrick & Yonge, 2004).

As part of their teaching as well, preceptors continuously model professional behaviors, critical thinking skills, and nursing competencies (Myrick & Yonge, 2001). Their actions directly impact the student's behaviors. For example, one student reported the following scenario exemplifying how her preceptor assumed the role of head triage nurse in emergency. The relative of a potential patient repeatedly expressed to the preceptor that things were moving too slowly. The preceptor acknowledged this person's feelings and explained the process of triaging. The student was impressed with the preceptor's patience and respect for this person especially when such respect was not reciprocated by the patient. Another approach preceptors may use in teaching is to allow the student to choose any method to complete a nursing intervention with a caveat that they give a rationale as to why and what they are doing. Preceptors may use scenarios as a way to work with students around "what if" questions. Such questioning not only provides a way to guide students in important unit issues, for example, how to contend with a patient whose airway is obstructed, but also serves as a means by which to assess the student's critical thinking abilities. Depending on the resources available on the unit, students may be expected to review videos, or familiarize themselves with articles, or Web-based standards of care for certain interventions such as pain management or bladder irrigation prior to their actual participation.

THE EVALUATION TRAJECTORY

Evaluation is an extremely complex skill that requires numerous data sources based on learning objectives, faculty, student, and preceptor expectations, as well as available resources. Also, there are always gradients within the evaluation process whereby students may perform a nursing intervention with confidence but may forget a part of the intervention. A classic example is the situation in which a student proceeds to change a patient's dressing but neglects to interact with the patient. The preceptor thus cannot rate the student's change of dressing skill as outstanding, even though the technical component of the procedure may have been completed at a high level of competency for the assigned clinical area.

Intrinsic to the evaluation process are evaluation forms which also provide special challenges. Preceptors may state that the forms are not always relevant to their specific agency. Usually the faculty/school of nursing uses the same form for all students regardless of the location of the clinical area. Enterprising preceptors will use the education-generated form and create another form specific to their clinical area. Preceptors believe the evaluation form should be brief and highly specific to their practice.

Students want and need a positive evaluation from their preceptor. Given that a preceptorship experience is usually at the completion of the program, they believe they should be functioning at an extremely high level. If the preceptor's evaluation is perceived by the student as unwarranted, the student may in turn question the preceptor's ability to evaluate a student. While there are times when there may be some merit to this perception since evaluation is a complex and time-consuming activity, for the most part, preceptors are not educated as to how to engage in the evaluation process including completion of the form. More specifically, they rarely have time or the luxury to engage in orientation to the evaluation process. Others on the health care team need to support the preceptor by assisting with the workload thus affording preceptors more time to learn the evaluation process.

Faculty play a pivotal role in the overall evaluation process. It is they who introduce the evaluation process to the preceptors at the commencement of the practicum. Because the course and the related learning objectives are the cornerstone of a student evaluation in the preceptorship model, each objective that is written by a student must undergo a process of discussion and dialogue to ensure its accuracy and relevance. If it is found that a student quickly and easily meets self-identified learning objectives, it may be that the objectives are written too simplistically or are at a level that does not necessarily reflect the students' potential level of achievement. Additional objectives will then be formulated to guide the practice experience. It is the role of faculty, therefore, to meet with the preceptor on a regular basis and at each meeting, address how the students' objectives are being met.

Each preceptor may use the written objectives differently. For example, in one situation, a preceptor literally carried the objectives in her uniform pocket and checked with the student at the completion of every shift to determine progress. Another kept a journal. On one side of the page she recorded the student's behavior while on the other side of the page she entered the corresponding objectives. If the journal entry confirmed the student had met the objective, the preceptor marked the objective with a check. If the student continued to meet the objective, the preceptor did not record this. She was not concerned with the frequency of behavior, simply whether the behavior had ever occurred. Another preceptor kept the course syllabus outlining the objectives in her work mailbox and checked them every week to determine how the student was progressing.

Part of the evaluation also involves the completion of a baseline assessment of the student. Preceptors achieve this assessment primarily through their questioning of the student, observations, acquisition of information about the student from other team members, and formulation of a plan. Preceptors and students' expectations must be explicitly stated and explored. Preceptors will often take time away from the agency to meet with the student and work through both of their expectations thus ensuring congruent communication.

The evaluation process is formalized through the final written evaluation using an evaluation form. The process of evaluation is, however, threaded throughout the practicum. This process is embedded in the giving and receiving of feedback. The preceptor and student need to decide how, when, and where to give feedback. Students expect feedback; they are learners and will make mistakes. They want to enhance their nursing abilities. They also want to be acknowledged for their efforts. When students are preceptored for the first time, they may miss being taught by a clinical professor who is accustomed to giving constructive and frequent feedback. Part of the preparation for the preceptor and the student, therefore, are sessions regarding the giving and receiving of feedback. A typical strategy that is taught is called perception checking. To illustrate, the preceptor may state a perception such as, "I noticed that when Ms. Smith started to complain about her diabetic diet, you stayed silent." This is then followed with a check on the perception, "Did you not know what to say to her?" This strategy allows students to describe their perceptions of an interaction without being defensive.

The purpose of giving feedback is to generate a change in behavior. Students are thus required to integrate the feedback into their practice. If after repeated feedback, there is no change of behavior on the part of the student, the preceptor begins to question the teaching/learning relationship. At such a time, preceptors are well advised to seek input from their peers and faculty. A special meeting may need to be arranged with the student, faculty, and preceptor to discuss the student's and preceptor's perceptions of how the feedback was given and received.

Frequently, preceptors will indicate their lack of skills or disinterest in evaluating students. They may not have time to write anecdotes about the student performance preferring instead to use a quick checklist. If a student is not progressing well in the practicum and appears not to be responding to the feedback, the preceptor may feel frustrated by the demands of evaluation and possibly recommend failure. A failure could lead to an appeal process that would inevitably involve the preceptor, an involvement that may be perceived as an unfair expectation.

Regardless of the various issues arising, the majority of nurses when asked to assume the preceptor role again usually respond in the affirmative noting that benefits vastly outweigh disadvantages. The majority of preceptors tend to write positive student evaluations and although they state they would prefer a checklist, they write meaningful and insightful student-centered narratives. Indeed, preceptors display a level of diligence and conscientiousness when evaluating students reflective of their ongoing commitment to professional nursing practice.

THE PROCESS OF CLOSURE

As students complete the required number of hours for their practicum, both they and their preceptors begin to engage in "termination rituals." Preceptors inquire as to where students will be seeking employment and frequently offer them advice and tips on how to apply for a position. Preceptors may engage the preceptee in a practice job interview. If their agency is hiring staff, preceptors and students will often seek out more information about the job posting. Administrators look kindly upon hiring students precepted in the agency, particularly if they have demonstrated success while acquiring a sense of the context of the work environment. In fact, some specialty areas, such as the operating room or neonatal intensive care, participate in preceptorship programs for the express purpose of recruiting students as potential staff.

Students, when nearing the completion of the preceptorship practicum, frequently become quite anxious about relinquishing the student role. They question whether they are ready to assume the role of the registered nurse. This anxiety is coupled with their apprehension about writing their imminent national examinations. If they also have financial concerns, many will apply for jobs while studying for the national examinations and completing the practicum. All these factors are expressed in student fatigue. It is often the preceptor to whom the students will inevitably turn for support and reassurance that they can indeed be successful.

Preceptors are thus most supportive of the student at the completion of the practicum, particularly those who relate readily to the student experience. It is that preceptor support that resonates profoundly for the student at this juncture in their nursing career. As previously discussed, nursing students acknowledge the contribution of the preceptor in the form of a gift, but interestingly, preceptors too will often give a small gift to their students. They will either treat the student to lunch or dinner, offer to write a letter of reference, or sometimes give a personal gift such as a book or pen. They want to say good-bye to the student and to acknowledge what the relationship has meant to them.

SUMMARY

When exploring preceptorship pathways, many issues can arise throughout the course of the experience that either contribute to its success or impede its progress. Being aware of these issues is critical. Indeed, such awareness allows for anticipatory planning that can assist all players to effectively and efficiently resolve any issues that may arise. Faculty are in a position to act as an ongoing resource to the student and preceptor. A keen understanding of the nature of preceptorship and its pathways affords the faculty, students, and preceptors the potential for ensuring a rewarding experience. Strengths can be maximized, conflicts resolved, and relationships empowered because of the confidence that such understanding engenders. Through discussion and insight into these pathways, faculty, students, and preceptors can more readily work together in a true spirit of collegiality. Ultimately that spirit benefits not only the individual players themselves, but on a more macro level it also influences the ongoing relationship between those in the educational and practice environments which in turn can serve to invigorate the nursing profession in general.

LEARNING ACTIVITY

EXPLORING WAYS OF THINKING AS A PRECEPTOR BY USING DE BONO'S SIX THINKING HATS

Robin M. Scobie, RN, MScN

Context: This learning activity is designed to be used with a group of preceptors as part of a preceptor workshop. It is my belief that every preceptor wants each student they work with to be successful. But what does the preceptor do when there are feelings of anxiety or distress about a student? How can the preceptor explore different ways of finding new perspectives on the situation? I suggest this learning activity might be one way to explore different ways of thinking about a challenging student situation.

Edward de Bono developed a "game of thinking" (1985, p. 30). He uses six thinking hats, each of which has a color related to its function. I have listed the reference at the end of this learning activity and I suggest it would be most useful if the facilitator for this activity read the book to gain further understanding about the different colored hats. There is also an interesting De Bono Web site: http://www.innovatraining.com/meeting-mgmt.htm.

A brief summary of the thinking of each of the six hats is listed below, taken directly from De Bono's book *Six Thinking Hats.* As you read each of these descriptions think about how preceptors will use that specific lens for exploring different practice situations that may arise with students.

White Hat. White is neutral and objective. The white hat is concerned with objective facts and figures.

Red Hat. Red suggests anger (seeing red), rage, and emotions. The red hat gives the emotional view.

Black Hat. Black is gloomy and negative. The black hat covers the negative aspects—why it cannot be done.

Yellow Hat. Yellow is sunny and positive. The yellow hat is optimistic and covers hope and positive thinking.

Green Hat. Green is grass, vegetation, and abundant, fertile growth. The green hat indicates creativity and new ideas.

Blue Hat. Blue is cool, and it is also the color of the sky, which is above everything else. The blue hat is concerned with control and organization of the thinking process.

de Bono suggests each person is usually more comfortable with one type of thinking than another. By having preceptors experiment with a new hat, a new way of thinking, they may see the situation with the student in a new light, using new roles and thus new ways of knowing.

For those who have been preceptors already, they may have a story to share of a challenging situation with a student. The facilitator may wish to use one of these stories as the case scenario. Otherwise please use the following case scenario:

- Divide participants into six groups with no more than five to six people per group.
- Have each group take *one* colored hat.
- Read the case scenario aloud. Give each group their own copy with identifying characteristics about their own colored hat listed.

Case scenario: *You have spent 3 weeks working with Janet on an acute medical unit. Despite your ongoing feedback, she is having persistent problems organizing and prioritizing her care. For instance, she is not sure which of her patients to assess first at the beginning of shift. Furthermore, she seems to be unsure of the significance of many of the medications that she is administering.* (With thanks to Patricia Rodney, RN, PhD, for permission to use this scenario.)

1. Instruct participants to make a list of the issues this case scenario raises for each of them. Have each person offer their own views, then discuss issues arising within the group but *only* from the thinking perspective of the group's specific colored hat. Write the main points of the discussion on a flip chart. Note that only the person wearing the hat can speak so please take turns wearing a hat.
2. In each group, choose one reporter to wear the group hat while presenting ideas, perspectives, and questions evident in your group's discussion; that is, *your group's thinking*, to the large group. In discussion, the large group will respond to your group's report on how a preceptor with your particular thinking hat on might approach this situation with Janet.
3. Summarize the discussion with a view to exploring new ideas that arose from the whole group. Then, lead a discussion designed to envision a new plan of approach with Janet based on newfound awareness and ideas.
4. Evaluate how this activity worked for the preceptors in the room. Did they gain new awareness? Do they feel this might be a useful approach when they next have a challenging issue with a student?

Source: de Bono, E. (1985). *Six thinking hats*. Markham, ON: Penguin Books Canada Ltd.

RESOURCES FOR EDUCATORS

PLANNING THE TEACHING/LEARNING EXPERIENCE

Questions to Support a Thoughtful Reading

1. What are the best methods to prepare students, preceptors, faculty, and the agency for the preceptorship experience?
2. What would an ideal preceptorship experience be like?
3. How will the preceptor orient, guide, coach, teach, and then evaluate the student?
4. Describe the roles of the preceptee, faculty, preceptor, and agency staff.
5. If a student is not progressing, what might explain this behavior?
6. What needs to be considered when evaluating preceptees?

EVALUATING THE TEACHING/LEARNING EXPERIENCE

Questions to Elicit Feedback from Students on Their Learning

1. Compared to other clinical practica, how was the preceptored practicum different and similar?
2. What was it like to have a one-to-one relationship with a preceptor?
3. As a result of this experience, will you volunteer to be a preceptor?

Reflective Questions for the Educator

1. Before a placement is chosen, ask why this placement for this student?
2. What stress is inherent in this type of program for preceptees, preceptors, faculty, and agency personnel?
3. What is the most effective way of acknowledging preceptors? Should preceptors be given academic credit? How can this type of teaching be sustained?

References

Andrews, M., & Chilton, F. (2000). Student and mentor perceptions of mentoring effectiveness. *Nurse Education Today*, *20*(7), 555–562.

Beeman, R. Y. (2001). Educational innovations. New partnerships between education and practice: Precepting junior nurses in the acute care setting. *Journal of Nursing Education*, *40*(3), 132–134.

Birx, E., & Baldwin, S. (2002). Nursing staff-student relationships. *Journal of Nursing Education*, *41*(2), 86–88.

de Bono, E. (1985), *Six Thinking Hats*, Markham, ON: Penguin Book, Canada, Ltd.

Byrd, C. Y., Hood, L., & Youtsey, N. (1997). Student and preceptor perceptions of factors in a successful learning partnership. *Journal of Professional Nursing, 13*(6), 344–351.

Corlett, J. (2000). The perceptions of nurse teachers, student nurses and preceptors of the theory-practice gap in nurse education. *Nurse Education Today, 20*(6), 499–505.

Ferguson, L. (1996). Preceptors' needs for faculty support. *Journal of Nursing Staff Development, 12*(2), 73–80.

Freidburger, O. A. (2001). A tribute to clinical preceptors: Developing a preceptor program for nursing students. *Journal for Nurses in Staff Development*, *17*(6), 320–327.

Goldenberg, D., Iwasiw, C., & MacMaster, E. (1997). Self-efficacy of senior baccalaureate nursing students and preceptors. *Nurse Education Today*, *17*(4), 303–310.

McGregor, R. (1999). A precepted experience for senior nursing students. *Nurse Educator, 24*(3):13–16.

Myrick, F. (1988). Preceptorship: A viable alternative clinical teaching strategy? *Journal of Advanced Nursing, 13*(5): 588–591.

Myrick, F., & Barrett, C. (1992). Preceptor selection criteria in Canadian basic baccalaureate schools of nursing: A survey. *Canadian Journal of Nursing Research, 24*(3), 53–68.

Myrick, F., & Yonge, O. (2001). Creating a climate for critical thinking in the preceptorship experience. *Nurse Education Today, 21*(6): 461–467.

Myrick, F., & Yonge, O. (2003). Preceptorship: A quintessential component of nursing education. In M. H. Oermann & K. T. Heinrich, (Eds.). *Annual Review of Nursing Education* (Vol. 1, pp. 91–107). New York: Springer.

Myrick, F., & Yonge, O. (2005). *Nursing preceptorship: Connecting practice and education.* New York: Lippincott Williams & Wilkins.

Neal, L. J. (1999). Teaching strategies. Preparing students to practice in the home. *Nurse Educator, 24*(3), 13–16.

Phillips, E. (2002). On the job: Legal matters. Managing legal risks in preceptorships. *Canadian Nurse, 98*(9), 25–26.

Souers, C. (2002). Teaching strategies. Comprehensive performance review: Preparing students for a preceptor experience. *Nurse Educator, 27*(1), 9–12.

Trevitt, C., Grealish, L., & Reaby, L. (2001). Educational innovations. Students in transit: Using a self-directed preceptorship package to smooth the journey. *Journal of Nursing Education, 40*(5), 225–228.

Yonge, O., Myrick, M., Ferguson, L., & Haase, M. (2003). Faculty preparation for the preceptorship experience: The forgotten link. *Nurse Educator, 28*(5), 210–211.

Yonge, O. (1997). Assessing and preparing students for distance preceptorship placements. *Journal of Advanced Nursing, 26*(4), 81–816.

Additional Resources

Myrick, F., & Yonge, O. (2004). *Nursing preceptorship: Connecting practice and education.* New York: Lippincott Williams & Wilkins.

Council of University Teaching Hospitals, 260–575 West 8th Avenue, Vancouver, BC., V521C6. Web site. Available at: www.couth.bc.ca.

Chapter 19

Living Curricular Concepts: Opening Pedagogical Spaces

Anne Bruce

The class is abuzz as we go around the room sharing introductions. Anthony, 34, has a degree in history and lived in Japan teaching English for 4 years before entering the nursing program 2 years ago. Anthony returned to Canada with his Japanese wife and now has an 18-month-old daughter. He is looking forward to finishing his studies and getting into the nursing work world. Jo, 29, a mother of two, has struggled with the multiple demands of family and school and wonders why students cannot do the nursing program part time. Amy, 20, is soft spoken and emigrated with her family 6 years ago from Korea. She lives with her parents and works part time in the family store. The class of 26 is diverse with students bringing a breadth of life and academic experiences.

INTENT Drawing on curriculum theorist Ted Aoki's (1993, 2003) practice of **lived curriculum**, an emphasis on curricular landscapes that attend to learners' lived experience is explored. Complex and unpredictable health care environments call nurse educators to revisit educational processes that support and prepare students to engage with critical reflection and discernment within current health care arenas. How learners and educators move from experience to learning within gender/racial/social pedagogical spaces is considered alongside critiques and challenges when using experientially-oriented curricula.

OVERVIEW

INTRODUCTION

In al ll traditions of adult learning, experience is accorded a privileged position as the source of learning and center of knowledge production (Usher, Bryant, & Johnston, 1997). During the following 13 weeks, Anthony, Jo, Amy, and the rest of our class examined an array of nursing concepts that included health, health promotion, community, and social determinants of health. In the context of a third-year baccalaureate course, we explored marginalization, race, and empowerment. Even though there was a push from some students and clinical organizations toward an instrumentalism and knowing-how, the challenge was to foster **pedagogical spaces** where these curricular concepts opened and shifted from abstract ideas into lived experiences related to the fullness of learners' lives. However, in doing so, their realities also included increasing stress related to academic, financial, and personal demands and the dissonance they experienced between what is being taught by promoting health and empowerment and what is experienced in their university life (Young, Bruce, Turner, VanderWal, & Linden, 2001).

In this chapter, an approach of lived curriculum introduced by curricular theorist Ted Aoki (1993, 2003) holds considerable promise for exploring experience within pedagogical spaces. While specific strategies for engaging experiential learning are addressed elsewhere in the literature (Lee, 2003; Oermann, 2004; Wheeler & McLeod, 2002), an emphasis on opening curricular spaces for learning is examined here. How can we understand experience as an ongoing process calling forth living concepts in our pedagogy? How might we shift from privileging curriculum as content to be covered to engaging curriculum as relationship happening among students and between teachers/students—however it may be manifest. And finally, how can we understand content and process not as separate entities in opposition but as an interplay that shifts away from holding too tightly to predetermined plans toward a response-ability to what is happening in each educational situation? Although focusing on content and process as interlinked phenomena is not new, revisiting notions of curriculum and pedagogical spaces may open new possibilities beyond oppositional thinking of content versus process, learner and teacher, or health and illness. As with any view, these perspectives are not unproblematic; therefore, historical and ideological misgivings of experientially and process-focused learning are also considered.

LEARNING AND EXPERIENCE

Learners bring diverse experiences to the classroom and clinical settings. Many experiences are evident as students share past understandings along with immediate classroom experiences all enmeshed within their cultural and historical **locations**. Other student experiences are less visible yet equally diverse based on gender, culture, and history. These include the subtle effects of formal academic settings or the impact of unspoken rules and invisible expectations for successful completion of university studies (Anderson, 2001). However, experience alone does not necessarily translate into learning.

Making Meaning

Mezirow (2000) suggests that in order for learning to occur we must make meaning from our experiences. Each student brings their unique social and material **situatedness** as the context in which meaning making occurs. Although Mezirow theorizes about **transformative learning**, his perspectives provide a useful understanding of how learning can arise from experience. In brief, Mezirow suggests that experience becomes interpreted through our frame of reference which is composed of two dimensions. First is our habits of mind that are sets of assumptions about the world that filter our interpretation of experience and second is the points of view resulting from these habitual assumptions. Our habits of mind become expressed as points of view and are often below our conscious awareness.

Frames of reference shape experience and interpretation as this anecdote from a colleague illustrates:

> *A friend and I were driving to go kayaking. En route, we stopped at a light. I, as a mother, drew attention to the group of children walking by all dressed in red T-shirts and hats. He, as an electrical engineer, drew attention to a man who was working on an electrical box up on a pole. We laughed because I did not notice the man, and he did not notice the children. Yet, we were sitting in the same, yet different, landscape.*

As this story demonstrates, our unique situatedness in gender, professional, and social frames of reference both includes and excludes how we live and understand our world. In addition, this situatedness also shapes how we are understood (or not) by others who also live and interpret through their unique frames of reference.

According to Mezirow (2000), our understanding, consisting of habits of mind and ensuing points of view, are embedded in assumptions. For example, in this chapter, assumptions about teaching and learning are written into the language used to describe the students Anthony, Jo, and Amy introduced in the opening paragraph. Reflecting on my assumptions as an educator and author, there is a belief that sharing personal stories and getting to know students' as adults with life histories is integral to learning in nursing and therefore should be fostered. Another assumption includes valuing personal connection with course concepts so that learning becomes useful in our lives as individuals, citizens in society, and as nursing professionals. On quick reflection, these assumptions are apparent (and readers may have different interpretations) along with inevitable values and beliefs that I am unaware of without deeper reflection.

> *Our values and sense of self are anchored in our frames of reference. They provide us with a sense of stability, coherence, community, and identity. Consequently they are often emotionally charged and strongly defended. Other points of view are judged against the standards set by our points of view. Viewpoints that call our frames of reference into question may be dismissed as distorting, deceptive, ill intentioned, or crazy. . . . Learning tends to become narrowly defined as efforts to add compatible ideas to elaborate our fixed frames of reference. (Mezirow, 2000, p. 18)*

Situatedness

Pedagogy that focuses primarily on mastering course concepts through developing well-supported arguments may narrowly limit learners to those efforts of strengthening already fixed frames of reference. In contrast, learning that is transformative, according to Mezirow (2000), goes beyond solidifying what we already assume to know and challenges, reconstructs, or elaborates our habits of mind and points of view. Understandably, this process may be unsettling and emotionally charged. Periods of uncertainty and confusion may be evoked as learners' sense of stability and identity come into question. However, avoiding the pitfall of oppositional judgments by too rapidly seeking certainty through finding empirical evidence to support one's position when faced with frames of reference different from our own is recommended. Pedagogical openings recognize student vulnerability, uncertainty, and not knowing as natural processes in learning that can also be valued. Therefore, trusting in these open spaces (i.e., pedagogical openings) allows room for critical reflection, analysis, and insight to occur. These pedagogical moments are what Homi Bhabha calls "third space," a space of potentiality for something new, (Rutherford, 1990) and what David Jardine (1992) calls sites of "original difficulty" where the challenge of ambiguity and uncertainty simultaneously holds promise of possibilities and hope (cited in Aoki, 2003).

Supporting spaces for Jardine's (1992) notion of original difficulty also means leaving room for dialogue to continue. If, as Jardine claims, we convey the message that there is only one definition or one perfect way of doing things, then the conversation ends. Such definitive clarity is closed. There is nothing more to say and the goal for students often becomes figuring out what normative standard (frame of reference) individual faculty want to hear. With the exception of specific skills and particular practical knowledge, little knowledge in nursing need fall into closed clarity.

Some may argue that there *are* specific curricular concepts and substantive knowledge that student nurses need to master in order to be safe competent practitioners. This is not at issue; rather, the intention suggested here is opening spaces for learners to experience the partial and political nature of knowledge so that it becomes their own while realizing the impact of holding particular interpretations. For example, a common experience of dying patients is often identified as delirium. Delirium is a medical diagnosis and kind of knowledge generated within a biomedical view of reality. However, in caring for Aboriginal or First Nations families, such end-of-life experiences have other meanings that may include assumptions about the spirit world and other realms of reality. Ways of engaging pedagogically to support students' understanding of knowledge as contextual and always changing becomes important if we are to avoid recognizing only one kind of knowledge. Identifying the impact on the care patients and families receive when nurses do not acknowledge other ways of interpreting experience becomes a pedagogical challenge. Critical reflection identifying the assumptions of our situatedness and that of others in gender, history, culture, social stratification, and professional discipline is one way of meeting this challenge.

Kasl and Elias (2000) suggest that, in addition to surfacing uncritically assimilated beliefs about the world and its inhabitants, learning also happens through a process of discernment. Discernment begins with an open attitude of receptivity and appreciation where patterns of relational practices can be seen. In keeping with the above example of end-of-life care, nurses who hold an attitude of openness and appreciation will try to learn how each unique patient and family understands and makes meaning of their experience without generalizing from knowledge about Aboriginal beliefs and practices. In lieu of critical reflection and analysis, through discernment one transcends old frames of reference about what delirium is as new frames emerge that include other possibilities. Although critical reflection is well known as an important activity for learning in nursing, the process of discernment seems more subtle requiring attention to **experiential textures** and one's relationship to the learning process itself.

EXPERIENTIAL TEXTURES IN CURRICULA

Experience is rarely isolated but happens in relation—in relating with our physical or emotional environments of thoughts and feelings or relating with other people. Two highly significant relationships in learning are those between students and with students and faculty. This seems particularly relevant in nursing where the centrality of caring, respectful relationships with patients and families, goes virtually undisputed. Therefore, it is to be expected that Em Bevis and Jean Watson (1989) go beyond conventional notions of curriculum as a body of courses offered in an educational institution (McCutcheon, 1995) and circumscribe curriculum as "the interactions, oral, and written, that occur between students and faculty and among students" (Bevis & Watson, 1989, p. 12). This relational perspective locates curriculum within what these authors term an "educative-caring" wherein curriculum is not a planned, predetermined outline of course outcomes but a lived experience between students and teachers. Further, I am suggesting that through attending to these experiential textures with receptivity and appreciation, the development of discernment as described by Kasl and Elias (2000) can occur. This view of curriculum as relationship shifts the foci from an oppositional emphasis on message and medium toward an interdependence of content and process with capacities to critically engage, to discern, and to relate openly with situations and people. This demands from faculty a willingness and capacity to also be vulnerable as we ask students to take risks in not knowing. While thoughtfully preparing for each educational session, faculty must also be willing to let go of fixed expectations and engage with the immediate content of each class as it manifests. From this view, curricular content is uniquely configured in each class by learners' understandings of substantive knowledge, clinical experience, and their lived experience in the moment. As educators we skillfully prepare our class plans but must also learn to be open and receptive to the unplanned that is present in pedagogical spaces.

Lived Curriculum and Curriculum as Plan

> *Lived curriculum of students is, of course, not the curriculum as laid out in a plan but a plan more or less lived out. (Aoki, 1993, p. 257)*

Resonating with Bevis and Watson, Aoki's (1993, 2003) distinction between plan and lived experience is apparent. **Curriculum as plan** corresponds to conventional notions of curriculum as course content that usually originate outside the classroom either in the work of curriculum planners or in teachers' predetermined course syllabi. In contrast, living engagement that arises with the unique elements of each class is embedded in Aoki's notion of lived curriculum.

For educators this manifests in the face-to-face living with each student within a classroom collective (Aoki, 1993). With unique student–teacher relationships, teachers relate with each student (each curricula). This does not mean that educators will know or retain the personal histories and circumstances of every student, but that each engagement in the classroom or clinical setting will be unique and open. Lived curriculum is "really a multiplicity of curricula that . . . [students and the teacher] experience" (Aoki, 1993, p. 598). Teachers become alert to the interplay of lived and planned curricula; "and know that there are many lived curricula, as many as there are self and students, and possibly more" (p. 258). Juxtaposed with the curriculum as plan, a curriculum-as-lived happens in the spaces between what is planned and what is being lived out where colearners meet.

> *An educated person, first and foremost, understands that one's way of knowing, thinking, and doing flow from who one is. Such a person knows that an authentic person is more than a mere individual, an island unto himself or herself, but a being-in-relation with others and hence is, at core, an ethical being. (Aoki, cited in Pinar, Reynolds, Slattery, & Taubman, 1995, p. 428)*

Attending to and following with students as they are being-in-relation with assigned readings, the responses and comments of fellow students and teacher, and the class energy offers what Aoki (1993) calls a "retextured landscape, populated by a multiplicity of curricula, disturbing the traditional landscape with its single privileged curriculum as plan awaiting implementation" (pp. 258–259). It is in the unsettling of the planned curricular landscape where opportunities for **reflexive** critical engagement can occur for faculty and students. Critical engagement is used broadly here to link with the aims and values of critical theorists who examine taken-for-granted assumptions about how some knowledge is privileged over others, and how students/teachers may unwittingly perpetuate structures of power and inequity in classroom and clinical settings (Kincheloe & McLaren, 1994). In accepting these aims of critical engagement, the unsettling of the planned curriculum opens opportunities for examining these issues as they are lived in-the-moment in educational settings.

In/visible Agendas

How best can the fullness of students' experience be linked to curricular concepts, even when the experience is of dissonance between what is espoused in class and what is lived by learners? Drawing on the prevalence of stress reported among student nurses as an example, the dialectic of health and high levels of stress will be used to address this question. **Dialectic** is used to infer a tension between seemingly opposing forces of health and student stress where the tension itself becomes the site of interest rather than the binary poles of stress or health. Although the issue of student nurse stress is of importance for educators, it will not be specifically addressed in this chapter yet is used to exemplify possible outcomes when the dialectical tensions of learners' experience are examined. Further, by using learners' experience, such as stress, as the basis for understanding a broad range of curricular concepts, students develop capacities in making links between personal experience and theoretical concepts that are genuinely their own.

Student stress is an expected aspect of any academic experience. However, research suggests that student nurses have additional stressors within clinical experiences that differentiate the nursing population from other academic and health-related disciplines (Beck, Hackett, Srivastava, McKimm, & Rockwell, 1997). Stress and its effect on school performance among nursing students have been investigated extensively (Haack, 1988; Jones & Johnson, 2000; Lindop, 1999). Jones and Johnson (2000) reported that nursing students' sources of stress were frequently related to the academic environment and to financial and personal factors, while Beck, et al. (1997) implicate relationships with faculty as main sources of stress for student nurses. The contradictions become disheartening as key curricular concepts such as health and therapeutic relationships are lived through the tension of their presence and absence within student nurses' experience.

As suggested earlier, the tension of student health and stress/disease is only one of many contradictions students experience in classroom and clinical settings. It follows, then, that nursing education would be strengthened through modeling processes that foster understanding of these contradictory student experiences. Through Aoki's (2003) lived curriculum lens, one approach is to acknowledge the tensioned and complex nature of such contradictions and begin learning how to understand and negotiate one's way through them. Through being able to acknowledge and address lived realities of student stress, a space can be opened to examine and understand what is happening—what personal, political, social, and institutional forces are at play. In doing so, inevitable differences among students and the concepts espoused in the course content will arise and in turn will inevitability invite diversity, difference, and complexity. As educators alert to both the flow of personal experience and evidence-based resources available, the pedagogical call is in provoking students to think and make links between experience and curricular concepts. If we accept that each student is unique with particular understandings and responses to course and pedagogical processes, then difference becomes an expectation. Although the foci here may seem to privilege individual student experience, it is not intended to minimize the situatedness of individual students within social and academic forces.

Similarly, nurses make decisions in clinical practice drawing on a variety of data sources (empirical, theoretical, and personal) often in ambiguous and complex situations. In the same way, ambiguity can be invited into the classroom embedded in opportunities for each student to make meaning of curricular concepts in their own way, valuing differences inherent in learners and learning styles. By accepting difference as an anticipated norm, the inconsistencies students' experience between what is taught and what is experienced in the classroom or clinical setting can be addressed openly as difference (or inconsistency or hypocrisy). That is, the inevitability of other agendas/curriculum is the starting point and the learning process entails making visible what was previously invisible. Once revealed, unspoken curriculum or agendas become negotiable and visible to all participants including educators and learners (Anderson, 2001). In turn, exposure "allows change, defence, and improvement of—or at least informed dialogue about—formal educational processes and structures" (p. 28). If student stress is acknowledged openly with encouragement to critically explore links between learners' experience of stress and curricular concepts of marginalization, power, and health, then what is taught about health and what is learned will, at the least, be examined openly. At the risk of sounding naive, this process assumes a level of integrity and self-awareness from faculty in truly valuing difference and not simply paying lipservice while expecting uniformity from students. For educators with clear expectations of student behavior and performance who wish to engage in lived curriculum, an awareness of the frames of reference employed in determining these expectations must be articulated for students to scrutinize and make their learning decisions accordingly.

Living Curricular Concepts

Using Aoki's (2003) lens of lived curriculum, the experiences of disconnect or tension becomes part of the classroom texture that may be named by students, or arise indirectly through student behavior. In this curricular situation, educators alert to the interplay of lived and planned curricula can create spaces where the tension can present itself. For example, in class discussions addressing power and marginalization as determinants of health, student perspectives of excessive academic workload or uncertainty of course expectations may arise as their concerns relate to the concepts of power and marginalization in their academic lives. Through attending to visible and invisible processes with receptivity and acceptance, patterns of personal, institutional, and social relations can be identified. Critical reflection of beliefs and current habits of mind can be surfaced.

Educational and clinical institutions are complex multilayered spaces permeated with tensions and gaps that are sometimes enriching, sometimes unacceptable, and often inevitable. The challenge rests with faculty and students to recognize these tensions while developing capacities of critical reflection and discernment. Learning to read and hear pedagogical spaces means learning to rest in the situation as it is . . . in the tension between living by a plan *and* in the plan as it is currently lived. Dwelling in the tension between plans and what is actually happening necessitates an openness and appreciation of the present moment and a capacity to use such tension as a force for critical insight and new possibilities (Aoki, 1993).

WHY IS LIVED CURRICULUM IMPORTANT IN NURSING EDUCATION?

How curriculum is understood becomes important when looking at the kinds of nurses we hope to graduate and how best to prepare students for health care environments that are multifaceted, unstable, and often are sites of conflict and change. Increasingly, cultural and ethnic diversity within classrooms and work settings requires renewed examination of difference and valuing diverse ways of being, knowing, and learning. Moreover, how one defines curriculum informs how nurses view their work, how nursing work becomes evaluated and valued, and how research and scholarship are acknowledged (Bevis & Watson, 1989). As reflected in changing clinical settings, the desirability for faculty to control and predict the learning environment is diminishing under learner-centered and experiential-based pedagogies (Bilimoria & Wheeler, 1995). A new approach to curriculum that embraces process and indeterminacy and consequently is more complex, pluralistic, and unpredictable was foreseen by curricular theorists a decade ago (Doll, 1993). Why is change then so slow? Are educators too steeped in content-oriented curricular experience to be willing or able to embrace process on an equal pedagogical footing?

HISTORICAL AND IDEOLOGICAL BARRIERS

Nursing has been highly influenced by the frame of reference of structuralism characterized by a penchant for categorizing all phenomena. Structuralist beliefs can be spotted in nursing models, research, and curricular plans that are "conceived and legitimated by order and rationality" (Pinar, et al., 1995, p. 486). Although a shift away from structuralist perspectives has been occurring with the integration of adult education principles in nursing over the past 20 years, it is a gradual transition. By privileging behaviorism and rationality, alternative forms of knowledge that look not only at what we know but our way of knowing have often been minimized. Bevis and Watson (1989) present a historical overview chronicling the emergence and integration of Tyler's behavioral rationale that has contributed enormously with its emphasis on measurable, outcome objectives and paved the way for a smoother transition into an evidence-based ethos in nursing. However, without diminishing these contributions, behaviorist and structuralist frames of reference are also limited by what they leave out.

Pinar et al. (1995) in *Understanding Curriculum* present a comprehensive exploration of curricula from a poststructuralist perspective and the barriers experienced in applying these viewpoints to pedagogical practice. Although barriers to change remain, the assumption that classrooms, teacher–student relations, textbooks, and assignments are politically and socially constructed remains at the root of the change. From this standpoint, the question is not how do we create neutral learning environments, but rather, how can nurse educators foster curiosity and analysis into the political/gender/racial experiential nature of classrooms and curricular concepts? Educational efforts question not only what a phenomenon such as stress is, but what causes and conditions are at play to construct different understandings? This poststructuralist position suggests that any perspective is always temporary, conditional, and can be challenged. Curriculum must now also model and prepare students for social, political, and clinical situations that are complex, pluralistic, and unpredictable. The shift does not neglect so-called fixed information such as anatomy and physiology but privileges processes—learning how to learn, how to discern with discrimination, how to think critically, how to reflect on experience and re/construct frames of reference and meanings, how to hold the tensions of difference.

CRITIQUES

As with any view, there are limitations and contesting voices. For some educators, an experiential and process-oriented focus raises concerns when the now of the present is viewed as if carved off from the history of what has come before (Pinar, et al., 1995). Smith (as cited in Pinar, et al.) writes in response to such concerns, "when I look at a classroom situation, I do not see it as 'present'; I see it as 'presently' expressing its history while at the same time as embodying within itself a sense of hope for the future" (p. 422). Nevertheless, a caution against fixation on the personal in-the-moment to the detriment of shared or group experiences of class or culture is justified. Similarly, Usher and Edwards (1994) caution that experience has been conceptualized within a liberal, humanist frame of reference where learners are seen as autonomous agents who independently make meaning of their experience. Other critiques include recognizing that personal experience is not generalizable and therefore it is limited when theorizing more broadly. Brookfield (1998) also questions the romantic assumption that all experience is useful for learning by virtue that it is our own. Without critical reflection, sharing experiences may lead to "an uncritical celebratory swapping of war stories and anecdotes in which all stories possess equal value, merit, and significance" (p. 130). Focusing too heavily on individualism while ignoring the sociopolitical nature of experience is also a challenge educators using experiential learning must face.

FOSTERING PEDAGOGICAL OPENINGS

Teacher flexibility and openness in these curricular landscapes invites a willingness to take actions that are beyond our habitual habits of mind and learning style—into spaces of risk without knowing what might happen. Learning to trust the learning process and students' capacity to work with in-the-moment experience is needed if we are to foster learning opportunities that cannot be planned or foreseen. The importance of sensitivity to changing classroom textures is emphasized in the literature (Borich, 1998; Wheeler & McLeod, 2002) in order to experience in the classroom what is important and transferable into clinical settings. As educators in relation with students and the unique contextual elements of each class situation, our willingness to engage with complex, diverse, and unpredictable in-the-moment pedagogical situations demands that we also engage critically and self-reflexively with the invisible tensions within our classrooms.

Notwithstanding these challenges and critiques, lived curriculum as constituted by Aoki (1993, 2003) emphasizes experiential approaches that strive to open curricular spaces for learning. Sites of learning arise in between plans and the realities of the moment where colearners meet. Educators and students whose learning of nursing is guided by curriculum as lived experience, come to know the tensions of curricular concepts such as stress, health, and power through an interplay of content and process.

SUMMARY

Learners bring a breadth of diverse experience into nursing programs that reflect their situatedness in gender, previous education, culture, and political orientation. Through engaging curriculum as relationship among students and between teachers/students (Aoki, 1993)—student experience can provide opportunities to think critically about what they are learning, how they are learning it, and how this learning is inevitably political and multifaceted. Student nurse stress embedded in the dissonance between what is taught and what is experienced in the classroom exemplifies contradictions that are inevitable in educational and clinical institutions. Process-oriented curricula can provide pedagogical openings for understanding the complexity of these tensions and how to influence change. Further, this approach highlights the constructed nature of human experience and knowledge within an everchanging context of history, culture, and social politics. Increasingly complex and unpredictable health care environments call for nurses with broader views and capacities in order to effectively negotiate within arenas of difference and possibility.

LEARNING ACTIVITY

SENTENCE STEM WRITING ACTIVITY

This brief 3- to 5-minute freewriting activity is adapted from Peter Elbow (1998) and can be used by teachers at the beginning of class. The activity provides opportunities for individual reflection and a means of focusing students' attention. Begin the activity with instructions about how long students are to freewrite and coach learners to keep their pens on the page and write whatever they wish in response to a sentence stem provided. Students are encouraged to write spontaneously without judgment or concern for coherence or grammar.

Sentence stems may address the content and process of the course or can be solicited from the class. Examples include:

- Health promotion is . . .
- I find the contradictions of . . .
- The most stressful . . .

Following the writing, sharing in dyads or large group may be appropriate.

RESOURCES FOR EDUCATORS

PLANNING THE TEACHING/LEARNING EXPERIENCE

Tips for Developing a Student-Centered Learning Environment

- Practice listening and leaving spaces.
- Encourage cross-discussion among students rather than directed at instructor.
- Model how to critically surface assumptions and invite input.

Questions to Support a Thoughtful Reading

1. What most struck me about the text we read for the discussion today was . . .
2. The question that I'd most like to ask the author(s) of the text is . . .
3. The idea I most take issue with in the text is . . .
4. I interpret the author(s) privilege located in . . .
5. I interpret the readers' (my) privilege located in . . .

EVALUATING THE TEACHING/LEARNING EXPERIENCE

Questions to Elicit Feedback from Students on Their Learning

1. What new questions does this evoke?
2. What have I learned or relearned today?
3. How can I apply what I've learned today in practice?

Reflective Questions for Educators

1. What assumptions did I make about how students responded or participated?
2. How did the discussions privilege particular groups or perspectives?
3. What perspectives were left out? What factors contribute to that?
4. Who spoke most? Who was silent?
5. How were student perspectives solicited?
6. In what ways was power shared during class?

Sample Evaluation Strategies

1. As a learner, how have you experienced moments of pedagogical openings? Reflect on what was happening to support or impede your learning.
2. Contemplate and discuss dominant habits of mind as described by Mezirow (2000) in relation to your teaching and learning patterns.
3. How can educators recognize the flow of what is happening in a learning environment? How is this experienced in clinical practice?
4. Reflecting on your practice, have you ever experienced an unexpected situation in the classroom that was unsettling? Was this seen as an opportunity for learning or a dreaded situation to be controlled? What values and beliefs underlie each interpretation?

References

Anderson, T. (2001). The hidden curriculum of distance education. *Change, 23*(6), 28–35.

Aoki, T. (1993). Legitimating lived curriculum: Towards a curricular landscape of multiplicity. *Journal of Curriculum and Supervision, 8*(3), 255–268.

Aoki, T. (2003). Locating living pedagogy in teacher "research": Five metonymic moments. In E. Hasebe-Ludt & W. Hurren, (Eds.). *Curriculum Intertext* (pp. 1–9). New York: Peter Lang.

Beck, D., Hackett, M. B., Srivastava, R., et al. (1997). Perceived level and sources of stress in university professional schools. *Journal of Nursing Education, 36*(3), 180–186.

Bevis, E., & Watson, J. (1989). *Toward a caring curriculum: A new pedagogy for nursing.* New York: National League for Nursing.

Bilimoria, D., & Wheeler, J. V. (1995). Learning-centered education: A guide to resources and implementation. *Journal of Management Education, 19*(3), 409–428.

Borich, G. D. (1998). *Observational skills effective teaching.* Upper Saddle River, NJ: Merrill.

Brookfield, S. (1998). Against naive romanticism: From celebration to the critical analysis of experience. *Studies in Continuing Education, 20*(2), 127–142.

Doll, W. (1993). *A postmodern perspective on curriculum.* New York: Teachers College Press.

Elbow, P. (1998). *Writing with power: Techniques for mastering the writing process.* (2nd ed.). New York: Oxford University Press.

Haack, M. (1988). Stress and impairment among nursing students. *Research in Nursing and Health, 11*(2), 125–134.

Jardine, D. (1992). The fecundity of the individual case: Considerations of the pedagogic heart of interpretive work. *Journal of Philosophy of Education, 26*(1), 51–61.

Jones, M., & Johnson, D. (2000). Reducing distress in first level and student nurses: A review of the applied stress management literature. *Journal of Advanced Nursing, 32*(1), 66–74.

Kasl, E., & Elias, D. (2000). Creating new habits of mind in small groups. In J. M. Associates, (Ed.), *Learning as transformation: Critical perspectives on a theory in progress* (pp. 229–252). San Francisco: Jossey-Bass.

Kincheloe, J., & McLaren, P. (1994). Rethinking critical theory and qualitative research. In N. Denzin & Y. Lincoln, (Eds.). *Handbook of Qualitative Research* (pp. 138–157). Thousand Oaks, Ca: Sage.

Lee, M. (2003). Engaging the whole person through the practice of collaborative learning. *Journal of Lifelong Education, 22*(1), 78–93.

Lindop, E. (1999). A comparative study of stress between pre- and post-Project 2000 students. *Journal of Advanced Nursing, 29*(4), 967–973.

McCutcheon, G. (1995). Curriculum theory and practice for the 1990s. In A. Ornstein & L. Behar, (Eds.). *Contemporary issues in curriculum.* Boston: Allyn & Bacon.

Mezirow, J. (2000). *Learning as transformation: Critical perspectives on a theory in progress.* San Francisco: Jossey-Bass.

Oermann, M. (2004). Using active learning in lecture: Best of "both worlds." *International Journal of Nursing Education Scholarship, 1*(1), 1–9.

Pinar, W. F., Reynolds, W. M., Slattery, P., et al. (1995). *Understanding curriculum: An introduction to the study of historical and contemporary curriculum discourses.* (Vol. 17). New York: Peter Lang.

Rutherford, J. (1990). *Identity, community, culture, difference.* London: Lawrence and Wishart.

Usher, R., Bryant, I., & Johnston, R. (1997). *Adult education and the postmodern challenge: Learning beyond limits.* London: Routledge.

Usher, R., & Edwards, R. (1994). *Postmodernism and education.* London: Routledge.

Wheeler, J., & McLeod, P. L. (2002). Expanding our teaching effectiveness: Understanding our responses to "in-the-moment" classroom events. *Journal of Management Education, 26*(6), 693–716.

Young, L. E., Bruce, A., Turner, L., et al. (2001). Student nurse health promotion: Evaluation of mindfulness-based stress reduction (MBSR) intervention. *Canadian Nurse, 97*(6), 23–26.

Additional Resources

Educational Insights. This is an electronic journal based at the University of British Columbia Web site. Available at: http://ccfi.educ.ubc.ca/publication/insights/.

Diekelmann, N. (2003). Thinking-in-action journals: From self-evaluation to multiperspectival thinking. *Journal of Nursing Education*, 42(11), 482–484.

Habits of Mind Web site. Available at: http://www.habits-of-mind.net/.

Jumashiro, K. (2004). Uncertain beginnings: Learning to teach paradoxically, *Theory into Practice*, 43(2), 111–115.

Marshall, M. (2003). Creative learning: The mandala as teaching exercise. *Journal of Nursing Education*, 42(2), 517–519.

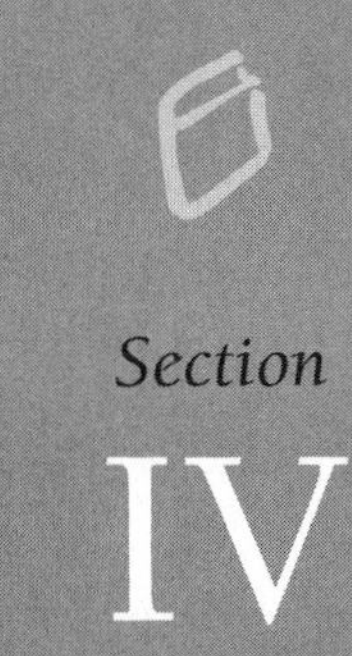

Section

IV

STUDENT-CENTERED TEACHING: CHALLENGES AND ISSUES FOR FACULTY

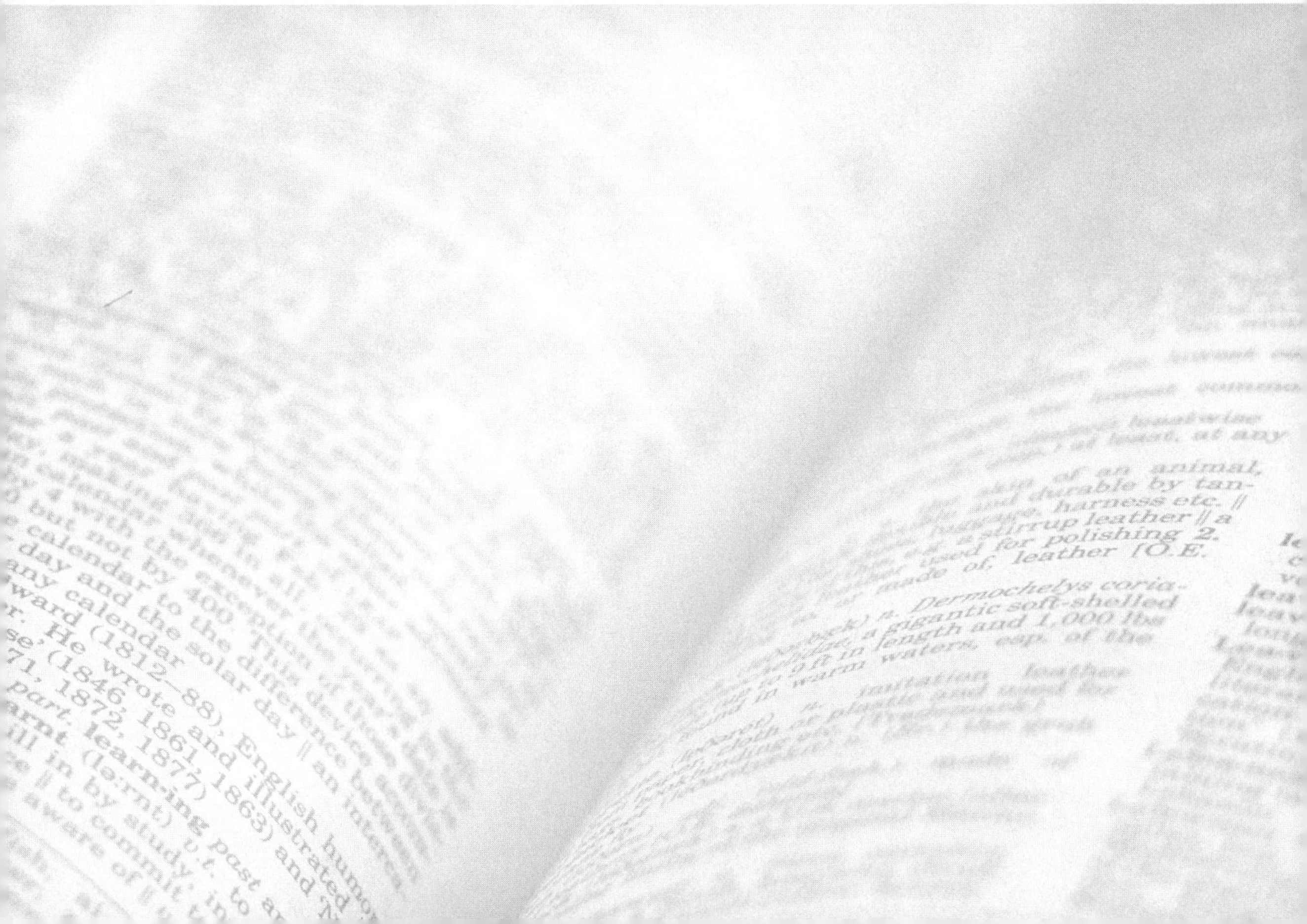

Chapter 20

Racing Around the Classroom Margins: Race, Racism, and Teaching Nursing

Colleen Varcoe
Janice McCormick

Last summer I[1] had the wonderful opportunity of teaching a course titled "Culture and Health" to fourth-year nursing students. I had advocated long for such a course. Although culture and context are central concepts within the nursing curriculum we teach, **culture** was usually treated in a "culturist" manner; that is, as something that is about values and beliefs held by groups and individuals rather than something that is deeply intertwined with power and **structural inequities** such as sexism, poverty, and racism. In developing and teaching this course I had new opportunities to deal openly and directly with issues related to **race**, **racialization**, and **racism**, and to explore and model ways racism can be named and interrupted in the classroom and practice.

Two days into the five full-day course, a student confided to me that she had not disclosed that she was Aboriginal. I found her choice of words jarring. I associate disclosure with stigmatizing conditions and understand that being seen as Aboriginal exposes a person to racism and stigma. Although I am often seen as White, my father is Aboriginal and I have experienced such racism and stigma myself; but I had not thought of these experiences in relation to disclosure before. I had no further conversation with this woman, but the next day noticed that her demeanor had changed. She seemed angry, did not join in class discussion (as she had previously), and seemed to be avoiding me personally. Over the next day her participation continued to wane. When I tried to speak with her, she left, and did not return for the final day.

I sent her a note inviting her to contact me, both immediately after the course and after I had submitted the course grades. She did not contact me, however, she did contact an advisor to the program with her concerns, a fact that I discovered accidentally. I am not sure what I did, but I can guess. Anonymous evaluations of the course revealed one student who was dissatisfied—rating almost every aspect of the course as "poor." In particular, I was disturbed by comments from one person that the course "only had one focus—Aboriginal."

In my zeal to foster understanding, I had packed the course with what I thought were interesting readings and speakers. None of the more than 20 readings addressed Aboriginal issues, but two of five guest speakers did. One was an Aboriginal woman

[1] The first-person "I" in this section is that of author Colleen Varcoe.

from an HIV/AIDS organization and another was a professor who does research in Aboriginal mental health. And I shared my research on violence against women that involves Aboriginal participants. I do not think the problem was volume; I think that through my choices, I had inadvertently reinforced stereotypical and negative understandings of Aboriginal people, emphasizing victimization rather than capacity. Since then, I have tried to preface any work I do with the ideas behind Razack's (1998) warning that:

> *culture talk is clearly a double-edged sword. It packages difference as inferiority . . . yet cultural considerations are important for contextualizing oppressed groups' claims for justice, improving their access to services, and for requiring dominant groups to examine the invisible cultural advantages they enjoy.* (p. 58)

As Razack suggests, even in our most well-intentioned efforts, we can breathe life into **racism**. Engaging in talk about culture, race, racism, and **marginalization** always both risks reproducing and reinforcing stereotypes and offers opportunity to contest and counter stereotyping, discrimination, and institutional inequity. Thus each teaching/learning moment requires careful scrutiny and reflexivity.

INTENT The intent of this chapter is to discuss how teachers can explicitly deal with race and racism in teaching and learning spaces. We argue that in doing so, teachers leave these spaces less open to stereotypical thinking—**Eurocentrism**, **ethnocentrism**, and racism. We suggest that building community in the classroom and focusing on difference are vital strategies for nurse educators to participate in the important work of unlearning racism and fostering social justice and ethical nursing practice.

OVERVIEW

Taking Up the Challenges of Racism in Teaching Nursing
Racism, Health Care, and Nursing
Challenges and Tensions: Dichotomies and Individualism
Challenges and Tensions: Language as Context
Western Society as Context
Nursing and Health Care as Context
Teaching as Context
Traps for Students and Teachers
Implications and Strategies: Building Community and Working with Difference

- Reflexivity: Begin With Yourself
- Expanding: Seek and Become Allies
- Talking: Expand Language Practices
- Centering: Rethink Safety
- De-centering: Introduce Marginalized Knowledge
- Re-"framing": Work the Context
- Relevance: Offer Experiential Opportunities

TAKING UP THE CHALLENGES OF RACISM IN TEACHING NURSING

As racism, ethnocentrism, Eurocentrism, **classism**, **patriarchy**, **heterosexism**, and **homophobia** characterize contemporary Western societies, they also pervade nursing education. Although their influence is always present and unavoidable, nursing educators can choose the extent to which they explicitly address these issues (Puzan, 2003). Over the past several years we have come to believe that without direct attention to the existence and effects of racism (inextricably intertwined with other forms of oppression), we, by default, allow our learning spaces (classrooms, online courses, and clinical settings) to be more open to discriminatory and stereotypical thinking, leaving extant power dynamics unchallenged. We purposefully draw on theory arising from Anticolonialism, **postcolonial theory**, and **antiracist pedagogy** to try to create teaching and learning spaces in which it is possible to constructively examine oppression and particularly racism. We have found this goal elusive and a struggle to achieve.

This chapter explores some of the tensions we have encountered between and among those teaching and learning nursing in multiethnic, multicultural, diverse settings.[2] Set against the historical backdrop of nursing as a class-based and racialized profession, we identify some of the challenges that we and others have faced. We consider the specific oppression of racism as it intersects with other forms of oppression in the content and process of nursing education. We discuss how the particular contexts of nursing, health care, and teaching shape the ways in which teachers and students take up the language and ideas that dominate Western societies. Readers will be asked to consider the challenge of struggling with the power inherent in the position of teacher and the privileges that often accompany such positions. Then, the issue of facilitating learning in an environment where some people have significantly more social **privilege** and "voice" than others will be considered. We draw upon bell hooks' book *Teaching to*

[2] We do not believe that these tensions are lessened or are of lesser importance in more monocultural settings; indeed hooks (1994) points out that addressing race in such settings is of critical importance. Rather, we are simply drawing on our experience in ethnically diverse settings.

Transgress (1994) and other writers to suggest ways that teachers might engage in practices that are actively critical of and counter to oppression, discrimination, and in particular, racism. We suggest that rather than focusing on safety and overlooking difference, building community and focusing on difference as an analytic tool can join people with diverse identities and social locations in common purpose.

RACISM, HEALTH CARE, AND NURSING

Racism is of specific and continuous concern in nursing. Racism, particularly as it intersects with poverty, profoundly determines health (Krieger, 1999; Krieger & Gruskin, 2001; Nazroo, 1998), and racism, again particularly as it intersects with poverty, shapes health care (Anderson & Kirkham, 1998; Browne & Fiske, 2001; Chow, Jaffee, & Snowden, 2003; Henry, Tator, Mattis, & Rees, 2000b; Jiwani, 2000). Health care access, resources for health care, and experiences of health care are shaped by such inequities. Although racism has been denounced as contrary to nursing's mandate, ethics, and commitment to social justice, studies have found racism to be a component of discrimination directed at both patients and nurses (Condliffe, 2001; Shaha, 1998).

Although little research has focused explicitly on racism and nursing, nurses have been observed to label patients and provide differential care on the basis of ethnicity (Browne, Johnson, Bottorff, Grewal, & Hilton, 2002; Stevens, 1992; Varcoe, 2001, 2002). In the United States, Stevens found that differences in the quality of care could be attributed to discrimination based on gender, class, race, and culture and included excessive waiting time, less thorough diagnostic evaluations, withholding indicated treatments, inappropriate and degrading interventions, and decreased access to care. In their Canadian study of clinical encounters between health care providers and South Asian women patients, Browne et al. (2002) found that although the women were reluctant to express their concerns, they experienced being distinguished as "other" (e.g., by references to "our women" and "their women"), being avoided, or inappropriately treated. In interviews, the health care providers expressed discriminatory attitudes, with well-intentioned remarks revealing stereotypical thinking. Notably, nurses recognized the problems the women encountered with the health care system, but expressed their frustration toward the women. In a study of emergency nursing, Varcoe (2001, 2002) observed that nurses tended to anticipate that women from particular racialized groups would be victims of intimate partner violence, whereas women from the dominant white population were presumed unlikely to be victimized, which diminished the quality of care for all. Studying nursing practice in relation to children with chronic conditions, McCormick (1997; McCormick, Rodney, & Varcoe, 2003) found that nurses were more likely to label those parents and families who were poor, racialized, immigrant, Aboriginal, or who did not speak English as neglectful. While in the hospital, children from such families were more likely to be thought of by the nurses as better off in the hospital where they could get the attention they needed (McCormick, 1997; McCormick, et al., 2003).

Nurses also experience racial discrimination. Das Gupta's (1996) study of nursing in Ontario, Canada, illustrated that health care reform is not color blind. She described how individual Black nurses' experiences of harassment, scapegoating, and infantilizing were linked to the racial segregation of the workforce (wherein most managers are White, and most women of color are staff nurses). Within this context, changes in employment practices disproportionately affected women of color, compounding their underemployment, lack of promotion, and deployment in heavier units. Hagey, Choudhry, Guruge, and Turrittin (2001) studied nine female nurses of color in Ontario who had filed discrimination grievances with their employers. The women argued that they were denied privileges that White nurses were allowed and were subject to "petty harassment," excessive supervision, and "punitive reprimands" from their supervisors for the same kinds of activities in which White nurses engaged without similar penalties. Furthermore, although the nurses had from 7 to 33 years experience, they were subjected to surveillance of routine nursing practices; their charting was monitored, and their decisions questioned. The study also drew attention to the association between experiences of discrimination, a lack of knowledge in nursing regarding diversity, and White dominance of the higher levels of the nursing profession. These studies occurred within the wider Canadian context where activists and scholars have noted a backlash against equity programs despite some headway against racism and discrimination (Hankivsky, 1996).

Racial discrimination by peers is also a problem in nursing. Researchers have shown that bullying or horizontal violence is a significant problem for nursing (McKenna, Smith, Poole, & Coverdale, 2003; Freshwater, 2000; Rn, 2001; Randle, 2003). Although the racial dynamics of such violence rarely has been explicitly explored, in a study of nurses in New Zealand, McKenna et al. (2003) found that inappropriate racial comments and gestures were a component of horizontal violence for some nurses. Randle (2003) notes more generally that strategies to deal with horizontal violence and bullying in nursing do not always account for historical and contextual factors. Given the pervasiveness of horizontal violence in nursing and of racism in society more broadly, it is likely that these social processes overlap considerably, particularly in multiethnic environments.

Nursing has begun to look more closely at its attitudes and practices and to work toward more inclusive approaches by embracing cultural diversity, difference, and cultural sensitivity in theory and education. However, despite inclusive rhetoric, a veil of assumptions and expectations of nursing being predominantly White and female clings to nursing, with the underlying assumption being that nursing students should learn to adopt the values and behaviors of the dominant culture (Paterson, Osborne, & Gregory, 2004). As Paterson et al. show, overt messages teachers may give regarding equality may be contradicted by students' experiences. Their recent institutional ethnographic study illustrated "largely unwritten and invisible expectations" in discourses of equality and cultural sensitivity in clinical nursing education. Simultaneous with overt messages about equality, clinical teachers gave unspoken messages that tended to take issue with differences and construct difference as being less than the expected norm. Paterson et al. noted that the complex and contradictory experiences of difference and homogeneity to which students were exposed contributed to the perception of cultural diversity as a problem. They theorized that this occurred because of the "macro" influences that shaped how teachers and students experienced diversity, and challenged nurse educators to examine their attitudes, beliefs, and assumptions about inclusivity.

The dominant approach to issues of race in nursing has been congruent with the tenets of multiculturalism that focus on sensitivity and tolerance for minority groups by dominant groups, approaches that underlie the problematic construction of diversity in clinical education described by Paterson et al. (2004). The ideas of multiculturalism do not address **everyday racism** or the structures and practices that support institutional racism. Nursing scholars have shown that in nursing, as in the wider world more generally, multiculturalism and such ideas as cultural sensitivity do not take "difference" and structural inequities into account (Browne & Fiske, 2001; Culley, 1996; Hartrick-Doane & Varcoe, 2005a, 2005b; Swendson & Windsor, 1996). If racism is to be addressed, it is not sufficient to ignore difference, to pretend that differences do not exist, or to tolerate difference. However, it is tough and challenging to actively and explicitly engage in antiracist pedagogy.

CHALLENGES AND TENSIONS: DICHOTOMIES AND INDIVIDUALISM

In teaching situations, engaging in conversations about race and racism seems a risky business. As in the opening scenario, such conversations can construct people from positions of relative disadvantage as victims or worse, as inferior. Such conversations can position students as representatives of certain groups, placing them in defensive positions as either privileged or victimized. Examining these tensions more closely, it is clear that they arise, at least in part, from constructing oppression as a dichotomy: oppressor/oppressed. These tensions also arise in part because racism (and other forms of oppression) is individualized rather than being seen as a pervasive feature of Western society. When the focus is on individual behavior, and when individuals are divided into either oppressed or oppressor categories, the stage is set for individual students to feel scrutinized, judged, and seen as representatives of particular positions of power.

Dichotomous thinking pervades Western reasoning (Derrida, 1978) and is often traced to Descartes' splitting of body/mind.[3] Following McConaghy (2000), Anderson (2004) argues that in relation to diversity and racism "it is no longer useful, for ***analytic*** purposes, to think in terms of dichotomous categories" such as "Aboriginal/non-Aboriginal; immigrant/nonimmigrant; heterosexual/gay and lesbian; oppressed/oppressor" (p. 12, emphasis in original). Rather Anderson argues that we need to examine specific oppressions at specific sites within specific contexts. She notes that "those of us constructed as the 'marginalized' by virtue of the category in which we are placed, might see this as our right

[3] René Descartes (1596–1650) was a French philosopher from whose name the word "Cartesian" is formed. Considered by many to be the principal founding father of philosophy (Scrunton, 1995), he was instrumental in shaping Western philosophical thought. Descartes wanted to establish a foundation for philosophy that would be based on statements known to be true. His famous quote, "I think, therefore I am," was an expression of his belief that there was at least one piece of knowledge that all humans have and cannot doubt—hat we know we exist because we are able to think. He declared that knowledge is defined by thought, and the "I" that thinks (the mind) is distinct from the mechanical structure of human existence (the body). According to this view, the mind is a substance that is essentially different from bodily substance, and Descartes clearly privileged the mind. Thus began a centuries-long ontological split between the mind and the body that continues to this day. The body/mind split was only the first of a long series of similar binarisms—terms that are defined in opposition to each other, but also depend on each other for their existence and meaning.

to lay claim to a moral superiority by virtue of our 'oppression' and in so doing, may perpetuate even more virulent forms of oppression" (p. x). Conversely, those constructed as the oppressor or racist may experience this as an impetus for guilt, anger, or defensiveness. Further, use of dichotomous categories may foster assumptions that members of groups defined by presumed shared identities also share similar experiences and ideological commitments. Thus, in line with Anderson's recommendations, rather than thinking about individuals as oppressors or oppressed across contexts, the specific oppression (racism) needs to be examined at the specific site (nursing) within a specific context (nursing education).

Dichotomous thinking also fosters the process of "**othering**;" that is, the process of defining self against an exoticized "other," dividing the world into us and them. Indeed Said (1979) argues that the West was only created in opposition to the exoticized Eastern oriental other, meaning that the notion of the Western world is reliant upon racializing processes. Taussig (1993) notes that the opposition between self and other is a relationship, not a thing in itself. In the context of nursing "individuals may be designated as the 'other' based on a variety of reasons and circumstances, including the color of their skin, their gender, sexual identity, and social class; and whether or not they are homeless, refugees, illegal immigrants, addicted to drugs or alcohol, experience a disability, are HIV positive, have a diagnosis of tuberculosis, experience a mental illness, or are imprisoned" (Peternelj-Taylor, 2005, p. 133). Peternelj-Taylor argues that othering as a form of engagement is contrary to ethical nursing practice.

Dichotomies are a feature of Western thinking that is congruent with individualism, the idea that people are autonomous actors that make independent decisions based on self-interest. Individualism is a main characteristic of liberalism, the liberal ideology underlying Western thinking. Browne (2001) argues that "in nursing the central tenets of liberal political philosophy—individualism, egalitarianism, freedom, tolerance, neutrality, and a free-market economy" (p. 118)—are primarily manifested in (a) an individualistic focus in nursing science; (b) a view of society as essentially egalitarian and equitable; (c) a preference for politically neutral knowledge development; and (d) "knowledge development that supports rather than challenges the status quo" (p. 118). When used in nursing practice and education, these assumptions foster ignoring racism (in the belief that society is essential equitable), treating racism as a problem of individual behavior (in congruence with individualism), and ignoring the larger social and cultural sources of inequities that sustain racism, classism, and sexism. Consequently, nursing fails to develop knowledge regarding racialization and racism, thus perpetuating the status quo. In contrast, exposing rather than ignoring these assumptions offers the opportunity to analyze dynamics of difference, racialization, and racism in nursing educational and practice settings. Such exposure can begin with turning attention to language, including the ways that both individualism and dichotomies are embedded in language.

CHALLENGES AND TENSIONS: LANGUAGE AS CONTEXT

Language is important in dealing with racism because language both obscures and sustains racism. Poststructuralist understanding of language suggests that we inherit the language of the society into which we are born, and thus we are able to share meanings with other members of the society. However, the language we use is a fundamental constraint to what is and can be known. In telling our stories, we draw on the language available to us, and the narratives we use are shaped by the purpose of the narratives and the contexts within which they are told (Hardin, 2003). Language does not merely reflect reality, it constructs reality by substituting words for direct experience. For example, we read a story in a newspaper about events we did not experience firsthand, but use words to construct what we think of as knowledge of the events. Through language we also develop our understanding of who we are, what our values are, and what we believe in—thus creating our *selves*.

In relation to racism, then, we are limited by the language available (e.g., dichotomies such as black and white), draw on the language available (e.g., by using racializing categories such as "Asian"), choose certain stories in line with our purposes and interests, and thereby create certain selves and realities. Bell (2003) illustrates how narratives are shaped by the purpose for which and the context within which they are told. Her analysis of stories of racism told by a sample of college educated adults in the United States shows how those stories told by people of color and some White people focused on the enduring features of racism and the slow pace of change, whereas the stories told by the majority of White people in the study were almost a mirror opposite. In keeping with other studies that show how we use language to show our selves in the best light with regard to racism (Gillespie, Ashbaugh, & DeFiore, 2002; Levine-Rasky, 2000; Schick, 2000), bell's analysis was that most stories tended to "minimize racism, trumpet dramatic progress, and portray [U.S.] society as either color blind or compensating almost to the point of 'reverse racism'" (p. 22) in ways that positioned the people telling the stories as good, fair, and progressive. Indeed Dlamini (2002), Schick, and Gillespie et al. illustrate that superficially admitting to one's privilege can function as a strategy to distance oneself from racism and complicity. Bell goes on to point out, however, that with analysis, such stories open up possibilities for examining contradictions, creating **race cognizance** and imagining new stories.

Language also has a performative aspect; it can accomplish changes in status and/or actively create entities. An example of the performative function of language is the Christian wedding service in which the priest or chaplain declares, "I now pronounce you husband and wife" and the couple utters the words "I do." The performative function of language brings about conceptual entities such as culture and society; these do not exist outside of the ways in which we talk about them or participate with others in social and cultural spaces. For example, racializing people, that is, distinguishing and labeling people on the basis of physical characteristics or arbitrary ethnic or racial categories, and dealing with people based on beliefs related to those labels (Agnew, 1998) has a performative aspect. Labeling individuals or groups (Vietnamese, Chinese, Aboriginal, and so on) centers their identity on race and creates and sustains racial categories. While we need ways of referring to particular contexts and the experiences of groups and individuals, we need to search for and create alternative ways of speaking. Keeping the *person* in the foreground, rather than the *label*, and *being accurate* regarding the experience in question are two important strategies. Rather than using the category of "Indocanadian" in developing a diabetes program, nurses began to talk about "people who emigrated from India." In doing so, the nurses realized that they actually were concerned about people with diabetes who spoke Punjabi or Hindi as their first language and who could not access the existing diabetic clinic offered in English only. Speaking in this way helped the nurses center the concerns of language, access, and diabetes, rather than centering identity on race. Doing so helped focus on barriers to health care access rather than upon the patients as "deficient."

Most pertinent for discussion of race, racism, and diversity in the nursing classroom, is this idea that conceptual entities such as culture or society do not exist outside of the ways in which we talk about or participate in them. Allen and Hardin (2001) demonstrate that "social structure is an *effect* of taking up practices and reproducing and modifying them" (emphasis in original, p. 163). In this view, culture and society are daily performances by all members of the group(s) constituting society. Each day we recreate or reproduce society in our interactions. Although society may seem fairly static or unchanging, attitudes and behaviors do shift over time. This means that both teachers and students have daily opportunities to change our collective reality by consciously changing how we interact as colearners/coteachers, and how we interact with the substantive professional materials that shape our work. Because society does not exist out there as a real entity, we have daily opportunities to shape social interaction by what we say and do. Thus, alternative discourses, languages of resistance, and space for alternative discourses and diverse voices are central to antiracist pedagogy.

WESTERN SOCIETY AS CONTEXT

Working and living within Western society, we are shaped by particular dominant ways of thinking about and living out the ideas of race. Despite extensive critique of racism and wide acceptance of the idea that race is a social construction, race is experienced and lived as a social–cultural reality and has profound influences on us all. Particularly important to this discussion of nursing education are the ideology and practices of color blindness. Henry, Tator, Mattis, and Rees (2000a) describe color blindness as a powerful liberal discourse in which people "insist that they do not notice the skin color of a racial-minority person" (p. 27). In this way of thinking, we are all the same; experiences of inequity based on race (as it intersects with gender, class, and so on) are overlooked, and attention is diverted away from difference and privilege. And as argued earlier, people in positions of racial privilege (including most importantly in North America, **White privilege**) can position themselves in blameless ways. Thus, rather than promoting equity, color blindness supports seeing the world from dominant perspectives. For example, in their study of Anglo Australian nurses, Blackford and Street (2002) found that treating all people the same hid cultural differences and the imposition of dominant perspectives and led to inequitable nursing care. Nurses saw the need for interpreters as disruptive and treated the care (such as baby baths) in medicalized ways so that migrant women lost confidence in their own abilities.

In Western societies, white skin confers unearned privilege. However, dominance and uncritical acceptance of White privilege sustain racism, not Whiteness per se (Gillespie et al., 2002). And uncritical acceptance of White privilege is taken up not only by White people. Re'em (2001) illustrates this effectively in his study with black

Christian U.S. school children. In the context of color blindness and a focus on their Christian identity, the children crafted identities of themselves that associated them with "White and normal" in contrast to Jewish people as "dark and other" (p. 381). The children expected Jewish people, including those in the Bible and Re'em himself to be dark skinned and were surprised to find that he was "normal" or "a regular guy" despite the fact that he was white skinned. Re'em argues that color blindness goes hand in hand with what King (1991) calls **dysconscious racism**, the habit of uncritically justifying inequity and exploitation by accepting inequity and exploitation as just the way things are.

Color blindness is not blind to color, but to inequity. Henry et al. (2000a) argue that in Canada color blindness facilitates what they call liberal democratic racism, in which Canadian values for fairness, equality and social justice coexist with discrimination and institutionalized racism. This democratic racism encompasses a variety of other interrelated discourses such as the discourses of equal opportunity, of reverse racism, of White victimization, and importantly, multiculturalism. Multiculturalism pervades Canadian society (Brown & Kelly, 2001; Henry, et al., 2000a; Ng, 1995) and is a fundamental idea underlying most public policy related to culture and race in Canada. Multiculturalism depends on color blindness and the assumption that we are all equal and that we all exist on a level playing field. Of course, we are all not equal in terms of life chances, opportunities, and resources, and this view overlooks such structural inequities and the impact of colonization, conditions of immigration (including historical and ongoing slavery and human trafficking), and racism. Multiculturalism is synchronous with liberal individualism. Given the liberal ideology which also pervades Western society, individuals are held responsible for their life chances and opportunities, for their successes and failures, and structural inequities are ignored. Therefore, a person who is disadvantaged by racism (say, for example, poverty due to lack of employment opportunity) is held accountable for these disadvantages and race rather than racism is implied as the cause, thus blaming the victim (Henry, et al., p. 384). In fact, Henry et al. argue that through such dynamics, multiculturalism actually serves to keep certain ethnic groups on the margins of Western societies. If everyone is seen to have similar opportunities, then failure to achieve is the individual's fault and there is no commitment to correcting structural inequities.

NURSING AND HEALTH CARE AS CONTEXT

How, then, do these dynamics play out in nursing and health care? As Browne (2001) notes, liberalism and its predominant feature, individualism, are so interwoven into the fabric of Western society that it is almost impossible to recognize the extent to which it shapes our social, political, and scientific assumptions and practices. Multiculturalism has become policy in Canada and other places with diverse populations and liberal agendas, including the United Kingdom (Culley, 1996; Foolchand, 2000) and Australia (Swendson & Windsor, 1996). Widely disseminated in state organizations, including health care settings, it has profound but often invisible effects on organizations and individuals. Henry et al. (2000b) argue that under multiculturalism, racism is institutionalized in human service organizations through ethnocentric and monocultural

(English only, expert-driven and science-driven) values and programs, the devaluing of minority practitioners, lack of minority representation in decision-making positions, and inadequate funding for, and thus little access to, ethnoracial community-based services. These authors argue that these dynamics encourage nurses to treat all patients the same, obscuring differences and inequities.

REPEAT ABORTION

One year I was teaching a clinical course in which students were to complete change projects in various community health care agencies. Students selected projects with the guidance of field guides, typically leaders within the agency. Two students assigned to an abortion clinic reported back that the clinic staff asked them to complete a project on "Repeat Abortion and South Asian Women," based on the idea that such women were "repeaters" at the clinic. When the students reported this in class, I was aghast. And although the pair of students did not seem to have any reservations about the project, I could see that other students (particularly those who might be racialized as "South Asian") were disturbed. I tried to respond in a way that would address the stereotypes and assumptions that would underlie such a project. "Who are they calling South Asian?" I asked. "What is the basis for identifying this as a concern?" The students quickly realized that the staff included diverse women in this category (women who immigrated from many countries, women born in Canada, women who spoke at least 10 different languages including English as their first languages) and that the staff did not have any evidence that some women were more likely to experience repeat abortion than any other. No statistics were kept and no record of ethnicity of women was ever made. In the course of the project, staff had directed the students to consult with several ethnic-based health care organizations. Personnel at one of these organizations were openly angry at what they saw as a project based on racist assumptions. In the face of these reactions, the students were disturbed at their own complicity, and initially wanted to request a clinical placement change. With support, they compromised and completed a project on repeat abortion generally, analyzing influential factors such as health care access and the role of violence and abuse in reproductive decision making. They prepared research-based resource materials for the clinic staff to promote understanding of these issues. I met with the clinic staff and students to facilitate this shift in the project and tried to walk a fine line between sharing our concerns (the students, mine) and alienating the clinic staff and the otherwise valuable clinical placement.

The students in this case felt that they had a profoundly important learning experience, and felt that they had carried out their work in an ethical way. However, a year later, field guides from the same clinic asked other students to carry out the exact same project.

This story reminded us of the importance of taking into account how nursing education and practice occur within a wider, powerful social context. This wider context shapes not only ourselves, students, and practice settings, but the nature of nursing and nursing education.

Western nursing is often talked about as a gendered profession, but rarely acknowledged to be both class based and raced. The particular histories of diversity, racism, and antiracism within the nursing profession vary with specific contexts. In western Canada, registered nursing[4] has been predominantly occupied by lower and middle income White women. However, over the past few decades the ethnic diversity of staff nurses has burgeoned. A cursory glance reveals that this diversification has not yet significantly affected leadership or teaching roles, where White women still predominate.

In addition to a lack of diversity among teachers, racism can be institutionalized in nursing education through the use of ethnocentric and monocultural knowledge, theories, and learning approaches and the underuse or devaluing of educational resources from ethnically and racially diverse sources. In a study of the portrayal of African Americans in nursing fundamentals textbooks in the United States, Byrne (2001) found that few African American leaders were included, and racial bias and stereotyping were apparent. Byrne concluded that differences were often discussed using Eurocentric norms and that language tended to minimize racism and emphasize assimilation. Browne (2001) argues that nursing knowledge has been developed within the political ideology of liberalism, thus promoting understanding that maintains current positions of dominance, including racial privilege. The liberal focus on individuals and the ideas of free choice and responsibility for decisions are integral to many nursing theories used in Western nursing curricula such as theories by Newman, Parse, Mitchell, and Cody (Browne, 2001; Hartrick-Doane & Varcoe, 2005a). Such ideas are based on Eurocentric models of individuals, families, and communities, and do not take systematic inequity and privilege explicitly into account. Therefore, such theories do not serve nurses adequately in contexts (such as the contexts of Aboriginal health) where more communal understandings of individuals, families, and communities pervade, and where understandings of systematic inequity are fundamental to understanding health. Similarly, concepts widely used in nursing are often congruent with such ways of thinking. For example, Murphy and Canales (2001) point out that the idea of compliance is most often accepted uncritically in nursing literature. The idea that individuals (as patients) should act in their own best interests and that this usually involves following expert advice (e.g., by taking medications) is consistent with liberal ideas and overlooks inequities (such as poverty and unemployment intersecting with racism) that might prevent compliance (such as the ability to afford medication). Even attempts to develop knowledge in nursing about people who are marginalized paradoxically may be **marginalizing** through stereotyping and overlooking dehumanizing and marginalizing environments (Meleis & Im, 1999). For example, the idea of risk behavior is used widely in nursing, and can be applied to individual behavior (e.g., sexual practices and risk for HIV or other infections) without taking into account how racism and other inequities create risk,

---

[4] Other forms of nursing that pay less, have less prestige, or require fewer years of education, such as license practical nurse or care aides or psychiatric nurse—may be more accessible to racialized individuals (Puzan, 2003). For example, for several years now, English-speaking nurses with baccalaureate degrees who immigrate from counties such as the Philippines have not been permitted to practice as registered nurses in Canada; however, they are allowed to work in some other (usually lower paying) category of nursing, or may be offered domestic work such as child care. At the same time because there was a nursing shortage in Canada, nurses from countries such as England and Australia were being actively recruited to work in major American and Canadian hospitals. This is an example of the way that job segmentation can discriminate against workers. For example, segmentation has been used to create separate categories within the nursing staff with variable salaries. These practices have been used to pay nurses of color less than their White counterparts and assign nurses of color to heavier units such as long term care (Das Gupta, 1996; Glazer, 1991).

such as through despair, incarceration, or poverty that requires sex in exchange for survival (Krieger, 1999; Zierler & Krieger, 1997; Zierler, et al., 2000). Nursing knowledge also can be used in ways that maintain rather than challenge racism and inequity. For example, using an example of Black women and crack cocaine use in an uncritical manner in teaching could inadvertently reinforce stereotyping and discrimination.

Only recently have decolonizing and antiracist perspectives joined critical and feminist views in North American nursing literature. Curricula vary greatly from school to school, but it is probably safe to claim that nursing does not draw routinely on the rich postcolonial, anticolonial, and antiracist literature available in fields such as education, philosophy, and cultural studies. However, the increasing diversity of voices in nursing literature offers hope for a widening of perspectives. For example, Banks-Wallace (2000) offers an important contribution to the ways of knowing discourse in nursing, "womanist ways of knowing," which are ways of knowing developed from understanding of the intersections of African American women's gendered, classed, and *raced* experiences. Taylor (1998, 2000, 2002) takes a similar perspective in her work with African American women who experience male partner violence, illustrating how a "womanist" approach to research creates knowledge that is in contrast to dominant understandings, but relevant and useful to African American women. In another example, a group of researchers have conducted analyses of how race is used in nursing research (Drevdahl, Taylor, & Phillips, 2001), with a view to fostering more critical interpretation and conduct of nursing research. In their review of research published in the journal *Nursing Research*, race and ethnic variables were rarely defined, race and ethnic labels were often intermixed, and the majority of studies provided no information about how categorization of the participant's race or ethnicity was made. In addition, there was relatively little growth in the number of studies that had racial/ethnic groups, other than Whites, as the majority of the sample.

If nursing as a profession is to take difference and race seriously, we can begin by analyzing the Eurocentric roots of our theories. We can refuse to offer only a Eurocentric vision by using articles and books and assignments that draw on a diversity of ideas, ways of knowing, and authors. For example, with rare exceptions, in Western nursing literature and texts, most references to nursing history begin with or emphasize Florence Nightingale and her disciples. Where would we begin if not with Nightingale? That is, what are the alternatives? Lynne Young (editor of this collection) searched for alternatives while presenting on curricula in Japan. The nurses with whom she spoke did not have alternatives. However, a physician directed her to a story of Iwa Uryu, a woman born in Kitakata in 1829. From the limited information Young was able to obtain, she learned that prior to the mid-1800s, nursing in Japan was carried out by women in families. Iwa Uryu nursed wounded soldiers during the Boshin Civil War and raised children who were orphaned by that war. She apparently established an organization to help orphans and children from poor families, built a hospital, and established a training school for nurses. Young saw the fact that the nurses could not provide her with an alternative to Nightingale as an example of the power of colonialism. Failing to actively seek alternatives not only "distorts and excludes [the] histories, contributions, and lived experiences" (Brown & Kelly, 2001, p. 501) of many students, teachers, and future patients, but also constrains and limits our curricula and our vision for nursing.

TEACHING AS CONTEXT

Teaching/learning spaces always involve unequal power dynamics, and are thus a potent medium within which to discuss race/racism. Teaching is always a political act, even if the teacher claims to be neutral or is not critically aware of power dynamics. Regardless of commitments to power sharing approaches to teaching (commitments both authors of this chapter share) teachers are always in positions of power relative to their students. As teachers our power is not limited to assigning lower or higher grades, or to passing or failing a student in a given course. Rather, because of our responsibilities to our profession and ultimately to patients, and because of our participation in generally hierarchical educational institutions, our power often extends to facilitating entry or baring access to a student's chosen profession.

To engage students in conversations about race and racism is an exercise of power. And such an exercise of power must be undertaken cautiously. Despite Audrey Lourde's (1984) maxim that the oppressor is in all of us, it is far easier to point to the oppressive practices of others. This, we think, extends to teachers pointing out the oppressive acts of students while failing to examine their own practices. In this, we agree with bell hooks (1994) who explains that she will not expect students to take risks that she herself will not take.

■ WRIGGLING OUT

A few years ago I[5] *taught for the first time a course titled "Self and Others." It was one of three courses that focus on the nurse in relation to others; this particular course incorporated concepts of collaborative group work, largely based on Peggy Chinn's (2001) feminist model. Assignments and learning activities were designed to help students reflect on "who they bring to practice"—the social, cultural, and familial patterns that shaped them into the people they are today, how these factors affected the kind of person they had become, and in turn, how this affected their practice. A major purpose in exploring these issues was to create awareness in students of their own biases, prejudices, blind spots, and to help them recognize how these can affect their relationships with patients and families in practice.*

Our campus is located in one of the most ethnically diverse areas of Canada, and the classroom and practice settings reflect this diversity. Students routinely share stories of their experiences of racism in practice settings (directed at staff, patients and families, and the students themselves). When exploring these stories, I often asked students what they said or did in response. The most common response from students was "I didn't know what to say so I didn't say anything." If pressed, most students said that they were "just students" and that the person making the racist remarks had more power and authority than they did (sometimes it was an instructor) and furthermore they were concerned that speaking out might jeopardize their clinical rotation. Often students said something like, "I just wanted to finish that course and move on. I didn't want any trouble." Discussions in class included exploration of why silence or not speaking might be interpreted as silent assent to the racist remarks or behaviors. Reasoning that part of the problem was that these situations occur without

[5] The first-person "I" in this section is that of author Janice McCormick.

warning, and that when they occurred, students were shocked and unprepared, course writers created an assignment to give students an opportunity to rehearse a "script" that would enable them to register their disagreement with what was happening, while maintaining relationships with people such as preceptors and instructors. The assignment was a group project called "Interrupting Racism," widely regarded as important by instructors who had taught the course previously.

Prior to this assignment (which was near the end of the course), I reviewed the syllabus in detail, including going over the assignments. The written instructions for the assignment were:

> *Working in groups of six to seven, students create an unscripted videotaped vignette examining an aspect of interrupting racism within nursing practice. Each scenario will be about 5 minutes in length and your critique of the scenario will be about 10 minutes in length. While intentions are important, it is not enough for a critique of your scenario. You need to create a scenario where you actually act out your positive intentions. Keep in mind that this assignment is about practicing the new skills that you are learning from this course, not just demonstrating previous learning from other communication courses. The idea is to get you to use the content of this course and begin to introduce it into your nursing practice. You will likely find that you discuss many of the ideas that we've talked about in class.*

In the 2 weeks before the assignment was due, I spent time in class clarifying the assignment, answering students' questions, and providing examples of what constitutes racism, and what "interrupting racism" meant. Students also had time in class to work on their group assignments. The assignment involved demonstrating how the student nurses interrupted the racism, rather than simply keeping quiet or talking about the people involved behind their backs.

During one class when students were working on their assignments, I went around to each group to discuss what scenario they planned to use for their video. Of the six groups, three had selected a scenario that did not involve race or racism. One group wanted to present a scenario that featured a female patient who refused to have a male nursing student care for her; another group's scenario involved a nursing manager who automatically assumed that a Jewish staff member would not mind working on Christmas Day because "It's not her holiday;" the third group wanted to look at the idea that female nurses tend to expect male nurses to do the heavy lifting on the unit.

I was struck by the fact that three groups had ignored the explicit instructions to address the issue of racism in practice. When I commented on this and asked for dialogue, the groups that ignored the instructions regarding racism defended their choices, arguing that the issue of importance was discrimination, and racism was just one form of discrimination. Some students became quite angry and argued with me when I tried to explain the importance of maintaining the focus on racism. In addition to several students whose families had immigrated from China or India, there were also three women in the class who identified as African Caribbean and one man who was an immigrant from Africa. At first none of these students spoke, but after several minutes of heated discussion between myself and other students, two of the African Caribbean women spoke up saying that they believed that it was important to talk about racism and not be diverted to the more general (and potentially less difficult topic) of discrimination. Ultimately, I said that I would not accept other scenarios, and insisted that all groups address racism in their videos.

Initially what was interesting to me was how angry some students were that they had to address racism, and how vigorously they tried to wriggle out of the issue of racism. I began to wonder why these students found it so difficult to approach this subject and why they tried to choose other topics, even in groups well represented by people of color. I am struck now by my implied assumption that students of color would have spoken up in their groups and actually disagree with their fellow classmates. I do not think that students of color are less likely to be biased or even racist, as I acknowledge that we are all born into a racist society and inherit unspoken (and frequently unexamined) assumptions about others. I know that often students are reluctant to openly disagree with others, especially popular, outgoing, outspoken students, in class. I think this is made more difficult by the dynamics of racism. At the time I saw the refusal to participate in "interrupting racism" as part of a larger societal reluctance to critically examine collective racism. Now I see possibilities that could be opened up through a frank exploration of the issues. This, in itself, can strengthen a sense of community in the classroom. Unlearning racism is difficult work; it requires that we all be self-reflective about our decisions and actions, and work as learners together. This work is never completed; as teachers, learners, and as human beings, we are always "in process." Such examination can be an effective tool for self-reflection and growth.

What was interesting to me[6] were the power dynamics between Janice and the students. She was able to assign the project, to decide what counted as racism—excluding discrimination against a Jewish person, and to insist on changing scenarios. I see this situation as an example of a hot spot where there is something different we could do in our teaching. This story left us both wondering what the students learned from this forced experience. We think the students' reactions suggest that they were not ready to produce such a video, that perhaps more time and work could be spent working on biases and perspectives. I think that it also points to a much larger curricular issue; racism is being presented in the curriculum (through this assignment) as a one-time concern and only attended to in one course rather than as a fundamental concept throughout the curriculum. I had a similar experience.

■ ALL "-ISMS" ARE NOT EQUAL

At the end of a course I was teaching on Women's Health, we were ready to focus intensively on commitments and action to counter various forms of oppression. I asked students to decide how we should proceed: if they wanted to work in large groups, small groups, or if they wanted to focus on populations (perhaps rural communities versus urban). Although we had been using the idea of **intersectionality** *throughout the course, the students elected to divide in groups according to -isms with which we had been working throughout the course. The sexism, heterosexism, ageism, and sizism groups filled up fast; no one, regardless of ethnicity, wanted to tackle racism.*

[6] The first-person "I" is that of author Colleen Varcoe.

I could have interpreted this as another instance of wriggling out, which I suppose it was. However, I now see this as problematic in at least two other ways. First, in my perhaps somewhat misguided commitment to student empowerment, I did not interrupt this. At the time I saw my choices as being to let it go, as the students had been given and made this decision, or to force students to deal with racism. I now see that I could have shifted discussion to focus our attention on the decision-making process and what we could learn from the avoidance of racism in that process. Second, I see this as a failure on my part to have adequately laid the ground work—the impacts of our racial histories and experiences and the philosophical underpinnings of intersectionality.

Both of these experiences point to the missed potential of using the opportunity to focus on difference as an analytic tool. In what has been called **border pedagogy** (Aveling, 2002; Giroux, 1991; Jackson, 1997; King, 2004) teachers can use differences as a focus to analyze the power relationships between and among teachers and students. Instead of insisting that students focus on racism in the video activity, Janice could have examined the students' resistance to the directions and the power to insist. Instead of going along with groups that avoided racism, Colleen could also have focused on the power dynamics in which she was more concerned with being seen to be egalitarian than with fostering critical analysis.

TRAPS FOR STUDENTS AND TEACHERS

From the analysis of our experience we think that there are some common traps that derail our attempts to develop race cognizance, unlearn, and counter racism. Many of the traps are related to the discourses of liberal democratic racism. For example, color blind ideas and sentiments such as "I'm not racist" or "I treat everyone the same" can be used by teachers and students alike to wriggle out of engaging with the real and ever present dynamics of racism. A major trap for us has been the discourse of multiculturalism. As a reasonable idea that appeals to a sense of fairness, and works with liberal individualism and common sense, it is difficult to counter. Multiculturalism focuses attention on the values and beliefs of others against an unspoken norm. And focusing on others lets everyone "off the hook" for considering their own privilege. Conversely, as Nairn, Hardy, Parumal, and Williams (2004) point out, as antiracist approaches may overlook culture, rather than favoring one or the other, exploring the tensions between multiculturalism and antiracism may be most fruitful.

As this suggests, there are traps even when teachers explicitly engage in antiracist efforts. First, behaviorism leads to the idea that learning can always be seen, heard, read, and measured, and that behavioral change equals learning. Thus, as teachers we seek evidence of students' transformation, in written assignments, videos, group work, and the like. Second, and closely related, is the idea that transformation should be immediate, or at least soon enough so that the teacher feels some satisfaction. I[7] was

[7] The first-person "I" is that of author Colleen Varcoe.

immensely relieved to read bell hooks' (1994) admission that she had to surrender her desire to have that positive and immediate feedback from all students. Dealing with racism will be uncomfortable and challenging, may not result in positive feedback for teachers, and may result in anger and student resistance to the teachers' plans. However, this opens a space for educators to work with tensions, a process that has potential to foster rich learning. This brings us to a third trap, that is, the idea that a teacher can create safety for all. This idea relies on the myth that the classroom is a neutral space, somehow isolated and protected from the larger world—a neutral space in which students can choose to act freely without fear of repercussions outside of the classroom. These traps and myths mean that each and every teaching strategy needs to be considered carefully. When we engage in antiracist pedagogy, challenging our own and students' assumptions and attitudes, the classroom may not be a comfortable place. Anger, defensiveness, and resistance all can occur as teachers and learners negotiate difficult learning tasks together.

JELLY BEANS FOR VOICE

When we began to struggle with antiracist and anticolonial pedagogy, we were told a fable about a teacher who used jelly beans to deal with the unequal participation in classrooms where White students typically dominated and students of color were often silent. The idea was that each student would begin with the same number of jelly beans (or some similar token), and could consume or give away a jelly bean for each contribution in class. Each person was to use all of his or her jelly beans, and when all of one's beans were gone, the person was expected to listen rather than speak.

Over the years, we have often tossed that fable around. Does this strategy focus on silence rather than silencing? Would doing this trivialize the challenges students, and particularly racialized students, face? Would it overlook the need for safety to speak? Does it equate voice with speaking, and is this adequate? Are other forms of expression valid? Does it overlook how we may "learn from spaces of silence"? (hooks, 1994, p.175) Does it overlook how classroom participation is contiguous with participation in the wider social world? Rather than focusing on silence, verbal participation, and safety per se, we take up the ideas of hooks. hooks says that rather than focusing on safety, teachers would do better to build community (p. 40). What follows are some of our evolving ideas regarding how to do so.

IMPLICATIONS AND STRATEGIES: BUILDING COMMUNITY AND WORKING WITH DIFFERENCE

How, then, should one go about building community that takes racism into account? What strategies can teachers use to encourage students to discuss what is going on for them? How can teachers learn to appreciate learning that may occur without the standard evidence? How can feelings of anger, guilt, or resistance be attended to constructively? How can conflict be lived through?

Reflexivity: Begin With Yourself

As hooks (1994) notes, "Teachers must be actively committed to a process of self-actualization" (p. 15). Beginning with yourself as a teacher does not mean a one-time inventory of your social locations and privileges. Rather, we believe that aiming to teach from an antiracist stance demands continuous self-reflection and action on the self. As we continue to live in societies laced with racist imagery and discourse, we need to be vigilant and active in our choices. How are we taking up and living these various discourses? We have found that being explicit about our agenda of actively dealing with race and racism, and being honest about our challenges and our privileges serves us best in creating an atmosphere in which we are comfortable teaching. Sharing your reflexive work with students models praxis, contributes to countering power imbalances between teachers and students, and sets the stage for risk taking by all.

Beginning with ourselves necessarily involves exploring the impact of our own racial identities and histories. As Dlamini (2002) demonstrates, classroom identities are negotiated by all involved, including students and teachers. Articles by Dlamini, a black woman educator who teaches students who identify themselves predominantly as White, and Gillespie et al. (2002), White women educators who also teach students who identify themselves predominantly as White, clearly illustrate how the racial identities of teachers matter. The experiences described in these two articles clearly present different but interrelated challenges. For example, Dlamini describes students challenging her as "biased against White students" (p. 63) and challenging her authority as a teacher; Gillespie et al. describe being accused of "White bashing" and saw themselves as relying on White skin privilege to gain credibility with their students.

Beginning with ourselves is prerequisite to assisting students to begin with themselves. Cook (2000) describes considerable success in helping students develop critical race cognizance through journaling based on the principles of border pedagogy. We offer another learning activity aimed at helping students tune into their own responses as a component of developing reflexivity. Although it is posed as a learning activity for students, we have found it useful as teachers (Box 20.1).

Expanding: Seek and Become Allies

Although we might begin with ourselves, we do not need to do this work alone. Few of us have had preparation in antiracist teaching, so regardless of our own identities and experiences, the wisdom of others is important. Seeking allegiances with others—through workshops, networks, meetings, and interested colleagues—offers sources of wisdom, support, and practical strategies.

Talking: Expand Language Practices

If you begin with yourself and share your reflexive work with students and allies, you can offer alternative language and discourses in advance of conversations that become problematic because they draw on racializing discourses and stereotypical thinking. For example, we have found it important to discuss what we mean by othering,

BOX 20.1 USING EMBODIED EXPERIENCE TO EXAMINE REACTIONS TO RACISM IN THE CLASSROOM

In order to help students identify embodied knowledge in relation to racism, ask students to reflect on what they are feeling in their bodies when discussions are occurring on various topics in class. Specifically, when topics that are often avoided or dealt with in a cursory manner are being examined in the classroom, including an exploration of the feelings that such conversations elicit can provide another source of knowledge or understanding. Topics such as racism often make people feel uncomfortable. Encouraging students to get in touch with these feelings can help them understand bodily rather than intellectually. Artz (1993) states that strong feelings are messages the body is sending about what one values the most—about what is most important to a person. As such, these messages are important sources of knowledge. Through reflection, individuals can enhance understanding of what the body is "saying" through these emotions.

QUESTIONS TEACHERS MIGHT ASK

It is important to keep the focus on feelings, and resist going to analysis or purely intellectual processes too early in this exercise (the final step is analytical).

- How did you feel when we talked about racism today? What feelings or emotions did you experience?
- Where did you feel it? (If no response: cues can be used such as—we often say that we know something in the gut, in the heart, or even in the bones. Was anyone nervous? How do you know you were feeling nervous? How did you feel when we ended the conversation about racism?)
- Identify one important insight that you got from this experience.

intersectionality, oppression, race, racialization, and racism before engaging in conversations that involve these ideas. Reflexively examining the stereotypes, myths, and assumptions that underlie our thinking and language invites new and more diverse ways of seeing the world.

Centering: Rethink Safety

As explained, we believe that hooks' (1994) directive to focus on building community offers more potential for constructive classroom relationships than trying to ensure safety. Whereas safety tends to imply danger, and may marginalize some individuals as at risk from others, dichotomizing oppressor and oppressed, building community fosters different dynamics of responsibility and relationship. Engaging all in the process of building community potentially can draw everyone into the center. Thus, the idea of safety may have most value as a point of discussion toward building community in the classroom. What does safety mean? Does it mean no risk? Does it mean never moving out of your comfort zone? Is it possible to engage in conversations about racism without ever feeling unsafe? Indeed we think that acknowledging the nonsafety inherent in the classroom and the world more widely may be a useful strategy.

In order to engage everyone, inclusive of all identities, and in order not to dichotomize, paradoxically, teachers must deal with "White defensiveness" (Aveling, 2002; Roman, 1993). As others have done, (Gillespie, et al., 2002) we have found it useful to emphasize that it is racism, dominance, and uncritical acceptance of privilege that is problematic (not Whiteness per se), and to focus on how racism is institutionalized and embedded in language. And we stress that individuals are not representative of particular power positions or social identities or locations.

Focusing on building community while taking difference seriously, rather than focusing on trying to ensure safety, helps to acknowledge the range of people's experiences of privilege and oppression without depoliticizing and overlooking the suffering that the most marginalized endure (Anderson, 2004). Thus, students who have experienced poverty, but also are privileged based on race, can have the fullness of their experience acknowledged without overlooking privilege. Students who have lived with racism on a daily basis can be seen as more than victims, and their privileges and capacities acknowledged.

De-centering: Introduce Marginalized Knowledge

Critical analysis of Eurocentric theories sets the stage for introducing other ways of knowing and for uncovering and reclaiming previously marginalized and subjugated knowledge (Battiste, 2000; hooks, 1994). Examining and critiquing the Eurocentric roots of theories and clinical tools can be accompanied by the exploration of alternative forms of knowledge. For example, a student recently pointed out to Colleen that an alcohol abuse screen she was using asked if close family or friends ever expressed concern about the person's drinking. The student pointed out that the screen was based on the assumption that some alcohol was acceptable, whereas, in her ethnic and religious communities any use of alcohol would be abhorred. She said that if she had even one drink, her mother would be horrified. What then, might be an alternative basis for identifying alcohol abuse?

Dei (1996) urges educators to consciously draw on more nonWestern theories, narratives, ways of knowing, perspectives, and ways of being, as well as history from subjugated knowledges and stories from the vanquished rather than the victors (who usually get to tell all the stories). In his book on antiracism pedagogy, Dei observes that what is considered knowledge in Canadian schools is an extremely narrow sample of the world's wealth of knowledge. Examination of this canon reveals an overwhelming emphasis on the history and perspectives of Western Europeans. Such approaches result in the de facto acceptance of Western knowledge, ways of thinking and viewpoints as the only acceptable pedagogical practice. The events that are seen as important, historically, socially, and culturally, are events that relate to the exploits of Europeans who are almost universally White males. Furthermore, this practice ensures the reproduction of Western, Eurocentric approaches to knowledge and knowledge development. For students of color, one of the unspoken messages received through such educational experiences is that it is only the White race that has created knowledge, explored the oceans and continents, and made the important decisions. Knowledge, theories, and perspectives of other nations and peoples are either ridiculed or ignored. Dei proposes that one way of correcting this imbalance is to introduce Afrocentric discourse and knowledge. Introduction of these knowledges and ways of thinking could help not only students of color, but all students identify the unique thinking and knowledge of various peoples, and can foster the pride of all and help to balance the current narrowness of perspective.

These insights have encouraged us to consider these ideas within a nursing context. Not only do students largely come to nursing education with these prior Eurocentric experiences; we realize that we have largely accepted the current canon of nursing knowledge, including the fact that virtually all of the nursing theories or models of nursing we know and study in North America were created by a handful of White, middle aged, middle class to upper class women, almost all of whom are from the United States. This prompts us to ask, "How are differently-centered (e.g., Afrocentric) knowledges being used to theorize nursing? What nonAmerican nursing theories exist? How do these differ from current dominant nursing theories? What would happen if we asked students to locate an alternative nursing theory, to describe it, show how it differs from the mainstream North American theories? How might expansion of inquiry into different countries and cultures affect students' perceptions of knowledge and knowledge development in nursing?"

Reclaiming marginalized knowledge is not mere altruistic inclusiveness; it may be essential to the survival of the human race. For example, indigenous knowledge is being reclaimed, not only by indigenous peoples in service of their own survival, but also by many who seek a more harmonious coexistence among people and their environments (Battiste, 2000; Battiste & Youngblood Henderson, 2000). Drawing on the knowledge and history of various groups is not a matter of inserting stereotypes into learning or treating such knowledge as an add-on. For example, teachers developing a nephrology nursing course used case studies, but by linking certain health problems (drug use, diabetes) to certain groups, invited stereotypical thinking rather than understanding. Instead, drawing on marginalized knowledge means drawing on more diverse sources in teaching including articles and other forms of knowledge by diverse authors, stories of strength, and health among all groups and interrogating the basis of inclusion or exclusion of such knowledge. Such reclaiming can be done in a range of nursing contexts: a pharmacology course might attend to relationships between traditional use of herbs and other natural substances and current drugs; a nursing ethics or a nursing theory course might draw on a wider range of philosophers. As racism pervades our societies, such knowledge is salient to every course and classroom.

Re-"framing": Work the Context

Suggesting that racism ought to be addressed in every aspect of curriculum means taking action outside of particular classrooms. Lobbying for racism to be dealt with as a pervasive feature of our social world requires rethinking curriculum concepts such as context and culture. It requires efforts to promote the diversification of teachers and leaders in practice, and of the student body. It also requires working toward equity in policy, both within educational and health care settings.

Arguing that racism is a pervasive feature of our social world requires turning attention to the social world beyond the classroom. First, we must recognize that the lives of our students within the classroom are continuous with the rest of their lives. As Brown and Kelly (2001) argue, students come with histories, values, and perceptions that shape the classroom, their reading of the curriculum, and their learning. For example, students' actions within the classroom can result in repercussions outside the classroom, within themselves, from fellow students, and from others. Numerous students have told us of going home after class and "seeing" their family or friends in a new light which sometimes created disorientation and distress for the student. Second, urging our students to action outside the classroom, for example, in clinical settings, must take into account their positions within that context. As our repeat abortion story suggests, the context of practice shapes possibilities in powerful ways.

Relevance: Offer Experiential Opportunities

Rather than talking about racism in the abstract, we have found experiential learning to be most powerful. King (2004) builds on the work of others arguing that service experiences are important learning experiences within border pedagogy. King describes service experiences wherein students literally cross national borders, but within nursing the same potential may be tapped by helping students cross borders into places beyond the usual purview of health care providers. Indeed we have found that nontraditional experiences facilitate the development of race cognizance. We offer an experiential learning activity that invites students to cross borders in other ways (Box 20.2).

BOX 20.2 REFLECTIVE FIELD WORK: EMPIRICAL KNOWING

In this assignment, you are asked to do an observational exercise. You are asked to choose a public location where you might observe culture in action. You are asked to record your observations over 30 minutes, and then to analyze those observations in terms of race, racism, and health. Here is how to proceed:

(a) Choose a location in a public setting where you can observe a variety of people.

(b) Spend 30 minutes in the location of your choice purposefully observing. Observe the world around you in careful detail, and record your observations. What are you seeing, hearing, smelling, and feeling? Record your observations on one half of your paper divided vertically.

(c) Analyze your observations. What did you pay attention to, and why? What does this tell you about culture, race, racialization, and racism? And what does this tell you about how you are participating in your culture?

Identify one important insight you have had from this experience.

QUESTIONS TEACHERS MIGHT ASK

- Ask students to ask themselves *how* they knew what to call or label what they were observing, or how they knew to use the label they did for the analysis part of the exercise.
- Ask students one way in which they think their observations and analysis were shaped by their own racial histories.

Humility: Work With Conflict

Teaching can seductively pull us into positions of authority, power, and expertise. And dealing with race and racism seems invariably to create tension and conflict. Rather than dealing with such conflict by asserting power, however, we have found it more constructive to take a stance of humility. First, we have found it useful to claim our own struggles. Second, we have found it useful to follow the advice of hooks (1994) and others to acknowledge pain and anger; the pain that racism causes us all in individual interactions, in the classroom, in institutions, in acts of genocide, and subjugation between nation states. Indeed, Audre Lourde (1984) says that any discussion of racism must include the recognition of and use of anger. Finally, we are striving to use anger, conflict, and student resistance to our agendas as points for learning, for ourselves and not just our students. In keeping with the ideas of border pedagogy we look to these experiences as opportunities to examine power and difference and create new knowledge. If resistance arises, we now search for the roots of that resistance, not just in the students, but in ourselves and our teaching practices. As hooks so eloquently describes, we work to surrender our desire for immediate affirmation of good teaching. I (Colleen) find this difficult. Negative comments in evaluations of teaching painfully stand out. For example, "Don't dump too much on White bashing," or "address the dominant culture in a respectful way so that they do not feel guilty" or "it would be nice to have more discussion around the various cultures and some specific differences between them." But, she tries to engage with each of these as a slightly different opportunity for learning about teaching. We recognize with others (Aveling, 2002; Gillespie, et al., 2002) that such work will always be demanding of our emotional labor. And as Dlamini (2002) points out, we cannot assume that all students given the right conditions will join with us in our quest to end racism.

SUMMARY

Teaching nursing from an explicitly antiracist stance infuses our work with purpose, challenge, and hope. It requires careful examination of the ideologies of liberalism and multiculturalism, and the introduction of alternative discourses and ideas such as intersectionality and racialization. Weaving such work into nursing requires developing a critical awareness of the Eurocentric and liberal ideological roots of our theories and ideas, and working toward alternatives. In the process, we believe that we must begin with a stance of humility and ongoing examination of our own biases and perspectives. It requires introducing alternative language, conceptual tools, and previously subjugated knowledge, building community rather than focusing on safety in the classroom, and extending that building of community beyond the classroom to the wider context.

We have the immense privilege and opportunity of teaching the most amazing, diverse, vibrant students. We have the opportunity of continuously learning how to live the curriculum goal of being fully colearners and coteachers with our students, learning to let go of the desire to have all the answers, and to hold all the power. We have the opportunity to learn, to listen as well as speak and to follow as well as lead.

LEARNING ACTIVITY

McIntosh (1998) suggests the following learning activity as a process to help students explore their relative positions of privilege and oppression in a possibly safe and familiar context (small group discussions with fellow students). The proposed exercises move from the easy to address (one's disadvantages), to those more risky (one's positionality in privilege). The process she suggests is:

1. Working with a group of four or five students, and adhering ***strictly*** to a rule of equal time for every student, name and describe some effects of **one** *unearned disadvantage* you have had in life. Anyone who takes more time than is allotted may be privileging himself or herself.
2. Next, still adhering to the rule of equal "air time," name an *unearned advantage* you have had in your life (that has not been already mentioned by another student).
3. Discuss a way you have seen White privilege at work in particular contexts. (Here we think preparatory work on institutionalized versus individual privilege is essential.) We suggest asking students to focus on practice settings and the classroom. The rule of equal air time still applies.
4. Name one way in which you can use your power to share power in your context or use privilege to weaken systems of unearned privilege. The rule of equal air time still applies.
5. Have each person discuss some frustrations, difficulties, and/or payoffs in structuring the uses of time in this way during these discussions. McIntosh notes that she hopes people will begin to understand that time use habits will be seen as one more aspect of privilege and that when everyone takes equal time this represents a sharing of power.

RESOURCES FOR EDUCATORS

PLANNING THE TEACHING/LEARNING EXPERIENCE

Instructions for Educators

One especially pivotal idea we have been working on is the stance that race, racialization, and racism cannot be add-ons—just another topic we toss into the class every once in a while. Rather, these ideas need to be integrated into the whole curriculum. This spurred Janice to use topics of racism as examples in the research class she was teaching. For example, she posed the question of why race is such a pervasive fact of life, but we avoid the topic in our research. Racism is evident in the stories students tell of their experiences in health care settings, but we do not talk about it or design studies to explore its features or how we can dismantle the structures that keep it firmly in place.

When Janice related this story to Colleen later, she remarked that it would have been interesting to ask students what their embodied experiences of that interaction were; what did they experience in their gut or heart? During the next class, Janice posed this question to the class. Two students said they felt mildly anxious when she began to talk about racism. One student said, "I thought, 'oh! Where is she going with this?'" Another said she felt her stomach tense a bit as we were involved in the discussion. Janice noticed that not one student looked bored during this discussion; they were all alert, interested, and involved. Her interpretation is that as issues of racism and racialization reflect the everyday reality for many students, the discussion was pertinent to their lives and their practice as nurses. Furthermore, as the teacher she felt interested and involved in the class, and had a sense that the class had engaged in a meaningful discussion on a relevant topic. As a follow up, Janice encouraged students to be more aware of what they are feeling and to reflect on what their bodies are "telling them." This kind of reflection, engaged in thoughtfully and regularly, can become a way of knowing (Artz, 1993). Artz shows how feelings can be a window into understanding one's values. For example, feeling badly about something one has done (or neglected to do) is a clue that one may not have lived up to one's beliefs or values, or that others have violated one's values in some way.

EVALUATING THE TEACHING/LEARNING EXPERIENCE

Reflective Questions for Educators

1. How is your own social location at the intersection of systems of privilege such as gender, class, and ability, shaped by race? For example, if you have had access to education, safe housing, and food security (examples of privileges), how is that access shaped by race?
2. How do the social locations and privileges of your students vary, and how do they compare to yours? What might the consequences of differences or similarities be?
3. How does the power of the teacher influence classroom dynamics? What role does race play in these power dynamics? How might your position of power interact with student subject positions in ways that supplant silence, and even oppress?
4. How do we promote a culture in the classroom that encourages teachers and learners to learn from each other?
5. How do we create a sense of community in the classroom across ethnic, cultural, gender, class, religious, and ideological differences?

Questions to Elicit Feedback from Students on Their Learning

1. How have race, racism, and racialization been dealt with in your previous teaching/learning experiences?
2. What range of reaction can you imagine that you and your fellow learners might have in response to explicit analysis in the classroom of race and racism?
3. What are the risks and dangers of such explicit analysis? Of no explicit analysis?
4. Think of an example from practice in which race and racializing processes played a role, what were the dynamics and how are they related to health promotion and ethical practice?

Sample Evaluation Strategies and Tools

Signs of boredom can help you identify when you need to change what you are doing:

1. Pay attention to the way students appear in class. Are they alert? Do they participate in class? (i.e., do they attempt to answer when you pose a question?) Do they look bored? (i.e., head in hands, looking around, or talking to colleagues?)
2. Pay attention to what you are feeling. If you feel tense or experience silence, ask yourself why.
3. In your own style, share your observations with the class. For example, you might say, "I am noticing that there seems to be a lack of energy today. Shall we try something different?" Perhaps the students were up late completing a paper, or perhaps you are not being engaging. In any event, recognizing student responses, and being sensitive to their experience in class, you can recognize earlier when you need to switch topics, end the lecture or "talking to" part of the class, and ask students to participate in a small group learning activity that engages them in a task.

References

Agnew, V. (1998). *In search of a safe place: Abused women and culturally sensitive services.* Toronto: University of Toronto Press.

Allen, D. G. (1999). Knowledge, politics, culture, and gender: A discourse perspective. *Canadian Journal of Nursing Research, 30*(4), 227–234.

Allen, D., & Hardin, P. K. (2001). Discourse analysis and the epidemiology of meaning. *Nursing Philosophy,* 2(2), 163–176.

Anderson, J. (2004). The conundrums of binary categories: Critical inquiry through the lens of postcolonial feminist humanism. *Canadian Journal of Nursing Research, 36*(4), 11–16.

Anderson, J., & Kirkham, S. R. (1998). Constructing nation: The gendering and racializing of the Canadian health care system. In V. Strong-Boag, S. Grace, A. Eisenberg, et al. (Eds.), *Painting the maple: Essays on race, gender, and the construction of Canada* (pp. 242–261). Vancouver, BC: University of British Columbia Press.

Applebaum, B. (1997). Good liberal intentions are not enough! Racism, intentions, and moral responsibility. *Journal of Moral Education, 26*(4), 409–421.

Artz, S. (1993). Feeling as a way of knowing. *Journal of Child and Youth Care, 8*(4), 1–11.

Ashcroft, B., Griffiths, G., & Tiffin, H. (2000). *Post-colonial studies: The key concepts.* New York: Routledge.

Aveling, N. (2002). Student teachers' resistance to exploring racism: Reflections on "doing" border pedagogy. *Asia-Pacific Journal of Teacher Education, 30*(2), 119–130.

Banks-Wallace, J. (2000). Womanist ways of knowing: Theoretical considerations for research with African American women. *Advances in Nursing Science, 22*(3), 33–47.

Battiste, M. (Ed.). (2000). *Reclaiming indigenous voice and vision.* Vancouver, BC: University of British Columbia Press.

Battiste, M., & Youngblood Henderson, J. (2000). *Protecting indigenous knowledge and heritage.* Saskatoon, SK: Purich.

Bell, L. A. (2003). Telling tales: What stories can teach us about racism. *Race, Ethnicity & Education, 6*(1), 3.

Bhabha, H. (1994). *The location of culture.* London: Routledge.

Blackford, J., & Street, A. (2002). Cultural conflict: The impact of western feminism(s) on nurses caring for women of non-English speaking background. *Journal of Clinical Nursing, 11*(5), 664–671.

Brewer, R. M. (1993). Theorizing race, class and gender: The new scholarship of Black feminist intellectuals and Black women's labor. In S. M. James & A. P. A. Busia (Eds.), *Theorizing Black feminism: The visionary pragmatism of Black women* (pp. 13–30). London: Routledge.

Brown, R. M. (1974). The last straw. In C. Bunch & N. Myron (Eds.), *Class and feminism* (pp. 14–23). Baltimore: Diana Press.

Brown, D., & Kelly, J. (2001). Curriculum and the classroom: Private and public spaces. *British Journal of Sociology of Education, 22*(4), 501–518.

Browne, A. J. (2001). The influence of liberal political ideology on nursing practice. *Nursing Inquiry, 8*(2), 118–129.

Browne, A. J., & Fiske, J. (2001). First Nations women's encounters with mainstream health care services. *Western Journal of Nursing Research, 23*(2), 126–147.

Browne, A. J., Johnson, J. L., Bottorff, J. L., et al. (2002). Recognizing discrimination in nursing practice. *Canadian Nurse, 98*(5), 24–27.

Byrne, M. M. (2001). Uncovering racial bias in nursing fundamentals textbooks. *Nursing and Health Care Perspectives, 22*(6), 299–303.

Chinn, P. L. (2001). *Peace & power: Building communities for the future* (5th ed.). New York: NLN Press.

Chow, J. C.-C., Jaffee, K., & Snowden, L. (2003). Racial/ethnic disparities in the use of mental health services in poverty areas. *American Journal of Public Health, 93*(5), 792–798.

Collins, P. H. (1993). Toward a new vision: Race, class, and gender as categories of analysis and connection. *Race, Sex & Class, 1*(1), 25–45.

Condliffe, B. (2001). Racism in nursing: A critical realist approach. *Nursing Times, 97*(32), 40–41.

Cook, I. (2000). "Nothing can ever be the case of 'Us' and 'Them' again": Exploring the politics of difference through border pedagogy and student journal writing. *Journal of Geography in Higher Education, 24*(1), 13.

Culley, L. (1996). A critique of multiculturalism in health care: The challenge for nurse education. *Journal of Advanced Nursing, 23*(3), 564–570.

Das Gupta, T. (1996). *Racism and paid work.* Toronto: Garamond.

Dei, G. J. S. (1996). *Anti-racism education: Theory and practice.* Halifax, NS: Fernwood.

Derrida, J. (1978). *Writing and difference.* London: Routledge & Kegan Paul.

Dlamini, S. N. (2002). From the other side of the desk: Notes on teaching about race when racialised. *Race Ethnicity and Education, 5*(1), 51–66.

Drevdahl, D., Taylor, J., & Phillips, D. (2001). Race and ethnicity as variables in nursing research, 1952–2000. *Nursing Research, 50*(5), 305–313.

Essed, P. (1990). *Everyday racism: Reports from two cultures.* Amsterdam: Hunterhouse.

Essed, P. (1991). *Understanding everyday racism: An interdisciplinary theory.* London: Sage.

Foolchand, M. K. (2000). The role of the Department of Health and other key institutions in the promotion of equal opportunities: Multi-cultural and anti-racist issues in nurse education. *Nurse Education Today, 20*(6), 443–448.

Freshwater, D. (2000). Crosscurrents: Against cultural narration in nursing. *Journal of Advanced Nursing, 32*(2), 481–484.

Gillespie, D., Ashbaugh, L., & DeFiore, J. (2002). White women teaching white women about white privilege, race congnizance and social action: Toward a pedagogical pragmatics. *Race Ethnicity and Education, 5*(3), 237–253.

Giroux, H. A. (1991). Democracy and the discourse of cultural difference: Towards a politics of border pedagogy. *British Journal of Sociology of Education, 12*(4), 501–519.

Giroux, H. A. (1992). *Border crossings.* New York: Routledge.

Glazer, N. Y. (1991). "Between a rock and a hard place": Women's professional organizations in nursing and class, racial, and ethnic inequalities. *Gender & Society, 5*(3), 351–372.

Gray, P., Kramer, M., Minick, P., et al. (1996). Heterosexism in nursing education. *Journal of Nursing Education, 35*(4), 204–210.

Hagey, R., Choudhry, U., Guruge, S., et al. (2001). Immigrant nurses' experiences of racism. *Journal of Nursing Scholarship, 33*(4), 389–394.

Hankivsky, O. (1996). Resistance to change: Exploring the dynamics of backlash. London: Centre for Research on Violence Against Women and Children. Available at http://www.crvawc.ca/docs/pub_hankivsky1996.pdf.

Hardin, P. K. (2003). Constructing experience in individual interviews, autobiographies and on-line accounts: A poststructuralist approach. *Journal of Advanced Nursing, 41*(6), 536–544.

Hartrick-Doane, G., & Varcoe, C. (2005a). *Family nursing as relational inquiry: Developing health promoting practice.* Philadelphia: Lippincott Williams & Wilkins.

Hartrick-Doane, G., & Varcoe, C. (2005b). Toward compassionate action: Pragmatism and the inseparability of theory/practice. *Advances in Nursing Science. 28*(1), 81–90.

Henry, F., Tator, C., Mattis, W., et al. (2000a). *The colour of democracy: Racism in Canadian society*. Toronto: Harcourt Brace.

Henry, F., Tator, C., Mattis, W., et al. (2000b). Racism and human-service delivery. In *The colour of democracy: Racism in Canadian society* (pp. 207–227). Toronto: Harcourt Brace.

hooks, b. (1984). *Feminist theory: From margin to center*. Boston: South End Press.

hooks, b. (1994). *Teaching to transgress: Education as the practice of freedom*. New York: Routledge.

Humm, M. (1990). *The dictionary of feminist theory*. Columbus, OH: Ohio State University Press.

Jackson, S. (1997). Crossing borders and changing pedagogies: From Giroux and Freire to feminist theories of education. *Gender & Education, 9*(4), 457–468.

Jiwani, Y. (2000). *Race, gender, violence and health care: Immigrant women of colour who have experienced violence and their encounters with the health care system*. Vancouver, BC: Feminist Research, Education, Development and Action.

Johnson, A. G. (1995). *The Blackwell dictionary of sociology*. Oxford: Blackwell.

King, J. E. (1991). Dysconscious racism: Ideology, identity and the miseduation of teachers. *Journal of Negro Education, 60*(2), 133–146.

King, J. T. (2004). Service-Learning as a site for critical pedagogy: A case of collaboration, caring, and defamiliarization across borders. *Journal of Experiential Education, 26*(3), 121–137.

Krieger, N. (1999). Embodying inequality: A review of concepts, measures, and methods for studying health consequences of discrimination. *International Journal of Health Services, 29*(2), 295–352.

Krieger, N., & Gruskin, S. (2001). Frameworks matter: Ecosocial and health and human rights perspectives on disparities in women's health—The case of tuberculosis. *Journal of the American Medical Women's Association, 56*(4), 137–142.

Levine-Rasky, C. (2000). Framing whiteness: Working through the tensions in introducing whiteness to educators. *Race Ethnicity and Education, 3*(3), 271–292.

Lourde, A. (1984). *Sister Outsider*. Freedom, CA: The Crossing Press.

Macey, D. (2000). *The penguin dictionary of critical theory*. London: Penguin.

McConaghy, C. (2000). *Rethinking indigenous education: Culturalism, colonialism and the politics of knowing*. Flaxton, Australia: Post Pressed.

McCormick, J. (1997). *The discourses of control: Power in nursing*. Vancouver, BC: University of British Columbia, unpublished doctoral dissertation.

McCormick, J., Rodney, P., & Varcoe, C. (2003). Re/interpretation across studies: An approach to qualitative meta-analysis. *Qualitative Health Research, 13*(6), 933–944.

McIntosh, P. (1988). *White privilege and male privilege: A personal account of coming to see correspondence through work in women's studies* (Working paper #189). Wellesley, MA: Wellesley College Center for Research on Women.

McIntosh, P. (1998). Images of Euro-Americans: White privilege, color, and crime: A personal account. In C. R. Mann & M. Zatz (Eds.), *Images of color, images of crime* (pp. 207–216). Los Angeles: Roxbury Publishing Company.

McKenna, B. G., Smith, N. A., Poole, S. J., et al. (2003). Horizontal violence: Experiences of Registered Nurses in their first year of practice. *Journal of Advanced Nursing, 42*(1), 90–96.

Meleis, A. I., & Im, E.-O. (1999). Transcending marginalization in knowledge development. *Nursing Inquiry, 6*(2), 94–102.

Murphy, N., & Canales, M. K. (2001). A critical analysis of compliance. *Nursing Inquiry, 8*(3), 173–181.

Nairn, S., Hardy, C., Parumal, L., et al. (2004). Multicultural or anti-racist teaching in nurse education: A critical appraisal. *Nurse Education Today, 24*(3), 188–195.

Nazroo, J. Y. (1998). Genetic, cultural or socio-economic vulnerability? Explaining ethnic inequalities in health. *Sociology of Health & Illness, 20*(5), 710–730.

Ng, R. (1995). Multiculturalism as ideology: A textual analysis. In M. Campbell & A. Manicom (Eds.), *Knowledge, experience, and ruling relations: Studies in the social organization of knowledge*. Toronto: University of Toronto Press.

Paterson, B. L., Osborne, M., & Gregory, D. (2004). How different can you be and still survive: Homogeneity and difference in clinical nursing education. *International Journal of Nursing Education Scholarship, 1*(1), 1–13.

Peternelj-Taylor, C. (2005). An exploration of "Othering" in forensic psychiatric and correctional nursing. *Canadian Journal of Nursing Research, 36*(4), 130–147.

Puzan, E. (2003). The unbearable whiteness of being (in nursing). *Nursing Inquiry, 10*(3), 193–200.

Razack, S. (1998). *Looking white people in the eye: Gender, race and culture in courtrooms and classrooms.* Toronto: University of Toronto Press.

Re'em, M. (2001). The politics of normalcy: Intersectionality and the construction of difference in Christian-Jewish relations. *International Journal of Qualitative Studies in Education (QSE), 14*(3), 381–397.

Randle, J. (2003). Bullying in the nursing profession. *Journal of Advanced Nursing, 43*(4), 395–401.

Rn, B. T. (2001). Identifying and transforming dysfunctional nurse–nurse relationships through reflective practice and action research. *International Journal of Nursing Practice, 7*(6), 406–413.

Roman, L. (1993). White is a color too! White defensiveness, postmodernism, and anti-racist pedagogy. In C. McCarthy & W. Chrichlow (Eds.), *Race, identity and representation in education.* New York: Routledge.

Said, E. (1979). *Orientalism.* New York: Vintage.

Schick, C. (2000). By virture of being white: Resistance and antiracist pedagogy. *Race Ethnicity and Education, 3*(1), 83–102.

Scrunton, R. (1995). *A short history of modern philosophy: From Decartes to Wittgenstein* (2nd ed.). London: Routledge.

Shaha, M. (1998). Racism and its implications in ethical-moral reasoning in nursing practice: A tentative approach to a largely unexplored topic. *Nursing Ethics, 5*(2), 139–146.

Stephenson, P. (1999). Expanding notions of culture for cross-cultural ethics in health and medicine. In H. Coward & P. Ratanakul (Eds.), *A cross-cultural dialogue on health care ethics* (pp. 68–91). Waterloo, ON: Wilfried Laurier University Press.

Stevens, P. E. (1992). Who gets care? Access to health care as an arena for nursing action. *Scholarly Inquiry in Nursing Practice, 6*(3), 185–200.

Swendson, C., & Windsor, C. (1996). Rethinking cultural sensitivity. *Nursing Inquiry, 3*(1), 3–12.

Taussig, M. (1993). *Mimesis and alterity: A particular history of the senses.* New York: Routledge.

Taylor, J. Y. (1998). Womanism: A methodologic framework for African American women. *Advances in Nursing Science, 21*(1), 53–64.

Taylor, J. Y. (2000). Sisters of the Yam: African American women's healing and self recovery from intimate male partner violence. *Issues in Mental Health Nursing, 21*(5), 515–531.

Taylor, J. Y. (2002). Talking back: Research as an act of resistance and healing for African American women survivors of intimate male partner violence. *Women & Therapy, 25*(3/4), 145.

Varcoe, C. (2001). Abuse obscured: An ethnographic account of emergency nursing in relation to violence against women. *Canadian Journal of Nursing Research, 32*(4), 95–115.

Varcoe, C. (2002). Inequality, violence and women's health. In B. S. Bolaria & H. Dickinson (Eds.), *Health, illness and health care in Canada* (3rd ed., pp. 211–230). Toronto: Nelson.

Young, I. M. (1990). *Justice and the politics of difference.* Princeton, NJ: University of Princeton Press.

Zierler, S., & Krieger, N. (1997). Reframing women's risk: Social inequalities and HIV infection. *Annual Reviews of Public Health, 18*, 401–436.

Zierler, S., Krieger, N., Tang, Y., et al. (2000). Economic deprivation and AIDS incidence in Massachusetts. *American Journal of Public Health, 90*(7), 1064–1073.

Additional Resource

Diversity Gateway—Canadian Policy Research Networks Web site on the changing face of Canada. Available at http://www.cprn.org/en/diversity.cfm.

Chapter 21

Barriers to Student-Centered Teaching: Overcoming Institutional and Attitudinal Obstacles

Carol Jillings

It is 1974. A young, soon-to-be-graduated university nursing student, under the influence of a particularly inspirational teacher, voraciously reads the Postman and Weingartner classic, *Teaching as a Subversive Activity* (1969) and Carl Rogers' *Freedom to Learn* (1969). Both books build a case for teaching that attends to learners' needs, motivations, and approaches to learning. Fast-forward 30 years. This same nurse, now an educator with over 25 years of experience, begins to construct a chapter on "student-centered teaching," and muses that despite the passage of time, many issues in nursing education remain unchanged. Indeed, the compelling arguments of the 1970s continue to resonate. Why?

INTENT In this chapter, categories of barriers to student-centered teaching are examined. The chapter begins with some definitions of "student-centeredness" as a basis for discussing the multiple contexts wherein this view of education may be impeded or facilitated. Following the discussion of actual and potential barriers, proposals are advanced for translating these factors into facilitators of student-centered teaching.

OVERVIEW

Introduction
- Definitions and Related Concepts
- Constructivist Approaches
- The "Proof of the Pudding": Barriers and Facilitating Factors

Elements of Student-Centered Teaching

Barriers to Student-Centered Teaching
- The Institutional Context
- The Curricular Context
- The Instructional Context
- The Faculty-Related Context
- The Learner-Related Context
- The Nursing-Related Context

From Barriers to Facilitators

Specific Recommendations: Facilitating Student-Centered Learning

INTRODUCTION

The concept of student-centered teaching—and its close relative, student-centered learning—has been introduced in this textbook as encompassing approaches to teaching that actively engage the learner. Inherent in student-centered teaching is a focus on the learner, rather than a preoccupation with content and teacher-driven strategies for its structure and delivery. Numerous textbooks and Web site resources in general education describe student-centered teaching and learning, extolling the virtues of this shift in pedagogical approach and describing the underlying core values, beliefs and strategies. In a similar vein, literature in nursing education embraces and describes concepts at the core of student-centered instruction and articulates numerous teaching orientations and strategies that promote the goal of placing and maintaining the learner at the center of the educational process. This chapter will explore the elements of student-centered teaching and their links to structures and processes in nursing education. Barriers and facilitators in relation to student-centered teaching will be discussed in relation to six contexts: institutional, curricular, instructional, faculty-related, learner-related, and nursing-related.

Definitions and Related Concepts

As has been noted earlier, there are many definitions for student-centered teaching and learning. General definitions include the ideas of student choice, (Glasgow, 1997; University of Washington, 1998) student control and engagement, (University of Colorado, Boulder, 2004) and active participation of students in the learning community (Weast & Davis, 2004). McCombs and Whisler (1997) expand a basic description of learner centeredness to include consideration of metacognitive/cognitive, affective, developmental, and personal/social factors, as well as individual differences, arriving at a definition that synthesizes core principles:

> *The perspective that couples a focus on individual learners (their heredity, experiences, perspectives, backgrounds, talents, interests, capacities, and needs) with a focus on learning (the best available knowledge about learning and how it occurs and about teaching practices that are most effective in promoting the highest levels of motivation, learning, and achievement for all learners). (p. 9)*

A number of discussions about student-centered teaching and learning go beyond the mere definition of the notion to describe synonymous or analogous concepts: problem-based learning, collaborative learning, developmental learning, cooperative learning, and communities of learning. Still other conceptions of student centeredness frame the idea in terms of alternative delivery methods such as online or distributed learning. The essence of the definition, however, is the break from teacher-driven approaches to mere content delivery and the introduction of learner-as-focal-point; thus, learning needs, styles, choices, and motivations drive the material to be learned and the experiences wherein learning will be constructed and consolidated.

Constructivist Approaches

Chapter 1 positions student-centered teaching within constructivism; that is, the core beliefs and values underpinning student-centered pedagogy acknowledge the processes of individual meaning making and the social and relational processes involved in acquiring knowledge. Knowledge is not transferred or transmitted in a unidirectional approach from teacher to student; rather, it is built through engagement and interaction with one's learning environment. Constructivist education moves away from didactic student–teacher interactions to a more active and collaborative process of learning that is "internally controlled and mediated by the learner" (Technology Assistance Program, 1999, p. 1). It consists of knowledge building through interaction, transformation, and inquiry (Sandholtz, Ringstaff, & Dwyer, 1997, p. 14)—processes of *con*struction, rather than *in*struction. Nurse educators recognizing the challenges of promoting learning in a practice profession that is client-focused, have embraced constructivism as a critical orientation to teaching and learning that places the student of nursing at the core of the learning process (Chapter 1). Recognition of the learner as the mediator of the learning process is essential if nursing curricula are to achieve their goals of producing knowledgeable and accountable professionals who engage in evidence-based practice.

The "Proof of the Pudding": Barriers and Facilitating Factors

Academic nursing has long valued innovation in education. Theories and concepts in the broader field of general education have been applied to the context of university nursing education throughout its history, and educators have been keen to adopt and adapt trends in curriculum development, instructional design, measurement and evaluation, and orientations to pedagogy. Student-centered teaching, as an idea whose time has come, is at the forefront of current educational discourse and yet, most educators would be quick to acknowledge that many barriers or obstacles exist which can and do impede the successful implementation of this approach. Conversely, factors that facilitate student-centered approaches can be identified and enhanced in nursing education. Subsequent sections of this chapter will address principles and strategies at the core of student-centered teaching and learning and their link to contexts of nursing education.

ELEMENTS OF STUDENT-CENTERED TEACHING

Before examining the nature of specific barriers and facilitators to student-centered learning, it is helpful to examine principles that are foundational to student-centered teaching and their relationship to specific educational strategies and styles. This will provide the backdrop for considering the various contexts and for discussing issues specific to nursing education. The literature abounds with presentations and dialogue surrounding learner-centered principles that, when applied by educators, should facilitate (and indeed embody), best educational practices.

The discipline of psychology posits 14 principles "intended to deal holistically with learners in the context of real-world learning" (APA, 2004, p. 2). These principles encompass cognitive and metacognitive factors, motivational and affective factors, developmental and social factors, and individual differences; together they comprise a foundation for educational reform that puts the learner at the core of curricular and teaching processes. In a similar vein, Chickering and Gamson (2004) describe seven principles at the core of "good practice in undergraduate education":

> *encouragement of contact between students and faculty; development of reciprocity and cooperation among students; encouragement of active learning; transmission of prompt feedback; emphasis on time "on task"; communication of high expectations; and respect for diverse talents and ways of learning. Each of the aforementioned principles locates the student/learner at the center of the teaching process. Attention is given to individual variables, environmental and contextual factors in the learning situation, processes of engagement and communication, and timeliness of learning activities and feedback. Underlying values concerning respect for learners and acknowledgement and acceptance of diversity are clear. The principles, as foundational to student-centered teaching, are put forth as integral to the improvement of education. (p. 1)*

Beyond principles, numerous authors in the educational field describe specific teaching strategies and styles that are conducive to student centeredness. Ornstein and Lasley (2004) examine historical perspectives, personality types, and specific teacher behaviors, noting that both product-oriented and process-oriented research have contributed to the understanding of effective teaching approaches. They argue that expert teachers attend to several main areas that are learner driven, rather than content driven: information about students; student cues; starting points; planning; students themselves; and self-focus (pp. 79–80). Each of these areas provides a focal point on the learner: expressions of learning needs (questions and concerns, for example), indications of priority or urgency, experiences and expertise that students bring to the situation. The current plethora of educational trends and buzzwords—critical thinking, problem-based learning, group and cooperative learning, learning communities—reminds us of the multifaceted nature of both teaching and learning and of the need to expand educational horizons beyond the delivery and consumption of content. In the context of academic nursing, Norton (1998) describes a learning, as opposed to instructional, paradigm that includes a learning environment and learning experiences that are "learner-centered and learner-controlled" (p. 211). This orientation is intended to move nursing education away from traditional content-focused and skill-focused curriculum and instructional designs. A change in teaching approaches is mandated, grounded in beliefs and values emphasizing the primacy of the student and in the application of holistic approaches to planning, implementing, and evaluating the activities inherent in nursing education.

Clearly, teaching principles and their manifestations in particular teaching strategies and styles are worthy of attention as nurse educators strive to prepare competent practitioners for their professional roles. Student centeredness is a concept that has great appeal for nursing, since it fits with our client orientation and our attentiveness to processes of engagement and communication. Psychological and educational principles, theories, and frameworks all have the potential to guide our activities and to produce program outcomes that reflect cognitive, affective, and behavioral attributes expected of nursing graduates. Yet, as has been indicated, while concepts and principles give clear direction for how learning may be facilitated, barriers to their successful application and enactment are numerous. The ensuing discussion will explore six contexts of relevance for nursing education. By examining various contextual factors, a framework for addressing obstacles to student-centered teaching can be proposed.

BARRIERS TO STUDENT-CENTERED TEACHING

Six contexts in the realm of nursing education can be identified: institutional, curricular, instructional, faculty-related, learner-related, and nursing-related. Each of these gives rise to specific factors or issues that may enhance or impede the implementation of a student-centered philosophy of teaching.

The Institutional Context

Historically, the mandate and culture of the university have revolved around teaching and research. Depending on the size and structure of the university (for example, the commitment to undergraduate and/or graduate education, professional programs, and high profile research faculties), teaching may occupy a prominent place in the institution, or it may play "second fiddle" to research. While many postsecondary institutions now place greater value on teaching (even to the point of emphasizing teaching excellence), the university's reward systems have been slow to accord the same import to educational processes as to the business of knowledge creation. The advent of specialized departments or institutes devoted to teaching and learning is indeed a sign of positive change, as is the recognition of the entity known as teaching scholarship. However, putting teaching—and *student-centered teaching*—into vital strategic documents such as mission and vision statements does not ensure that resources for faculty development will be put into place and made accessible or mandatory for all.

Attention to teaching is not synonymous with student centeredness, however. While some university planning processes go beyond giving lip service to the concept by recommending action and allocating resources for student-centered teaching (California State University, Chico, 1997), the difficult task of helping faculty to articulate and live a philosophy that values constructivist approaches to knowledge and learning remains. Nursing in the academy, having relatively recently earned its stripes as a credible, viable, and productive contributor to the research enterprise, often does not create opportunities to discuss or debate educational values, orientations, or strategies. Often, undergraduate teaching is delegated to faculty junior in rank and experience or to expert clinicians, working on a sessional or contractual basis without the requisite orientation and ongoing support for their development as educators. Without a thorough grounding in the curriculum or valuable role modeling, teachers of nursing may find it tempting to revert to teacher-centered models of content delivery and skill teaching. In addition, in the current climate of fiscal restraint, time and monetary resources may not be provided for important activities such as ongoing programs of orientation and teacher development. The pace in many schools and faculties of nursing is currently so frenetic that colleagues see each other "on the fly" without adequate quality time for consultation and mentoring. Furthermore, nursing faculty may not have the time, energy, or inclination to participate in the intellectual and cultural milieu of the university—the substance of which ought to shape reflective constructivist educational practice.

The Curricular Context

The curriculum is the blueprint for teaching and learning that incorporates the core concepts and the arrangement of courses making up an educational program. The curriculum is, of course, at the core of the educational process, providing the cornerstones and conceptual structures for the organization of teaching and learning.

Nursing curricula have evolved from historically rigid, content-laden entities steeped in biomedical and traditional science models to integrated, reflexive structures built around nursing knowledge. Nursing has emulated the discipline of education in describing and prescribing its approaches to curriculum design, first drawing on the work of scholars such as Tyler (1949), Taba (1962), and Beauchamp (1975), and later embracing poststructuralist perspectives. The first curriculum revolution of the 1960s and 1970s incorporated meticulous activities in conceptual framework development (using core nursing concepts as organizing centers) and the articulation of behavioral objectives (National League for Nursing, 1974). The second wave of the 1980s brought the curricular focus back to the core nursing value of caring (Bevis and Watson, 1989) and drew attention to the critical importance of teaching and learning processes and partnerships in learning. This latter movement could be considered as heralding a commitment to student-centered teaching, since it raised the consciousness of the nursing education community concerning educational process (as opposed to structure). Although this shift in orientation provided a valuable reawakening to the importance of process, it has diverted educators' attention in many cases from important aspects of curriculum structure and the potential synergies of form and function. At present, nursing curricula are somewhat eclectic in their focus, due in part to the diverse student population and the everchanging landscapes of nursing knowledge, clinical practice environments, and technology.

Eclecticism, on face value, ought to facilitate student-centered teaching, since it is less rigid and more accommodating than traditional curricular approaches. However, there exists a danger that faculty may pay less attention to the overall curriculum intent and structure and to the articulation of the parts of the curriculum; this may result in individual teachers "doing their own thing" and conveying a less-than-cohesive or redundant approach to students. Time and resources surface once again at the heart of this potential problem. As enrollments increase in response to the nursing shortage, the need to rapidly and efficiently produce graduates may overtake the desire to develop students as learners and to directly engage them with learning. Hence, the curriculum as a facilitating force in student-centered teaching may suffer from a lack of critical attention and the periodic fine-tuning necessary to maintain its relevance to nursing practice and unity.

Beyond the various philosophical underpinnings and educational theories that set the curricular stage for nursing, it is important to consider specific aspects of the curriculum and how these might create impediments to student centeredness. Traditionally, components of the nursing curriculum have included the program philosophy, the conceptualization of the recipient of nursing care, terminal outcomes, a conceptual framework, and the design (comprising core concepts, elements of content, and their sequential arrangement across years and/or levels of the program). These elements have been seen by educators to create a unified and often integrated whole, providing a blueprint for teaching (hence, student learning). In the early days of the integrated nursing curriculum, each foundational piece was explicated so that the interface between core concepts and outcomes was linked, often through meticulously stated behavioral objectives that reflected "threads" and their structural or process orientations. As educators, under the influence of poststructuralist thought, became disenchanted with behaviorist approaches, the detail of the blueprint became more relaxed and less dependent on objectives as a driving force. Regardless of the approach taken, however, each aspect of the curriculum has the potential to govern the strategies selected for promoting teaching and learning. The curriculum framework, made up of core concepts and subconcepts describing nursing, health and illness, the environment (or main ideas similar to these) has the potential to drive teachers to consider content in great detail, to the possible exclusion of the processes involved in its understanding, application, and mastery. Similarly, the curricular design—the configuration of nursing and support courses and their grouping across years or semesters—can be construed as a directive for content, rather than as a provider of parameters for student learning and for the development of core competencies. Although the content/process balance is not a new challenge for nurse educators, consideration needs to be continuously given to the interplay between curricular structures and guideposts and the concomitant educational approaches that will facilitate a student-centered orientation.

The Instructional Context

The context of instruction is perhaps the most complex enhancer of or detractor from student-centered teaching, for it is here that curricular variables converge and have their greatest impact. Despite the best laid curricular plans, the classroom, laboratory and clinical settings, and the pragmatics of resources give rise to issues that can greatly influence the application of teaching approaches that are student centered. The design of instruction and its implementation merit consideration in the analysis of factors and issues contributing to student centeredness.

Instructional design takes into account variables such as content, context of clinical nursing practice, and resource-related factors such as setting, teacher/student ratios, time, and teaching/learning technologies. Content and context of practice may be spelled out in the curriculum, but resources influence the degree to which learner-centered strategies are uppermost or even feasible. Norton (1998, pp. 165–166) describes a number of resource constraints that have an impact on the selection and implementation of learning activities: time, funding, classroom facilities, and technology for teaching in classroom and laboratory simulations, and clinical practice settings. Each of these has the potential to limit or expand the use of possible teaching strategies. Time, for example, may dictate the degree to which the nurse educator can individualize instruction, reinforce content, or debrief following clinical experiences. Classroom environments that are crowded may impede the use of small group activities or student presentations. Technological limitations may not allow for individual pacing or repetition. Instructional design and lesson planning may specify general goals and processes, but cannot account for all possible ranges of ability, readiness to learn, and applicability. Increasing enrollments in schools of nursing have magnified these issues: class sizes have grown, making seminar learning less feasible from both space and faculty perspectives; clinical agencies have limited student numbers in both inpatient and community settings as a result of their own restructuring and greater patient acuity; learning resources (equipment and audiovisual/computer technology) may be subject to cost constraints because departmental budgets have not grown in proportion to student numbers. Thus, the design of instruction, while attempting to embrace the ideals of critical thinking, reflexivity, and change may be constrained by the realities of resources as well as by the ever present tension between conveying knowledge and allowing time for learning.

The implementation of instruction involves many teaching strategies, some of which may be dictated by course design or lesson plans and others of which revolve around faculty variables (to be discussed later in this chapter). Faculty orientation to teaching may be student centered or not. As Rogers (1969) notes, "the facilitation of learning [is] the aim of education" (p. 105) and "teaching and the imparting of knowledge make sense in an unchanging environment" (p. 104); both of these orientations, in his view, are at the core of the interpersonal relationship between teacher and learner. The introduction of novel and innovative teaching strategies also bears consideration: concepts of cognitive rehearsal (Northam, 2000), learning communities (Churchill, Reno, & Batchelor, 1998), problem-based learning (Glasgow, 1997), and other emerging educational trends may be explicitly built into instructional design within a student-centered philosophy, but their uptake may be contingent on faculty familiarity with and ability to adopt new approaches in lieu of more traditional ones. Once again, resource limitations may hamper the introduction of change and the creation of student-centered environments. According to hooks (1994), "If classes became so full that it is impossible to know students' names, to spend quality time with each of them, then the effort to build a learning community fails" (p. 204). This statement serves as a reminder of the complexities involved in implementing instruction that is consistent with curricular ideology, however innovative. Some specific illustrations of current instructional challenges may be helpful at this point. Class sizes in nursing, as an example, have expanded due to the enrollment surge aimed at countering the nursing shortage. Greater numbers of students have made it difficult to implement student centered approaches such as small group learning or seminars, and laboratory learning groups have become larger. Faculty have therefore begun to struggle to be student-centered in large lecture settings that detract from interactive and personalized teaching styles. An additional problem that has been alluded to in the discussion of the institutional context is staffing patterns that do not promote teacher engagement with the curriculum or continuity of faculty across courses and clinical teaching settings. These examples are but two of the many that illustrate the challenges that may hamper curricular implementation and instructional process.

The Faculty-Related Context

The faculty context of student-centered teaching, like the design and implementation of instruction, is where "the rubber hits the road." Faculty preparation for teaching, their orientation to nursing practice and teaching praxis, their understanding of their multiple roles, and their investment in, and commitment to, their ongoing development as teachers are at the core of this context.

The individual teacher's philosophy of education is crucial to the ability to be, become, or remain learner centered. Often, nurse educators enter the field without having had the opportunity to ponder or articulate their underlying values and beliefs in relationship to teaching and learning. When challenged to do so, the ensuing struggle involves reflection on their own experiences as learners and often, as novice practitioners of nursing. Theories, concepts, and principles from the broader field of education may stimulate teachers' thoughts about knowledge and about learning and its facilitation. The individual educator's perspective on teaching and learning may evolve along lines that could be considered traditional (imparting or transmitting knowledge to the "empty vessel") or more contemporary (facilitating critical thinking and problem solving). Pratt (1998) describes five perspectives on the teaching of adults, noting that "if we are to understand our personal perspectives on teaching, we must consider other ways of thinking and believing about teaching, alternative ways of constructing learning, knowledge or skill, and multiple roles for instructors" (p. 34). Exposure to, and consideration of, various teaching/learning perspectives is critical to faculty preparation for teaching and ongoing development, especially if educators are to move beyond teacher-centered approaches in nursing education.

The faculty member's orientation to both nursing and teaching practice is also significant. Chapter 1 alludes to the parallels between client-centered practice and student-centered pedagogy, noting that nurses have long been focused on individual client needs, responses, and outcomes, making learner centeredness a natural and logical extension of practice. The learner-centered model depicted by McCombs and Whisler (1997, p. 12) provides a holistic perspective that integrates factors—metacognitive, cognitive, affective, developmental, personal, social, and individual—into and in with the learner and learning, not unlike many holistic models of nursing. Following a faculty member's teaching philosophy, such an orientation provides a foundation for student-centered teaching and for approaches to selecting content and strategies that will promote this.

The notion of "roles and rules" comes into play in the faculty context. Nursing programs are, by their nature, highly structured with clearly developed systems and policies for student evaluation and progression. Faculty, in addition to facilitating learning in myriad contexts, settings, and situations, must also determine students' achievements of outcomes at various intervals, both formative and summative. The power gradient that exists in the evaluative context is undeniable. Although student input into evaluation and self-appraisal may be encouraged, true student centeredness may be overshadowed because of faculty accountability for preparing practitioners who are safe to practice and because unlimited time for learning may be practically unrealistic. If these factors cannot be changed, at the least faculty should be aware of their existence and of their impact on student-centered approaches.

Faculty development is a final consideration in this category. Norton (1998, p. 163) discusses several faculty-related constraints to achieving curriculum outcomes, including lack of experience, personal attributes, and problems understanding students' knowledge and skills. Schaefer and Zygmont (2003), in a study examining teaching styles of nursing faculty, note that although participant scores reflected teacher centeredness, their expressions of teaching philosophy indicated a motivation toward becoming more student centered; however, participating nurse educators were uncertain of how this might be accomplished. The related implications for the ongoing preparation and development of nurse educators are clear. This is further supported by Lang, McBeath, and Hebert (1995), who discuss approaches to becoming an effective teacher, and by Aaronsohn (1996), who identifies several factors related to teacher conservatism (hence, to the inability to foster student centeredness): feeling vulnerable to the judgment and power of administrators, parents, and the community; feeling isolated from one another; feeling overworked; focusing "on the immediacy of the day-to-day interactions with their classes" (pp. 8–9). It is not surprising that one of the greatest challenges to student-centered teaching rests with the growth of teachers themselves.

The Learner-Related Context

Volumes have been written concerning learners and learner-centered variables. The task here is not to reiterate values, beliefs, and discourses, but to capture the relevant considerations in the nursing educational context. As described earlier, many learner-centered characteristics and processes have been identified in literature reflecting educational theory and practice, ranging from motivation to attitudes to developmental factors to social and cultural diversity. Nurse educators have become increasingly cognizant of the diverse nature of the student population and of the need to attend to this diversity by gearing teaching approaches to meet individual needs and learning styles. The challenges inherent in attending to diversity are numerous, however, and can be daunting.

Cultural diversity is a characteristic of the current population of nursing students in the North American context. Nursing curricula value diversity and multicultural or transcultural approaches to the provision of client care and by extension, to the teaching of nursing; yet a recent study by Paterson, Osborne, and Gregory (2004) indicates that student perceptions of difference and homogeneity can have an impact on clinical nursing education. These authors encourage a greater understanding of the meaning of cultural diversity "within a wider context of the social relations in both the educational and clinical institutions and within the nursing profession" (p. 11). In order to become student centered, then, nurse educators must go beyond giving lip service to the notion of cultural diversity and ensure that approaches to teaching embody the values and principles of understanding and acceptance.

Another aspect of the learner context pertains to learning style. Proponents of student-centered teaching exhort educators to consider not only individual orientations to learning, but to incorporate and account for these differences in the selection of approaches to content and learning experiences. Indeed, many individual and collective philosophies of education address stylistic differences/diversity among learners and propose that teaching approaches be modified or tailored in order to address these. This challenge becomes problematic, however, as indicated in Chapter 4. Firstly, learning style theory has its limitations from a conceptual point of view; secondly, constant attempts to stretch-and-fit strategy with style may not be time or cost effective, nor will they encourage students to approach learning in new and different ways. Once again, it seems that educators must balance theory and practice, accounting for everyday reality and responding to learning style considerations judiciously.

A final dimension of the learner-related context revolves around issues at the core of socialization into a practice profession. The teaching of nursing involves the interaction of students with care recipients, often in highly charged clinical environments. Students must fulfill and achieve roles and competencies specified by professional regulatory bodies and their learning of these core elements of nursing takes place in hands-on situations. It is, therefore, no surprise that learning in nursing involves stress and anxiety on the part of students, who must internalize and apply content in the immediacy of the clinical environment, often when it is still "hot off the press." Similarly, the knowledge at the center of most nursing courses, although evidence based, is everchanging such that a finite curriculum and instructional package is impossible to produce and deliver. Student centeredness demands that teachers remain sensitive to, and knowledgeable about, the complexities of learning *what it is to be a nurse* and assist students with the challenges of learning and practicing in an ever changing environment.

The Nursing-Related Context

The final context giving rise to barriers (and their companion facilitators) to student-centered teaching is that pertaining to the profession of nursing in its broadest sense. The roles and competencies at the core of professional practice have already been mentioned. In addition to demonstrating these, graduates of nursing programs must meet standards of practice that span many clinical settings and client contexts. It is difficult to maintain student centeredness while at the same time factoring in expectations for practice that are all-encompassing (and not left to the orientation or style of the individual nurse). Daley (1999) explores the concepts of novice and expert learning in clinical nursing practice, noting that while novice learning relates to concept formation and assimilation, expert learning is a constructivist process involving self-initiated strategies (p. 1). If student-centered approaches are founded on constructivism, how might educators reflect on the novice contexts wherein students find themselves? Clearly, the nursing profession at large creates a paradox when attempting to address barriers to student-centered teaching. Professional standards and competencies dictate, at least to a degree, core content, learning experiences, and outcomes of nursing programs. This fact compels educators to structure learning in ways that ensure coverage of fundamental concepts and skills—a practice that is more teacher-driven than student-driven. How can educators assist students to define, understand, and apply concepts in ways that capture the realities of clinical nursing practice while at the same time nurturing their abilities to engage in the self-directedness that is characteristic of the expert practitioner? Perhaps partnerships between educational institutions and practice settings could develop strategies for orientation and mentorship that acknowledge that the transition from student to practitioner unfolds over time as experiential knowledge evolves.

The profession's regulatory parameters also create some different issues within the broader nursing context. Approval and accreditation processes typically set out standards and criteria that must be met by nursing programs preparatory to nurse registration. These, combined with entry-level competencies that delineate core knowledge and skill sets, can potentially constrain the nursing curriculum and processes of education by leading faculty to structure content and learning experiences according to externally imposed standards. Although such standards are a crucial component of the accountability of the educational enterprise, they may fly in the face of student-centered approaches to teaching and learning and contribute to a potentially uniform or regimented curriculum. Educators must continually strive for a balance between their mandate to the professional body (and the public) and their quest for unique and learner-focused teaching strategies.

FROM BARRIERS TO FACILITATORS

The previous sections of this chapter have focused on categories giving rise to barriers to student-centered teaching. These contexts are not mutually exclusive, nor are they particularly surprising or novel. They have been selected as focal points, however, for examining obstacles that arise from institutional structures and processes, or from attitudinal sources more linked to the individuals in the teaching/learning encounter. The institutional variables are evident from the mission statement and philosophy of the university or college and from those of the department, school, or faculty of nursing. These in turn influence the construction of the curriculum and the selection of the foundational educational theories and concepts. The discipline of nursing provides the overlay of core values and the related concepts concerning the client, health and illness, and the practice of nursing. Faculty and students are at the core of the educational process, wherein precepts and concepts are given life and translated into learning. In each of these contexts, one may (and indeed, the writer does) identify barriers which prevent student centeredness from being a prime consideration or a value that is made manifest in the selection of teaching strategies; however, one may turn to the antitheses of barriers and find facilitators, or those variables, qualities and orientations that promote student-centered teaching and learning. By considering these factors in their larger context, a focus is provided, with the goal of creating change in educational praxis in nursing.

In the institutional context, it is noteworthy that many colleges and universities have renewed a commitment to excellence in teaching by acknowledging its importance in their mission statements and strategic planning documents. Indeed, many institutions of higher learning have established centers or institutes that promote teaching excellence through programs of faculty development and opportunities for dialogue on evidence-based education. Including such bodies within the college or university infrastructure—with the concomitant resource allocation—is an admirable beginning. However, this foundation is only useful if other institutional structures and processes (promotion and tenure criteria, for example) value and address teaching scholarship. While according credibility to teaching is only one step in promoting a student-centered environment, it signals support for a constructivist philosophy of education within and across disciplines.

In the curricular and instructional contexts, nursing has an impressive history of student centeredness. Historically, the values and beliefs that have been foundational to the nursing curriculum have acknowledged student diversity and promoted the active engagement of the learner in the process of learning. Yet, as has been noted, the nature of nursing introduces complex variables which can impede student centeredness: the vast amount of knowledge to be presented, integrated, and applied; rapidly changing technologic advances that must be factored into the teaching of clinical competencies; increasingly stretched and stressed clinical resources; the cumulative nature of learning and its assessment through formative and summative evaluation; the temptation (mandate?) to "cover it all" when helping students to learn about clients, health, and illness in numerous contexts and settings. The current enrollment increases, aimed at addressing the nursing shortage, compound these challenges by adding student numbers to a context where resources are already constrained. Nursing faculty can attempt to respond to these issues by ensuring that teaching and learning are at the core of curricular discussions, so that strategies for promoting student centeredness are explored concurrently with the elaboration of core curricular concepts, the selection of content, and the design of learning experiences. Faculty dialogue and debate are crucial to the design and implementation of the nursing curriculum and teaching must be a focal point that is equally weighted with content. Faculty must develop both a tolerance for multiple strategies of teaching and a zeal for trying novel approaches. Similarly, they must engage in ongoing scrutiny of instructional processes to determine what is reasonable and realistic in terms of learning and evaluation styles.

The contexts alluded to above create a direct linkage to faculty and to their ongoing development as teachers, and continuing learners themselves. The barriers of time and opportunity that are often cited as detracting from opportunities for faculty development can be transformed into a reorientation of teaching. The investment of days or hours for institutes or seminars focused on faculty development ultimately pays dividends in the growth of faculty as teachers and engaged colleagues.

What of the learner-related context? It may be difficult to prescribe solutions for addressing student variables, since students will invariably always arrive at our institutional doorsteps with their individual experiences, styles, and orientations to learning. In this context, perhaps the wisest approach is to continue to build in mechanisms for engaging with learners, not only to determine learning style or the diverse social and cultural variables that may have an impact on learning, but to establish a climate for working in partnership, with ongoing validation of learning needs, activities, and outcomes.

Finally, the larger context of nursing and the complexities it creates for learning and for ongoing professional development must be addressed. For this, the author does not have a magical suggestion, except to say that open communication and the resultant notion of partnership between educational and service institutions must be facilitated. Mutual awareness of and respect for the complexities of both nursing education and practice can shape the necessary strategic collaboration that will promote student centeredness and its ultimate consequence, nurse centeredness.

SPECIFIC RECOMMENDATIONS: FACILITATING STUDENT-CENTERED LEARNING

The final section of this chapter will enumerate several recommended considerations for transforming barriers into factors that facilitate student centeredness. As the preceding discussion has indicated, each particular context gives rise to opportunities for expanding attention on students and for moving away from traditional teacher-driven or content-driven approaches to learning.

THE INSTITUTION AS STUDENT-CENTERED

- Beyond valuing student-centeredness in the mission and vision, the college or university should establish dedicated centers or units focused on teaching and learning. These resources can provide a forum for discussion and debate and deliver programs for ongoing faculty development. Expert teachers from across various disciplines can contribute to ongoing programming for orientation and mentorship for new faculty and for the development of teaching scholarship.
- Research in teaching and learning should be valued to the same degree as basic and applied disciplinary research. Forums for communicating research issues and findings should be established in order to showcase teaching scholarship. Centers of excellence focused on teaching and learning should be developed and funded and students should play an integral role in their development, evolution, and evaluation.
- Criteria for tenure and promotion should recognize the teaching component of the faculty role and acknowledge that, for some faculty, teaching scholarship may outdistance research scholarship.
- The synergy between research and teaching should be examined and promoted as a valued form of knowledge dissemination, transfer and exchange.

THE CURRICULUM AS STUDENT-CENTERED

- The nursing curriculum should clearly articulate the philosophy of teaching and learning. Faculty should have input into this aspect of the curriculum and have regular opportunities for discussion of their teaching philosophy. Students should be aware of values and beliefs underpinning the curriculum and have an opportunity to discuss these with faculty.
- Curricular materials—course outlines, syllabi, and, learning materials—should be constructed in such a way that student learning activities are clearly articulated. Options for learning activities, geared to different learner preferences, interests or styles, should be considered.
- Opportunities for faculty–student dialogue should be provided, so that students may express learning needs and priorities. The curriculum committee or senior administrators should facilitate this process.
- Flexibility should be provided where possible, in consideration of students' learning needs and the realities (personal, family, financial) of contemporary student life.

INSTRUCTION AS STUDENT-CENTERED

- Strategies for teaching and learning should be multiple and varied, encouraging student engagement with course material. Teaching approaches that stimulate discussion, debate, and critical reflection should be included. Validation of student learning and satisfaction with teaching approaches should be done regularly. For example, reliance on lecture or didactic instruction may not allow students opportunities for questioning, clarifying, or application; on the other hand, in some situations, students may prefer a didactic presentation followed by a hands on opportunity for practicing a new skill.
- Learning experiences should be tailored, where possible, to student interests and styles of learning. For example, in one laboratory learning group, several different approaches may be possible for learning and demonstrating competence with a clinical nursing skill. Also, in a clinical learning group, students may express the need to care for a client with a particular health concern, in order to expand their knowledge or apply new material.
- Self-evaluation should be an integral component of learning experiences and involve active discussion with the teacher in order to plan for new learning.

FACULTY AS STUDENT-CENTERED

- Faculty should "walk the talk." Often, curricular documents pay lip service to student centeredness while faculty continue to structure and control teaching and learning activities.
- Faculty should have opportunities to discuss issues encountered with student-centered teaching. For example, areas of the curriculum may be prescriptive of necessity (ensuring basic clinical competencies, for example); faculty should be able to discuss strengths or limitations of learning experiences and debate ways of building greater student centeredness into the program.
- Faculty should explore and discuss the evidence base for their teaching practices and formulate research questions out of issues that arise.
- Faculty should engage with teachers from other disciplines to share ideas and explore strategies for student-centered learning.
- Faculty should reflect on their own teaching practice and areas for further growth and development.

SUMMARY

Student-centered teaching is not a new idea. The educational debates surrounding the placement of the learner at the heart of the learning process have existed for decades, and nurse educators have enthusiastically built concepts and strategies for student-centered teaching and learning into curricula and instructional designs for a comparable period of time. What is new is perhaps the great number of challenges faced by contemporary educators, who must balance demand and constraint, complexity and simplicity. Each barrier to student-centered teaching, however, can be turned around and transformed into a potential facilitator, given the appropriate value system and positive spin. Nurse educators are encouraged to rise to this challenge, with the aim of not only promoting and achieving excellence in nursing education but also of improving clinical nursing practice and producing a positive impact on client care.

LEARNING ACTIVITY

In a small group, consider and discuss the following questions:

1. Consider the interplay of structure (how the curriculum and its components are laid out) and function (how teaching and learning actually occur) in the promotion of student-centered learning. In the institutional and curricular contexts, who can structure and contribute to student centeredness? What happens if too much attention is paid to structure, or if too much attention is paid to function? Reflect on some strategies that nurse educators can use to promote a balance in this regard.
2. Some learners may actually prefer teacher-centered approaches to learning, based on their own style of learning or on past experiences in teacher-centered programs. How might the educator address this issue?

RESOURCES FOR EDUCATORS

PLANNING THE TEACHING/LEARNING EXPERIENCE

Questions to Support a Thoughtful Reading

1. In your learning journey, have you noticed any changes at the institutional level designed to foster student-centered learning?
2. What aspects of the curriculum that now guides your nursing education is designed to foster student-centered learning?
3. Identify a teaching strategy that you have experienced as student centered. How did this strategy support your learning?
4. Have you observed faculty members developing skills with student-centered teaching? If so, what do you see as their greatest challenge?

EVALUATING THE TEACHING/LEARNING EXPERIENCE

Sample Evaluation Strategies or Tools

1. Use the Learning Activity as a basis for an in-class debate on the merits and drawbacks of attending to structure and function in a nursing fundamentals course.
2. Have learners reflect on their discussion and then design specific approaches to address the issues. They could, for example, propose a role for the departmental curriculum committee in response to Learning Activity question #1. For Learning Activity question #2, they could debate the merits of trying to convert the student to a new style of learning.

References

Aaronsohn, E. (1996). *Going against the grain: Supporting the student-centered teacher.* Thousand Oaks, CA: Corwin.

American Psychological Association. (2004). Learner-centered psychological principles: A framework for school design and reform. Retrieved November 7, 2005, from www.apa.org/ed/lcp.html.

Beauchamp, G. A. (1975). *Curriculum theory.* (3rd ed.). Wilmette, IL: The Kagg Press.

Bevis, E. O., & Watson, J. (1989). *Toward a new curriculum: A new pedagogy for nursing.* New York: National League for Nursing.

California State University, Chico. (1997). Report of the Provost's Task Force On Student-Centered Learning. Retrieved November 7, 2005, from www.csuchico.edu/vpaa/report.html.

Chickering, A. W., & Gamson, Z. F. (2004). Seven principles for good practice in undergraduate education. Retrieved November 4, 2005, from http://honolulu.hawaii.edu/intranet/committees/FacDevCom/guidebk/teachtip/7princip.htm.

Churchill, J., Reno, B., & Batchelor, N. (1998). The learning communities concept: Increasing student involvement. *Nurse Educator, 23*(6), 7–8.

Daley, B. J. (1999). Novice to expert: An exploration of how professionals learn. *Adult Education Quarterly, 49*(4):133–148.

Glasgow, N. A. (1997). *New curriculum for new times: A guide to student-centered, problem-based learning.* Thousand Oaks, CA: Corwin.

hooks, b. (1994). *Teaching to transgress: Education as the practice of freedom.* New York: Routledge.

Lang, H. R., McBeath, A., & Hebert, J. (1995). *Teaching strategies and methods for student-centered instruction.* Toronto: Harcourt Brace.

McCombs, B. L., & Whisler, J. S. (1997). *The learner-centered classroom and school: Strategies for increasing student motivation and achievement.* San Francisco: Jossey-Bass.

National League for Nursing. (1974). *Unifying the curriculum: The integrated approach.* New York: NLN.

Northam, S. (2000). Cognitive rehearsal. *Nurse Educator, 25*(1), 19–20.

Norton, B. (1998). Selecting learning experiences to achieve curriculum outcomes. In D. M. Billings & J. A. Halstead, *Teaching in nursing: A guide for faculty.* (pp. 151–169). Toronto: Saunders.

Ornstein, A. C., & Lasley, T. J. (2004). *Strategies for effective teaching.* Toronto: McGraw Hill.

Paterson, B. L., Osborne, M., & Gregory, D. (2004). How different can you be and still survive? Homogeneity and difference in clinical nursing education. *International Journal of Nursing Education Scholarship 1*(1), 1–13.

Postman, N., & Weingartner, C. (1969). *Teaching as a subversive activity.* New York: Dell.

Pratt, D. D. (1998). *Five perspectives on teaching in adult and higher education.* Malabar, FL: Krieger.

Rogers, C. R. (1969). *Freedom to learn.* Columbus, OH: Charles E. Merrill.

Sandholtz, J. H., Ringstaff, C. & Dwyer, D. C. (1997). *Teaching with technology: Creating student-centered classrooms.* New York: Teachers College.

Schaefer, K. M., & Zygmont, D. (2003). Analyzing the teaching style of nursing faculty: Does it promote a student-centered or teacher-centered learning environment? *Nursing Education Perspectives 24*(5), 238–254.

Taba, H. (1962). *Curriculum development: Theory and practice.* New York: Harcourt, Brace & World.

Technology Assistance Program. (1999). *TAP into learning: On the road to student-centered learning.* Southwest Educational Development Laboratory. Retrieved November 5, 2005 from http://www.sedl.org/tap.

Tyler, R. W. (1949). *Basic principles of curriculum and instruction.* Chicago: University of Chicago.

University of Colorado, Boulder. (2004). Culture of a student-centered learning environment. Retrieved November 7, 2005, from www.colorado.edu/sacs/stu-affairs/centered/concept.html.

University of Washington. (1998). What is student-centered learning? Retrieved November 7, 2005, from http://www.washington.edu/uwired/outreach/teched/using/stcntr.html.

Weast, W., & Davis, J. (2004). *Student-centered learning: A manual for liberal arts educators in the 21st century.* Unpublished manuscript, State University of New York, Fredonia.

Chapter 22

Challenges, Issues, and Barriers to Student-Centered Approaches in Distance Education

W. Dean Care, Cynthia K. Russell, Margaret T. Hartig, Victoria S. Murrell, and David M. Gregory

Daniel is a new tenure track faculty member in a university school of nursing. He has been assigned to teach a course by computer-mediated instruction using a WebCT platform. Daniel teaches a class of diverse learners including several minority students, a sight impaired learner, and students who have no previous experience in a distance course. As a graduate nursing student, Daniel participated in a videoconference course that connected with other students living in remote communities. While he performed well in this course, instructional and technical problems prevented it from being a positive learning experience. He experienced a sense of isolation from his fellow nursing students and faculty. The remotely located students were often intimidated by the more vocal on-campus students. Some students withdrew from the course because of feelings of frustration and isolation. Moving forward in time, Daniel now has concerns about meeting the criteria for tenure and promotion. He finds teaching by distance time-consuming and one of the many academic responsibilities he faces in the coming years. Daniel realizes he will need to address numerous challenges and issues in making this an optimal learning experience for himself and his students.

INTENT At the completion of this chapter, the reader will be able to describe the issues and challenges facing students and faculty participating in a distance learning environment. Possible administrative and teaching strategies for dealing with challenges associated with distance education will be explored. Strategies for promoting a student-centered approach in distance education will be examined. Through focused learning activities, the reader will begin to apply student-centered approaches to distance education within their own personal situation.

OVERVIEW

BACKGROUND AND CONTEXT

This chapter is written at a time of increasing demand for distance learning opportunities in postsecondary institutions including nursing education programs. The rapid evolution of distance delivery, particularly Web-based courses, has generated tremendous excitement for its potential to attract new students and alleviate classroom space pressures (Volery, 2001). This movement is particularly important in light of increasing enrollments in colleges and universities. Predictions of significant enrollment increases in the next 3 to 5 years (Jones, 2003) will place considerable strain on human, infrastructure, and fiscal resources in institutions of higher education and schools of nursing. Many institutions are turning to distance education (DE) as a viable alternative to addressing the enrollment situation. However, this is often carried out in the absence of a well thought out strategic plan for DE development. As Bates (2000) suggests, perhaps "the biggest challenge [in distance education] is the lack of vision and the failure to use technology strategically" (p. 7). These challenges and others will be examined in relation to the promotion of student-centered approaches relevant to teaching and learning at a distance.

A recent survey by the United States Department of Education (2003) found that 56% of colleges and universities offer distance courses, with an additional 12% planning to offer distance courses in the next 3 years. While this represents a positive, rapid development in the DE enterprise, it also raises some serious questions about the ability and capacity of institutions and faculty to manage this growth. The current trend in DE is movement toward the use of **asynchronous Web-based instruction**. Educational institutions are migrating away from other DE modalities such as print-based and videoconference delivery. According to the U.S. Department of Education (2003), of those offering DE courses, 90% of postsecondary institutions now offer online courses with 88% planning to promote and market the use of this medium as a primary delivery method. Another important trend is the increased use of **hybrid or "blended" instruction models** where faculty incorporates computer-based learning into traditional classroom settings (Barker, 2003). While the teaching context is different, this trend includes similar challenges experienced by faculty who teach and students who learn at a distance.

Distance education has evolved to the point where it is now closer to being mainstream than many faculty and administrators in universities thought it ever would. However, distance students differ from their traditional counterparts in important ways. Today's distance learner tends to be older and have more life experiences than conventional students. They are likely to have completed more credit hours and have higher grade point averages than traditional students (Diaz, 2002). For example, Diaz found that students enrolled in online courses received twice as many As as traditional students and half as many Ds and Fs. This researcher suggested that DE formats appeal to students with independent styles of learning and that these styles are well suited to DE. Furthermore, this generation of **information age** learners prefers "doing to knowing, trial-and-error to logic, and typing to handwriting" (Howell, Williams, & Lindsay, 2003, p. 4). Multitasking and staying connected are essential to today's students. Nursing faculty who teach by distance need to be aware of these trends in order to design and deliver courses that match their students' learning styles and personal characteristics.

Even with the aforementioned challenges and issues, there are several reasons why universities and other educational institutions decide to employ distance teaching modalities. The three most commonly cited reasons include enhancing the quality of instruction and learning, maintaining competitiveness with other educational agencies, and improving access to education (Bates, 2000).

CHALLENGES AND ISSUES TO TEACHING AND LEARNING AT A DISTANCE

This chapter employs Cross' (1981) model for describing barriers to participating or persisting in structured learning activities. This model, based on the works of Boshier (1973), is a useful organizational framework for examining issues and challenges experienced by nursing students and faculty in a distance education environment. Cross describes obstacles to participation and learning under three general headings: situational, institutional, and dispositional challenges.

Situational challenges are those arising from one's situation in life at any given time. These include socioeconomic factors, family and home responsibilities, and technical problems, as well as unique challenges facing minority students and students with disability. Institutional challenges include those that are "subconsciously erected by providers of educational services" (Cross, 1981, p. 104). These "providers" can be facility-related, for example, technological supports and faculty workloads or faculty related aspects such as faculty development activities. Dispositional challenges are those related to attitudes, personality, feelings of self-confidence, and gender-related issues.

TABLE 22.1 CHALLENGES AND ISSUES

Situational
• Socioeconomic factors.
• Technological challenges.
• Learners with disabilities.
• Minority students.
Institutional
• Faculty workload.
• Incentives and recognition.
• Course ownership.
• Faculty development.
Dispositional
• Attitudes toward innovation and change.
• Feelings of isolation.
• Gender differences.

Conceptual tools and practical strategies for addressing each of these challenges are presented. This chapter emphasizes the need for a comprehensive, systemwide approach in promoting and sustaining a learner-centered approach to distance learning in nursing education. Table 22.1 provides an overview of the challenges and issues to be discussed in this chapter.

Situational Challenges

In a rapidly evolving information age, those living at the margins of society will become even more marginalized unless corrective action can be taken to remove technological obstacles. Kenway (1996) summarizes this concern as follows: "The information revolution makes promises about society and cultural riches and opportunities. However, it can only keep these promises to a fortunate few. For many it spells disaster. . . . It points the way to dangerous economic and social polarization and accelerating disenfranchisement of major sections of the population" (p. 229). That is, those in our society who are already technologically disadvantaged because of situational conditions will fall even further behind the mainstream. This is especially true for remotely located and economically disadvantaged nursing students and those living in the inner core areas of urban centers. The commonly called "**digital divide**" will continue to drive a wedge between the "haves" and "have nots" in our society unless solutions can be found. This widening gap could have a profound effect on the social and economic viability of such minority groups as Aboriginal people of Canada, Native Americans in the United States, or other disenfranchised groups, including those located in rural areas or persons of lower socioeconomic status. According to Greenall and Loizides (2001), "there is a significant danger that Aboriginal peoples will be left behind and disenfranchised as the pace of technology adoption and integration in the economy increases" (p. 7).

Solutions to this complex issue require systematic and sustained efforts from many levels including government, educational institutions, and faculty. The challenge will be to narrow the digital divide by attending to the economic, cultural, technological, and pedagogical needs of marginalized groups in our respective countries.

SOCIOECONOMIC FACTORS

While motivational factors affecting participation and persistence in higher education are complex, there is no question that students' socioeconomic conditions affect their ability to learn effectively. As educational institutions become more technologically advanced, it becomes more costly for students to engage in distance learning. These expenses may range from required travel, to audio conference or videoconference sites, to the costs for computer and software upgrades that allow learners to access courses through the Internet and university resources. Furthermore, some institutions charge higher tuition fees for distance courses to help offset increased overhead costs. Additionally, Internet access fees or long distance telephone charges may represent a significant barrier to those students wanting to study at home.

Studying at a distance, while providing important opportunities, can simultaneously exact unanticipated demands on students. Increased access allows students to remain in their home communities and close to their families; however, school work is one more demand to add to the long list of tasks required of one attending to family, home, and school responsibilities. The multitasking required under such circumstances may interfere with successful course or program completion for some students. The extent of family responsibilities is often closely aligned with the socioeconomic condition of people—particularly women. This becomes an issue in nursing where the vast majority of students are women who traditionally shoulder major responsibility for the home and family.

Socioeconomic and family challenges are complex and not easily resolved. A student-centered approach to distance education, however, takes into consideration these factors during course design and implementation phases. Three such approaches are included in Box 22.1.

BOX 22.1 CONSIDERATIONS FOR STUDENT-CENTERED DISTANCE EDUCATION

- Anticipate that most remotely located students do not have ready access to technical supports. Faculty need to be sure that problem-solving instructions are clearly stated and readily available to learners. Having easy access to help desks through toll-free numbers can reduce feelings of isolation among remotely located nursing students.
- Keep synchronous (real time) instruction to a minimum. This mode of delivery interferes with the time flexibility needs of distance students with families.
- Assist students to form tech-support groups in their local communities.

TECHNOLOGICAL CHALLENGES

Closely aligned with socioeconomic factors is the fact that information and learning technologies are advancing at a rapid rate which challenges learners' capacities to keep pace with technological changes. While institutions of higher learning often provide the financial and human resources to make continuous improvements to information and learning technology infrastructures, learners working at home alone may lag behind in this ability given the lack of human and technological resources. Thus, for many there is a risk that faculty may introduce innovative and high tech teaching strategies that unintentionally create barriers for learners and student-centered approaches to learning. The more "bells and whistles" that are introduced to an online course, the greater the potential for difficulty in accessing and retrieving course materials. This is particularly true for students who live in remote communities without the benefit of high speed Internet connections. The limited bandwidth of ordinary telephone lines reduces the ability to send audio and video materials to online students. Similarly, when courseware and course-authoring systems are too complex, it can lead to frustrated faculty. Faculty development activities and technical support personnel may be required to support the distance enterprise of the facility.

Recognition of the need for readily available technical and academic supports is paramount. Educational facilities and faculty must develop awareness of the limits of the technology and technical supports for students in remote program sites. Designing courses with advanced instructional technologies beyond the capacity of the remote site and the learner's economic situation could lead to student frustration and increased attrition. A few suggestions for dealing with these technological challenges are included in Box 22.2.

LEARNERS WITH DISABILITIES

One of the fastest growing cohorts in higher education consists of students living with disabilities (Moisey, 2004), yet they represent a group that is not well attended to within the context of distance education. In the United States, disability services for

BOX 22.2 SUGGESTIONS FOR DEALING WITH TECHNOLOGICAL CHALLENGES

- Faculty and administrators should explore the availability of technological supports in students' communities, including local libraries, hospitals, and community centers. Involving the community in the educational process will provide a sustainable infrastructure for future programming and student success.
- Faculty should avoid becoming overly enamored with high tech instructional delivery methods. Greater complexity often leads to student frustration and an increased need for more technical supports.
- Instructional technology should be a functional tool, simple to operate (for students and faculty), user friendly, visually appealing, and easy to navigate.

students are mandated by legislation. As such, support services are commonly found in postsecondary institutions. In Canada, the lack of similar legislation has slowed the introduction of support services in higher education. Fichten, Asuncion, Barile, Robillar, and Lamb (2003) estimate there are 100,000 postsecondary students in Canada living with disabilities, but fewer than half receive the necessary support services. Although few students with disability enter nursing at this time, rapid advances in instructional and adaptive technologies will create greater opportunities for entry in the future.

For many students with disabilities, traditional approaches to education are largely inaccessible (Kinash, Crichton, & Kim-Rupnow, 2004). If not thoughtfully designed to provide "**reasonable accommodation**," distance courses may inadvertently present significant challenges to this group of already disadvantaged learners. Nursing students may present themselves with various degrees of auditory, visual, tactile, and learning abilities. Often the faculty member will not have prior knowledge of these students and their disabilities and thus not enact accommodation of their DE learning needs. These challenges may be exacerbated inadvertently by the type of educational medium employed.

Designers and instructors of distance courses need to be cognizant of the impact of various distance and instructional technologies on the abilities of some students to access information and learn in these environments. There is tremendous potential for computer-mediated applications to enhance the learning of those with disabilities if appropriately applied. For example, visual disabilities include those with limited vision, color impairment, and degrees of blindness. Each group has a specific set of learning needs and requires a different set of adaptive technologies to address these needs. For example, a legally blind learner may use a screen reader to read the content of the Web page aloud while a student with low visibility may need the content presented in large print.

There are many **adaptive technologies** available for the distance learner with disability. Some of these options include:

- Screen enlargement software.
- Speech control and dictation programs.
- Audio Web browsers.
- Braille printers.
- Text-to-speech software.
- Modified keyboard.
- Large screen monitors.

Options for accommodating the learning needs include: taped or electronic versions of course textbooks, Braille versions of printed materials, tape recorded tests, extended time to complete assignments or tests, and alternative forms of testing to name a few.

There are many other ways to adapt a distance course for students with disability, but they depend on the distance method used and the type of disability experienced. One suggestion is to enlist the services of a student with disability or educational specialist on the design team of the course or program. They will know best how to modify the educational medium to enhance learning. O'Connor (2000) calls online learners with disabilities "early adopters" because they often take advantage of technology-enhanced learning methods well before the general student population, leading the way for other learners to follow. "When we encourage the use of adaptive technology in accommodating the needs of learners with disabilities, we also serendipitously make positive strides in addressing the diverse learning styles of students without disabilities as well" (Cook & Gladhart, 2002, p. 1). As such, when nursing faculty teaching at a distance attend to or accommodate the needs of students with disabilities, they are more likely to incorporate learner-centered approaches into their distance courses.

MINORITY STUDENTS

It is well known that minority groups are underrepresented in professional programs such as nursing. The reasons for this are multiple and complex, and may include socioeconomic factors, and low numbers of minority faculty. The many challenges or barriers that minority students face in postsecondary institutions may be exacerbated in a distance learning environment.

For the most part, university and college curricula represent the dominant Anglo-Saxon, middle class culture of our society. According to Crow (1993), the culture of higher education is dominated by competition, time-oriented expectations, and individual effort. These characteristics are often viewed as being in direct opposition to a learner-centered approach to education and may not suit the needs of minority students.

Padilla, Trevino, Gonzalez, and Trevino (1997) describe a model for encouraging success of minority students using a construct known as "**heuristic knowledge**" also known as informal knowledge of academia. Findings of their study focus on the need for minority students to learn the rules of the academic world because these often conflict with their known cultural values and norms. Barriers to participation and persistence in minority students are often related to feelings of being marginalized, lack of being nurtured, and feelings of powerlessness (Padilla, et al., 1997). This finding was validated in a study by Care (2003) where remotely located Aboriginal learners studying in a videoconference environment described the need to first "learn the rules" in this new learning experience. These rules related to knowing when to speak out in class, how loud to talk, and when to ask a question. Videoconferencing was a totally foreign experience for the participants. The Aboriginal nursing students felt "awkward and disoriented" until new rules of behavior were learned. Classroom interactions were often dominated by more assertive students at the main university campus. Aboriginal students felt a lack of connection with their on-campus counterparts. They reported feeling "separated and left out" of discussions. As such, they were hesitant to share their knowledge and experiences in this videoconference format. Dickerson, Neary, and Hyche-Johnson (2000) describe this disconnectedness as "being on the fringe" of the learning environment and is consistent with the marginalization felt by other minority groups in distance settings.

In contrast to a videoconference class setting, Web-based learning appears better suited for the learning needs of minority students. In this learning environment, minority students have a degree of anonymity that protects them from feelings of being marginalized and powerless. They are less likely to be negatively impacted by the more verbal and assertive students of the dominant culture group. This is largely because of the asynchronous nature of Web-based delivery. Students find they have time to ponder and carefully consider the posted questions. Because they have more time, learners can consult the literature, formulate their thoughts, and compose their responses before posting to the discussion forums. This tends to be a less threatening environment for many students. It is clear that developing student-centered approaches to the Web-based environment enhances the learning experience for minority students.

An effective strategy to reduce feelings of isolation in Aboriginal students in distance courses is the use of case studies. This approach is consistent with the value placed on storytelling and being open to discuss issues in a safe group environment. These case discussions capture the multiple perspectives of the group members and allow students to share their different viewpoints.

Institutional Challenges

Because the success of any institutional distance program depends on the attitudes and abilities of faculty, understanding and addressing those issues that concern distance faculty is a significant priority for program administrators. There is increased pressure being placed on educational institutions to introduce pedagogical practices that will address the future needs of society. These pressures are often felt most directly by the faculty who feel underprepared or unwilling to fulfill this evolving role. In no small way, the development of innovative instructional technologies has affected the way faculty members teach and communicate with their students. Not only does the introduction of distance courses require faculty to learn about new instructional technology, it also requires a paradigm shift in how faculty facilitate the learning process (Hassenplug & Harnish, 1998). This section will address the institutional barriers that hinder the paradigm shift from an instructional (teacher-centered) to a student-centered approach to education.

FACULTY WORKLOAD

There has been escalating pressure on nursing faculty to incorporate teaching with advanced instructional modalities into already heavy workloads. However, there is conflicting evidence whether or not the use of technology contributes to increasing faculty teaching workloads.

Teaching at a distance represents a significant shift in faculty roles and responsibilities. In the distance environment, the instructor migrates more toward a mentor or facilitator role (Clay, 1999). The use of instructional and information technology in course design and teaching tends to be poorly understood by many faculty. This results in an increase in the initial, upfront time required to develop and deliver a distance course. Bates and Poole (2003) concur that "all forms of technology-enhanced teaching need more preparation time for teachers" (p. 115). Although it is speculated that after a period of adjustment, the preparation time needed in distance courses is the same as face-to-face courses.

The most commonly cited barriers to developing and teaching distance courses are those related to faculty workload and time. This is illustrated in a qualitative study by Care and Scanlan (2000) in which most faculty reported that "course design for distance delivery was carried out in addition to their regular teaching assignment" (p. 124). Conclusions drawn from a National Education Association survey suggest that "teaching a distance learning course does, in fact, require more time than teaching a traditional course" (NEA, 2000, p. 49). Furthermore, a study by Pachnowski and Jurczyk (2003) suggests faculty who engage in Web-based instruction require far more preparation time than those who teach with videoconferencing. This is not surprising since the latter method is more closely aligned with traditional face-to-face delivery than Web-based approaches.

Unfortunately, many faculty feel that this additional investment of time does not result in an adequate return in terms of support, recognition, or compensation. In contrast, more recent empirical evidence does not support the widely held belief that distance courses require more work than traditional classroom offerings (DiBiase, 2000). A more serious concern is the impact of this perception on the ability to attract faculty willing to teach by distance. The most qualified faculty may choose not to participate because of the workload involved, thus undermining the delivery of quality programming to those students most in need. The DiBiase study does not support the commonly held belief that teaching an online course requires more effort than teaching comparable classroom courses, refuting an NEA claim of higher workloads as being based on anecdotal evidence. It was found that while students in distance courses require more frequent attention, the total teaching and maintenance time per student was actually less than required of traditional classroom courses. These results are not universally accepted by nursing faculty. While it is understood that course design affects delivery, further research is needed to find ways to design distance courses that use faculty time more efficiently.

The change from traditional teaching to student-centered learning approaches requires additional knowledge and skills. This often requires a period of growth and adjustment on the part of faculty. When nursing faculty are adequately compensated for the workload and time involved, they are more likely to embrace this type of teaching in their distance courses.

INCENTIVES AND RECOGNITION

A major institutional barrier to faculty agreeing to teach by distance is the lack of incentives and recognition. This issue is closely aligned with the value placed on teaching in a university environment. While teaching and scholarly work, like research, are normally considered to be equally weighted for tenure and promotion purposes, the underlying ethos of the institution suggests that research productivity is a dominant factor in that environment. In Reinert and Fryback's (1997) study, faculty reported having little or no time for research and publication when they were involved in developing courses for distance delivery. Furthermore, much of the teaching by distance is often invisible to peers. These represent serious challenges since faculty may be reluctant to take on teaching by distance if tangible incentives are not provided. There needs to be a concerted effort to recognize the development of courses or teaching by distance as a bona fide scholarly activity. One approach to addressing this challenge is to include the development of technologically enhanced courses in the criteria for tenure and promotion of the teaching unit. This will heighten the visibility and value of teaching by distance within the university and faculty community. This should serve, in part, as an incentive for nursing faculty to take on this important activity. Adopting the Boyer (1990) model of scholarship would allow for a broader definition of research and scholarly activity within a nursing faculty. This model includes a scholarship of teaching category where application of teaching and learning theories and processes into distance courses would be considered scholarly work.

Another inhibiting factor is the lack of financial incentive to take on distance teaching. Schifter (2000) surveyed administrators about their perceptions of motivating factors affecting faculty participation in distance delivery. Three of the top five incentives identified included monetary support, credit toward tenure and promotion, and **release time**. In contrast, a literature review conducted by Parker (2003) found most faculty develop and deliver distance courses for little or no financial remuneration. The granting of release time is a popular incentive. This is important to consider as initial development time for distance delivery is almost twice that of face-to-face classes (McKenzie, Mims, Bennett, & Waugh, 1999). An alternative to release time for faculty is the establishment of course design teams. Care and Scanlan (2000) elaborate on this idea further when they suggested that faculty needs were best served with a multidisciplinary team approach to course development. This team should include an instructional designer, faculty member as content expert, technical support personnel, and an administrative person assigned to coordinate this multidisciplinary group. It has been found that the formation of such a team is a tangible support strategy that is less costly than providing release time for faculty (Marriot, 2003).

In a literature review conducted by Parker (2003), the following intrinsic motivators were cited as being attractive incentives to teaching by distance:

- Personal satisfaction.
- Flexible scheduling.
- Reaching a wider audience.
- Intellectual challenge.
- Ability to use new technology.

External motivators such as monetary stipends, decreased workload, and release time to develop and teach distance courses are seen as sources of encouragement for teaching by distance. Additional incentives include access to personal laptop computers, personal digital assistants (PDAs), and Internet connections. The introduction of these incentives needs to be considered in light of the budgetary situation of the educational institution.

COURSE OWNERSHIP

The issue of ownership is a sensitive matter for nursing faculty who prefer having control over their own courses being offered by distance delivery. At the heart of the ownership matter is who pays for the development of this scholarly work. Faculty members invest considerable time and energy into course design and delivery especially if it involves a student-centered approach. They want to maintain the right to make changes to their courses. It becomes more complicated when the design of distance courses is undertaken by a hired consultant external to the agency, an instructional designer from another university unit, or a multidisciplinary team. These approaches may be seen as detracting from clear ownership of the distance course. As such, educational administrators must attend to the following questions: What are the institutional policies regarding intellectual property? What happens if the course author leaves the institution? Can the course author sell or lease the course to others? and Can alternate faculty be assigned to teach the distance course designed by another (Link & Scholtz, 2000)? Unless these course ownership issues can be adequately resolved, it will remain a barrier to the distance learning movement in higher education. In the absence of institutional policy, it is recommended that contractual agreements be developed with course developers and faculty that clearly outlines ownership and intellectual copyright of distance courses and instructional materials.

FACULTY DEVELOPMENT

Implementing student-centered approaches in distance courses requires a change in faculty roles and responsibilities. This not only entails a set of specialized skills and strategies, it also necessitates that faculty must plan ahead, be highly organized, and interact with their students in new and creative ways. Distance faculty must be skilled in communication because of the increased demands for student-to-teacher interaction (NEA, 2000). Faculty members are also being called on to be facilitators of learning in this more student-centered environment. For many, this is a strange and untested climate in which to teach.

Some faculty members, in attempting to adapt to the new way of teaching, initially try to use their traditional classroom methods at a distance. This leads to frustration when these attempts are unsuccessful (Dasher-Alston & Patton, 1998). One avenue to alleviate this frustration is to participate in faculty development activities geared toward teaching with technology. This training and skill acquisition is seen as a precursor to lowering resistance to change and encouraging success when teaching by distance (Pajo & Wallace, 2001). Such training needs to be viewed as an investment in the future of individual faculty and the promotion of the goals of educational institutions.

Dispositional Challenges

Dispositional barriers to student-centered approaches in distance education are based on fears, feelings, and how people relate to each other. This section of the chapter will explore the impact of these challenges on the development of student-centered approaches to distance education.

ATTITUDES TOWARD INNOVATION AND CHANGE

Despite the growing acceptance of technology in higher education, there still remains a degree of skepticism over the adoption of innovative approaches to teaching. Bates (2000) summarized the issue by suggesting that while technology changes rapidly, human beings tend to change slowly. This issue is compounded when one considers that many institutions of higher education are slow to adapt and change from their traditional roots and ethos. How faculty embrace and accept technology is a determining factor in its integration into the teaching enterprise.

Each person reacts differently to change. Our ability to adapt to technological innovations is based on factors such as prior experience with change; the number, magnitude, and pace of the change; our individual coping mechanisms; and our trust in the change agent. A suitable framework for examining common responses to change is Rodgers' (1983) Diffusion of Innovation Theory. Bushy and Kamphuis (1993), building on the work of Rodgers, identified behavioral categories commonly seen in response to change:

- Innovators.
- Early adopters.
- Early majority.
- Late majority.
- Resistors.

Each will be applied to the issue of instructional technology.

Innovators are those who readily adopt change. They are the first in line to try out new instructional technologies. These are individuals who thrive on change and innovative ideas. *Early adopters* are receptive to new ideas, but less so than innovators. They are willing to implement new technologies before most others. The *early majority* prefers the status quo, but will adopt new innovation technologies after a "wait-and-see" period of time. *Late majority* individuals are the followers. They are skeptical about new ideas and do not hesitate to express their negative views. This group tends to adopt the technologies late and often as a result of peer pressure. *Resistors* actively oppose or reject innovative instructional technologies. They encourage others to do so as well. Change and innovation leave them suspicious and often immoveable in their views. While the late majority and resistor groups will undoubtedly cause concern to administrators, they need to be attended to since there may be valid reasons for resisting the introduction of the new technology into their workplace.

Education administrators who understand the multiple layers of resistance and adoption will go a long way to changing faculty and student attitudes toward technological changes in higher education. It is clear that organizations must adopt a flexible set of strategies that address the variety of responses to change (Pajo & Wallace, 2001). These strategies should include technical support, addressing workload issues, providing training, recognizing and valuing distance education, and facilitating a smooth transition from traditional to innovative teaching approaches.

In keeping with this dispositional barrier is the fear by some faculty "that an increase in the use of distance education technologies may decrease the need for teachers" (Muilenburg & Berge, 2001, p. 7). While the reality of technology replacing humans has been largely unfounded, for some, the fear or perception serves as a significant barrier to the development of quality student-centered course offerings.

FEELINGS OF ISOLATION

The inherent nature of DE includes the geographic separation of students from faculty and from other learners. This can often contribute to feelings of social and psychological isolation in DE environments. Moore and Kearsley (1996) coined the phrase "**transactional distance**" to describe the psychological distance that occurs in learners. This transactional distance is often caused by miscommunication and psychological gaps occurring between the learner and the instructor. In a traditional classroom, students are in touch with the nuances of nonverbal communication. Their presence in class

BOX 22.3 STRATEGIES FOR PROMOTING A COMMUNITY OF LEARNERS

- Jointly formulate goals for learning.
- Negotiate guidelines for online discussions.
- Post student introductions and learning expectations.
- Form teams and posting guidelines for their performance.
- Encourage the sharing of real life experiences.
- Ask questions that promote group discussion.
- Share responsibility with students for facilitation of online discussions.
- Expect that students will provide constructive feedback to each other.
- Encourage students to share additional learning resources with others.

contributes to a sense of community with other students and the instructor. In a virtual classroom, faculty must make a conscientious effort to bridge the psychological distance experienced by learners. This can be achieved by promoting the establishment of a **community of learners** among students. Strategies for promoting a community of learners in a distance environment have been proposed by Palloff and Pratt (1999) and are included in Box 22.3. Faculty who establish communities of learning are promoting a student-centered approach to distance education. It fosters the development of strong social connections among students and encourages them to be actively engaged in the learning process.

Similar to their students, faculty may also experience feelings of isolation when teaching in a distance environment. The physical separation from students may affect faculty satisfaction, motivation, and long-term commitment to distance teaching. These feelings of isolation may be offset by working with a peer in a cooperative teaching arrangement or through a multidisciplinary team approach to course design and implementation.

GENDER RELATIONSHIPS

Over the past 10 to 20 years, a great deal has been reported on gender bias in traditional classroom settings where male students were perceived to have experienced higher quality education than their female counterparts (Gougen, 1998). Deborah Tannen (1990) has studied the impact of socialization of men and women on their patterns of communication. Her work has shown that men generally feel a primary need for recognition, identity, and status while women generally feel a primary need for personal connection and interaction. Women meet this need by creating intimacy with others. This is achieved by building "symmetrical relationships" where similarities are emphasized. In contrast, men tend to establish independence from others, where "asymmetrical relationships" or differences are the norm. Gougen summarizes this point by stating that "females generally interact in a manner where there exists horizontal or equal alignment among others whereas males generally interact in a manner where they "one-up" and others are "one-down" in alignment" (p. 5). When applied to Web-based learning, these relationship patterns potentially contribute to males dominating the online discussion forums.

BOX 22.4 CRITERIA FOR ONLINE PARTICIPATION

The following criteria will be used to assess your degree of online participation:

- Participates in online discussion on a regular basis (3 times a week minimum). This should include posting responses to required Learning Activities and responding to one to two postings by other students.
- Shows respect for the comments and perspectives of others.
- Is open to divergent points of view.
- Demonstrates application of course content in responses.
- Discussions are thoughtful and relevant to the topic.
- Engages in critical thinking around issues and posted "threads".
- Considers the topic (thread) from a different perspective.
- Initiates discussion with other students and/or instructor.
- Discussions are timely, i.e., not discussing a topic or "thread" several weeks after it has been thoroughly discussed by other students.
- Reads other students' postings and comments accordingly.
- Engages in reflective thinking, i.e., share with the instructor how the course content has influenced your thinking.

It has been suggested that Web-based courses provide the necessary structure to support an egalitarian, student-centered approach for online learning (McAllister & Ting, 2001). As such, providing for interactivity, reflectivity, and collaboration in online activities can contribute to a gender-neutral atmosphere. Creating this egalitarian learning environment also requires a concerted effort on the part of faculty. McAllister and Ting believe "the fact that discussion items are designed and mandated as activities in a credit-bearing course may be a 'leveling' factor in terms of how often students choose to participate" (pp. 15–16). This is best achieved by requiring a minimum number of postings to the discussion area per week as well as setting clear criteria for participation. Learners will be particularly attentive to these criteria if a portion of the course grade is based on these expectations. Box 22.4 provides an example of participation criteria that promotes a learner-centered, egalitarian approach to online learning.

SUMMARY

The ability to address the issues, challenges, and barriers to student-centered education is the hallmark of quality DE programming. The complex nature of delivering distance learning opportunities requires a complex set of strategies. Increasing demand for distance learning opportunities will pressure faculty and administrators to find creative solutions to the myriad of barriers presented in this chapter. An overarching goal will be to design distance courses to prepare students for participation in knowledge-based economies. The traditional faculty-centered educational model has been found not suitable for the emerging field of distance education. Student-centered approaches to distance learning will result in empowered students who have learned how to learn.

LEARNING ACTIVITY

CRITICAL THINKING

Refer back to the case scenario at the beginning of this chapter and respond to the following questions:

1. How could Daniel prepare himself to teach the computer-mediated course and the challenges it presents? For assistance refer to: Barker, A. (2003). Faculty development for teaching online: Educational and technological issues. *The Journal of Continuing Education in Nursing, 34*(6), 273–278.
2. Daniel will be challenged by having students with disabilities in his distance course. What strategies could he employ to address their learning needs? For assistance refer to Coombs, N., & Banks, R. (2000). Distance leaning and students with disabilities: Easy tips for teachers. Proceedings of the Technology and Persons with Disabilities Conference, March 20–25, California State University at Northridge, Los Angeles, CA. Retrieved May 10, 2004 from http://www.csun.edu/cod/conf/2000/proceedings/0119 Coombs.htm.

RESOURCES FOR EDUCATORS

PLANNING THE TEACHING/LEARNING EXPERIENCE

Instructions for Educators

Case studies can be an effective online teaching strategy. They provide the learner with insight into the context of a problem and encourage application of theoretical concepts to solutions generated. The following are suggestions for planning this intervention.

- The case study should relate to the subject matter being discussed.
- Assign roles to students such as facilitator, process observer, and "devil's advocate" in order promote collaborative problem solving.
- In large classes, assign learners to working groups of four to six students per group.
- Ensure the discussion questions challenge the students to think critically and apply course content to the case study.
- The faculty member should serve as moderator of the discussion forum to pose follow-up questions, seek clarification, and encourage application of content to the case.
- A summary of the discussion should be provided to all students by faculty or an assigned student.

Questions to Support a Thoughtful Reading

1. Based on your experience and/or what you have learned in this chapter, should teaching assignments or workload be adjusted when teaching distance courses? Why?
2. Think about a time when you were faced with technological change. How might you use knowledge of the behavioral categories of change and/or change theory to influence acceptance or reduce resistance to the innovation?

3. Think about a time when you were resistant to a change in your work environment. Which of the previously listed characteristics best describes your reaction to this change?

EVALUATING THE TEACHING/LEARNING EXPERIENCE

Questions to Elicit Feedback from Students on Their Learning

1. How might you incorporate criteria for online participation into your own course(s)? What percent of the course grade would you allocate for participation? Is it the same as you would allot for a traditional classroom-based course?
2. How might the criteria for online participation be used to support a learner-centered approach?
3. How would you develop a learning exercise or assignment that incorporates these criteria?
4. How should faculty members guide students in addressing real or potential socio-economic factors?

References

Barker, A. (2003). Faculty development for teaching online: Educational and technological issues. *The Journal of Continuing Education in Nursing, 34*(6), 273–278.

Bates, A. W. (2000). *Managing technological change: Strategies for college and university leaders.* San Francisco: Jossey-Bass.

Bates, A. W., & Poole, G. (2003). *Effective teaching with technology in higher education: Foundations for success.* San Francisco: Jossey-Bass.

Boshier, R. (1973). Educational participation and dropout: A theoretical model. *Adult Education, 23*(4), 255–282.

Boyer, E. (1990). *Scholarship reconsidered: Priorities for the professoriate.* Princeton, NJ: The Carnegie Foundation for the Advancement of Teaching.

Bushy, A., & Kamphuis, J. (1993). Response to innovation: Behavioral patterns. *Nursing Management, 24*(3), 62–64.

Care, W. D. (2003). The learning experiences of First Nation nursing students in a distance education environment. In J. Oakes, R. Riewe, A. Edmunds, et al., (Eds.). *Native Voices in Research* (pp. 82–93). Winnipeg, University of Manitoba: Aboriginal Issues Press.

Care, W. D., & Scanlan, J. M. (2000). Meeting the challenges of developing courses for distance delivery: Two different models for course development. *The Journal of Continuing Education in Nursing, 31*(3), 121–128.

Clay, M. (1999). Development of training and support programs for distance education instructors. *Online Journal of Distance Learning Administration,* 2(3). Retrieved November 5, 2005, from http://www.westga.edu/~distance/clay23.html.

Cook, R. A., & Gladhart, M. A. (2002). A survey of online instructional issues and strategies for postsecondary students with learning disabilities. *Information Technology and Disabilities, 8* (1). Retrieved November 5, 2005, from http://www.rit.edu/~easi/itd/itdv08.htm.

Cross, K. P. (1981). *Adults as learners: Increasing participation and facilitating learning.* San Francisco: Jossey-Bass.

Crow, K. (1993). Multiculturalism and pluralistic thought in nursing education: Native American world view and the nursing academic world view. *Journal of Nursing Education,* 32(5), 198–204.

Dasher-Alston, R. M., & Patton, G. W. (1998). Evaluation criteria for distance learning. *Planning for Higher Education,* 27(1), 11–17.

Diaz, D. P. (2002). Online dropout rates revisited. *The Technology Source.* Retrieved December 22, 2004, from http://technologysource.org/article/online_drop_rates_revisited/.

DiBiase, D. (2000). Is distance teaching more or less work? *The American Journal of Distance Education, 14*(3), 6–20.

Dickerson, S. S., Neary, M. A., & Hyche-Johnson. M. (2000). Native American graduate nursing students' learning experiences. *Journal of Nursing Scholarship, 32*(2), 189–196.

Fichten, C., Asuncion, J., Barile, C., et al. (2003). Canadian postsecondary students with disabilities: Where are they? *Canadian Journal of Higher Education, 33*(2), 71–113.

Gougen, T. D. (1998). Gender sensitive instruction: A distance education issue. Paper presented at the Annual Meeting of the American Association for Adult and Continuing Education (Phoenix, AZ, November 20 1998). Educational Resources Information Center (ERIC), ED 428 269.

Greenall, D., & Loizides, S. (2001). *Aboriginal digital opportunities: Addressing Aboriginal learning needs through the use of learning technologies*. Ottawa, ON: The Conference Board of Canada.

Hassenplug, C., & Harnish, D. (1998). The nature and importance of interaction in distance education credit classes at a technical institute. *Community College Journal of Research and Practice, 22(6)*, 591–606.

Howell, S. L., Williams, P. B., & Lindsay, N. K. (2003). Thirty-two trends affecting distance education: An informed foundation for strategic planning. *Online Journal of Distance Learning Administration, 6*(3). Retrieved November 4, 2005, from http://www.westga.edu/~distance/ojdla/fall63/howell63.html.

Jones, R. (2003). A recommendation for managing the predicted growth in college enrollment at a time of adverse economic conditions. *Online Journal of Distance Learning Administration, 6*(1). Retrieved November 4, 2005, from http://www.westga.edu/~distance/ojdla/spring61/jones61.html.

Kenway, J. (1996). The information super highway and post-modernity: The social promise and the social price. *Comparative Education, 32*(2), 217–242.

Kinash, S., Crichton, S., & Kim-Rupnow, W. S. (2004). A review of 2000–2003 literature at the intersection of online learning and disability. *The American Journal of Distance Education, 18*(1), 5–19.

Link, D. G., & Scholtz, S. M. (2000). Educational technology and the faculty role: What you don't know can hurt you. *Nurse Educator, 25*(6), 274–276.

Marriot, M. (2003, January 12). Technology: Beyond the blackboard. *The New York Times*, 4A–19A.

McAllister, C., & Ting, E. (2001). Analysis of discussion items by males and females in online college courses. Paper presented at the Annual Meeting of the American Educational Research Association, Seattle, WA. (April 10–14, 2001). Educational Resources Information Center (ERIC), ED 458 237.

McKenzie, B. K., Mims, N., Bennett, E., et al. (1999). Needs, concerns, and practices of online instructors. *Online Journal of Distance Learning Administration*, 2(3). Retrieved November 4, 2005, from http://www.westga.edu/~distance/ojdla/fall33/mckenzie33.html.

Moisey, S. D. (2004). Students with disabilities in distance education: Characteristics, course enrollment and completion, and support services. *Journal of Distance Education, 19*(1), 73–91.

Moore, M. G., & Kearsley, G. (1996). *Distance education: A systems view*. Belmont, CA: Wadsworth.

Muilenburg, L., & Berge, Z. L. (2001). Barriers to distance education: A factor-analytic study. *The American Journal of Distance Education, 15*(2), 7–22.

National Education Association. (2000). A survey of traditional and distance learning higher education members. Retrieved November 4, 2005, from http://www.nea.org/he/abouthe/dlstudy.pdf.

O'Connor, B. (2000). E-learning and students with disabilities: From outer edge to leading edge. Keynote address for NETworking 2000 Conference, Flexible Learning, November 1–4, Australia. Retrieved November 4, 2005, from http://www.flexiblelearning.net.au/nw2000/summary/sum_Key.htm.

Pachnowski, L. M., & Jurczyk, J. P. (2003). Perceptions of faculty on the effect of distance learning technology on faculty preparation time. *Online Journal of Distance Learning Administration, 6*(3). Retrieved November 4, 2005, from http://www.westga.edu/~distance/ojdla/fall63/pachnowski64.html.

Padilla, R., Trevino, J., Gonzalez, K., et al. (1997). Developing local models of minority student success in college. *Journal of College Student Development, 38*(2), 125–135.

Pajo, K., & Wallace, C. (2001). Barriers to the uptake of web-based technology by university teachers. *Journal of Distance Education, 16*(1), 70–84.

Palloff, R. M, & Pratt, K. (1999). *Building learning communities in cyberspace: Effective strategies for the online classroom*. San Francisco: Jossey-Bass.

Parker, A. (2003). Motivation and incentives for distance faculty. *Online Journal of Distance Learning Administration, 6*(3). Retrieved December 22, 2004, from http://www.westga.edu/~distance/ojdla/fall63/parker63.html.

Reinert, B. R., & Fryback, P. B. (1997). Distance learning and nursing education. *Journal of Nursing Education, 36*(9), 421–427.

Rodgers, E. (1983). *Diffusion of innovations*. New York: The Free Press.

Schifter, C. C. (2000). Faculty motivators and inhibitors for participation in distance education. *Educational Technology, 40*(2), 43–46.

Tannen, D. (1990). *You just don't understand: Women and men in conversation*. New York: Ballantine.

Volery, T. (2001). Online education: An exploratory study into success factors. *Journal of Educational Computing Research, 24*(1), 77–92.

U.S. Department of Education, National Center for Education Statistics. (2003). *Distance education at degree-granting postsecondary institutions: 2000–2001*. (NCES2003-17). Washington, DC: Author.

Additional Resources

A Survey of Online Instructional Issues and Strategies for Postsecondary Students with Learning Disabilities. Available at: http://www.rit.edu/~easi/itd/itdv08n.htm.

Americans with Disabilities Act. Available at: http://www.usdoj.gov/crt/ada/adahom1.htm.

The Chronicle of Higher Education. Available at: http://chronicle.com/indepth/distance/.

Cultural Issues and the Online Environment. Available at: http://www.csu.edu.au/division/celt/resources/cultural_issues.pdf.

Disabilities and Distance Education: DO-IT Project, University of Washington. Available at: http://www.washington.edu/doit.

Distance-Educator.com. Available at: http://www.distance-educator.com/.

Institute for Higher Education Policy. (2000). *Quality on the line: Benchmarks for success in Internet-based distance education*. Washington, DC: Author. Available at: http://www.ihep.org/Pubs/PDF/Quality.pdf.

Journal of Distance Education. Available at: http://www.athabascau.ca

Meta-Analysis of the Effectiveness of Teaching and Learning with Technology on Student Outcomes. Available at: http://www.ncrel.org/tech/effects2/index.html.

National Education Association. Available at: http://www.nea.org/he/abouthe/distance.html.

Resources for Distance Education. Available at: http://www.ccc.commnet.edu.

Chapter 23

Demonstrating the Scholarship of Teaching: A Sample Course Portfolio

Beverly Williams

A memo from the Provost appears in all faculty mailboxes one morning, announcing that from now on every candidate for tenure and promotion must submit a teaching portfolio along with the usual research documentation. Faculty reaction is swift and divided. Some faculty see the requirement as an indication that the administration is finally starting to take teaching scholarship seriously, while others view it as just another demand for their time that will not accomplish anything and could actually hurt them. Either viewpoint could be correct depending on how the program and process are handled (adapted from Felder & Brent, 1996).

INTENT A central premise of this chapter is that constructing knowledge about teaching in nursing is a scholarly activity. It is the scholarship of teaching that links the scholarship of discovery with the scholarship of integration and application. **Scholars of teaching** in nursing are excellent and expert teachers, and they advance the knowledge of teaching within the discipline through peer reviewed publications. In this chapter **teaching portfolios** and **course portfolios** are compared in relation to their respective utility in demonstrating the scholarship of teaching in nursing. A nursing course portfolio that has been externally peer reviewed is offered as an example of how the scholarship of teaching can be exemplified.

OVERVIEW

INTRODUCTION

Demands for faculty to demonstrate their scholarship in teaching, as exemplified in the previous situation, can be traced back to the work of Boyer (1990) who identified four categories of scholarship: discovery, integration, application, and teaching. He indicated that it is the interconnections among the four categories that are essential for the generation and sharing of knowledge within a discipline such as nursing education. Boyer further suggested that all four categories of scholarship should be recognized and rewarded by universities. Although the distinction associated with modern universities is built on the scholarship of discovery, knowledge alone remains incomplete without the insights of scholarly teachers who can demonstrate how to integrate and apply it in professional practice. When the scholarship of teaching is conceptualized within the discipline of nursing, it can be described as the scholarship of how to best prepare practitioners who will demonstrate excellence in nursing practice through reflection, collaboration, use of evidence, and continuous learning (Riley, Beal, Levi, & McCausland, 2002).

SCHOLARSHIP OF TEACHING IN NURSING

The scholarship of teaching has been conceptualized in a variety of ways in the literature (Kreber & Cranton, 2000). In relating these conceptualizations to nursing education, the first perspective contends that teaching scholarship in nursing is demonstrated through systematic study of teaching and learning and the related dissemination of findings through academic journals and conferences. This perspective is congruent with scholarship as discovery. A second perspective that is more congruent with scholarship of application suggests that teaching scholarship in nursing is synonymous with teaching excellence as measured by either peer review or learner ratings of nursing instruction. A third perspective, consistent with scholarship as integration, suggests that teaching expertise in nursing is evident when faculty members reflect on and use knowledge gained through research within the context of their own teaching. Kreber (2002) would describe scholars of teaching in nursing as excellent teachers, as well as expert teachers, but in addition, they share their knowledge and advance the knowledge of teaching and learning within the discipline of nursing through publication in peer reviewed journals.

Scholarship in teaching nursing is conceptualized somewhat differently by Glanville & Houde (2002) who suggest that scholarship of nursing involves having knowledge of the discipline, knowing about teaching and learning in nursing, demonstrating that knowledge in teaching practice, and reflecting on the teaching process and learning outcomes. Learning about teaching and learning in nursing, they say, is best achieved by reflecting on the interaction of one's actual teaching practice in light of research-based knowledge about teaching and learning. Then the process of disseminating that knowledge contributes to knowledge development about teaching and learning in nursing as it becomes public and is available for critical review and evaluation by members of the scholarly community.

Some suggest that the quality of teaching scholarship in nursing can best be assessed on the basis of documented evidence. The rich and varied materials that the individual scholar assembles over time should demonstrate direct links between the literature on nursing education and the educator's work (Glassick, Huber, & Maeroff, 1997). It takes imagination, discipline, and critical reflection to present evidence that is research based, has clear purpose, and links methods to learning outcomes reflective of nursing practice. Teaching scholars in nursing need to be clear about the pedagogical goals of their work, ensuring that the learning goals are realistic and achievable. They should be able to demonstrate an understanding and application of the existing knowledge related to teaching and learning in nursing. By effectively selecting and using teaching and evaluative methods appropriate to the learning goals, teaching scholars in nursing are more likely to be able to help learners achieve significant outcomes related to desired competencies in nursing practice. Teaching scholars in nursing think deeply about what they are doing while they are doing it. Insightful reflection guides the nurse scholar's thinking about what went right, what went wrong, what opportunities were taken, and which ones were missed. However, teaching scholarship in nursing remains incomplete unless insights are shared through informal and formal seminars, conferences, and publications.

TEACHING PORTFOLIOS IN NURSING

Following their inception in the 1980s, (Shore, 1986) teaching portfolios have been conceptualized as one way to demonstrate excellent and expert teaching in nursing (Glanville & Houde, 2004; Reece, Pearce, Melillo, & Beaudry, 2001; Riley, et al., 2002). Through the process of developing a teaching portfolio, teachers reflect on their teaching and become more conscious of the theories and assumptions that guide their teaching practice. This has the potential to alter their teaching practice to facilitate optimal learning (Zeichner & Wray, 2001).

The teaching portfolio is described as a collection of information from students, colleagues, and the faculty member's own files which results in a comprehensive profile of teaching effectiveness. Each teaching portfolio is unique and represents teaching expertise and excellence for the individual faculty member. The teaching portfolio generally includes a reflective statement that explicates the individual's philosophy about teaching and learning as well as goals and objectives that contribute to the evaluative mechanisms chosen. Examples of course work (courses developed, course materials, and evaluations), involvement in curricular design, evaluation and revision, peer reviewed publications/presentations, faculty practice, learner advisement and teaching awards are often included in a teaching portfolio (Felder & Brent, 1996; Reece, et al., 2001; Seldin, 1997).

Teaching portfolios in nursing are currently used primarily for formative and summative evaluation of faculty and are rarely peer reviewed beyond the institutional evaluative process. In the case of formative evaluation, portfolios can be used to facilitate faculty development through identification and remediation of teaching concerns. When portfolios are used for summative evaluation they are used to evaluate teaching performance as a rational basis for decisions about promotion and tenure (Felder & Brent, 1996). Whether used for formative or summative evaluation, there are several challenges in both the preparation and review of teaching portfolios (Burns, 1999).

The preparation of a teaching portfolio entails a great deal of time and energy expenditure on the part of faculty in collecting and analyzing the wide variety of materials that comprise the portfolio. Furthermore, in order to maximize the utility of a teaching portfolio, it must be reviewed and revised on a regular basis. Since teaching portfolios are meant to present a comprehensive profile of teaching effectiveness, it follows that the faculty member's emphasis in creating the teaching portfolio is likely to be on successes (Burns, 1999; July, 1998). This means that the portfolio may not provide a balanced view of the faculty member's teaching performance (Abrami, d'Apollonia, & Rosenfield, 1997). The internal review of the portfolio also entails a great deal of time and energy on the part of reviewers who may or may not be using common criteria to evaluate the portfolio.

When teaching portfolios are to be used for promotion and tenure decisions, it is suggested that they be prepared with consideration of several basic aspects according to Felder & Brent, 1996:

- Relevant—elements selected for evaluation are clearly linked to established criteria for effective teaching.
- Reliable—ratings from different colleagues are reasonably similar.
- Practical—portfolios are well-organized, clear, and concise.

Once a portfolio is submitted for review, it is recommended that several people independently evaluate it and rate it according to predefined categories and a predefined rating system. Widely divergent evaluations should be reconciled and a weighted average rating should be calculated. The final evaluation would be a collective rating (Burns, 1999; Felder & Brent, 1996; Quinlan, 2002). Since there is still little research on the reliability and validity of using portfolios to evaluate teaching for the purpose of promotion and tenure, it is suggested that faculties using portfolios for such decisions closely monitor the portfolio development and review process (Burns, 1999; Centra, 1993).

COURSE PORTFOLIOS IN NURSING

In thinking about teaching in nursing as scholarly inquiry, it is beneficial to conceptualize the portfolio as a qualitative and quantitative representation of the work of a particular nurse educator, usually presented within a specific time frame, and associated with a particular course (Kreber, 1999). A course portfolio is briefer than a teaching portfolio. The focus of a course portfolio includes rationale for course design, evolution of teaching strategies, and learner outcomes. Qualitative descriptions often relate to learner and faculty reflection on various aspects of learning process and outcomes. Quantitative aspects often include specifics related to learning outcomes and comparisons of outcomes from previous renditions of the course.

A course portfolio can be used to highlight teaching scholarship when it is published following internal and external peer review (Cerbin, 1994, Weimer, 1993). Through a course portfolio, individual faculty members document the design, evolution, and execution of a particular course. Utilizing accountability through an internal and external peer review process, teaching can be understood and presented as a form of scholarship. In this way course portfolios can be used to:

1. Increase the variety of methods for assessing teaching effectiveness.
2. Set standards for excellence in documenting effective teaching/learning practice.
3. Raise expectations for documenting teaching effectiveness (Brassell & Robinson, 2001).

The process of designing a course portfolio facilitates: reflection on pedagogy and teaching activities; recognition of elements critical to learner success; documenting learning outcomes; showcasing innovation and excellence; longitudinal studies of effectiveness of changes in teaching methods and practices; and external independent assessment of teaching and evaluation through the peer review process.

A course portfolio generally contains the following components:

- An introduction to the teaching philosophy of the individual faculty member.
- A description of course design including a statement of the goals, objectives, and content.
- A description of teaching strategies based on sound pedagogy.
- Evidence of learning outcomes.
- Most importantly, a reflective narrative addressing the relationship of philosophy, course goals, teaching strategies, and learning outcomes (Brassell & Robinson, 2001; Cerbin, 1994).

When a course portfolio is used to demonstrate the scholarship of teaching the same guidelines required in any other scholarly work apply. Those guidelines include clarity of purpose, original ideas, effective use of evidence, significant conclusions, replicability, and potential contribution to current empirical and theoretical literature (Diamond, 1995). In this way, a course portfolio can be utilized as a model of exemplary teaching practice and as a resource for information about the effectiveness of specific teaching approaches.

Nursing course portfolios are most commonly reviewed internally within the faculty and sometimes externally by faculty members in other disciplines on the same campus. Weimer (1993) suggests that external review by nursing peers outside of one's academic setting may be more rigorous than internal review by those in other disciplines within one's own academic environment. Similarly, external review by peers from other disciplines outside of one's academic setting may be more rigorous than internal review by those in other disciplines within one's own academic environment. Sharing with faculty from other disciplines and on other campuses establishes a broad dialogue that facilitates the exchange of ideas and helps identify successful approaches to learning. Through continued development and revision, course portfolios become an iterative account of an individual teacher's inquiry and can serve as a generative tool for the professional development of other nursing faculty. The consistent use of course portfolios has the potential to provide a systematic way to ensure that evidence-based teaching occurs in nursing education.

SAMPLE COURSE PORTFOLIO

The following course portfolio is an example of how I[1] set up a description of my teaching as evidence that my teaching is scholarship. In particular, I focus on my work as an undergraduate educator teaching a specific course, NURS 394 Nursing in Context. NURS 394 is the last theory course in the third year of a four-year undergraduate baccalaureate program in nursing.

Course Description

The goal of the course is to continue the development of concepts related to health, health promotion, professional nursing, and human responses across the lifespan. The focus is on care of clients (individuals, families, and groups) located in institutions and communities who are experiencing acute and complex variances in health.

(University of Alberta Collaborative Baccalaureate Nursing Program, 2003)

Course Objectives

1. Discuss issues (poverty, elder/nurse abuse, respite, case management, institutionalization) related to the delivery of health care and implications for registered nurses.
2. Discuss roles and functions (delegation, decision making, case management, resource allocation) of registered nurses in acute and complex settings.
3. Discuss roles of multidisciplinary health professionals.
4. Apply concepts of primary health care in acute and complex practice situations.
5. Analyze selected nursing and interdisciplinary models and theories.
6. Analyze knowledge related to biological, psychological, sociological, cultural, and spiritual dimensions of the human response to acute and complex variances in health.
7. Demonstrate competence with self-directed, context-based, small group learning.
8. Demonstrate competence in using additional information technology (finding nursing research) to support scholarly activity.

(University of Alberta Collaborative Baccalaureate Nursing Program, 2003)

Teaching Philosophy

I believe that learners need to graduate from undergraduate nursing programs with retrievable disciplinary knowledge that they can transfer to a variety of situations and continuous learning skills to extend their knowledge base in order to remain professionally competent. The faculty of nursing has chosen to use a context-based learning (CBL) approach to facilitating learning in all nursing courses. (For further detail on CBL, please refer back to an earlier discussion in Chapter 9.) CBL is a learner-centered approach to learning and is based on a constructivist theory of learning (Savery &

[1] The first-person "I" is that of author Beverly Williams.

Duffy, 1995). Constructivists believe that learners create new knowledge by actively interpreting and processing information within the context of prior knowledge (Duffy & Cunningham, 1996). Real professional practice situations are used as an initial activity to stimulate learning rather than as a culminating activity following faculty presentation of content. The faculty member or tutor becomes an advisor and facilitator rather than a transmitter of information. Learning processes (e.g., identification of learning needs, seeking out resources, analyzing/evaluating information, and sharing it with colleagues) and learning outcomes (e.g., knowledge, critical thinking, leadership, collaboration, self-direction) are addressed equally during CBL, and it is my view that socialization into the discourse and practice of nursing as a discipline can be accomplished using this approach. The theory underlying CBL supports my beliefs that learners want to do their best if they are in a supportive environment, have control of the learning process, are actively involved in learning, receive feedback, and perceive that learning is relevant.

My role as faculty tutor is to create a supportive environment, encourage inquiry through critical scrutiny of assumptions, values, and behaviors, provide helpful feedback, and draw attention to the connections between theory and practice. I consider myself a resource with specific expertise in nursing as well as a facilitator who can guide learners to meet course and program outcomes.

Teaching Approach

As a tutor, I meet with my group of 15 learners for 3 hours twice a week for 6 weeks. Each week we discuss one of the following learning packages: "Nursing Organizations," "The Jacobs," "The Webbs," "Matt Boychuck," and "The Inmates." Each learning package consists of general learning goals and a description of an authentic nursing practice situation. Specific concepts from nursing and support courses from other disciplines are integrated into each of the learning packages. Learners are required to carry out independent research to support their learning.

Nursing Organizations is a package designed to engage learners in considering how nursing and nursing education are organized at the local, national, and international levels, and how the professional organizations interface with governments at all levels. In addition, learners discuss practice standards, continuing competency, balancing nursing labor supply and demand, collective bargaining, and entry to practice issues. In the learning package, The Jacobs, learners encounter a family experiencing a high risk pregnancy. They discuss causes of high risk pregnancy, premature birth, ethical issues related to right to life, patient advocacy, and parental and sibling grief related to an infant death. Matt Boychuck introduces the learners to the trauma care of an adolescent involved in an alcohol-related motor vehicle accident. Learners discuss rural versus urban health care, life-threatening neurological and musculoskeletal injuries, levels of prevention, and prevention programs. In addition, they are encouraged to explore issues related to life support, sudden death, and organ donation. The Webbs is a case description that introduces an elderly couple who have a number of chronic health concerns. Learners examine issues pertaining to a family with adult children caring for frail elderly parents. They discuss homecare nursing, caregiver burden, elder abuse, respite care, decision making, and how to conduct a family meeting.

The following is a sample learning package LP 3.2.5 from The Inmates:

> *Learning Goals:*
> This learning package is designed to introduce learners to the application of principles of program planning for inmates in a correctional institution. Learners will be able to explore values, beliefs, and strategies for working with clients and aggregates who are experiencing addictions, HIV, HepC, and TB.
>
> *Scenario:*
> You are employed as a registered nurse in a correctional institution for male offenders. This institution has 600 inmates, is located close to a major highway, and is 30 kilometers from a city of 60,000 people.
>
> The following (2 out of 4) descriptions have been drawn from the current population in this institution:
>
> Jaime (21) grew up on a farm in Saskatchewan. He did not use drugs or alcohol when he was growing up. He moved to Calgary when he was 18 and began to use marijuana heavily. Jaime committed several robberies and was apprehended. He has approached you saying, "There's a bunch of guys in here that I know have HIV and hepatitis. I'm terrified of them and I'm not the only one who feels this way".
>
> Tom is from a minority cultural group and has been using drugs and alcohol for many years. He has always used clean needles until he began living with Mary and sharing "rigs." Although Tom didn't know it, Mary was HIV positive. He didn't find out that he was HIV positive until he asked to be tested in jail because he was suffering from night sweats.
>
> (University of Alberta Collaborative Baccalaureate Program, 2003)

During the initial tutorial, learning is stimulated by brainstorming or verbal exploration of the situation outlined in the learning package. Existing knowledge about the situation is discussed, and through guiding and challenging questions from their peers and me, learner needs for learning are identified. For example, in relation to the inmates, I might ask:

> What do you already know about HIV?
>
> What will you say to Jamie? How does your response reflect your values?
>
> What does society say about providing inmates with condoms and clean needles?
>
> How do we differentiate risk behaviors from risk groups? Why is this important?
>
> Do health care personnel have legitimate reasons for knowing if someone is HIV positive? Do patients have to disclose their HIV status to health care personnel/employers?

With further guidance from their peers and me and through self-reflection, learners are able to begin to clearly identify their learning needs and to discuss relevant resources that could be used to help them learn unfamiliar information. Learners use the learning time between one tutorial and the next to engage in self-directed study, addressing learning needs, either in pairs or independently.

During a follow-up tutorial, written information is distributed to members of the tutorial group and discussed in relation to the situation identified in the learning package. This process provides an opportunity to evaluate the quality of the information, credibility of resources used to retrieve the information, creativity used in sharing the information, the learners' understanding of the situation, and their capacity to articulate the role of the professional nurse in the situation.

An optional weekly resource session, which takes the form of a guest/faculty lecture/discussion, is offered to learners. These sessions provide an opportunity for learners to extend their knowledge about the particular situation under study. For example, when we worked with The Inmates package, the HIV clinical nurse specialist from the hospital and an HIV positive volunteer from the correctional institution came to speak to the learners. Through telling their stories and answering questions that learners had, they were able to greatly enrich learning.

Learners engage in self-reflection and reflection on peer and tutor participation in the tutorial process following each learning package discussion. Using the tutor as a role model, learners are encouraged to offer constructive criticism of themselves and their colleagues using specific criteria in the areas of critical thinking (e.g., synthesizes information from a variety of references, including evidenced-based references), communication and respect (e.g., provides direct, honest, constructive feedback), self-direction (e.g., demonstrates formal and informal leadership ability), and group process (e.g., actively facilitates group discussion). Learners will often pick names at the beginning of each scenario, watch the chosen individual closely for the week and then during tutorial they will provide both written and verbal feedback to the individual. The written feedback becomes evidence that each learner must incorporate into her own written self-evaluation for both midterm and final course evaluations.

Evidence of Learner Understanding

Formal NURS 394 course evaluation is based on the following: (1) Tutorial participation: 30%, (2) Content examination: 40%, and (3) Scholarly writing: 30%.

Tutorial Participation

To arrive at a tutorial participation grade, learners rank themselves and are ranked by me in the following areas: critical thinking, communication and respect, self-direction, and group process. Through self-evaluation, learners must provide specific examples of their tutorial behavior as evidence of having met the criteria, and I do the same. Learners have been creative in using resources and sharing information with their colleagues. Increasingly, I find the majority of learners will use at least two or three resources; however, only about half of any group will use evidence-based references. Many learners comment that "they are using more resources than they ever have before, including while obtaining other degrees." Almost all learners will try to demonstrate creativity in sharing their information. The following are examples of their work:

1. A telephone interview with a nurse who worked at a correctional institution. The following are a sample of questions that the learner asked: Can you describe your role as nurse and how the scope of your practice is influenced by your environment? What are the challenges/rewards of working with this type of high risk population? What are the effects of the institutionalization on health? What types of health promotion strategies are utilized within the institution for inmates/staff? There is much debate in the literature about protecting confidentiality. In your experience should staff be informed about the HIV status of inmates? Should other inmates be informed?
2. Retrieval of a Federal Report on HIV and Prisons. Based on the report, the learner was able to provide current information on the incidence and prevalence of drug addiction, HIV and TB, HIV testing, educational programs, issues of confidentiality, a candid description of the inmate social system, and incidence of violence and exploitation to peers.
3. A poem that was written by a gentleman who was experiencing early onset dementia at the time he was writing the poem.
4. An extensive list of credible Web sites for explaining death to a child.
5. A model (plastic bag filled with 415 grams of water in a light stocking) to represent the size of a 28-week-old infant who was small for her gestational age.
6. Pretest and posttest quizzes for their classmates.

Learners have demonstrated thoughtful reflection in their self-evaluations. For example:

> I do ask the group questions to promote discussion, but I would like to facilitate more discussion and also be more creative when sharing my information. I can be more alert to the cues of others' lack of understanding and at times I need to wait for others to finish speaking before I begin. I can work on giving more constructive feedback—the feedback I give tends to be only positive.

Learners are able to provide direct honest feedback to each other even though they still find it uncomfortable. For example:

> I appreciate your attentiveness to others when they are speaking. Your information is complete. Although you read points off your sheet, you elaborate on the topics by asking questions to stimulate discussion. I encourage you to speak up more in class—we all have a responsibility to each other to contribute in order to maximize our learning and critical thinking.

Generally, the tutorial participation marks within a single tutorial group reflect a range of skills and ability (11–19 out of a possible 20 marks).

Examinations

The NURS 394 examination includes multiple choice questions (MCQ), as well short and long answer questions. As a reflection of CBL, each series of MCQ is preceded by a short description of a client/patient situation. The multiple choice questions used on NURS 394 exams are comparable to those I used for a case-based course that I taught in the previous traditional program. The mean range for learners in the traditional course was 66 to 68% and the mean range for CBL learners on the same questions was 68 to 77%. Clearly, CBL learners are learning content considered relevant to nursing practice. A sample long answer question might be:

> You are the only nurse in a small community without a physician. Since your arrival a month ago, you have observed that unemployment is high. During your first visit to the school, the Grade 5 teacher, Ms. Lewis, expresses concern that she thinks some of her learners are experimenting with alcohol and solvents. She asks, "What can we do?"
>
> First, how will you respond to Ms. Lewis? Then, using the Population Health Model, outline how you will determine the issues of priority for the school/community and how you respond to identified needs.

Scholarly Writing

Scholarly paper topics usually focus on exploration of a current issue related to health care and the implications of the issue or resolution for professional nursing. For example, learners may be asked to "discuss the effects of privatization on healthcare of Albertans" or "argue that employing baccalaureate nurses is beneficial to the health of Albertans." Although the following represents a conclusion to a paper graded as "excellent," it is still a struggle for many learners to clearly and logically identify an issue, outline possible solutions including the pros and cons of each, arrive at an informed conclusion, and identify the implications for the nursing profession.

> On one hand, physicians as gatekeepers of the health care system have served Canadians well. Continuous, comprehensive care has been maintained. On the other hand, accessibility to healthcare and the individual's right to self determination in choice of healthcare practitioner have been violated and interdisciplinary/intersectoral collaboration has been minimal. The individual's right to self-determination in maximizing use of the nation's healthcare resources make it imperative that barrier-free multiple entry points to the healthcare system be optimized. Legislative changes and healthcare reform are necessary. Nurses have an obligation to become politically active in order to. . .

Achievement of Level Outcomes

By the end of NURS 394, learner achievement of the third-year level outcomes related to self-directed learning and critical thinking is evident. In their self/course evaluations, learners provide evidence to support their descriptions of themselves as developing the characteristics of self-directed learners as outlined in the literature. They recognize the sense of responsibility they are developing in being able to work with others. Learners indicate they are confident in their ability to identify their learning needs, select and use a variety of resources, choose relevant information, and share their information in creative ways. They acknowledge that they are learning how to effectively question each other, deal with ambiguity, and value a diversity of viewpoints. Learners comment that through regular self-evaluation and peer evaluation they are developing a deeper awareness of themselves and others and are increasingly able to communicate their observations of each other. Finally, learners indicate that they are developing the skills that will enable them to continue to learn once they are practicing professionals. As one learner said, "I don't know too much about _____, but if there is one thing I learned from the course, it is that I know how to learn." This is evidence of my scholarship of teaching as it pertains to applying self-directed learning strategies. I am currently engaged in a study that will compare learners' self-directed learning readiness at the beginning and end of 4 years in the CBL undergraduate nursing program.

Learners demonstrate the ability to think critically when making clinical decisions as confirmed by their comments on self/course evaluations, their answers to examination questions, their scholarly writing, and the clinical decision-making assessment completed prior to them being hired as senior nursing learners. A colleague and I are currently engaged in a study using Facione and Facione's (1994) *Holistic Critical Thinking Rubric* that will compare learners' critical thinking abilities at the beginning and end of the four-year undergraduate program.

Reflection on Instructional Practice

It is important for me to get to know each of my learners personally, and for them to get to know one another at the beginning of our teaching–learning relationship. During the first tutorial, learners are asked to interview one of their classmates and then introduce that person to the group. Learners as a group interview me as their tutor. I prepare myself for tutorial interaction by reviewing the learning goals for the current learning package, ensuring that I know how these goals interface with the course and curriculum as a whole. I often review content theory and the most recent professional literature that pertains to current topics learners have identified. I think generally about questions I might ask the learners to challenge their understanding, as well as stories from my practice that I might share. Learners comment that I am "knowledgeable and well prepared" for tutorial discussions and am able to "assist them in understanding complex concepts."

When I first started as a tutor, my questions tended to guide the learners to discussions about pathophysiology, pharmacology, and general nursing care. In a short period of time I realized that they would learn this information on their own and what they needed help with was professional practice integration and application. The following are examples of the types of questions I might ask to bring forward such issues: "As the RN in charge on evenings, what would you need to know in order to effectively delegate activities to the two licensed practical nurses who are working with you? How would you inform the Jacobs of the hospital policy regarding resuscitation of infants with a birth weight below 500 grams? How would you respond to Matt's mom when she tells you that she and Matt discussed organ donation when he received his driver's license? Who should initiate discussion about organ donation if the family does not? How? Could the Webbs benefit from a family meeting? How would you conduct one, who would you invite, what observations might you share, what questions might you ask?" It is this type of questioning, I believe, that has prompted learners to comment that I encourage them to "think why things are the way they are" and to "dig deeper to understand."

It is an ongoing challenge for me to find different ways to ensure that the content is relevant, that learners maintain control over their learning, and that all learners are equally involved in the learning while trying to consider the various learning styles among learners. It is important that learners in nursing develop the ability to think critically in order to arrive at sound clinical judgments. Initially, I used the strategy of questioning almost exclusively, however, over time I have developed a repertoire of strategies to use with CBL. Although I still use questioning (e.g., What do you already know about this situation? How do you know _____? Why do you think _____? Is there a relationship between _____ and _____?), I also use role playing (You are the nurse in this situation. What will you do/say? How will you respond if I say _____?). I also challenge with hypothetical situations (What are the possible outcomes? What would happen if _____?), and I use stories and poetry from popular and professional literature as well as use examples from my own professional practice.

Learners respond that they "feel respected, look forward to tutorial, even at 8 in the morning and are stimulated to get involved." They consistently report how much they appreciate the questions that I ask to help "challenge the depth of their understanding and their ability to apply what they are learning to actual practice." Learners indicate that when I encourage them to "actively engage in critical thinking," they feel "confident that they are meeting the learning goals for the course and for the program" while still pursuing theory that is relevant to them. They indicate that within the structure of CBL I have achieved the essential balance between "telling them nothing" and "telling them everything." It has taken me some time to reach this balance. Learners who I tutored in second year and subsequently in third year commented that I was "more a part of the group, less reserved, and controlled my nonverbal communication better."

One of the most challenging aspects of teaching is helping learners continue to develop by giving feedback that recognizes the strengths of each individual as well as the areas that each learner can develop further. There is an art to providing this kind of feedback publicly to learners and in helping learners develop the skill to provide direct and honest feedback to each other in a public forum. I sometimes find myself pondering how best to share my thoughts and suggestions to ensure that the learners' self-confidence remains intact. It is important that they understand that I am commenting in writing and/or verbally because I value each of them and want to help them become the best that they can be. I consider myself a role model and coach as well as someone who is there to support them if they need it. Learners have commented that they have "grown so much through the feedback" and "for the first time are able to provide feedback to colleagues and significant others in their personal lives.

Conclusion

The evidence strongly suggests that at the end of NURS 394, learners generally have achieved the level outcomes. In their self/course evaluations, learners provide evidence to support their descriptions of themselves as developing the characteristics of self-directed learners outlined in the literature. They recognize the sense of responsibility they are developing in being able to work with others. Learners indicate they are confident in their ability to identify their learning needs, select and use a variety of resources, choose relevant information, and share their information in creative ways. They acknowledge that they are learning how to question each other effectively, deal with ambiguity, and value a diversity of viewpoints. Learners comment that through regular self-evaluations and peer evaluations they are developing a deeper awareness of themselves and others and are increasingly able to communicate their observations of each other. Finally, learners indicate that they are developing the skills that will enable them to continue to learn once they are practicing professionals. I believe that effective learner outcomes have become more evident since I started using a CBL approach to my course.

COURSE PORTFOLIO AS EVIDENCE OF TEACHING SCHOLARSHIP

This particular course portfolio has been through an internal and external review that was conducted by the PBL Peer Review Portfolio Project supported by Samford University and the Pew Charitable Trusts. A preliminary review was conducted by the Project Director to ensure that the portfolio met the minimum standards for the project. Since those standards were met it was sent out for review by an expert in the discipline of nursing at Samford University. Following the internal review, the portfolio was sent out to two experts in disciplines outside of nursing at Samford University and one of these individuals was an expert in teaching and learning strategies. The portfolio was judged for its adherence to the following guidelines for scholarly work: clarity of purpose, original ideas, appropriate use of evidence, replicability, significant conclusions, and potential to contribute to theoretical and empirical literature related to nursing education. After suggestions for revisions were made, the portfolio was published on the Samford University Web site as an example of teaching scholarship using CBL.

SUMMARY

Constructing knowledge about teaching in nursing is a scholarly activity. It can be achieved by nursing faculty when they reflect on the interaction between their teaching practice and research-based knowledge on teaching. Constructing knowledge involves learning more about teaching and demonstrating that knowledge through evidence-based documentation. The course teaching portfolio can be used to document this synthesis and when presented for public review, can be considered teaching scholarship. If portfolio programs are well designed they will have an impact on disciplinary teaching quality and should enhance faculty dialogue, learning, and morale thereby avoiding the skepticism alluded to at the beginning of this chapter.

LEARNING ACTIVITY

TEACHING PREFERENCE

Every teacher represents a unique way to be an excellent teacher. Self-awareness is one of the most significant factors involved in teaching excellence. Excellent teachers understand their discipline, their approach to teaching, and their learners.

Cranton (1998) proposed eight teacher preferences based on psychological type theory. If teachers reflect on who they are as people and how that affects how they work with learners, they can develop their own unique way of being an excellent teacher.

The following activity is designed to encourage this reflective process. Using the table as a context, please work through the questions that follow it.

TEACHER PREFERENCES

	MORE EXTROVERTED	MORE INTROVERTED
THINKING	DIRECTING	REFLECTING
	1. Do I enjoy lecturing, explaining, and directing a class?	3. Do I reflect on my teaching after every class?
	2. Do I like to organize and structure my teaching?	4. Do I especially enjoy teaching theory and models?
FEELING	COLLABORATING	PERSONALIZING
	5. Do I prefer that learners collaborate in groups?	7. Do I have intense personal feelings about teaching?
	6. Do I especially care about the sense of harmony in class?	8. Do I prefer working closely with individual learners?
SENSING	EXPERIENCING	OBSERVING
	9. Do I enjoy real, concrete, and practical experiences?	11. Do I like to sit back and notice the details in class?
	10. Do I especially like an action-filled class?	12. Am I especially sensitive to what happens in class?
INTUITION	REFORMING	ENVISIONING
	13. Am I enthusiastic about education as a means of reform?	15. Do I have inexplicable hunches about works in class?
	14. Do I see opportunities for learning around every corner?	16. Do I have a sixth sense about teaching?

A preference for thinking in teaching prompts the teacher to create a carefully organized, planned, and structured environment with a choice of methods and strategies based on logical judgment. The feeling teacher emphasizes harmony and collaboration among learners. A teacher who prefers sensing focuses on concrete reality and practical experiences in the teaching/learning process. An intuitive teacher is interested in alternative possibilities, change, and reform. Each of these preferences may include either an introverted or extroverted dimension (Cranton, 1998). Most teachers embody elements from all preferences but usually prefer to use one or two over others.

It is important that you recognize your individual teaching preference(s). Because your learners also have preferred ways of learning, it is critical that you develop your teaching preference by expanding and adding to your repertoire in a way that is congruent with you as an individual.

RESOURCES FOR EDUCATORS

PLANNING THE TEACHING/LEARNING EXPERIENCE

Questions to Support a Thoughtful Reading

1. Does the idea of scholarly teaching appeal to me?
2. Would I classify myself as an excellent teacher?
3. Would I classify myself as an expert teacher?
4. Would I classify myself as a scholarly teacher?
5. How would I demonstrate the scholarship of teaching?

EVALUATING THE TEACHING/LEARNING EXPERIENCE

Reflective Questions for Educators

1. Why did I decide to become a teacher?
2. What personal needs does my teaching fulfill?
3. What do I like and dislike about teaching?
4. Am I a good teacher? What makes me think so?
5. How do my learners view and value teachers?
6. How have I developed my knowledge of teaching?
7. How often do I think about teaching?
8. What are the most important things I know about teaching?
9. What do I do to foster learning?
10. Where would I like to expand my knowledge about teaching?

References

Abrami, P., d'Apollonia, S., & Resenfield, S. (1997). The dimensionality of student ratings: What we know and what we do not. In R. Perry & J. Smart, (Eds.), *Effective teaching in higher education: Research and practice,* (pp. 321–367). Edison, NJ: Agathon.

Boyer, E. (1990). *Scholarship reconsidered: Priorities for the professoriate.* Princeton, NJ: Carnegie Foundation for the Advancement of Teaching.

Brassell, S., & Robinson, J. (2001). *Peer review of teaching and course portfolios.* Bloomington, IN: Indiana University.

Burns, C. (1999). Teaching portfolios and the evaluation of teaching in higher education: Confident claims, questionable research support. *Studies in Educational Evaluation*, *25*, 131–142.

Centra, J. (1993). *Reflective faculty evaluation.* San Francisco: Jossey-Bass.

Cerbin, W. (1994). The course portfolio as a tool for continuous improvement of teaching and learning. *Journal of Excellence in College Teaching, 5*, 9–105.

Cranton, P. (1998). No one way: Teaching and learning in higher education. Toronto: Wall & Emerson.

Diamond, R. (1995). *Preparing for promotion and tenure review.* Bolton, MA: Anker Publishing.

Duffy, T., & Cunningham, D. (1996). Constructivism: Implications for the design and delivery of instruction. In D. H. Jonasssen, (Ed.), *Handbook of research for educational communities and technology* (pp. 170–198). New York: Simon & Schuster Macmillan.

Facione, P. A., & Facione, N. C. (1994). *Holistic critical thinking scoring rubric.* Millbrae, CA: California Academic Press.

Felder, R., & Brent, R. (1996). If you've got it, flaunt it: Uses and abused of teaching portfolios. *Chemical Engineering Education, 30*, 188–189.

Glanville, I., & Houde, S. (2004). The scholarship of teaching: Implications for nursing faculty. *Journal of Professional Nursing, 20*, 7–14.

Glassick, C., Huber, M., & Maeroff, G. (1997). *Scholarship assessed: Evaluation of the professoriate*. San Francisco: Jossey-Bass.

July, F. (1998). The teaching portfolio in nurse faculty evaluation. *ABNF Journal, 9,* 11–13.

Kreber, C. (1999). A course based approach to the development of teaching scholarship: A case study. *Teaching in Higher Education, 4*, 309–325.

Kreber, C. (2002). Teaching excellence, teaching expertise and the scholarship of teaching. *Innovative Higher Education*, 27, 5–23.

Kreber, C., & Cranton, P. (2000). Exploring the scholarship of teaching. *Journal of Higher Education, 71*, 476–496.

Quinlan, K. (2002). Inside the peer review process: How academics review a colleague's teaching portfolio. *Teaching and Teacher Education, 18*, 1035–1049.

Reece, S., Pearce, C., Melillo, K., et al. (2001). The faculty portfolio: Documenting the scholarship of teaching. *Journal of Professional Nursing, 17*, 180–186.

Riley, J., Beal, J., Levi, P., et al. (2002). Revisioning nursing scholarship. *Journal of Nursing Scholarship, 34*, 383–389.

Savery, J., & Duffy, T. (1995). Problem based learning: An instructional model and its constructivist framework. *Educational Psychology,* Sept-Oct, 31–38.

Seldin, P. (1997). *The teaching portfolio*. Boston: Anker Publishing.

Shore, B. (1986). *The teaching dossier: A guide to its preparation and use*. Montreal: Canadian Association of University Teachers.

University of Alberta Collaborative Baccalaureate Program (2003). NURS 394 Course Outline: Edmonton: University of Alberta.

Weimer, M. (1993). The disciplinary journals on pedagogy. *Change, 25*, 44–51.

Zeichner, K., & Wray, S. (2001). The teaching portfolio in US teacher education programs: What we know and what we need to know. *Teaching and Teacher Education, 17*, 613–621.

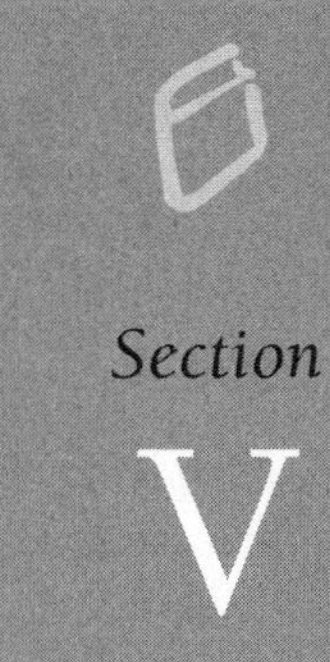

Section

V

TOWARD A NEW FUTURE

Chapter

24

Career Development: What New Faculty Members Need to Know, See, and Do

Janet L. Storch

Dr. Jolan Herzog was appointed to the Faculty of Nursing at Excellence University in part because of her expertise in distance education. Her faculty colleagues had been struggling to implement several distance learning technologies and they believed Dr. Herzog was the answer to their desire to mount a quality distance education program. Dr. Herzog is quite aware of these expectations. She has also been given some wise advice by her doctoral supervisor and mentor that she, as a new academic member, needs to mark out time for her own scholarly work so that she can develop research grants and continue her writing for publication. She knows that she needs protected time to become the faculty member and scholar she wants to be; and that her scholarship is critical to her ability to gain tenure and promotion at Excellence University. Prior to her starting date she talks to the director and speaks to her new faculty members about their scholarly commitments and her own need for some protected time for her scholarship. They agree on her work plan and promise to support her in her scholarship.

INTENT

The focus of many of the previous chapters has been on what nurse educators need and can do to provide student-centered teaching. One of the contextual elements that determine in part how nurse educators like Dr. Herzog will teach is the nature of the institution in which they teach. In this chapter, the ideology, culture, and political structure of universities that influence a nurse educator's ability and willingness to teach in a student-centered manner will be highlighted. While the focus is on universities as places of teaching and learning, community colleges bear many similarities to this setting, although some elements (such as ideologies and reward systems) are often quite different.

Universities are particular and peculiar places to work. They are like other organizations, but they are most notable for their differences. In few other organizations does one see employees operating in such a self-directed, sometimes seemingly self-focused manner. Rarely do employees challenge their supervisors or directors as openly as they might in the university setting. Faculty rarely punch a time clock, yet most faculty members are committed and accountable for their time and their role in teaching and service, while also addressing a wider accountability for the generation of knowledge, for maintaining their currency in teaching, and for using their knowledge and university position to contribute to society. New faculty members need to understand the university, its structure, prevailing ideologies, and the faculty and staff mix that supports or constrains them in their work, and ways to push back against false beliefs. Using the analogy of theater, this chapter is intended to provide a focus on the context in which faculty are expected to enact their role, the conditions, the set of players they will engage with, and the importance of maintaining a balance in their positions.

OVERVIEW

INTRODUCTION

During the next 5 to 10 years, the need for nursing faculty members at universities, university colleges, and colleges is anticipated to be intense. The extreme shortage of nurse faculty members is impacting schools of nursing and is surpassing the shortage of staff nurses in health agencies, since higher numbers of nursing faculty are near the age of 60. Further, in North America and almost worldwide, the shortage of registered nurses is a serious problem (Aiken, et al., 2001; Ryten, 2002; Wieck, Prydun, & Walsh, 2002).

In 2002, Ryten updated and analyzed Canadian nursing statistics to provide a "cohorts" study demonstrating the seriousness of the nursing shortage that had resulted due to declining enrollments in nursing education entry to practice programs over time, and due to the effect of nurse retirements. Governments and health agencies have been alerted to these types of findings and have begun to take action to address the nursing shortage. These actions include increasing class sizes in nursing education programs, a recommendation whose effect accentuates the shortage of nursing faculty. In December 2004, for example, an American Association of Colleges of Nursing (AACN, 2004) press release indicated that more than 25,000 qualified applicants to entry-level baccalaureate programs were denied entry due primarily to a shortage of nursing educators. Since the majority of faculty members are recruited from masters and doctoral programs and since enrollments in these programs have not kept pace with demands for these graduates, ". . . fears that faculty shortages will worsen are not unfounded" (Bellack, 2004, p. 243). This means that there will also be a critical need to ensure that new nursing faculty members are well oriented to their positions and that their career development is carefully planned and guided. So what is it that new faculty members need to know? How might new faculty development be accomplished to facilitate uptake of their role? What are the challenges and the opportunities that await them?

Reilly and Morin (2004) note that "learning how to be a faculty member occurs in a variety of ways" (p. 520). These authors describe several career paths, such as beginning to assume a faculty role once a basic nursing education program is completed, practicing clinically for a number of years prior to choosing to entertain a faculty role, or moving to a faculty role directly after completion of a graduate program. Even in the latter instance, few nurses are well prepared to assume a faculty role since only a small percentage of graduate programs provide coursework that includes preparation for teaching in schools of nursing (Siler & Kleiner, 2001; Goldenberg, Andrusyszyn & Iwasiw, 2004). Yet, even this preparation needs to be augmented by a greater understanding of the faculty member's environment, role, and approach to teaching and learning.

Using the analogy of the theater (i.e., the performing arts), this chapter will focus on new faculty development through the lens of critical theory (Bottomore, 1984; Stevens, 1989; Wallace & Wolf, 1980). The societal context, the structure, and the ideology in which universities function (the theatrical stage) will be analyzed; the conditions that sustain the status quo at universities (the props) will be considered; and critical reflection on faculty roles (the cast) will be provided. Consciousness-raising for faculty (the rehearsals) and nursing faculty members' ability to take action in finding a balance in their multifaceted roles (the performance) will then be discussed. Finally, the importance of reflection on the new faculty capability (the postperformance notes) will conclude the chapter. It is hoped that this chapter will be of assistance to potential nursing faculty members considering this role, as well as new nursing faculty members recently recruited.

THE STAGE: CONTEXT, STRUCTURE, AND IDEOLOGY

The Context

Universities can be understood as a collective of faculty members, administrators, and students in the pursuit of knowledge. Universities provide opportunities for the creation and exploration of new ideas and changing thought. The mix of disciplines at universities offers a ripe ground for the generation of knowledge.

Ideally, the various approaches to knowledge development and transmission are valued collectively and equally by all. But in the author's experience, a tour of universities provides evidence that inequalities persist among various academic disciplines (as evident in the types of buildings dedicated to the pursuit of science and technology, engineering, medicine, business and management, and law). This suggests that the domination of science and technology, along with a leaning toward positivistic ways of thinking (empiricism) are a major aspect of most universities. These are traits the university board, senior administrators, and faculty members from "privileged" disciplines come to value and promote. Such promotion is reflected in university publications, public relations campaigns, and reward structures. Having served as faculty member, Director and Dean in Faculties of Medicine (13 years), and Nursing (29 years), the author has also observed that these inequalities are replicated in funding available to each unit, the availability of scholarships for students (both in number and amount of money) and increasingly, the salaries of faculty members. National research councils, who provide substantial funding to universities for their research, also lean toward supporting these values.

This all means that other units at the university (including the soft sciences, humanities and other "soft" professional disciplines) tend to experience being treated somewhat differently, regardless of enrollment size and pressing educational and research needs. Nursing is no exception to this situation.

Structure of Universities

Since most nurses work in organizations (e.g., hospitals, health units, etc.), it is important that they know something about the organization in which they work so they can appreciate where and how decisions are made and understand how to access resources they need. Dr. Jolan Herzog and her nursing faculty colleagues, for example, need to know that universities encompass a somewhat unique system of administrative and faculty governance, called the bicameral system of governance; essentially, having two parts that work together (deWolf, Gregg Harris, et al., 1997). Administratively, like most other organizations, there is a president (chief executive officer), a board, and an executive staff made up of vice presidents (normally a vice-president for academic affairs (the provost), and vice presidents for research, for operations/finance, and for public relations); and associate vice presidents, including an associate who serves as vice provost. Deans and directors answer to these administrative heads. In addition to this administrative system of governance, there is also a parallel system of faculty governance that includes a general faculties council (sometimes called a senate) with elected members of faculty, staff, and students comprising its membership. This latter body normally holds the power for approval of curriculum and programs, as well as for university policies relative to student admission, progression, and graduation. Further, in each academic department or school, there is also a parallel bicameral governance system with an administrative structure that emanates from the dean or director down through administrative staff (administrative governance), alongside a faculty or school council made up of faculty members who approve curricula, student progression, and other academic decisions that then move upward through that faculty governance structure, ending at the general faculties council or senate.[1] This means that the majority of decisions in the university must involve negotiated decision making. Union or framework agreements for faculty work, including faculty appointment, reappointment, tenure and promotion, and faculty leaves, add to the need for these negotiated decisions as well.

These structures would suggest that "shared governance," a concept most nurses support, is a reality. And to a large extent this is the case. But as in most organizations, the environment in which the university exists can often compromise the degree of freedom faculty members experience and the nature of equality among faculty members and faculty units. Further, the cherished ideology of academic freedom may be threatened by government directives that emphasize values quite opposite to faculty values and ideals (Huisman & Currie, 2004).

University Ideology

In this author's experience there appear to be two cherished but competing ideologies in the university: academic freedom (a well-articulated view) and competitive success (a less articulated view but a widely enacted value). At its most profound level, academic freedom represents the right of the university as a collective, and the right of individual faculty members, to speak out on issues, however controversial, without fear of censure or retribution. This is an important freedom, and one which nursing colleagues in practice rarely are able to enjoy to the extent of nurses in academia. Academic freedom also includes the ability of universities to offer programs and courses of their choosing, without being constrained by others or ordered to create a particular program.

Many university faculty members also claim the right to teach courses in a manner of their choosing. This means that faculty self-governance is an integral part of academic freedom. However, it is a freedom that has come under increasing tension (threat) and it cannot always be fully realized. With growing government intervention in targeting funds to certain academic programs, in requiring performance indicators that do not often match the faculty members' intended outcomes, and in focusing on student enrollments linked to funding to the exclusion of recognizing an ebb and flow in student numbers, institutions of higher education are under serious pressure to meet the funding agencies' needs or to find their own sources of funding. This pressure often preempts a concentration on student or research needs (Huisman & Currie, 2004; Miller, Bleich, Hathaway, & Warren, 2004). The valuing of competition, often at the expense of collaboration, is found in the use of bell curves for undergraduate student grading, in limitations on the availability of merit increments for faculty, and in the public relations applause for those who bring into the university the largest research grants.

[1] Note that the province of Alberta has a unique university structure that includes both a general faculties council and a separate body called the senate. This senate functions much like the Canadian government Senate in relation to the House of Commons, and is an artifact of a peculiar historical situation.

Most universities evolved to offer general advanced courses in philosophy, history, literature, science, art, and other studies along with some professional programs, yet government and industry continue to emphasize the importance of programs that lead directly to employability and productivity of university graduates (Molzahn & Purkis, 2004). Often this results in an overemphasis on skill development to the disadvantage of knowledge development. Nursing schools are particularly susceptible to this pressure because nursing is poorly understood by most university administrators, who may wish to appease governments on this directive in order to gain a greater advantage in another program area. While targeted funds for nursing programs are welcomed, nursing faculties need to guard against such easy solutions to funding difficulties since nurses, being relative newcomers to university education, can become easy targets for government or industry directives. This can lead both to a loss of academic freedom and an unhealthy competition for such funds.

THE PROPS: CONDITIONS THAT SUPPORT THE STATUS QUO

Most universities place a high priority on research; that is, the scholarship of discovery (AACN, 1999). Research is integral to the image of being a university because it represents knowledge development—a function regarded as a distinguishing feature of universities in comparison to other postsecondary educational institutions. Universities' traditional approaches to research often marginalize the scholarship of integration, of application, and of teaching (AACN, 1999; Bleich, 2004; Canadian Association of Schools of Nursing, 2004; Storch & Gamroth, 2002).

Traditional approaches to research are enshrined in universities where empirical rational approaches and quantitative research are normally valued to a greater extent than constructivist approaches and qualitative research. Along with these traditional approaches is the ideology of science as free of value biases (value free), and the responsibility of the scientist to be value neutral. These approaches differ markedly from the work and values of the majority of nursing faculty who may well engage in both quantitative and qualitative research, but who normally choose studies for the values that add to or are upheld in nursing work.

Then, too, research offices at universities, designed to support faculty research, place a high value on faculty grantsmanship and the numbers of grants submitted and obtained, as well as the size of grant awards. In most cases, unfunded research is considered of less importance than research funded through a grant. It is as if the award of a grant (or the failure to obtain a grant award) truly signifies the value of the particular research. This greater value seems to rest almost entirely on the presence of a monetary award as a proxy for peer review and therefore greater "goodness;" since as scholars have noted over time, we have limited evidence of the effectiveness of the peer review itself (Tilden, 2002), and much anecdotal evidence to suggest that many peer reviews are less than objective. This may create a dilemma for some faculty members since most appointment, tenure, and promotion processes are based on the value of holding grant funds. The fact that many nursing faculty buy into this entire system of evaluation without question only continues to support the dominant ideology.

THE CAST: EXPECTATIONS AND REALITIES OF NURSING FACULTY WORK

Historically, health professional schools were not part of the university and their entry into the universities was controversial since they represented knowledge for instrumental purposes (application) rather than the pursuit of knowledge as an end in itself. The location of schools of nursing within universities was particularly questioned at its inception when Ethel Johns became the first Director of Nursing of a university-based school of nursing in Canada (Street, 1973). Nursing's place within the university continues to be a topic of discussion among those who cannot imagine why nurses should need an advanced education to do the "work" of nursing. These sorts of questions are not limited to those outside the university. The work of many of the caring professions is also poorly understood by faculty members from the humanities and sciences. This means that, to some extent, nurse faculty members are still finding their rightful place within university structures.

Early in their appointment to a university, nursing faculty members like Jolan Herzog come to recognize significant differences between the expectations placed on them compared to the types of expectations of many other faculty members in nonprofessional schools. Until recently it has been unlikely that faculty members in nonprofessional schools would design, develop, or operate from a set curriculum and to have part of their program performance standards set by an external nonacademic body. Nursing schools must operate under a curriculum they have designed to meet professional standards, and which then dictates the content, sequence, and performance standard of the exiting student. Curriculum development, implementation, and revision require a substantial amount of nursing faculty time and nursing faculty members need to know something about development and implementation of nursing curricula. Only recently are faculty members in most nonprofessional programs expected to meet such external requirements and serve on nonacademic bodies locally, provincially, or federally. Considerable nursing faculty time is spent by nurses' participation in community agencies' work and/or the professional association's work. This work benefits the school and the faculty by helping to forge and maintain links to health agencies that are so essential to maintaining sound clinical placements; yet, rarely is this type of work acknowledged in proportion to the amount of faculty time it requires.

Recruiting individuals who can meet the expectations of new faculty is challenging. Normally, schools of nursing will be seeking nurses who are considered to be good teachers, well trained researchers, clinicians, and those who are service oriented. In regards to teaching, schools will want someone who is preferably experienced in teaching, enjoys teaching, works to constantly improve teaching, seeks new knowledge, updates courses, is innovative in use of teaching strategies, and is likely to be skilled in curriculum development. Of course, newly graduated doctorally prepared nurses are eagerly pursued and welcomed.

Schools of nursing will also be seeking individuals with clinical skills to provide clinical supervision for students. This work requires special competencies, not only in relation to knowledge and skill in clinical work, but also in teaching and evaluating students in such work. Diekelmann (2004) points out that faculty members recruited from clinical practice need assistance in dealing with the new culture of the university. They need a good orientation to pedagogical/androgogical literature, to shifts in thinking about nursing education over time, and to the curriculum (its potential for creativity as well as its constraints). They also need to learn how to give up a commitment to covering content in favor of emphasizing thinking (Diekelmann, 2002a; Tanner, 2004). These new faculty members need feedback and support in their teaching and evaluation. Subjective evaluation of nursing students requires extensive documentation to support the criteria being applied to evaluate students. This, too, is a high level skill of communication. In the school's search for complementary characteristics of being a strong clinician, many search and selection committees will hope for someone who has a well focused clinical career (years of experience), and who is credible and respected by the clinical environments in which they will serve.

Finally, on most school recruiting lists will be the requirement that the person to be selected should be a good team player. That means that the lone academic in the ivory tower is not well regarded in schools of nursing, since there is considerable teamwork involved in maintaining a well integrated curriculum, and ensuring the relevant details of progression through a planned program are observed and monitored for each student. These latter faculty requirements make schools of nursing somewhat different from most nonprofessional university or college programs where students may take a variety of courses to complete a baccalaureate degree. It is as if academics in different faculties and departments at the university operate from different "scripts" in their performance.

In addition to the above work, the growing numbers of students admitted and the increasing service needs of academia (committee work), along with the normal high pressure to "publish or perish," often creates serious stress among faculty members. In light of this situation, it is critical that we continue to reflect upon newer and better ways to assist faculty in career development. Lack of attention to these issues will undoubtedly have implications for recruitment and retention of a new generation of nurse educators, which will in turn have a major impact on the school's ability to promote and provide student-centered teaching.

THE REHEARSALS: CONSCIOUSNESS-RAISING FOR FACULTY

Even if recruitment ideals were met, successful uptake of an academic faculty position is not without challenges. As in the case of our star actor, Jolan Herzog, the expertise desired in the new recruit can lead to substantial demands on both the individual and his or her fellow faculty members in the school of nursing. Some of the spill-offs of the "right" casting of players (new faculty members) may include some of the following scenarios.

■ SCENARIO 1. THE NEED TO ESTABLISH REASONABLE BOUNDARIES IN TEACHING

The group of young, enthusiastic, and capable nurses who love teaching and can envision new and different ways to provide a solid education base for nursing, may stimulate extensive curriculum change and renewal of the present teaching strategies. While this action may well be needed and desired, successful curriculum revisions take time, and new teaching strategies may well involve considerably more time. For example, many current teachers and their students will know how journaling as a teaching strategy took hold in some schools of nursing without a clear understanding of the approaches teachers might take in "marking" journals. Another example is the quandary many nursing faculty now experience in managing their 24-hour availability in WebCT mail or e-mail. They need help in determining what guidelines need to be set, and how those guidelines impact on teaching effectiveness and faculty time. Difficulty in determining the boundaries around teaching time means that these faculty members will have difficulty making time for research and writing, which are also essential aspects of their positions.

SCENARIO 2. THE NEED TO MAINTAIN A BALANCED WORKLOAD

The demands on academic faculty to publish or perish are likely to be keenly felt by the nurse who loves research as the call he or she has been awaiting. The desire to make and continue grant applications can soon be the driving force in this faculty member's life. As grants materialize, there are new pressures to conduct the research, to write, and to apply for further grants. This means this faculty member is likely going to have limited time for the teaching that is also required as part of his or her position. As well, when several proposals are submitted with the sense that it is unlikely all will be funded and then numerous research grants are received, this nurse faculty member will find that time for other commitments is limited. The proverbial "feast or famine" of research grantsmanship can be problematic!

SCENARIO 3. THE NEED TO RECOGNIZE THE DEMANDS OF CLINICAL WORK

The nurse clinician who is welcomed by the school with open arms for his or her clinical ability, can find himself or herself enmeshed in planning, supervising, and evaluating students in nursing practice experiences. As noted previously, this can be rewarding but time-consuming work. With clinical placements that match the learning needs of students becoming ever more difficult to locate, the creativity required in making and keeping student placements relies heavily on faculty working with the staff person responsible for placing students in practice (i.e., administratively conducting the formal arrangements to do so). This nurse faculty member will also find himself or herself short of time to teach the theory courses he or she might want to teach, and to be engaged in an active scholarly study.

SCENARIO 4. THE NEED TO RECOGNIZE AND OFFSET COMMITTEE WORK

The team player who is service oriented will find that committee work in the school, the faculty, the university, the health region, and through professional associations, can easily fill the majority of time available in any one day. Nursing faculty members tend to be welcome on many committees outside of nursing because of their great ability to organize and to keep their commitments for follow through. Once again, over involvement in committee work reduces time available to develop good teaching practices, to be engaged in scholarship, and to be involved in clinical work.

In sum, these examples illustrate the difficulty for new nursing faculty members in finding a balance to university pressures. The requirements for teaching, scholarship/research, and for service are in themselves a challenge. But the addition of clinical knowledge and skill to this already overloaded list means that nursing faculty members have unique challenges in finding a balance in their work. They need to be assisted in creating such a balance and protected from both themselves (i.e., particular interests consuming their time) and from the demands of the school (i.e., the director and/or other faculty members who may inadvertently take advantage of their interests).

THE PERFORMANCE: A FINE SENSE OF BALANCE

Past Performances

While most recruits selected to become faculty members at universities, colleges, and university colleges begin their new careers with the best of intentions, the challenges they face in meeting the requirements of the policies of institutions of higher learning can be daunting to the point of precluding faculty from becoming what they had hoped to be. Independent action can often be constrained by the criteria required for merit increments and by the standards set for tenure and promotion. For example, the criteria for reappointment at one university specifies that a reappointment is granted on the basis of teaching effectiveness and service and professional activities since being appointed, as well as scholarly achievements during the individual's career. Since reappointments commonly occur after 2 to 3 years in the position, this means new faculty members like Jolan Herzog must scramble to ensure that meaningful and visible progress is being made in all three areas. As faculty members move on to tenure and promotions, the criteria for publications (quality and quantity), teaching effectiveness (including innovative teaching strategies), and service expectations continue to mount. In the end, the picture of faculty members after a few years in these positions often seems to be one of self-interest as they strive to meet university criteria, to the disadvantage of the collective interests needed to sustain good nursing programs and research in the school of nursing. What needs to occur for these new faculty is a greater sense of involvement in planning their activities with the faculty as a whole, and in being freed from the heavy emphasis on competition that tends to exist in the university. Returning to the analogy of the theater, actors who compete for attention on stage rather than working to ensure a smooth quality production of the play, often reduce the quality of the play with subsequent loss of audience interest and support, accompanied by negative press reviews. University programs, too, can suffer from buying into the competitive ideology in the university environment.

Current Performances

This all means that nurse faculty members must be actively involved in changing systems to address their scholarly needs, including systems of appointment, reappointment, promotion, and tenure (ARPT). Broadening the university's view of scholarship to include the Boyer (1990) model of scholarship, as has now been adopted by both the American Association of Colleges of Nursing and by the Canadian Association of Schools of Nursing, is one way to match reward structures in the university with the pursuit of nursing's theoretical and clinical knowledge. Curriculum development, for example, is not a brainless activity. It involves substantial knowledge of nursing and educational development; understanding of the progression of student learning to reach the goal of safe, competent, and ethical practice; and continued environmental scans to appropriately make additions and revisions to individual courses and curricula. Further, it requires a commitment to teamwork throughout planning, implementation, and evaluation. This scholarship of teaching is monumental work that merits full recognition in university processes. In some universities, nurses and a few other disciplines have been able to begin to modify merit reviews and ARPT processes to incorporate this type of scholarship, as well as the scholarship of integration and application.

Finding Sustaining Structures and Supports

While faculty members' own responsibilities for career development should not be underestimated, they also need supportive structures and a culture that encourages their development. New faculty members need to be mentored. In addition to a dean or director's mentorship, an experienced faculty member should be assigned to them to provide individual, ongoing professional support (Bellack, 2004; Boylston & Peters, 2004). New faculty recruits should also seek out other faculty members, beyond their assigned mentor, for advice and critique of their work, including manuscripts in preparation for submission to journals. There is no particular valor in going it alone. Seeking assistance from other faculty members opens opportunities to connect with them and learn from them (Diekelmann, 2002b). An additional bonus is that existing faculty members can become better acquainted with the new faculty member's interests and abilities, which may assist in connecting a new member with those members (within or outside the school) with similar interests. In effect, a community of scholars is developed through such consultation and sharing.

Individually new faculty members like Dr. Herzog should be encouraged to dovetail their work, so that they can maximize the benefits of any endeavor to both fulfill the scholarly need and to identify their work for merit review. For example, when a new faculty member is invited to give a keynote presentation, he or she should be coached to ensure that time is taken to develop that presentation for publication as well. Ideally, new faculty should be assisted in dovetailing their teaching, scholarship, and service so that each supports the other. A faculty member might teach in an area (either clinical or theory) in which he or she also does research, and he or she might choose to serve on community boards or committees that focus in that area. One example is an oncology nurse faculty member who teaches students in clinical practice in the care of oncology patients, is involved in the scholarship of integration in the care of persons with cancer, and serves on a committee of the cancer society.

An important element of faculty development for all nursing faculty, including new recruits, is a culture where unconstrained communication and dialogue can flourish. This means that oppositional thinking is welcomed to unveil practices that do not serve the school of nursing well, that debunks myths about how things must be, and reflects on ways to modify systems to help nurses maintain a healthy balance. Serious reflection on conditions of the workplace and an analysis of constraints is imperative (Stevens, 1989) for making good choices of potential actions and taking action on workable choices.

Naturally, no one set of supports for faculty development could be considered a "one size fits all," precisely because the size and experience of the faculty members will determine what is possible. Strategies to enhance career development will be suggested here with the hope that two or more combinations will assist faculty to develop to their full potential. In the theater, postperformance notes are initially given by the play's director following dress rehearsals to assist the cast to improve their performance. As the play goes into full production, stage managers, costume designers, lighting experts and others will continue to give postperformance notes from time to time. Similarly, nurse faculty members need to stop from time to time to seek feedback, individually and collectively, and reconsider their performance to see if they could do things in a better way to better meet their goals given the multiple demands on their time.

POSTPERFORMANCE NOTES: BUILDING CAPACITY

As a collective, nursing faculty can imagine and choose processes that allow them ways to plan for release time for grantsmanship and publication, while fulfilling their commitments to teaching and service. They can do so by experimenting and promoting policies that work. In most cases, this involves planning as a team, and it may involve planning within a team. In other words, workloads might be differently organized to accomplish a better balance of position requirements, to enhance collegiality, and to stimulate more collective action.

Working Differently

In some nursing education programs, instructors/professors are assigned specific courses that are considered "their course;" in other schools, there may be a few faculty-specific courses but the majority are core courses in which different faculty members, taking turns, become involved over a period of years. Often neither of these approaches is entirely satisfactory, but restrictions of contracts/faculty agreements may require set units of teaching each year with limited ways and means to modify teaching workloads. In medium to large schools, there can be ways to overcome limitations of contracts through better integration of teaching, research, and service. Nursing faculty members can work toward maximizing opportunities for self-governance by changing their own working relationships and by working to change university policies that restrict innovation. Two examples (both part of the author's experience) are provided next.

EXAMPLE 1: SELF-SCHEDULING THROUGH TEAMWORK

In one school of nursing, some inroads to integration of workload were accomplished by the faculty members who established themselves as teams based on their teaching and research interests and activities. One grouping was the adult health and illness group, another the family nursing group, and a third, the community health group who, in addition to their research, took responsibility for teaching a set number and type of courses and who also arranged that their group was represented on various committees in the school. Incorporated into their group scheduling were plans for coverage for their sabbatical leaves, maternity leaves, and other duties that in any given year might require offsetting another team member's working commitments. The benefit of these groupings was to allow greater self-governance; to align the work of research, teaching, and service; and to provide a collegial network into which faculty members could fit. The downside of such an arrangement can be some fracturing of the faculty as a whole unless careful attention is paid to ensure the group's boundaries do not allow them to become insular. Another challenge can be the structuring of group rewards; universities do not provide group rewards as a rule and ferreting out individuals' contributions can be difficult. Yet, reducing competition and promoting collaboration among faculty by promoting team rewards can be a new, different, and productive possibility.

EXAMPLE 2: SELF-SCHEDULING AND COLLABORATION IN A SMALL SCHOOL

For a smaller faculty group, subgroupings of faculty are not possible. But the faculty as a whole might still meet to self-schedule and plan for ways to economize on their teaching while maintaining quality in their programs. To augment their research capabilities, they might want to establish connections with another school of nursing. If a good fit can be found, this may stimulate both teaching and research. Collaborations of all types are common approaches to enhancing faculty expertise. Such collaboration is made much easier through advances in communications technology to enable good communication with each other over distances, such as through videoconferencing, computer conferencing, standard e-mail and listservs, and teleconference. Smaller faculties might also pursue the regular involvement of a visiting scholar to match their particular needs in any given year. Larger faculties with senior scholars can encourage their faculty to devote some sabbatical time toward this goal, and these arrangements could well be accomplished by the matching needs and opportunities through CASN, AACN, or other national nursing faculty organizations.

BUILDING A MORAL COMMUNITY

An important aspect of these two examples is a change in the balance of school governance. Rather than faculty members meeting only one-on-one with the director to discuss their career goals and their preferred assignments, they take back the power and responsibility to create a different environment to develop a community of scholars and a moral community that honors and supports each one in his or her career goals. That requires space, a commitment of time, interest, and trust in one another.

Developing this chapter has allowed this author to pause to reflect on the importance of developing a moral community[2] in a university faculty or school of nursing. A moral community in an academic setting would be a community of scholars who shared similar commitments, who cared about each other, who worked together for the good of the students and the school, and who "walked their talk." If the faculty group, for example, believes in emancipatory education, their interaction with their students and each other

[2] A moral community is a community in which there is coherence between what (an organization) publicly professes to be, that is, a helping, . . . caring environment that embraces the values intrinsic to the practice of healthcare, and what employees . . . and others witness and participate in (adapted from Webster & Baylis, 2000).

would clearly demonstrate that commitment. Faculty members would also feel connected to each other and would be able to engage in meaningful communication about both their successes and their shortcomings. This author's awareness of the need for a moral community in nursing schools and other academic units has been provoked by her involvement with faculty colleagues in the scholarship of discovery focusing on nursing ethics in practice.[3] As we have worked alongside nursing staff on the hospital units, we have become ever more focused on the importance of connection and communication to create a quality work environment where nurses' self-governance can be realized. It seems clear that doing so requires trust and commitment to each other and to the unit. And while academic faculty members who are part of the participatory action research team have been quick to realize the importance of a moral community as critical to the provision of safe, competent, and ethical nursing care, we have not focused attention on our own needs for a moral community where faculty can maximize their effectiveness in teaching, scholarship, and service. Engaging in a moral community requires visible action on the part of the school and the faculty members. A vital part of this action might include reclaiming space to interact with each other over coffee or lunch since all too often that space has been sacrificed for seminar or classroom use. It also requires making time available for others and perhaps, sacrificing a bit of academic freedom to engage with others rather than rarely appearing in the school.[4] We need to learn from practice settings the importance of a collective sense of being a moral community.

THE REVIEWS

The stage, the casting of the players, the props, and the performance for faculty in schools of nursing are in place. It seems clear, that like their colleagues in nursing practice, faculty members need to have some degree of management of their workload and control over their work, as well as strong leadership, good learning opportunities, and organizational support. Yet, faculty members seldom recognize their needs as similar to those of nurses they try to help (directly or indirectly) in the tumultuous atmosphere of nursing practice today. Greater recognition of faculty members' own needs, their vulnerabilities, and their opportunities can be a positive step in career development and career progress.

Given the high number of retirements from nursing education programs anticipated in the coming years, we will likely see a re-emergence of the nursing faculty dilemma we were just about to overcome; that is, that busy, fulltime faculty members

[3] Our nursing ethics research team includes Drs. Paddy Rodney, Colleen Varcoe, Gweneth Doane, and doctoral students, Bernadette Pauly and Helen Brown, as well as research assistants Chris Davis and Patty O'Shaungnessy. We have several research projects in motion, including one on nursing ethics in action, ethics in nursing education, and leadership in ethical policy and practice.

[4] Diekelmann (2004) provides narrative accounts of clinical nurses who became faculty members at a university. They commented on their amazement with how little faculty were around, that faculty were busy, and that they (the new faculty members) felt isolated and alienated in the "new culture" (p. 101). Diekelmann suggests that the stories of these experienced practitioners offer faculty members an opportunity to rethink the nature of academic communities. She suggests that the multiple demands of academic settings may be obscuring possibilities for creating caring communities.

will also be students working on graduate programs to enhance their knowledge and skills. Further, junior faculty members from our relatively new PhD programs may well be pushed into leadership positions within their faculties with insufficient academic experience, in effect, promoted ahead of their time. With these realities in mind, careful arrangements for mentoring of new faculty like Dr. Jolan Herzog, and the formation of faculty teams are likely to be more essential than ever as a way to further faculty development. Retaining senior faculty and professor emeriti as advisors and mentors may also be a useful strategy (Bellack 2004), and "borrowing" faculty may become a must.

Nurses entering nursing faculty positions have an important educational trust to carry forward. To accomplish this mission, they need to take responsibility for their professional development and they should expect and demand support from others. Structures in the university, such as reappointment and tenure requirements, may also need to be changed to recognize the importance of collective work toward the common end of excellence in nursing education.

Although this chapter has focused exclusively on schools of nursing and nurse faculty members' engagement with nursing, the broader context of the university cannot and should not be ignored. Schools are not islands unto themselves. They are part of a vital structure that allows faculty and students a wealth of opportunities for collaboration across disciplines. As increased emphasis is being placed on multidisciplinary centers, interdisciplinary research, and interprofessional education in the health disciplines; nurses are being sought after for their contributions to such multidisciplinary teams. These opportunities will be easier to maximize through team planning as discussed above.

SUMMARY

In this chapter, universities and their operation are described by comparing them to a theatrical performance; that is, with a stage, props, a cast, rehearsals, performance, and postperformance notes (evaluations of success and tips for improvement). The purpose of this analogy has in no way been intended to diminish the importance of university faculty, but to encourage the new and not-so-new faculty to stand back and reflect on the play itself. What happens at universities? How is academic freedom being used for good or for a self-centered purpose? What might be done to change the props? To improve performance? To build a community of players?

Woven into this description has been the importance of critical theory in increasing understanding about one's position in this setting, and in challenging false beliefs and other constraints to good teaching, excellent research and service, and ultimately relevant education for nursing practice. Emphasized in concluding the discussion is the need for faculty members at universities to reflect on their relationships with one another, including the importance of making time to build those relationships. Only through collective action can current ideologies that interfere with faculty function be challenged and reformed. More importantly, only through building relationships can faculty develop a moral community of nurse educators. Such a community can be a major underpinning in the goal of teaching in a student-centered manner.

LEARNING ACTIVITY

VISION STATEMENT

In this assignment you will have an opportunity to develop a vision statement that may be an inspiration for you in the next few years. In this assignment you are encouraged to turn your hand to aesthetic knowing to create the final product.

1. Draw a time line of your life indicating the ups and downs of your life; that is, times of difficulty and times of excitement and hope.
2. Of these up and down periods identify points that were defining moments; that is, moments or periods during which your life took a distinct turn toward who you are today.
3. Think carefully about values that you drew on to navigate your way through these challenging times. Write these down as they formulate in your mind.
4. What core values crystallized for you during these defining periods? Write down two to four core values.
5. Map these values relative to each defining moment. Did each core value come into play in each defining moment?
6. Think now about the life you would like to be living in 5 years. What are you doing? What fundamental values are operating in this future life? Write a paragraph or two about this.
7. Think about who has helped you in your journey to this future life. Think especially about mentors you have had, and the mentors you need in the academic environment. Think, too, about how important a community of support and a moral community would be to you.
8. What professional characteristics do you want people to acknowledge as vital to your performance? Write these down.
9. What core values would you want to transmit to nursing students and/or new graduates?
10. Take these values and characteristics and write a vision statement for yourself—one that draws on these values and characteristics and will serve as an inspiration for you as you journey through the next 5 years of your professional life. The vision statement could be a poem, a piece of art with an explanation, a narrative statement or a song. Please submit your vision statement with the time line (step 1), the map of values to defining moments (step 5), the paragraph or two that you wrote in response to the instructions for step 6, and the characteristics that you identified in step 8.

(Adapted from Covey, S. (1990). *The 7 Habits of Highly Effective People.* New York: Fireside.)

RESOURCES FOR EDUCATORS

PLANNING THE TEACHING/LEARNING EXPERIENCE

Questions to Support a Thoughtful Reading

In this chapter you are asked to think about career development in nursing education. Prior to beginning this reading, explore with a small group of classmates in a round table format the following:

1. Your vision for a career in nursing education.
2. The challenges of assuming the multiple roles of teacher, researcher, and practitioner as an academic nurse.
3. What is most attractive about teaching as a career in nursing?
4. What is least attractive about teaching as a career in nursing?
5. The culture of nursing education if you perceive that there is a culture of nursing education.
6. What is it like for nurse educators to juggle professional responsibilities with personal responsibilities?

EVALUATING THE TEACHING/LEARNING EXPERIENCE

Reflective Questions for Educators

1. What inspires you to take up a faculty position?
2. From the description and discussion above, are there any surprises for you about your expected position?
3. Are there aspects of a faculty position that you feel the need to know more about?
4. Do all aspects of the position appeal to you? How might you deal with those that are less exciting or interesting to you?
5. What do you see as your long term goals, and who will you enlist to help you attain them?
6. How do you envision your shorter term goals, and what types of mentors would you seek?
7. How important is being part of a community to you?
8. What advantages might there be to working toward a moral community?
9. What questions would you want to ask to determine the strength of the ideology of academic freedom and competition at the university? And by what means could you attempt to gain that information?
10. How might you determine the culture and political structure of the school of nursing or faculty of nursing? What resources might you tap to assess the school on these dimensions?

Sample Evaluation Strategies and Tools

Using Web sites and publications as vital sources of information, the students might be assigned to compare three universities on dimensions of structure and ideology, and focus in on the school of nursing to infer what it tells students about priorities in the school, as well as the culture of the school.

References

Aiken, L. H., Clarke, S. P., Sloane, D. M., et al. (2001). Nurses report on hospital care in five countries. *Health Affairs, 20*(3), 43–53.

American Association of Colleges of Nursing (2004). Enrollment increases at U.S. nursing schools are moderating while thousands of qualified students are turned away. Retrieved on November 15, 2005, from www.aacn.nche.edu.

American Association of Colleges of Nursing (1999). Position statement on defining scholarship for the discipline of nursing. Retrieved on November 10, 2005, www.aacn.nche.edu/Publications/positions/scholar.htm.

Bellack, J. P. (2004). Once solution to the faculty shortage—Begin at the end. *Journal of Nursing Education, 43*(6), 243–244.

Bleich, M. R. (2004). The scholarship of practice within the academic enterprise. *Journal of Nursing Education, 43*(2), 51–52.

Bottomore, T. (1984). *The Frankfurt School.* New York: Tavistock Publications.

Boyer, E. (1990). *Scholarship reconsidered: Priorities for the professorate.* Princeton, NJ: Carnegie Foundation.

Boylston, M. T., & Peters, M. A. (2004). Interim leadership in an era of change. *International Journal of Nursing Education Scholarship, 1*(1), Electronic press.

Canadian Association of Schools of Nursing (2004). Position statement on scholarship. Retrieved November 10, 2005, from www.casn.ca.

deWolf, G. D., Gregg, R. J., Harris, B. P., et al. (1997). *Gage Canadian Dictionary.* Toronto: Gage Canadian Publishing Company.

Diekelmann, N. (2002a). "Too much content. . . ." Epistemologies' grasp and nursing education. *Journal of Nursing Education, 41*(11), 469–470.

Diekelmann, N. (2002b). Engendering community: Learning and sharing expertise in the skills and practices of teaching. *Journal of Nursing Education, 41*(6), 241–242.

Diekelmann, N. (2004). Experienced practitioners as new faculty: New pedagogies and new possibilities. *Journal of Nursing Education, 43*(3), 101–103.

Goldenberg, D., Andrusyszyn, M. A., & Iwasiw, C. (2004). A facilitative approach to learning about curriculum development. *Journal of Nursing Education, 43*(1), 31–35.

Huisman, J., & Currie, J. (2004). Accountability in higher education: Bridge over troubled water? *Higher Education, 34*(4), 529–551.

Miller, K. L., Bleich, M. R., Hathaway, D., et al. (2004). Developing the academic nursing practice in the midst of the new realities in higher education. *Journal of Nursing Education, 43*(2), 55–59.

Molzahn, A., & Purkis, M. E. (2004). Collaborative nursing education programs: Challenges and issues. *Canadian Journal of Nursing Leadership, 17*(4), 41–53.

Reilly, L., & Morin, K. H. (2004). Faculty roles in supporting new deans and directors. *Journal of Nursing Education, 43*(11), 520–523.

Ryten, E. (2002). *Planning for the Future: Nursing Human Resource Projection.* Ottawa: Canadian Nurses Association.

Siler, B. B., & Kleiner, C. (2001). Novice faculty: Encountering expectation in academia. *Journal of Nursing Education, 40*(9), 397–403.

Stevens, P. E. (1989). A critical social reconceptualization of environment in nursing: Implications for methodology. *Advances in Nursing Science, 11*(4), 56–68.

Storch, J. L., & Gamroth, L. (2002). Scholarship revisited: A collaborative nursing education program's journey. *Journal of Nursing Education, 41*(12), 524–530.

Street, M. M. (1973). *Watchfires on the mountains: The life and writings of Ethel Johns.* Toronto: University of Toronto Press.

Tanner, C. (2004). The meaning of curriculum: Content to be covered or stories to be heard? *Journal of Nursing Education, 43*(1), 3–4.

Tilden, V. (2002). Peer review: Evidence-based or sacred cow? *Nursing Research, 51*(5), 275.

Wallace, R. A., & Wolf, A. (1980). *Contemporary Sociological Theory: Continuing the Classical Tradition*, (2nd ed.). Engelwood Cliffs, NJ: Prentice Hall, Inc.

Webster, G., & Baylis, F. (2000). Moral residue. In S. B. Rubin & L. Zoloth, (Eds.), *Margin of error: The ethics of mistakes in the practice of medicine* (pp. 217–232). Hagerstown, MD: University Publishing Group.

Wieck, K. L, Prydun, M., & Walsh, T. (2002). What the emerging workforce wants in its leaders. *Journal of Nursing Scholarship 34*(3), 283–288.

Chapter 25

Musings: Reflecting on the Future of Nursing Education

Barbara L. Paterson

The first time I heard about student-centered teaching in the 1980s, I was a student in a graduate course in higher education. Although the concept of student-centered teaching had immediate appeal for me because of its promise to address many of the issues about the diverse learning needs of various students, I was confused about how it differed from other concepts, such as active learning and student self-direction. I was also not sure that such an approach could be sustained, particularly in the context of the competing demands to produce self-reflective, critical thinking, competent practitioners who could pass their licensing exams. And I was somewhat skeptical that an approach that was demonstrated to be effective with students in the field of education could be neatly catapulted into the unique and tangled world of nursing education. As time passed, I became concerned that student-centered teaching was becoming a fashionable buzzword. I observed nurse educators who used the jargon but maintained teaching practices that contradicted the tenets of student-centered teaching. I once heard a colleague speak eloquently in support of faculty-student partnerships; yet, shortly after, she debated fiercely that we should insist that a student with extensive experience in health care attend demonstrations about nursing procedures the student already knew because "we must be consistent."

Then, in the early 2000s, I was part of an accreditation team for a university school of nursing. The curriculum was student centered. The faculty talked about their teaching as student centered and provided examples of how they achieved this. However, it was the students who convinced me that student-centered teaching was an achievable reality in that program. They made statements such as, "We see our teachers and they are friends with each other. They don't see things exactly the same but you can tell they like and admire one another. They treat us the same way too. We feel that we and the teachers are working together." The positive regard that these students had for their teachers, the program, each other, and their learning experiences was remarkable, particularly in contrast with students in other programs who expressed concern about their lack of voice and the degree of competition and exclusiveness in the education program.

INTENT

This book represents a creative, provocative, and often courageous, effort by several nurse scholars to unravel the complex and often confusing concept of student-centered teaching, as well as to provide definitive strategies to teach in this way. In this, the final chapter of the book, I will draw on what has been written in the preceding chapters to detail what I believe to be the most significant directions for the future of nursing education and research in regard to student-centered teaching. I will do this by centering the discussion on three themes that have dominated the text of the book; i.e., the skills of student-centered teaching, partnership in student-centered teaching, and the context of student-centered teaching.

OVERVIEW

INTRODUCTION

The authors of the preceding chapters have addressed all the issues that once concerned me about student-centered teaching. They have addressed the myriad of conceptualizations of self-directed teaching in a way that both clarifies and expands the current literature about student-centered teaching in nursing education. They have provided "the meat and potatoes" that has been missing from much of the previous discussion about student-centered teaching (Shulman, 1987) while at the same time recognizing that student-centered teaching occurs "across variations in personal style, philosophy, and venues for teaching and learning" (Chapter 3). They moved the discussion of student-centered teaching beyond that of a philosophical approach, a kit bag of teaching strategies and trendy discourse to a new and expanded understanding of what student-centered teaching is, how it can be enacted, and the challenges that student-centered teachers encounter as they attempt to teach in this way. In this chapter, I will extend the discussion of student-centered teaching as it has been discussed by the authors of this book by probing those areas that I believe are yet to be discovered or fully understood.

SKILLED STUDENT-CENTERED TEACHING

The discussion of teaching skill in nursing education has typically centered on skill as a natural outcome of experience, as dispositional (e.g., reflective ability) or as a checklist of effective teaching behaviors. In the field of teacher education, these models have been largely rejected as too simplistic to capture the complex variations and components of skilled teaching (Sternberg & Horvath, 1995). Sternberg and Horvath suggest that skill in teaching is best understood by comparing the features of the teaching of effective teachers to determine how they resemble each other in their teaching practices. Such a comparison will lead to the development of a prototype of skilled teaching as a method of stimulating research and debate in the field about what skilled teaching really is and how it is attained.

The authors of preceding chapters, all leaders in nursing education and committed nurse educators, have contributed central exemplars toward a prototype of skill in student-centered teaching in nursing education. There are three themes that are similar in the authors' descriptions of skilled student-centered teaching in nursing education. These are:

1. The nurse educator maintains a confidence in student-centered teaching and in self as a student-centered teacher.
2. The nurse educator focuses on how his or her teaching practices influence students' learning.
3. The nurse educator is critically reflective about his or her teaching practices, beliefs, and assumptions.

The themes reveal the features and the tacit knowledge that is integral to expert student-centered teaching.

It is apparent that student-centered teaching requires not only a commitment to the philosophical and theoretical foundations of student-centered teaching but specific skills. The authors have defined, perhaps for the first time, the behaviors and responses of quality teaching in accordance with the student-centered approach in nursing education. For example, Paterson and Pratt, in their discussion of student-centered teachers' application of learning style theory, illustrated the sophistication and complexity of the skills of student-centered teaching when they indicated that the educator must be able to discern what nursing situations demand specific learning strategies and how to support students in adapting new ways of learning to fit particular practice situations or their personal needs. The delineation of such skills will lead in the future to determining how best to assist nurse educators to develop expertise in student-centered teaching.

Confidence

The ability to teach in a student-centered way requires considerable confidence in one's professional knowledge, teaching skill, and knowledge of the learners (Smith & Strahan, 2004). A nurse educator who lacks confidence as a teacher is unlikely to relinquish control of the classroom to students (Smith & Strahan, 2004). The authors of this book attested to a confidence in their ability to enact student-centered teaching, despite the contextual and other constraints that exist. Several of the authors demonstrated a strong personal motivation and belief in student-centered teaching, as well as high self-efficacy as a student-centered teacher. For example, Brown and Rodney describe how traditional case studies can be revised to become narrative approaches centered on students' knowing themselves as they experience the real of the profession. They base this discussion largely on their personal mission to make visible the "invisible or inaccessible, the embodied and socially embedded nature of patient/client and family experiences and ethical practice." Several authors suggested that nurse educators develop confidence in student-centered teaching as they develop a "firm grounding in the pedagogy of the teaching/learning experience" (Chapter 13). Without such a foundation, nurse educators have a tendency to believe in the mode of teaching (e.g., lecture, distance education), rather than in their skill as student-centered teachers. Nurse educators grounded in the tenets of student-centered teaching know that the most significant thing about teaching is that students learn in the context of a learning partnership in which their voice is equal in importance to that of the teacher; the strategy that the teacher selects to present new learning is not the significant thing in student-centered teaching.

Focusing on Students' Needs

The authors of the preceding chapters present student-centered teaching as a journey of creative discovery of what teaching behaviors and responses will best meet the diverse needs and ways of various students. They highlight the need to make connections so that the learner will be able to engage and find meaning in the learning experience. Those connections occur by making the relationships between isolated content and the relevance to the practice of the profession explicit, by using a variety of teaching strategies that are tailored to a variety of learning styles and ways of viewing nursing knowledge, by planning and improvising their teaching to meet the needs of students, and by monitoring and providing feedback.

Young refers to student-centered teaching as focusing on students' needs, rather than imposing what the teacher believes is essential to learn, as "letting learn." The ideal of student-centered teaching is that rather than students expending energy determining what the teacher wants, they explore and discover what they want and need to know. But, as Jillings indicates, there are a number of contextual and mediating factors that determine both students' and nurse educators' ability to achieve such a goal. For example, nurse educators who completed their basic nursing education in programs that were content-driven have the tendency to prefer courses with previously defined content that measure learning in terms of the achievement of directly observable and measurable objectives (Pardue, Tagliareni, Valiga, Davison-Price, & Orehowsky, 2005). If the critical mass of faculty is similar in their allegiance to content coverage, nurse educators who wish to try new approaches, such as student-centered teaching, will be discouraged from doing so because of the resistance they encounter from other faculty members (Pardue, et al.).

Rather than relying on educational outcomes to determine teaching strategies student-centered nurse educators are committed to presenting the profession of nursing to students in a dialogical way that engages them in critical reflection about their assumptions and preconceptions. All teachers can recall cries by students to "just tell us what we have to do" and many a teacher has been frustrated when the culmination of a creative, reflective exercise has been, "But what will be on the exam?" Despite the teacher's desire to enact student-centered teaching, students, for a variety of reasons (e.g., culture, socialization to school in earlier years), may not view themselves as active participants in their own learning; therefore, they may inadvertently sabotage the student-centered teacher's efforts. Students who learn to embrace student-centered teaching must learn to take risks in the context of an unequal power balance between the teacher and themselves (Paris & Gespass, 2001). Such risk-taking requires a particular level of self-confidence and trust in one's ability (Paris & Gespass, 2001). It remains unclear however, how a nurse educator meets the needs of both students who are willing and able to embrace more autonomy and critical reflection in their learning and at the same time meet the needs of students who are not developmentally or otherwise ready.

Critical Reflection

An underlying assumption in much of the relevant literature in nursing education is that a critically reflective teacher who is committed to engaging students in reflection on their beliefs and preconceptions will achieve that goal. This book has contributed to this body of knowledge by illustrating not only how teachers might be able to inspire critical reflection among students by their enactment of particular teaching approaches, but by detailing why critical self-reflection must be the beginning point and ongoing commitment for student-centered teachers.

All authors in this book illustrated their ability to be critically reflective about their teaching practices and their assumptions about student-centered teaching and several explicitly noted the need for nurse educators to begin student-centered teaching with critical self-reflection (Chapter 20). For example, Young and others discussed the need for nurse educators to apply critical theories to examine the taken for granted and the rituals of teaching practice in order to improve and extend the uses of teaching strategies, such as lecture and case study, to be congruent with the tenets of student-centered teaching. Varcoe and McCormick, for example, point to how the act of engaging students in conversations about race and racism "is an exercise of power" that should be undertaken with great caution and self-awareness. Several authors pointed to challenges and questions about student-centered teaching that remain unresolved and some openly admitted consternation about the issues in regard to student-centered teaching that they encounter in their teaching practice. Young and others, for example, questioned whether critical reflection is compromised when the educator has neither the psychological space nor time to reflect on their teaching. Such space is necessary to produce the ongoing self-examination and humility that is necessary in student-centered teaching (Chapter 20).

Building learning partnerships with other faculty may enhance critical reflection in student-centered teaching. Self-reflection is much like looking into the mirror to comb our hair; we may be unaware that there is a hunk of hair that is sticking out of the back of our hair because our mirror has limits to what it can reveal. Likewise, self-reflection is limited to what we can see about ourselves. A learning partnership among faculty may provide a safe place and more comprehensive picture to reveal our biases, preconceptions, assumptions, and practices taken for granted in teaching.

LEARNING PARTNERSHIPS

Many authors referred to student-centered teaching within the book as occurring within a community or partnership of learners. Shared ownership and control of learning, and mutual respect underlay this discussion. Varcoe and McCormick quote bell hooks as saying "that rather than focusing on safety, teachers would do better to build community" (p. 456). The chapters in this book addressed a limitation of the relevant literature to date in that they provided descriptions about what it means to provide a safe environment for students to participate as partners in the teaching–learning process, and addressed "how to facilitate such an environment" (Chapter 2).

Although content is important in establishing learning partnerships, these authors emphasized that the processes of learning within partnership transcends mere content knowledge. Student-centered teaching entails being able to manipulate content knowledge into forms that "are pedagogically powerful and yet adaptive to the variations in ability and background presented by the students" (Shulman, 1987, p.15). In such a notion, students and teachers do not stand outside themselves to critically gaze at the world of the other, but engage one another in learning through understanding and knowing themselves (Chapter 7).

The authors of this book present the building of relationships as integral to developing a learning partnership. They presented relationship with learners as the context in which effective student-centered teaching occurs. They suggest that student-centered teachers develop relationships by spending time with students, getting to know about them as individuals, and being open to learning from them. Relationships with students have previously been discussed in the literature as resulting in enhanced student motivation and the achievement of learning outcomes (Smith & Strahan, 2004). In contrast, the authors of this book present relationships as a feature of skilled student-centered teaching. However, as Pratt and Paterson suggest, not all situations or students may require the same intensity and nature of student–teacher relationship.

The idea of a learning partnership is extended by some authors beyond teachers and students to others, such as members of the profession and patients and their significant others. Brown and Rodney, for example, describe the narrative approach as "bringing learners closer to the people they are caring for as the basis for developing ethical knowledge." Yonge and Myrick describe learning partnership between faculty, students, and preceptors as the essence of effective preceptorship in nursing education.

Recently, my friend told me a story that occurred when her husband became ill and was hospitalized. After several harrowing days, she asked a nurse who had cared for him, "What did you learn from us?" She said that the nurse was taken aback, because it had never occurred to her that she should learn from patients and family members. Student-centered teaching should ultimately result in nursing graduates who enact the tenets of student-centered teaching (e.g., active engagement, partnership) in their nursing practice and their interactions with others in their learning or workplace (Chapter 9). If student-centered teaching is to be actualized to the full extent of its possibilities, surely nursing students who have learned in a learning partnership with student-centered nurse educators will be open to learning from everyone they meet, including those who are traditionally viewed as the passive recipients of care. This will ultimately revolutionize the practice of nursing.

A learning partnership that was not extensively addressed in the book is nurse educators' learning partnerships with other faculty members. Researchers in teacher education have determined that peer support systems are vital to faculty's ability to sustain a personal mission to student-centered teaching (Smith & Strahan, 2004), but the development and associated outcomes of such partnerships has not yet been the subject of much inquiry in nursing education. Much of what has been identified as outcomes of learning partnerships has been anecdotal. For example, Williams and Day report employers' positive comments about nursing students who used context-based learning as evidence to support the efficacy of such partnerships.

A realization that I had in writing this chapter, one that I think typifies the difficulty of enacting learning partnerships, is that we did not fully enact learning partnerships in the writing of the book. Lynne Young and I drew on our relationships with various authors to engage in dialogue about what the chapters might look like and to provide feedback about what they had written. Lynne Young established a norm of being dialogical and supportive to authors in our interactions with them. However, many of the authors did not know one another and most did not have access to what the others wrote. Although I could argue that the procedures we used were both resource and time efficient, I cannot help but wonder how we could edit a book about student-centered learning and yet operate in such an editor-directed way. I imagine and wish for another way in which we bring all the authors together to share their thoughts and they co-own the book. This embarrassing confession reveals how even student-centered teachers who believe passionately in learning partnerships sometimes fall short of their aspirations.

THE CONTEXT OF STUDENT-CENTERED TEACHING

Despite the overwhelming support for student-centered teaching within nursing education literature, it is a dismal fact that not all nurse educators teach in this way. This book has reinforced the notion that one cannot address student-centered teaching without acknowledging that there are many contextual influences that determine nurse educators' ability and willingness to teach in a student-centered manner. Student-centered teaching in nursing education takes place in complex and everchanging social environments, and nurse educators both affect and are affected by that environment. Many contextual influences in student-centered teaching have been discussed previously in the book (see Chapters 10, 16, 21, 24); therefore, I will focus on those that I believe to be missing or those mentioned in the book but needing expansion.

The Institutional Context

Some authors of preceding chapters have pointed to the contradictions that exist between the goal of providing student-centered teaching and what is actually possible in the context of the educational institution. Brown and Doane, for example, discuss the dominance of objective knowledge in nursing education that emanates from a similar focus in the profession; i.e., objective data is perceived as more valid and trustworthy than subjective data. This results in nurse educators having to focus on only students' knowledge that can be tested or assessed in discrete and objective ways, such as exams and skills testing. This often precludes nurse educators from engaging students in reflection about the subjective meaning of experiences or from teaching strategies designed to enhance students' abilities as experiential knowers. Varcoe and McCormick openly admit that student-centered nurse educators who are aware that students may respond in diverse ways (e.g., anger) to effective student-centered teaching and have worked to "surrender our desire for immediate affirmation of good teaching" (p. 462) may be compromised in their attempts to secure tenure and promotion by students' negative assessments of their teaching.

LACK OF INCENTIVES

One of the reasons that educators do not use student-centered teaching methods in their teaching is that there is generally little incentive within the educational institution to do so (Felder, 2004). As Storch and others point out, the university typically rewards research and publication productivity over teaching. In nursing education, scholarship about teaching often has been viewed as less scholarly and worthy than publications and research that are based solely in the discipline. Although some universities offer tenure and promotion based on teaching competence, the dominant model is one in which outstanding research is expected, but the quality of teaching is not considered unless it is unsatisfactory. Newly hired educators at a university-based school of nursing are likely to prioritize their time and energy in the activities that help them to secure tenure and promotion. They probably will not be encouraged to expend similar energy and time in activities such as writing about improving teaching by using student-centered methods, or designing creative new ways to provide student-centered teaching to students (Felder, 2004). Professors who present their funded research in scholarly venues receive tenure, raises, and paid trips to exotic places. Few comparable perks are available for those whose priority is exceptional student-centered teaching.

Within the traditional structures of most educational institutions, there is a dominant model of pedagogy that is acceptable as scientific and credible. Such a model favors teacher-centered approaches to instruction and is skeptical, if not disparaging, about pedagogical approaches that are student centered and more challenging to assess in directly observable and measurable, or "scientific" terms. The measure of effective teaching in this model is students doing well in their licensing exams and being assessed by employers as clinically competent. The students' part in such achievements is not acknowledged and neither are the limitations of assessment by multiple choice exams or employer surveys. In addition, the individualistic and competitive culture of most educational institutions requires that nurse educators be evaluated on their teaching as individuals, not as co-learners. Some institutions demand that ratings of teacher effectiveness include the delineation of lead teacher or course leader, presuming that this individual has made a greater contribution to the course than either students or other faculty. If nurse educators publish about their student-centered teaching practices in refered journals, they are expected by most journals to identify the authors in hierarchical order. Currently, there are few alternatives to the tradition of publishing as first, second, and third author. Consequently, nurse educators who wish to enact student-centered teaching may not be supported by administrators or tenure/promotion committees for engaging in teaching that departs from the dominant model of teaching within that institution (Clark, 2005).

CONTRAVENING STRUCTURES AND PROCESSES

A reason why student-centered teaching is so difficult to achieve in nursing education is that educational institutions, such as universities and health care institutions that serve as clinical agency placements for nursing students, are typically dominated by authoritarian structures that serve to separate people into categories of worthiness (Clark, 2005). Thorne suggests some of the theoretical foundations that may have influenced the adoption of these structures in nursing education. Such structures prohibit faculty or students experiencing the connection and equity that is essential to learning partnerships. Rather than cocreated meaning, they establish silos and hierarchies that produce gaps and inequities between them. Nurses who are faculty members of universities, for example, are often segregated into groups, such as the teaching faculty or the researchers and researchers are often viewed as having more status because of their research productivity (Chapter 24). Nurse educators who share an interest in highly technological and acute forms of nursing, such as in emergency departments or intensive care, are often viewed as more credible than those who focus on fields of study that are less technical and acute, such as gerontology.

The hierarchical, competitive, and authoritarian nature of education institutions is translated to many nursing education programs, such as in the structure of the curricula (Chapters 14, 16, 17, 19). What content is relegated to the first years of the program is often revealing of the faculty's view of how complex and sophisticated this information is. Information is often presented as discrete chucks (e.g., a course in mental health nursing; one in maternal and child health) and it is often difficult to see the interrelationships between information and learning experiences in various courses (Clark, 2005). In addition, the grading and evaluation practices, including the review of faculty for tenure or promotion, of many schools of nursing reinforces the dominant model of the institution; i.e., students are at the mercy of teachers who grade and assess them and teachers are at the mercy of anonymous examiners (Clark, 2005).

The Learning Setting

Different learning settings pose challenges to nurse educators' intention to use student-centered teaching approaches. For example, the reality of most educational institutions today is that nursing is taught to students in large classrooms, often in lecture halls with immovable seats. This poses a considerable challenge to educators wishing to engage students in small group reflection or other group-based teaching strategies. Young proved that this is not an insurmountable challenge to student-centered teaching. She described story-based learning as a strategy for combating the challenge of providing student-centered teaching to large classes. In a similar vein, Oermann revealed how lecture could be used in large classrooms in a way that was congruent with student-centered teaching. However, there are other learning contexts that were not specifically addressed in the previous chapters.

Not many of the authors of this book have referred to the challenges inherent in clinical education in student-centered teaching and those who did discussed this somewhat obliquely. In my research on clinical teaching in nursing education, I have found that faculty who espouse to student-centered teaching in the classroom often resort to other, more teacher-centered approaches, as clinical educators. In the clinical setting, teachers tend to focus on isolated incidents of directly observable student behaviors in order to make evaluative judgments about the student's ability to be a nurse (Paterson, 1997). The reasons that faculty contradict what they believe about teaching in clinical education are numerous, such as the need to comply with the school of nursing's requirement to complete a standardized behaviorist evaluation form for all students, being "guests in the house" of a clinical agency in which neither teacher or students are bona fide members and the pressure from external forces, such as professional associations, to guarantee that graduates are safe competent nurses (Paterson, 1997, 1998). A nurse educator who attempts to introduce student-centered teaching in a clinical setting may be met with resistance by nursing graduates, now staff members, who have been socialized to the dominant view of pedagogy. Such a teacher may be viewed by them as not doing the job of clinical teaching and the nursing staff may engage in fault finding to provide evidence of the educator's ineptitude. In order to keep the peace in a clinical setting, nurse educators may abandon their desire to enact student-centered teaching and teach in more traditional ways (Paterson, 1997). Such inconsistencies between what one believes as a teacher and how one practices teaching serve to confuse students and to validate their assumptions about the authority of the teacher (Paris & Gespass, 2001).

Likewise, faculty who teach students in the clinical setting often resort to supervisory and evaluation practices that are congruent with the accepted institutional model of clinical education but contrary to student-centered teaching. Rather than evolving from the needs of specific learners, this model most often grows out of institutional policies, past negative experiences with students, and faculty's experience as students. It tends to be highly directive, focused on the teacher's evaluation of the student's work, and places the teacher in the position of expert authority. Such models tend to become hardened within educational institutions as they are replicated by faculty who have been socialized to them as the only acceptable way (Paris & Gespass, 2001). Interestingly, a similar phenomenon occurs in the supervision of graduate students in many university schools of nursing.

Other Contextual Influences

There are other contextual factors that influence nurse educators' willingness and ability to enact student-centered teaching. One of these factors that has not been discussed at any length by the authors of preceding chapters is the changing nature of our student population. Although those who wrote about distance education discussed the changing needs of students for access to higher education in other than courses requiring in-person classroom attendance, there are new and evolving nature and needs of students that have a significant impact on nurse educators' ability and motivation to teach in a student-centered manner. One of these changes is students' past experiences as they enter the nursing education program.

Many nursing education programs across North America have embraced an advanced standing concept for nursing students admitted to the program. These students have substantial university credits or a completed university degree in another discipline before they apply to the nursing education program. They have been socialized to the disciplinary perspectives of other faculties and disciplines. However, there is a tendency in nursing education literature to regard all students as homogenous and coming directly into nursing from high school. The needs and the nature of advanced standing students are rarely addressed. Prior socialization to another discipline may be both an advantage and a source of confusion in learning about nursing. If one has learned to think like a social worker, it may be difficult to think like a nurse simply because nurse educators demand it; students socialized to social work may require unlearning consistent with constuctivism or at the least, acknowledgement of differing perspectives, before they are ready to embrace being a nurse. Thorne presented a provocative portrayal of the philosophical foundations of nursing and their curricular applications. It would have been interesting to speculate how nursing students who have other degrees prior to entering nursing contribute to or confound the conceptualization of nursing practice. It also would have been fascinating to reflect on the ethics and efficacy of requiring such students to unlearn their previous socialization and the implications of blending multiple disciplinary perspectives in nursing education.

FUTURE DIRECTIONS

The chapters of this book have contributed valuable insights about the skills of student-centered teaching in nursing education, particularly in regard to the tacit knowledge that expertise in this field requires. Several authors have called for evidence-based assessment of student-centered teaching competence (Chapters 8, 10, 11). It is possible that the features of student-centered teaching as articulated within this book be translated into best practices for student-centered teachers in nursing education. This may lead to more effective ways of teaching in student-centered ways and for assessing and developing these skills among nurse educators.

It is possible that there may be additional features of excellent student-centered teaching that are not clearly articulated in the book and that can be discovered in the study of nurse educators' teaching practices. As well, some of the relationships between the features of excellent student-centered teaching are not yet clear and require further study. For example, how does nurse educators' reflective ability relate to their confidence as student-centered teachers and the relationships they build with students? Additionally, we can not yet clearly articulate the outcomes of student-centered teaching in a way that justifies the allocation of resources and curriculum change to support this approach. Although some authors have contributed to the identification of such outcomes, there is a need for study about how the graduates of nursing education programs that espouse student-centered teaching compare in their practice to graduates of teacher-centered programs, as well as research that determines what specific student and teacher outcomes are associated with skilled student-centered teaching.

The prototype of skilled student-centered teaching as presented in this book has challenged many of the myths of effective teaching that are common in the nursing literature, such as the teacher as expert authority, everything depends on the teacher, and teachers are self-made (Fenimore-Smith, 2004). While the first two have been addressed within the book, what is missing is an in-depth exploration of how nurse educators learn the skills of student-centered teaching. For example, there is a tendency in the nursing literature to conceptualize confidence as a personal attribute, rather than a behavior that is a feature of expertise in student-centered teaching. It is unclear how a novice educator develops that confidence, particularly in light of the multiple demands (e.g., developing a program of research) that many new educators face. In addition, although some authors mentioned the tension to ensure that students achieve suitable grades (Chapter 14, 20, 21), it is not entirely clear how student-centered nurse educators negotiate this tension in student-centered teaching. Nor is it clear how they assist students to come to terms with the lack of focus on educational outcomes when these outcomes are used to determine eligibility for scholarships, bursaries, and admittance to graduate school.

Williams reminds us that insights such as those contained in preceding chapters about skilled student-centered teaching are of little benefit unless they are effectively disseminated and translated among nurse educators. There is a need to develop and sustain effective networks of nurse educators who share their practices and their responses to relevant issues in student-centered teaching. Every school of nursing should identify at least one exceptional educator who will function as a mentor to junior faculty and graduate students considering an academic career, and act as a consultant to other faculty as required, in regard to student-centered teaching. In addition, there is a need for empirical evidence that delineates the best practices of student-centered teaching so that decisions about adopting or abandoning student-centered teaching approaches are evidence-based (Iwasiw, Goldenberg, & Andrusyszyn, 2005).

It is apparent within the book that partnership is integral to student-centered learning. However, there is also evidence that delineating partners as only nurse educators and students limits the possibilities of student-centered teaching; partnerships with other learners, such as other faculty and patients and their significant others should be considered in further discussions about student-centered teaching. In addition, it is important that we discuss openly among ourselves and with students about the nature of the student voice in nursing education programs. Do we extend the tenets of student-centered teaching to include students' direct involvement in the planning and development of curricula and educational policy, or is their participation by providing feedback about teaching, courses, and the curriculum given mere token status? There are examples of effective student partnerships in educational policy making in secondary schooling in Canada, such as the appointment of high school students as trustees on school boards (Critchley, 2003), that could perhaps be considered in an assessment of this issue in nursing education.

The realization of student-centered teaching in nursing education necessitates more than the support and commitment of individual nurse educators; it requires a contextual shift in attitudes, beliefs, values, practices, and incentives in regard to teaching and learning in nursing practice, nursing education and in higher education (Clark, 2005). Nursing faculty need opportunities to dialogue about how their goal to enact student-centered teaching can be realized within the particular institutional contexts that constrain this as a reality.

At times, the possibility of transforming the institutional and setting contexts of nursing education appear so daunting that nurse educators try to get around this challenge by doing their own thing within the dominant social system. They design innovative student-centered teaching strategies, form alliances with faculty who are like-minded in their commitment to student-centered teaching, and quietly endure the daily contradictions that arise as they try to bridge the disparate worlds of their teaching and the institution (Clark, 2005).

The solutions to the problems that I have listed in this chapter in regard to contextual influences are complex; there is not one simple answer. However, there are possible ways of addressing the negative or confusing influences of context to student-centered teaching. For example, faculty in schools of nursing should advocate for the equal treatment of research and teaching in decisions about faculty tenure, promotion, and appointment. It should be equally possible to advance on the basis of exceptional teaching as it is on the basis of research productivity. Excellent student-centered teaching should be a concurrent expectation with outstanding research for faculty of schools of nursing. Nursing educators in schools of nursing should dialogue about the reasons why student-centered teaching is inconsistent or does not exist in specific learning settings or situations, and discuss ways that these can be addressed or mediated. Another topic for dialogue is how can nurse educators effectively share their skilled practice as student-centered teachers with educational administrators and other faculty in a way that acknowledges the skills of student-centered teaching?

There has been a recent shift in research about effective teaching to consider the social contexts that best support such teaching practices (Quinlan, 2003). In turn, this has resulted in a new body of research to investigate what teachers learn and gain as they participate in different types of teaching. Although some authors made reference to the learning community that supports student-centered teaching in nursing education, there is a need for further study about what factors inspire and support nurse educators' intention to teach in a student-centered manner. As well, there is a need for investigation of the nature of outcomes, such as learning and personal satisfaction, that are associated with student-centered teaching in nursing education.

I leave you with a list of questions to consider in regard to the future of student-centered teaching. Their answers will provide direction for both the practice and study of student-centered teaching.

- What factors and methods foster or constrain nurse educators' willingness to integrate student-centered teaching in their teaching practice?
- How can teacher development programs help to develop and sustain nurse educators' competence as a student-centered teacher?
- Do nurse educators really attend to students' feedback or do they view the opportunity to provide feedback as sufficient evidence of their status as partners? And what is their accountability for letting students know what changes have been made because of their feedback?
- How do skilled student-centered nurse educators develop and maintain learning partnerships with nursing students, other faculty, and others (e.g., nursing staff in clinical settings)?
- How do nurse educators determine what student–teacher relationships are appropriate in particular learning situations or with certain students?
- What research is necessary to identify best practices in student-centered teaching, and to identify benchmarks of successful student-centered teaching in nursing education?

- How can nurse educators build into their work ongoing opportunities to question their assumptions and beliefs about teaching and learning?
- How can nurse educators best share their narratives about their experiences of student-centered teaching, including their victories and challenges, in scholarly and informal venues and in mentorship of other faculty?

CONCLUSION

Thorne begins her chapter with a description of her excitement as an observer of the "progression of thinking" within the nursing profession. In a similar vein, this book provides nurse educators with a rare opportunity to trace the past, consider the present, and envision the future of student-centered teaching. It has provided a basis to draw evidence to support the philosophical foundations, practices, and outcomes of student-centered teaching in nursing education. However, there is some truth to the statement that there has been much reform in the history of education in North America with little real change (Cuban, 1993). The issues that are discussed in the book about enacting student-centered teaching are much the same as they were several decades ago.

Unfortunately, as long as the context of nursing education remains unchallenged, nursing educators and students will continue to be discouraged and at times, compromised about making the tenets of student-centered teaching an actuality. One answer lies in the next generations of nurses, those who are current or future nursing students. If we are truly student-centered teachers, we will assist students to develop the skills to learn, to be open to new ways of doing and being as practitioners, to embrace uncertainty, and to form partnerships with others in learning. Such nurses will advocate for the contextual shift that is required to transform the context of nursing education so that student-centered teaching becomes an expectation and a reality.

References

Clark, C. S. (2005). Transforming nursing education: A partnership social system for alignment with philosophies of care. *International Journal of Nursing Education Scholarship, 2*(1). Retrieved November 7, 2005, from http://www.bepress.com/cgi/viewcontent.cgi?article/1100&context/ijnes.

Critchley, S. (2003). The nature and extent of student involvement in educational policy-making in Canadian school systems. *Educational Management & Administration, 31*(1), 97–106.

Cuban, L. (1993). *How teachers taught: Constancy and change in American classrooms 1890–1990.* New York: Teachers College Press.

Felder, R. M. (2004). Teaching engineering at a research university: Problems and possibilities. *Educación Química, 15*(1), 40–42.

Fenimore-Smith, J. K. (2004). Democratic practices and dialogical frameworks: Efforts towards transcending the cultural myths of teaching. *Journal of Teacher Education, 5*(3), 227–239.

Iwasiw, C. L., Goldenberg, D., & Andrusyszyn, M. A. (2005). Extending the evidence base for nursing education. *International Journal of Nursing Education Scholarship, 2*(1), 1–3.

Pardue, K. T., Tagliareni, M. E., Valiga, T., et al. (2005). Substantive innovation in nursing education: Shifting the emphasis from content coverage to student learning. *Nursing Education Perspectives, 26*(1), 55–57.

Paris, C., & Gespass, S. (2001). Examining the mismatch between learner-centered teaching and teacher-centered supervision. *Journal of Teacher Education, 52*(5), 398–412.

Paterson, B. (1997). The negotiated order of clinical teaching. *Journal of Nursing Education*, *36*(5), 197–205.

Paterson, B. (1998). Partnership in nursing education: Vision or fantasy? *Nursing Outlook*, *46*(6), 284–289.

Quinlan, K. M. (2003). Effects of problem-based learning curricula on faculty learning: New lenses, new questions. *Advances in Health Sciences Education*, *8*(3), 249–259.

Shulman, L. (1987). Knowledge and teaching: Foundations of the new reform. *Harvard Educational Review*, *57*(1), 1–22.

Smith, T. W., & Strahan, D. (2004). Toward a prototype of expertise in teaching. *Journal of Teacher Education*, *55*(4), 357–371.

Sternberg, R. J., & Horvath, J. A. (1995). A prototype view of expert teaching. *Educational Researcher*, *24*(6), 9–17.

Glossary

A

Accelerated programs. An option in baccalaureate education; 12-month to 16-month programs for learners with previous non-nursing degree or completion of all prerequisite courses.

Accommodators. These learners like to learn using concrete experience and active experimentation. They seek new experiences and adapt readily to new circumstances. They tend to solve problems intuitively but rely on others for information.

Achieving learning. An approach to learning in which the learner attempts to achieve the highest grade possible by whatever means is required to achieve this grade; therefore, the maximum grade is the end goal.

Active learning. A form of learning in which students are involved in the process rather than listening passively to the teacher present information.

Adaptive technologies. Those technologies that allow learners with disabilities to access and participate in distance education courses. These are designed to accommodate specific disabilities experienced by the learner.

Advanced interactive delivery. In contrast to low technology development and delivery of course materials, such as print and audiotape or videotape, this mode involves the use of the computer and Internet for developing and delivering course materials.

Androgogy. The art and science of helping adults learn. A prime contributor to most theories of adult learning, androgogy as set out by Malcolm Knowles emphasizes adults' capabilities to direct and motivate themselves, utilize past knowledge to assist learning, and evaluate the contents of training for relevance and quality.

Anticolonialism. "The political struggle of colonized peoples against the specific ideology and practice of colonialism. Anticolonialism signifies the point at which the various forms of opposition become articulated as a resistance to the operations of colonialism in political, economic, and cultural institutions. It emphasizes the need to reject colonial power and restore local control" (Ashcroft, Griffiths, & Tiffin, 2000, p. 14).

Antiracist pedagogy. An action-oriented strategy for institutional, systematic change to address racism and the interlocking systems of social oppression. Pedagogy refers to central aspects of teaching that do not relate directly to or address a specific subject or content area. "Anti-racist pedagogy explicitly names the issues of race and social difference as issues of power and equity rather than as matters of cultural and ethnic variety" (Dei, 1996, p. 9).

Apprenticeship perspective. This view assumes that learning is both an individual cognitive process and a collective social process.

Learning, therefore, is facilitated when students work on authentic tasks in real settings of application or practice and alongside other, more experienced, practitioners.

Assimilation and accommodation. In Piagetian psychology, the processes by which cognitive development occurs. In assimilation, a given phenomenon is interpreted in terms of the schemas of a person's existing concepts. In accommodation, a person's existing concepts are altered in response to incompatible phenomena.

Assimilators. These learners prefer to learn using abstract conceptualization and reflective observation. Also called theorists, they like to ask such questions as, "How does this relate to that?" They tend to be most concerned with practical applications of knowledge and abstract concepts.

Asynchronous activities. Activities that occur at different times and do not require faculty and students to participate at the same time.

Asynchronously. Occurring at different times; not together.

Asynchronous Web-based instruction. Instruction that allows learners to access educational materials at different and flexible points of time and at their convenience, i.e., anytime learning.

Attitudes. The feelings, beliefs, opinions, and values predisposing a person to behave in a certain way.

Audio conferencing. Use of a telephone conference call or voice over Internet protocol application (*see* VoIP) to unite one or more students with instructors for purposes of office hours, delivery of course content, and/or other discussions.

Authentic problem (also referred to as **problem**). Refers to a clinical problem or situation that is presented the same way that it occurs in real world clinical experiences. As such, the problem represents challenges, demands, and contexts that students will face in their professional careers as a registered nurse. Congruent with the real world, authentic problems allow students to integrate information from nursing and many other disciplines when solving clinical problems.

B

Behaviorists. Theorists who maintain that learning is based on appropriate use of stimuli and rewards.

Bellevue Study. A study published in 1936 in *Clinical Education in Nursing*; a review with recommendations to improve hospital training school educational programs.

BIASes in teaching. An abbreviation of beliefs, intentions, actions, and strategies. Collectively, biases make up perspectives on teaching.

Block curriculum pattern. Structured and sequential curriculum plan; similar to medical model, organizes courses according to specialty areas of practice, and possibly body system within these courses.

Blogs. A Web page that is an individual's publicly accessible personal journal; short for Web log.

Border pedagogy. Pedagogy refers to central aspects of teaching that do not relate directly to or address a specific subject or content area. Giroux suggested that *border* pedagogy is a process that is intent on challenging existing boundaries of knowledge and creating new ones. Border pedagogy offers the opportunity for students to engage the multiple references that constitute different cultural codes, experiences, and languages. This means educating students to both read these codes historically and critically while simultaneously learning the limits of such codes, including the ones they use to construct their own narratives and histories. "Students should engage knowledge as border-crossers, as people moving in and out of borders constructed around coordinates of difference and power" (Giroux, cited in Aveling, 2002, p. 29). While multicultural education is generally seen to be about the other and taught in ways in which the "dominating aspects of white culture are not called into question and the oppositional potential of difference as a site of struggle is muted, the aims of border pedagogy are to interrogate the histories, memories, and stories of the devalued others who have been marginalised from the official discourse of the canon" (Giroux, cited in Aveling, p. 120) and to examine how the "boundaries of ethnicity, race, and power make visible how whiteness functions as a historical and social construction" (Giroux, cited in Aveling, p. 120).

Broadcast media. Delivery of course materials using radio and/or television distance learning technologies.

C

Caring. The concept of caring has been a guiding principle and a philosophical foundation of caring curricula in nursing. Nursing theories of caring guide the development of each nursing course with different dimensions of caring articulated and actualized throughout the baccalaureate curriculum. Caring is considered to be both ontological and epistemological. That is, students are educated from a caring, pedagogical paradigm that facilitates the opportunity for nurses to "be" caring practitioners as well as to "act" in ways that promote just and ethical nursing practice. Caring is not a soft and sympathetic notion. Instead, it is the driving force behind all nursing actions. As such, the attitude and action of caring provides a moral, ethical, and just foundation on which to base all forms of nursing practice and is a guiding principle on which the profession of nursing is both recognized and actualized.

Caring curriculum. A pedagogical approach to curriculum development devised by Olivia Bevis and Jean Watson in their 1989 book, *Toward a Caring Curriculum: A New Pedagogy for Nursing.*

Cartesian view. A Cartesian view of knowledge directly arises from the works of the French philosopher and mathematician, René Descartes (1596–1650). He proposed that mathematical reasoning should be the basis of a new system of knowledge extending this idea to a theory about the human mind and its distinction from the body. This view claims that thinking and feeling are distinct and unrelated human experiences. A Cartesian view presupposes that all human experience is made up of two incompatible kinds of substance—mind or consciousness and physical matter such as human bodies—and this division claims that bodies have no part in our essence as thinking beings.

Case analyses. The process of learning through addressing a case that is a narrative that includes information and data related to a subject area. Nursing, for example. Good cases are drawn around problems or big ideas that warrant serious, in-depth consideration.

Case method teaching. The use of cases as a tool for teaching. There are many variations of this approach to teaching.

Categories. In Kant's philosophy of mind, categories are innate cognitive structures that enable human beings to interpret perceptual experience. The four basic categories are quantity, quality, relation, and modality.

Classism. An assumption of superiority in relation to a group of people of a given social rank or status (usually socioeconomic) in the community. Social class is one of the most important concepts in the study of stratification; it is a social distinction and division resulting from the unequal distribution of rewards and resources such as wealth, power, and prestige. The sociologist Max Weber identified three dimensions of class distinctions: (1) *Class*, which refers to life chances, or the ability of people to get what they want and need to survive and prosper; (2) Inequality in the distribution of *power*. Because power is bureaucratically organized in industrial societies, individuals are relatively powerless unless they have access to organizations such as corporations, governments, unions, and other institutions; and (3) The distribution of *prestige*, or the degree of social honor, status, or deference that people enjoy in relation to others. In particular, occupational prestige is a way of measuring social mobility. bell hooks noted that class struggle is inextricably bound to the struggle to end racism. hooks cites Brown, who urged women to explore the full implication of class, noting that "your experience (determined by your class) validated those assumptions, how you are taught to behave, what you expect from yourself and from others, your concept of a future, how you understand problems and solve them, how you think, feel, act. It is these behavioral patterns that middle class women resist recognizing although they may be perfectly willing to accept class in Marxist terms, a neat trick that helps them avoid really dealing with class behavior and changing that behavior in themselves. It is these behavioral patterns which must be recognized, understood, and changed" (Brown, 1974, p. 15).

Cognitive constructivism. Posits that learning is best understood as a process of individual meaning making or knowledge building.

Cognitive theory. A view of learning that focuses on processing information in order to generate knowledge.

Cognitivists. Those who develop and espouse cognitive learning theory.

Collaborative learning. Informed by constructivist principles, collaborative learning is a teaching strategy that encourages confrontation between students' conceptions and course material by directly involving them in the learning process. Engaging students in researching course material using reference materials and working together with the instructor on developing categorization strategies are two examples of collaborative learning.

Collaborative nursing care. Informed by the principles of health promoting nursing practice, collaborative nursing care is a practice in which the nurse and client work together in partnership toward resolution of health-related issues.

Community building. An example of a goal for a learning experience intended to reinforce the sense of community among students and instructors.

Community of learners. A group of distance students who share a common purpose and make a commitment to the well-being of each other and the group.

Committee on the Function of Nursing. The group whose study chaired by Dr. Eli Ginzberg criticized hospital training schools' educational programs and recommended that nursing education be a 4-year baccalaureate degree course of study.

Committee on the Grading of Nursing Schools. Formed in the 1920s to review hospital training schools.

Competence. A dynamic process of integrating and applying knowledge, skills, attitudes, and judgment required to perform safely within the scope of an educator's role. This process requires educators to gain meaning from their experience. As a dynamic process, competence is situational-specific and context-bound. Motivation, interest, energy, and commitment are required to help an individual deal with the internal and external factors that influence his or her state of being competent. Throughout the process of gaining and maintaining competence, feelings experienced by educators fluctuate between anxiety and tension, and a sense of comfort and empowerment.

Competencies. Descriptive statements about the knowledge, skills, attitudes, and judgment required to perform safely within the scope of an individual's nursing practice or in a designated role or setting.

Complexity science. Complexity science refers to a set of nonlinear approaches to understanding complex, adaptive systems, including both physical systems such as weather or urban development and human systems such as organizations or networks. It reflects the efforts of a wide range of disciplines to work out ways of studying phenomena for whom the questions we pose are too large and complicated to be addressed in a satisfactory manner by the scientific conventions of any discipline alone. In nursing, scholars have been attracted to complexity science because it offers insights into ways in which, for example, the human person and his or her health might be understood within the larger context of lives and human societies.

Concept map. A flowchart type of diagram that represents an individual's understanding of a set of concepts imbedded in a framework of propositions. The map is typically organized in a top-down hierarchical fashion with lines or links placed between concepts to show relationships. Terms are often placed on the links to show more meaning.

Concept mapping. Concept mapping is a technique for visually representing how concepts within a domain are interrelated and is based on Ausubel's theory of meaningful learning which stresses that learning new knowledge is dependent on what is already known.

Conceptual or **organizing framework.** Theories or essential elements of the curriculum design; provides guide to development; reflects mission, philosophy, etc.

Conceptualizing or **conceptual thinking.** Conceptualizing or conceptual thinking refers to an emphasis on representational or abstract thinking. Concepts are mental representations of abstractions that come to be signified using language conventions. Humans have the capacity to communicate with one another because of this ability to conceptualize, to inscribe certain words with layers of meaning. By locating all of the assumptions, properties, and characteristics inherent in an abstraction within a concept, we create the ability to build theories, generate propositions, and articulate relationships between ideas. In nursing, conceptual thinking demands critical reflection on how language is used toward creating shared understandings of such entities as clinical phenomena and health problems. Conceptual thinking allows nurses to work with ideas as ideas rather than as facts or truths, and to remember that it is our collective relationship to these ideas that confers them with meaning.

Constructivism. A theory of learning primarily based on contemporary developmental psychology that emphasizes the building or construction that occurs in people's minds when learning. According to constructivism, learning principally occurs when a human being's current conceptions of the world are forced to change owing to interactions addressing incompatibilities. Constructivism, as a philosophical underpinning to education, holds to the view that learning is a developmental or generative process.

Context-based learning. Context-based learning (CBL) is a philosophical variation of problem-based learning. CBL is a learner-centered approach to learning that involves the use of real professional practice situations as the initial stimulus for learning rather than as a culminating activity following faculty presentation of content.

Contextual. Relating to the physical, emotional, and sociopolitical environment within which agents are engaged.

Course design team. A group of experts involved in developing courses for distance delivery. This team may include a design specialist, technical support personnel, content specialist (faculty), and graphic designer.

Course management system. A software package designed to help faculty create quality online courses. Sometimes also called e-Learning systems, learning management systems (LMS), or virtual learning environments (VLE). Examples of CMS include Blackboard, Moodle, and WebCT.

Course portfolio. A course portfolio is briefer than a teaching portfolio. It is a collection of information that describes the design, evolution, and learner outcomes associated with a specific course.

Convergers. These learners like to learn using abstract conceptualization and active experimentation. Although called pragmatists, they tend to be unemotional and focus on the practical application of idea.

Creative capacity. The ability to engage in processes that spark hidden forces within us as teachers/learners, allowing us to tune into emotive and reasoned ways of knowing so that we are able to hone, limit, and clarify ideas and experiences to give form.

Critical reflection. The ability to assess the content, process, and/or premises of our efforts to interpret and give meaning to our experience through dialogue with others.

Critical relationship. Being in critical relation with an idea, theory, person, etc. calls our attentions to examine various modes of thinking feeling, knowing, valuing, and believing within particular contexts. Being in critical relation with knowledge requires unmasking taken-for-granted assumptions and working to see anew with new questions and meanings potentially arising. Engaging in thoughtful and purposeful inquiry requires attention to critical nuances of experiences, ways of knowing, acting, and reflecting, among other intellectual and embodied processes.

Critical social theory. Critical social theory refers to both a school of thought and to a process of critique. One of the fundamental beliefs underlying critical theory is that standards of truth or evidence, such as rules, habits, etc., are always created in a social context. In addition, it is believed that no aspect of social phenomena may be comprehended unless it is related to the historical whole and to the contextual structures that surround it. Critical theorists contend people communicate and create meaning in relation to domination and to transform constraining conditions.

Critical social theory addresses the unequal social, economic, and power relations that exist within society. Questions are raised regarding the prevailing hegemony, or the prevailing dogma and ideology. Through dialogue, there is a raising of collective consciousness that leads to conscientization. Social, economic, and political conditions are viewed as determinants of health. Action is viewed as an outcome of conscientization. As people become more conscious of oppressive situations within society, there is the potential to take action. Such action leads to liberation and emancipation for nurses and their client populations.

Critical thinking. An intellectually disciplined process of actively and skillfully conceptualizing, applying, analyzing, synthesizing, and/or evaluating information gathered from, or generated by, observation, experience, reflection, reasoning, or communication as a guide to belief and action. In its exemplary form, it is based on universal intellectual values that transcend subject matter divisions: clarity, accuracy, precision, consistency, relevance, sound evidence, good reasons, depth, breadth, and fairness. It entails the examination of those structures or elements implicit in all reasoning: purpose, problem, or question-at-issue, assumptions, concepts, empirical grounding, reasoning leading to conclusions, implications and consequences, objections from alternative viewpoints, and frame of reference. Critical thinking—in being responsive to variable subject matter, issues, and purposes—is incorporated into a family of interwoven modes of thinking, among them: scientific thinking, mathematical thinking, historical thinking, anthropological thinking, economic thinking, moral thinking, and philosophical thinking.

It is also the process of distinguishing between a good argument and a faulty argument by understanding its implications and consequences, the assumptions on which it is based, and its logical structure.

Culture. A relational experience that is deeply embedded within webs of power, economics, and politics. This is in contrast to definitions of culture as shared values, beliefs, and customs that belong to groups of people.

Curriculum-as-planned. Planned, predetermined outline of course content and learning activities.

Curriculum development or **design.** Defines composition and outcomes of the educational experience.

Curriculum revolution. A movement led by nurse educators such as Peggy Chinn, David Allen, Pat Moccia, and others in the 1980s where the purpose of nursing education was reconceptualized so that nursing was taken up in a more explicitly politicized way. The revolutionized nursing curriculum was altered to include education in social and political thought, with an aim toward repositioning nursing as a force for social change.

D

Decision-making skills. The skills necessary to make clinical and group decisions, involves skills of negotiation, prioritization, collaboration, and clinical judgment.

Deconstructing. A scholarly project focused on revealing/uncovering the ideological biases (gender, racial, economic, political, cultural) of human experience by interpreting human language or texts.

Deep learning. Approach to learning in which the learner attempts to define the significance of new information, to relate the information to previous learning, and to understand the information as a coherent whole for the purpose of self-development and because of an innate curiosity; therefore, the learning is the end goal.

The use of higher order cognitive thinking skills, such as analysis and synthesis, that results in an incorporation of new ideas with existing knowledge and personal experience, that is thought to result from intrinsic motivation.

Developmental perspective. In this perspective, effective teaching must be planned and conducted from the learner's point of view.

Developmental learning. Developmental learning is held to result from the use of learning activities consistent with constructivist principles.

Dewey, John (1859–1952). American philosopher and educator whose writings and teachings had profound influences on education in the United States. Dewey's philosophy of education focused on learning by doing rather than rote learning and dogmatic instruction, the current practice of his day.

Diagonal curriculum plan. A baccalaureate program where nursing courses begin during the sophomore year.

Dialectic. Relating to seemingly opposing views or forces and the tensioned space between opposites; i.e., relatedness between living and dying; teaching and learning; clarity and confusion.

Dialogue. The skillful exchange or interaction between people that develops shared understanding as the basis for building trust, fostering a sense of ownership, facilitating genuine agreement, and enabling creative problem solving.

Didactic. Intended to convey instruction and information. The word is often used to refer to texts that are overburdened with instructive or factual matter to the exclusion of graceful and pleasing detail so that they are pompously dull and erudite.

Digital divide. The widening gap between those who have access to information and communication technologies and those who do not.

Digital immigrants. People born before 1980, prior to the digital world, who have become fascinated by and/or adopted aspects of new technology.

Digital natives. Learners born between 1980 and 2000 who are "native speakers of the digital language of computers, video games, and the Internet" (Prensky, 2001a, p. 1).

Discipline of nursing. The accumulated explicit and implicit theoretical substance that shapes, knowingly and unknowingly, the value systems underlying educational curricula, models of practice education and preferred methods for resolving tensions that arise between nursing practice and nursing education when these are understood as distinct yet related activities.

Distance education. A set of teaching and/or learning strategies designed to meet the learning needs of students separate from the traditional classroom setting and sometimes from the traditional roles of faculty. Distance education requires that teachers and learners are separate from each other. Thus, this definition excludes activities where the teacher travels to an alternative site for delivery of traditional courses or classes.

Divergers. These learners like to learn using reflective observation and concrete experience. They like time to reflect and think about the subject. They tend to be imaginative, interested in people and emotions.

Dysconscious racism. The habit of uncritically justifying inequity and exploitation by accepting inequity and exploitation as just the way things are.

E

e-books. An electronic, or digital, form of a book. Advantages of e-books include rapid searching of text, ability to carry hundreds on a single device, readable in low light, user adjustment of type size and type face, easy backup, low-cost distribution, and use with text-to-speech software.

Ecomap. A visual tool that describes the social support networks of families.

Educational Preparation for Nurse Practitioners and Assistants to Nurses. 1965 ANA position paper about nursing education programs.

e-Learning. Training, education, coaching, and information that is delivered digitally either asynchronously or synchronously.

Embodied responses. Responses that are of the physical body.

Empiricism. A philosophical view according to which human beings' understanding of the world derives directly from the actual characteristics of the world as it is experienced independently of the perceiver.

Epistemology. The branch of philosophy dealing with knowledge. Central questions of epistemology are how to distinguish knowledge from mere belief and the origin of knowledge.

e-Teaching. Teaching delivered electronically.

Ethical knowledge. Knowledge of the good in practice. Ethical knowledge is drawn from formal theory, but also comes from other sources, including experience and emotion.

Ethical practice. Practice that is directed toward the good for patients, families, and communities. Such practice takes guidance from nursing codes of ethics and requires respectful, interdependent relationships between nursing and other health care team members.

Ethical principles. Moral guideposts that have been drawn from a variety of theoretical sources. The traditional ethical principles include autonomy, beneficence, nonmaleficence, and justice. More relational principles (or concepts) include fidelity and care.

Ethnocentrism. "The tendency to judge the characteristics and cultures of other groups by the standards defined or recognized by the observer's own ethnic group. Cultural judgments made on an ethnocentric basis are inevitably negative and pejorative, and serve to justify the denigration of other cultures and to promote racism. Both Eurocentrism and Afrocentrism are forms of ethnocentrism" in this view (Macey, 2000, p. 115).

Eurocentrism. The conscious or unconscious process by which European cultural assumptions are constructed as, or assumed to be, the normal, the natural or the universal. European colonization of the globe actively promoted Eurocentrism through exploration, conquest, and trade. The intellectual authority of colonial institutions such as schools and universities were established through the civil service and legal codes which constructed European systems and values as inherently superior to indigenous ones.

Evaluation. A process of acquiring information about nursing education programs and materials that is used to inform decision making. Evaluation can be formal or informal, systematic or occasional, formative or summative.

Everyday racism. Everyday habits and cultural meanings which intimate covert aversions against particular groups but of which people are for the most part unaware. While people in Western society are committed to equality and believe that group differences should not matter, unconscious gestures connoting inferiority are commonplace. Everyday racism includes the daily slights, assumptions, looks, ways of being addressed, being overlooked, or having people assume that you are less intelligent than others, receiving harsher judgments than others, and so on. These daily small reminders form a discourse of deservedness, the outcome of which is that people come to understand where they stand in their society. (See Applebaum 1997).

Evidence-based decision making. A reasoning process in which clinical decisions are based on evidence generated using large clinical trials.

Existing cognitive structures. The content of the mind—the relationships that the learner establishes among the concepts and strategies the learner uses in abstracting concepts and in organizing them in long-term memory.

Experiential. Learning through direct experience.

Experiential learning. Attributed to Kolb's theorizing of the centrality of starting with student experience; Kolb developed the cyclical pattern of learning from experience through reflection and conceptualizing to action, and on to further experience, reflection, or action.

Experiential learning is focused more on active doing rather than the passive being done to. Thus learners practice what they are learning so that change is maintained over time. Experience-based learning (action alone) becomes "experiential" when elements of reflection, transfer, and support are added to the base experience: *reflection*—purposefully examining the process of an experience enhances the awareness of learning and leads to changes in feeling, thinking, or behaving that derive from that experience; *transfer*—when change obtained in an experiential program shows up in the real life workplace: this transfer of experiential learning can be enhanced by the use of metaphors and isomorphs; and *support*—providing time, resources, and team or project opportunities that permit people to continue changing (or maintaining new learning) and allows them to lessen their resistance.

Experiential learning cycle. A model of how learning occurs, developed by Kolb. The cycle starts with a concrete experience; that is, it begins with being actively involved in an assigned task. The second stage in the cycle is reflective observation, meaning that the learner takes time out to reflect on what has been learned and experienced. Abstract conceptualization, the third stage, is the process of making sense of what has happened. It involves interpreting the information or experience and comparing this with what was previously known. The final stage of the learning cycle, active experimentation, is when the learner considers how to apply the new learning to practice.

Experiential textures. From a postmodern perspective, the term text is used more broadly to include life as living and embodied text. The notion of experiential textures points to an interplay of experiencing the flux of life in the classroom and interpreting (thinking about) the flow of experience as it moves and changes. With openness and discernment, patterns of relational practice can be articulated.

Extrovert learner. This type of learner is energized by working with things and people. Extroverts are action oriented and like working in groups to learn.

F

Facilitation. A goal-orientated dynamic process, in which participants work together in an atmosphere of genuine mutual respect in order to learn through critical reflection.

Faculty member. A teacher in a college, university, or school of nursing who coordinates and supports a preceptored program between students and preceptors. This person assists the student and preceptor with all levels of teaching. Usually this person is responsible for the evaluation and final grade on the preceptorship practicum.

Feeling learner. This type of learner values harmony and is empathetic to the needs of others. Feeling learners prefer to learn in warm, friendly environments. They regard new information subjectively and may take things personally at times.

Feminism. Historically, feminism focused on valuing women and confronting systematic injustices based on gender. Since that time, there are those that contend that feminism has developed into an inclusive model of liberation for all people, with particular attention given to the status of women. There are a number of differing feminist perspectives. Categories of feminism identified by Sherwin include liberal, socialist, cultural, and postmodern feminism.

A feminist philosophy attends to the reality of women's oppression. Traditionally, women have been oppressed, and nursing as a predominately female profession has been particularly affected by the oppression of women. Thus, from a feminist perspective, questions are raised about the power relations that have existed in the context of nursing. Feminist critique of the health care system, of relationships with other health care professionals, and the role of women in the helping professions are integrated throughout a post-modern curriculum.

Feminist. A person who is actively committed to the fundamental equality of men and women.

Feminist epistemology. The idea that women may have their own particular ways of conceptualizing the world distinct from, and possibly superior to, scientific methods.

Field dependent learner. This type of learner prefers concrete learning that is structured and occurs in interaction with others. The field dependent learner learns best when the content is relevant to his or her experience. This type of learner may learn to please others and consequently, can be deeply affected by criticism.

Field independent learner. This type of learner is self-directed and analytical. The field independent learner tends to learn new information for its own sake and not vulnerable to the emotional effects of criticism.

Flexibility of pace. The technology's support for student-paced progression versus delivery-paced requirements for progression.

Flexibility of place. The technology's support for the location in which students and/or faculty are required to be for any given learning activity; may range from user-determined, such as home or anywhere computer access may be, or from technology-determined, such as a centralized classroom for interactive television sessions.

Flexibility of time. The technology's support for students and/or faculty variability for when class activities are done; ranges from synchronous, or real time, same time, to asynchronous, or different times.

G

Goal-oriented process. A process that addresses how individuals will meet the goals of the course and individual.

GUI (graphical user interface). A term used to describe what the computer user interacts with to provide commands, e.g., a mouse click on a hyperlink.

H

Habits of mind. Sets of assumptions about the world that is part of the frame of reference that filters the interpretation of experience.

Handheld electronic devices. Pocket-sized computing devices carried by individuals, such as smartphones, PDAs, cell phones, and handheld game consoles that provide rapid access to information.

Harvey Project. An international collaboration of interactive, dynamic human physiology course materials on the Web, prepared by educators, researchers, physicians, students, programmers, instructional designers, and graphic artists. Materials produced by the Harvey Project are freely available to any educational institution.

Health promotion. The current consensus view of health has been transformed from one dominated by the disease-treatment model to one typified by the declaration by the World Health Organization (WHO) that health is now understood to be deeply rooted in human nature and societal structures. Within this broader framework, health has been defined as "the extent to which an individual or group is able to realize aspirations, to satisfy needs, and to change or cope with the environment" (WHO, et al., 1986, p. 1). In this context, health promotion is defined as "a process of enabling people to increase control over and to improve their health . . . a mediating strategy between people and their environment, synthesizing personal choice and social responsibility in health" (WHO, 1984). It is both a philosophy (or way of being) and a practice (or way of doing) and in essence is a relational practice.

Health promotion in nursing practice is "a transformative process in which the nurse as partner engages clients in consciousness-raising characterized by respect for the dynamic relatedness between people and their environment." (Young, L.E. (2002). Transforming health promotion practice: Moving toward holistic care. In L.E. Young & V.E. Hodges (Eds.), Transforming health promotion practice: Concepts, issues, and applications. (pp.3–21). Philadelphia: F.A. Davis).

Heterosexism. "One of many intersecting forms of oppression . . . its dynamics are similar to those of others oppressions. Heterosexism is the belief that the only right, natural, normal, god-given and therefore privileged way of relating to each other is (with a member of the opposite sex). To be heterosexist is to value and see as 'normal' prescribed male-female gender dichotomies and to devalue anything other, or to label as 'abnormal' that which breaks down those prescribed dichotomies" (Gray, Kramer, Minick, McGehee, Thomas & Grenier, 1996, p. 205).

Heuristic knowledge. Pertains to the use of the general knowledge gained by experience, sometimes expressed as a "rule-of-thumb." It is the knowledge that underlies the art of good guessing.

Highly refined materials. Course materials such as print, audiotape or videotape, interactive multimedia, and Internet resources that are produced through an ongoing refinement of content, as compared to audio conferencing or videoconferencing that relies on spontaneous generation of content.

Homophobia. The word homophobia means an irrational fear of lesbians and gay men (homosexuals). This fear extends to bisexuals, transsexuals, and transgendered persons.

Hospital training schools. Nursing education programs operated by individual hospitals.

Humanism. Humanism is a philosophical perspective based on the assumption that people have a tendency to develop all of their capacities that serve to maintain or enhance them. The movement toward self-actualization is believed to be part of people's organismic nature. Broadly speaking, a humanist approach seeks to facilitate the release of an already existing capacity in potentially competent individuals. Underlying a humanist approach is the belief that if certain definable conditions are present in people's human relationships, they will gradually allow their self-actualizing capacity to overcome restrictions they have internalized through their life experiences. The three relational conditions include: (1) genuineness or congruence, (2) empathic understanding, and (3) unconditional positive regard.

Hybrid or "blended" instruction models. Instructional models that employ two of more types of technology; for example, combining videoconference and Web-based instruction.

I

Ideology. A linked set of ideas and beliefs that act to uphold and justify an existing or desired arrangement of power, authority, wealth, and status in a society.

Independent learning. The individual student takes on responsibility for learning activities. The student's learning issues, learning preferences, and learning style determine these learning activities issues.

Independent study. Involves planned study, sometimes individualized, that is not available in a class setting or format.

Information Age. The period of time following the Industrial Age where the development, storage, retrieval, and dissemination of knowledge and information is paramount.

Information literacy. The ability to recognize a need for information, find, evaluate, and use that information in whatever format (print index, online database, Internet, etc.) it appears.

Information processing. The processes involved in attending to new information, comprehending it, and placing it in the memory, to be retrieved when needed at a later time.

Inquiry-based learning. A student-centered learning approach that requires students to actively seek knowledge and information necessary to resolve questions and/or issues. It is associated with the idea "involve me and I understand." One such variation of inquiry-based learning is PBL.

Institutional variable costs. The economies of scale for the institution occurring from the use of specific distance education technologies; with specific technologies an increase in production efficiency results from an increased number of materials produced, thereby lowering the costs of materials as the fixed production costs are shared over an increased number of materials.

Instrumentalism. A conception of education which holds that education should promote knowledge and understanding that is personally, socially, or economically useful.

Integrated approach (to lecturing). Occurs when active learning methods are interspersed within a lecture.

Integrated curriculum pattern. An approach to organizing learning experience that features concepts and themes as the organizing elements; antithesis to the medical model approach in which body systems organize learning.

Interactive media. Delivery of course materials by computer (CD/DVD) or Internet (audio conferencing or videoconferencing) that allows interactive dialogue with the content or among faculty and students.

Interactivity. Opportunities for verbal as well as nonverbal student interface with faculty, fellow students, and/or educational materials. Increased interactivity promotes students' engagement with course materials, instructors, and other students.

Intermental ability. An intermental ability is a function a person is able to perform in interaction with others.

Internet. A series of servers connected worldwide. There are many services available on the Internet, the most familiar of which are e-mail and the World Wide Web. Others include Telnet, FTP, and gopher.

Internet telephony. The technology that enables voice conversations to be held over the Internet instead of the dedicated voice transmission lines of the telephone service; also called IP Telephony or voice over Internet protocol (VoIP). The Web-based services enable integration of live video and Web conferencing to enable a rich multimedia environment for real time presentations and meetings.

Intersectionality. The interaction between forms of oppressions (such as racism and sexism) in ways that magnify one another; for example, being racialized is not an added form of oppression for a woman; rather it magnifies that oppression.

Intramental ability. An intramental ability is a function that a person is able to perform independently or autonomously.

Intrapersonal intelligence. Entails the capacity to understand oneself, to appreciate one's feelings, fears, and motivations.

Introvert learner. This type of learner is energized by the inner world of ideas, concepts, and abstractions. Introverts want to understand the world but they need time and space for reflection.

Intuitive learner. This type of learner prefers concepts and interpretations, rather than facts. Intuitive learners like variety in their work but may become bored if there is too much detail.

J

Judging learner. This type of learner is organized and efficient in completing tasks. Judging learners tend to dislike surprises, thus they need advanced warning when change is introduced.

Judgment. The intellectual process exercised in forming a conclusion, decision, and plan of action based on a critical analysis of relevant evidence.

K

Kant, Immanuel (1724–1804). German philosopher whose work in the philosophy of knowledge and perception laid the foundations for modern psychology. Kant's central contribution was to show that knowledge of the world does not directly reflect how the world is in and of itself. Instead, knowledge results from an interaction between the mind and perception.

Knowledge. Broadly interpreted to extend beyond information, facts, and "knowing about" to include cognitive, experiential, and intuitive sources of knowledge applied in nursing practice.

Knowledge workers. The term knowledge worker is widely attributed to Peter F. Drucker. Drucker discussed the societal shift from people who work with their muscles to people who work with their minds. His theory has been twofold: that knowledge work requires formal education and that knowledge workers work in teams rather than alone. Knowledge work is nonroutine and nonrepetitive and requires a great deal of cognitive activity.

L

Learning collaboratory. A learning environment tailored to individual learning needs of students so that they can master content and develop skills for lifelong learning and teamwork.

Learning curve. A concept that indicates the relationship between experience and efficiency; essentially, the more experience an individual has with an activity, the more efficiently the activity can be done.

Learning plan. An organizational tool used by students to individualize and prioritize their learning needs, set learning goals and objectives, determine resources to be consulted, and establish criteria for evaluation.

Learning style. Cognitive, affective, and physiological behaviors that serve as indicators of how learners perceive, interact, and respond to the learning environment.

Lecture. A teaching methodology comprised mostly of one or more teachers providing information verbally (sometimes with visual materials) to a group of learners.

Liberal progressive movement. An educational movement according to which the aim of general education is the liberation of human beings' innate tendency toward moral goodness in contrast with conservatism which holds that general education's aim is the containment of human beings' tendency toward moral badness.

Linguistic intelligence. Linguistic intelligence is sensitivity to the meaning of words, the order among words, sounds, rhythms, inflections, different functions of language, phonology, syntax, and pragmatism.

Lived curriculum. Living engagement in the class or clinical setting; the experience of learning plans and pedagogy as it is lived.

Locations. We are located in the world and by others in the world based on how we identify and are identified based on gender, class, occupation, political affiliation, etc. *See* situatedness.

Locke, John (1661–1756). English philosopher and main figure in the empiricist movement in philosophy. Locke's two important philosophical works are *An Essay Concerning Human Understanding* and *Two Treatises on Government*.

Low threshold applications. Low threshold applications (LTA) are teaching/learning applications of information technology that are reliable, accessible, easy to learn, nonintimidating, and (incrementally) inexpensive. Each LTA has observable positive consequences and contributes to important long-term changes in teaching and/or learning.

M

Marginal, marginalize, and marginalizing. bell hooks (1984) states that "to be in the margin is to be part of the whole but outside the main body" (p. x). She notes that when one lives in the margins, one develops a particular way of seeing reality—from the outside in, and from the inside out. Survival, she says, depends on knowing both the margins and the center. Unlike people living at the center of society who know little or nothing of those living at the margins, people at the margins have to know a great deal about the oppressor—know, for example, how to negotiate around the powerful (i.e., those who are located in the center) in order to survive. In addition to knowing the oppressor, people at the margins must understand how to relate to the marginalized with whom they live and interact on a daily basis (pp. ix–x). Marginalization describes the social and material reality of many women, as well as migrants, Blacks, and ethnic minorities. It is a philosophical construct meaning the irrational and the margins. Marxist writers argue that marginality is functional to capitalism; feminist theory argues that marginality is a relational concept, not a reified category, since what is perceived as marginal at any time depends on the position one occupies.

Sociologist Elise Boulding calls for a more positive interpretation of marginality, arguing that the marginality of women and their basic leverage points in the family provide position of social transformation (Humm, 1990, p. 127).

McGill model of nursing. A collaborative, client-centered, family-focused approach to nursing first developed by F. Moyra Allen at McGill University School of Nursing in the 1970s.

Medical model. Common approach to learning in hospital training schools where the curriculum is organized around body systems and specialty areas of care.

Merlot. A free and open resource designed primarily for faculty and students of higher education. Merlot contains links to online learning materials along with annotations about those materials, such as peer reviews and assignments. Merlot is an acronym for Multimedia Educational Resource for Learning and Online Teaching.

Metacognition. Higher level thinking that involves thinking about thinking—reflecting on a situation, reviewing what is known, creating hypotheses, deciding what needs to be learned/done, questioning new information, and deciding how new information fits with what is known.

Metaparadigm concepts. Patient, nurse, environment, and health are the four central concepts underlying all theories of nursing. These concepts have been consistently used by subsequent theorists as analytic structures to examine formal and informal nursing models and frameworks and to analyze their relationship to nursing practice and research. They are collectively cited as the core problems underlying nursing theorizing.

Mind map. A weblike diagram that provides a visual display of an individual's ideas and thoughts about a given topic area. The emphasis of mind mapping is placed on the understanding, organizing, and linking of ideas, as opposed to memorization.

Model. *See* social learning theory.

Moral agency. The ability for people to be capable of, and engage in, deliberate ethical action. Our views on moral agency are significantly influenced by feminist and contextual theorists who extend traditional understandings to one that posits moral agency as enacted through relationships in particular contexts.

Moral sensitivity. Acting ethically presupposes moral sensitivity—that is, the morally relevant features of a situation are recognized. It is a seeing and perceiving that shapes how one cares for another person. It is also defined as a capacity to be addressed by the morally significant aspects of a particular situation, such as being emotionally engaged and involved in another person's condition or experience. Moral sensitivity requires seeing how our intellectual or cognitive understandings are related to our emotions and feelings that arise in response to clinical experiences.

Multimedia. Consisting of more than one medium; for example, television is multimedia because it incorporates the media of sound and visuals.

Multi-User Virtual Environments (MUVEs). "MUVE applications incorporate computer graphics, sound simulation, and networks to simulate the experience of real-time interaction between multiple users in a shared three-dimensional virtual world. Applications for multi-user virtual environment technology include distributed training, simulation, education, home shopping, virtual meetings, and multiplayer games" (http://www.cs.princeton.edu/~funk/ring.html).

N

Narrative and stories. There are some subtle distinctions made between narrative and story in the wider literature. Stories tend to have a particular syntactic shape (beginning, middle, and end) whereas narratives are more often defined as a construction that we place over events of our life in order to create of them a coherent pattern. Thus, narratives are often described as less structured. A much quoted description of their interchangeability comes from Hunter (1991): "In using the word 'narrative' somewhat interchangeably with 'story' I mean to designate a more or less coherent written, spoken, or (by extension) enacted account of occurrences whether historical or fictional" (p. 306).

Stories and narrative are ways of making sense of experience and events over time and signify a perspective on those events. Thus, stories are a kind a narrative. Both can be historical or fictional and can be expressed or told differently depending on the context or the purpose. Stories and narrative both show how we understand our world. Stories and narratives may differ in structure but generally share a rootedness in time, place, and personal experience. Our cultural ways of living speak themselves through both narratives and stories. The value of both narrative and story is that they bring us into our own experience and those of others. They call forth emotional and physical responses in us as both listeners and tellers. For these reasons, narrating and telling stories bring us closer to our subjectivity, lived experience, and embodiment.

Narrative pedagogy. An approach to teaching and learning that evolves from eliciting for interpretation the lived experiences of teachers, clinicians, and students.

Noninstrumentalism. A conception of education which holds that education should promote knowledge and understanding for its own sake irrespective of any practical use it might have.

Nonlinear learning. Known as the hallmark of e-Learning, nonlinear learning supports students' decisions about how to progress through the material, whether by repeating material, skipping material, and beginning and ending at times of their choosing. Nonlinear learning is the opposite of linear learning, which is the characteristic of classroom-based instruction.

Normal science. Normal science is a term originated by Kuhn to refer to the routine work or puzzle solving of scientific experimentation within an established paradigm as compared to other forms of scientific work that actually test the science or challenge its fundamental assumptions.

Nursing models. Conceptual models for nursing, also known as nursing models, conceptual models, and conceptual frameworks, are depictions of the central foci of all nursing action. They represent a mental image of the way the discipline understands its client (whether that be an individual, a family or group, or a community or population). Further, they create a reasoning structure whereby nursing can understand that client within its context (environmental, social, physical and so on) and its aspirations (health, optimal well-being, etc.). For a generation, starting in the late 1960s, prominent nursing scholars took up the challenge of articulating the inherent complexity in excellent nursing reasoning using the nursing model as a conceptual device for articulating nursing's purpose, scope, and intent. By the 1990s, this form of theorizing (philosophizing) went out of vogue within the discipline, and many current curricula do little more than give lip service to acknowledging them. However, as nursing graduate students re-engage in a study of these models using their more modern frames of reference from postmodernism and complexity science as analytic tools, they discover that the nursing models actually do represent an era of powerful and comprehensive thought that has relevance for our current challenges.

Nursing for the Future. Published by Dr. Esther Lucille Brown in 1948; advocates that nursing education belongs in institutions of higher learning.

Nurturing perspective. This view assumes that long-term, hard, and persistent efforts to achieve come from the heart, not the head. Within this view, people are motivated and productive learners when they are working on issues or problems without fear of failure.

O

Objective structured tutorial evaluation. An objective summative evaluation method to assess learner participation in the tutorial process.

Objectivity. The position that the properties of an object are independent of any particular subject's viewpoint.

Online. Provided via a computer network.

Online discussion boards. Electronic media that provide opportunity for posting messages.

Othering. The process of defining self against an exoticized other; dividing the world into us and them. A process whereby people considered different in some way are constructed as being even more different (from us) than they really are.

Ontology. A branch of philosophy that examines idea of existence and what it means for a thing to exist.

Outcomes. The desired end result, or consequence, of an educational experience for students.

P

Paradigm. Worldview that is characterized by patterned values, beliefs, and assumptions.

Partnership. Refers to collegial and collaborative partnerships established between PBL tutors and students as they work together to learn. Such partnerships reflect the intentions of openness, honesty, respect, shared power, trust, and reciprocity. Tutors and students are regarded as partners in learning.

Passive learning. Student role as recipient of information from instructor; limited, if any, engagement with content.

Patriarchy. The literal meaning is the rule of the father but it is habitually used, particularly within feminism, to mean male domination. Since the position of father in the family is no longer the sole basis for substantial social power, there has been a shift or slide in male dominance from the position of father in families to positions outside the family, politics, economics, and other institutions. The new order of gender politics is *androcratic* (that is, based on the principle of male dominance), and *androcentric* (i.e., giving primary attention and importance to men and what they do often to the exclusion of women).

Pedagogy. The work of a teacher; the art and science of teaching; instructional methods and strategies.

Pedagogical spaces. Sites of learning.

Pen-based computing. Using a pen, rather than a keyboard and mouse, to interface with a computer. Pens allow for more expressive input to computers, such as handwriting, gestures, and sketches. Pen-based interfaces are used in PDAs and Tablet PCs. In some instances, the computing device is able to interpret handwriting and gestures as text and commands.

Perceiving learner. This type of learner prefers spontaneity and flexibility to order. The perceiving learner can procrastinate and be disorganized.

Perspectives on teaching. A set of beliefs, intentions, actions, and strategies.

Phenomenology. The central tenet of phenomenology is the understanding of human experience as it is lived. The aim in phenomenology is to gain a greater understanding of the meaning of experience. Rather than focusing on the facts of a situation, the emphasis in phenomenology is to understand what meaning those facts had for the person. This focus requires a phenomenological attitude that compels people to raise questions about the nature of human experiences in an effort to uncover the deeper meaning structures within them. It is understood that the meaning structures that are uncovered are integrally related to the knower. That is, in phenomenology, the knower and the known are not separate, and there is no objective truth. Rather, knowing is individual. At the same time, because we are all situated in the world, we can gain understanding of another's knowing because we share some common meaning. In this sense, phenomenology is both a "way of being" (ontology) and a "way of doing" (practicing nursing). As Ray suggests, phenomenology offers a means by which human phenomena or the lived experiences of nurses and the people with whom they interact can be understood.

Philosophical perspective. We are using these terms to specifically refer to how Hadot draws on philosophers of antiquity to redescribe philosophy as wisdom that cultivates attention to everyday living. Taking this view of philosophy as the exercise of wisdom means that we approach the chapter from this particular view or perspective. Such a perspective then becomes a way for us as educators to live and look at nursing education and nursing practice in new ways.

Philosophical thinking. Philosophical thinking represents a search for understanding deriving from speculative rather than observational means. In nursing, it represents a method for pursuing knowledge related to the values and reality of the discipline through analyzing the conceptual meaning and grounds for expressions of fundamental disciplinary belief. It represents a search for wisdom rather than factual knowledge, and is understood to complement and integrate the many other forms of thinking within which nursing engages.

Piaget, Jean (1896–1980). Founding figure of developmental psychology in the 20th century. His research, which focused on knowledge development in children, showed that cognitive structures human beings use to understand the world evolve according to a set developmental pattern. The significance of his work principally resides in having overturned the Kantian idea that the cognitive structures of the mind are fixed from birth.

Postcolonial. Refers to concern with the effects of colonization on cultures and societies. Postcolonial "as it has been employed in most recent accounts has been primarily concerned to examine the processes and effects of, and reactions to, European colonialism from the sixteenth century up to and including the neo-colonialism of the present day" (Ashcroft, et al., 2000, p. 188).

Postcolonial theories. A critique of colonialism a process in which the other is represented as inferior. Colonialism serves to maintain unequal international relations of economic and political power.

Postmodern theories. Theories that call into question core concepts of modernity or the Enlightenment such as the subject/object distinction, progress, empiricism, and the rule of law.

Poststructural theories. A subcategory of postmodern theories that call into question the central tenets of structuralism, an approach to social science that assumes that human beings and human societies are governed by a set of structures or laws similar to those governing the natural world. Poststructural theorists generally believe instead that the social world is best understood as a manifestation of unjust and historically contingent power relations.

Pragmatist tradition. Philosophers working in the pragmatist tradition can be traced to the works of C. S. Peirce in 1878 and later to William James and John Dewey. In their similar ways, pragmatists have put forth theories of truth that rest on the notion that ideas (and theories, concepts, etc.) become true just so far as they help us to get into satisfactory relations with other parts of human experience. How true a particular idea or theory is reflects its contribution to our ability to be effective or solve problems in everyday life.

Preceptee. A student who is learning about nursing in a designated area of practice under the direct guidance of a preceptor and indirect guidance of a faculty member.

Preceptor. A registered nurse who supports, guides, teaches, and coaches another in their designated area of practice for a specified period of time.

Preceptorship. When a professional takes on the added responsibility of teaching a student for a specified period of time.

Presage–process–product model of learning. Developed by Biggs, this model is a framework of stages of learning that should be considered in explorations of how teachers can enhance student learning. Presage refers to student and contextual factors that influence the learning that takes place. Process includes factors that are present during teaching and learning, such as interaction with peers; it focuses on the approaches to learning used by learners. The third stage, product, includes the outcomes of learning.

Privilege. In general terms, privilege is a benefit or advantage by one person or group over others. It is a right or power conferred by special law or historically based practices. Often the result of such relations of privilege is to confer unearned advantages to particular groups, who often come to see these privileges as theirs by virtue of their assumed superiority (i.e., greater intelligence, harder work, etc.).

Problem-based learning. Problem-based learning (PBL) is focused, experiental learning (minds-on, hands-on) organized around the investigation and resolution of messy, real world problems.

It refers to learning that results from the process of working toward resolving a problem. The problem is encountered first in the learning process and serves as the stimulus for the search for knowledge to better understand the problem and the application of reasoning skills in the search for resolution of the problem.

Process-oriented learning. An approach in which learning activities that occur in small groups are designed to concurrently support the mastery of course content and particular skills: information processing; problem solving; decision making; communication; management; assessment; teamwork; and, critical thinking.

R

Race. "Race is a socially constructed phenomenon based on the erroneous assumption that physical differences such as skin color, hair color and texture, and facial features are related to intellectual, moral, or cultural superiority" (Henry, Tator, Mattis, & Rees, 2000, p. 4). Race is a term for the classification of human beings into physically, biologically, and genetically distinct groups—a classification that is widely agreed to have no scientific validity. The notion of race assumes that humanity is divided into unchanging natural types, recognizable by physical features that are transmitted 'through the blood' and permit distinctions to be made between 'pure' and 'mixed' races. The term implies that mental and moral behavior of human beings can be related to racial origin (Ashcroft, et al., 2000, p. 198).

Race cognizance. Critical and conscious awareness of the dynamics of race, racism, and racializing processes. This is the third position of three in the process of moving from essentialist racism (position 1, where race is seen as a determinant and explanation of human behavior), to color and power evasion (position 2, the color-blind position), to a position that recognizes the complexities of context, the ways in which race can interact with socioeconomic status to predetermine the meanings and realities of one's identity and experiences (Gillespie, Ashbaugh, & DeFiore, 2002, p. 241).

Racialization. The process by which people are labeled according to particular physical characteristics or arbitrary ethnic or racial categories, and then dealt with in accordance with beliefs related to those labels.

Racism. Can be defined as a way of thinking that considers a group's unchangeable physical characteristics to be linked in a direct, causal way to psychological or intellectual characteristics, and which on this basis distinguishes between superior and inferior racial groups.

Rationalist approaches. Emerging from early modern thought, rationalist approaches to science and knowledge rely on the possibility of obtaining objective truth about the world. From this view, methods for obtaining truth are refined and applied to the world so as to produce a set of desired results. In ethics, a rationalist approach to moral truth implies that an objective understanding of morality exists and that we can come to discover it by applying ethical decision models in a given situation. In this approach to ethics, there is little or no attention paid to social context, relationships, subjectivity, and power dynamics.

Reasonable accommodation. Any modification or adjustment to a job, an employment practice, or a school environment that makes possible for a qualified individual with a disability to gain equal employment and/or educational opportunities.

Received knowledge. Knowledge that one acquires uncritically. Rote learning engenders received knowledge.

Reflective learning. Occurs when the learner allows new information to process in a thoughtful way (i.e., not in an active manner). An example would be thinking about an abstract concept in order to understand it.

Reflexive. To be aware of the process of thinking while cognitively engaging ideas, for example attending to our *situatedness* while interpreting experience.

Relational pedagogy. An educational approach that considers the relation of teacher and student, nurse and patient, and the self and world.

Relational. A way of seeing human beings as contextual, social beings who are always in relation to oneself, with others, and the world more broadly. A relational view of self suggest that our individual identities and ways of being in the world are always shaped by the others and the context within which such relations take place.

Relativism. The view that truths are dependent on the context in which they are considered rather than having inherent value in and of themselves. Although this is a philosophically problematic idea, it is one that has had some appeal for nurses in that it seems to represent a way of thinking about the diversity of values, beliefs, and assumptions that human beings present us with when we engage with them in the provision of individualized nursing care. Some nurses assume that an inherent valuing of diversity is therefore logically consistent with a claim that there are no inherent truths underlying our discipline. Others claim that we have a social and moral mandate to strive toward an understanding of nursing as deriving from fundamental truths about the nature of human experience.

Release time. Generally refers to removing teaching responsibilities from a faculty member in lieu of taking on other activities.

Role modeling. A term originating in the work of Bandura on social learning theory that when used in health education refers to learning by exposure to the attitudes, approaches, beliefs, affect and characteristics of the educator.

Rote learning. Rote learning is held to result from teaching strategies following the transmission model of learning.

S

Scenario. The context within which the health care problem and the client exist. There is usually more than one scenario in each paper problem package (a comprehensive learning package used to facilitate PBL which is related to clinical concepts and skills).

Scholars of teaching. Expert and excellent teachers who share their knowledge and advance the knowledge of teaching within the discipline through publication in peer reviewed journals.

Self-directed learning. An approach to the learning process that encourages students to identify their own objectives or learning needs through mutual assessment and participative decision making. This approach allows students to develop learning strategies to meet those needs (e.g., inquiry, independent student, and experiential techniques) and promotes an evaluation of individual and group progress toward the achievement of identified objectives. The self-directed method of learning involves independent study by each student, either alone or in collaboration with peers.

Self-monitoring. The conscious monitoring and application of reasoning activities.

Sensing learner. This type of learner likes facts and observations. Sensing learners like to solve problems but do not care for abstractions or unexpected complications.

Situated learning. Learning that occurs in contexts that would require the knowledge that is being acquired. There is a focus on problem solving that occurs collaboratively with others during small group work.

Situatedness. We are situated in a particular way in the world based on our gender, class, history, past experiences, beliefs, values, and education. Our situatedness or location evokes responses from others that also shape how we come to understand the world. Our situatedness also holds assumptions that accompany us in our nursing practice and teaching. While some people may believe that we can extricate ourselves as educators from ourselves as people, it is not always clear that we can or would even want to do this.

Skills. Actions or behaviors, in the performance of tasks, carried out with a reasonably adequate degree of proficiency or dexterity. Skills can be psychomotor (involving body movement and dexterity), cognitive (involving critical interpretation and decision-making), or relational (involving communication and being with clients).

Social constructivism. A theory of cognitive development based on the research of L. S. Vygotsky. According to social constructivism advances made in a child's development occur first in the course of social interaction. Only once a competency has been performed in a social context (intermentally) can it be called on and performed independently (intramentally).

Sociological constructionism. A theoretical viewpoint which holds that the knowledge accumulated in the natural and social sciences is not value free and objective but instead reflects the contingent social context in which that knowledge is developed.

Socialization. The process whereby an individual acquires the patterns of thought, feeling, and behavior of particular social groups such as a family, institution, professional milieu, or society as a whole.

Social behaviorists. Theorists who believe that the system of stimuli and rewards for learning are based in the social system of the learner.

Social learning theory. A theoretical approach to understanding human behavior that stresses learning through the observation of others seen as models.

Social reform perspective. From this perspective, effective teaching is intended to change nursing practice and/or society in substantive ways, while also educating students to be competent nurse practitioners.

Static media. Course materials in printed text and/or images that are delivered to students by faculty or that are required of students, such as scholarly papers.

Structural inequities. "Structural inequities refers to inequities that arise from and within the basic structures in society such as the state, local, and global political economies, globalization, racialization, and dominant institutions such as health, legal, educational, and government systems" (Browne, 2001).

Student-centered learning. A term used to describe a teaching/learning process that actively engages students in the development of knowledge rather than passive recipients of information transmitted by teachers.

Student-centered teaching. Teaching that focuses on the experiences of and interactions with the learners. The learner is in the forefront of the educational activity. The focus of teaching is on helping students' discover and construct new knowledge and understanding.

Student-directed learning. Students are responsible for directing their own learning.

Surface learning. An approach to learning in which the learner memorizes surface information in order to accomplish a requirement that is imposed by the teacher or is required to pass a course; therefore, avoiding failure is the end goal. The content is often forgotten by students shortly after the course ends. Motivation is extrinsic, primarily based on achieving high grades.

Synchronously. In real time.

Synchronous activities. Activities that occur at the same time, in real time. Thus, faculty and students participate at a set time.

Systematic thinking. Systematic thinking is that which is marked by thoroughness and regularity, such that analysis and synthesis are coherent and formulated on the basis of a body of ideas or principles. In nursing practice, systematic thinking relates to a comprehensive nursing assessment of the whole person and context such that the implications of various nursing intervention approaches can be considered, appreciated and, at times, predicted. In its most basic form, it reflects an understanding that the patient represents not simply an organ system or a body, but also a human person living a unique life within a larger social and situational context. Systematic thinking refers to the nurse's capacity to apprehend both systems and parts of systems simultaneously in an effort to provide nursing care that is contextualized, relevant, and meaningful. The underlying goal of all nursing models, frameworks, and conceptual structures is to create ways of learning to "think" nursing in a systematic manner.

T

Tablet PC. A computer that resembles a notebook, or laptop, but has the additional capability of being written on through the use of a touch screen or digitizing tablet pen. Some Tablet PCs are slates and have only a monitor, while others are convertibles or hybrids and include a keyboard.

Tacit knowledge. Knowledge that functions as a background knowledge that assists in accomplishing a task in focus—the knowledge of approaching discovery.

Tabula rasa. This metaphor, central to Locke's empiricism, captures the philosopher's idea that human beings have no innate ideas but rather all ideas are ultimately derived from experience. Accordingly, before birth a human being's mind is like a blank slate—a *tabula rasa*—waiting to be filled in by experience.

Teacher-centered instruction. Involves the presentation of content to the students who listen but are otherwise not actively engaged in the learning.

Teacher-centered teaching. Teaching that focuses on the instructor rather than on experiences of, and interactions with, learners.

Teaching portfolio. An extensive collection of information that results in a comprehensive profile of teaching effectiveness.

Technical nurse. Level of educational preparation from associate degree programs as envisioned by Mildred Montag.

Thematic organization. A strategy in which thematic units organize learning experiences. The thematic units focus on a particular topic, idea, author, or concept.

Theorizing. Theorizing is a term used in nursing to describe the act of working with or generating theories, which are certain ideas held in relationship to one another. Theories range from linked facts to abstract thoughts or speculations, and represent the mechanism by which humans work toward developing understandings of the world around them, both material and human. In nursing, although some of our science has involved systematic conjecture and hypothesis testing, much of what we typically refer to as theorizing is best described as an attempt to work out a plausible body of principles that explain the phenomena with which we are concerned. Thus, the conceptual structures by which early nursing scholars attempted to taxonomize the complexity inherent in excellent clinical reasoning were termed nursing theories.

Thinking learner. This type of learner is logical and rational. Thinking learners can easily discern illogical thinking patterns in others. They may be impersonal with others.

Transactional distance. A physical separation of learner and teacher that causes a psychological and communicative chasm.

Transformative learning. A theory of learning developed by Jack Mezirow based on transformational theory that focuses on learning to negotiate and act on our own values and purposes rather than those uncritically received from others.

Transmission model of learning/teaching. Based on empiricist assumptions, this theory's ideal of instruction is the transmission of the educator's knowledge to the minds of her student. This ideal stands in contrast to the constructivist ideal of creating learning conditions that are meant to foster the student's own understanding of course material.

Transmission perspective. A transmission teacher's primary responsibility is to deliver the content accurately and efficiently.

Tutor. A faculty member who serves as a facilitator of the learning process.

Tutorial. A regularly scheduled time for tutor and learners to meet to learn about learning and learn about nursing through discussion of real nursing practice situations.

U

Upper-two. A baccalaureate curriculum plan where nursing courses are taught in the final two years of the program.

V

Videoconferencing. A two-way, or multiway, session of faculty and students that incorporates synchronous audio and video. Until rather recently video conferencing required point-to-point expensive systems. Currently, IP (internet protocol) based video conferencing is becoming more prevalent because of decreasing costs of video cameras and fast Internet connections. More institutions and students with Internet connections and Web cameras are, therefore, able to take advantage of videoconferencing.

Vygotsky, L. S. (1896–1934). Early 20th-century Belorussian psychologist and author of the theory of cognitive development known as social constructivism.

W

Ways of knowing. An approach to the understanding of multiple intelligences, popularized by theorists such as Howard Gardner, which espouses the idea that intelligence is not one measure but multiple measures of different traits.

White privilege. White privilege includes unearned privileges or advantages that are granted to people with white skin or those who can pass as White. In her 1988 paper on White privilege, McIntosh listed 46 "conditions" or ways that she, as a White woman, enjoyed benefits and perquisites that her colleagues of color did not. A decade later, McIntosh's list had grown by an additional 62 conditions (1998, pp. 207–211). Due to "inherited systems of systemic over-advantage granted to people with white skin," McIntosh said she had "come to see White privilege as an invisible package of unearned assets that I could count on in each day but about which I was meant to remain oblivious. White privilege is like an invisible, weightless knapsack of special provisions, maps, passports, codebooks, visas, clothes, tools, and blank checks" (p. 207). One result of these special, unearned privileges is that those with white skin often enjoy a "head start" in life and are able to achieve more than other groups who do not enjoy such privilege. The result of such relations of privilege is to confer unearned advantages to particular groups, who often come to see these privileges as theirs by virtue of their assumed superiority (i.e., greater intelligence, harder work, etc.).

World Wide Web. A system of Internet servers that support specially formatted documents. The documents are formatted in a markup language called HTML (*HyperText Markup Language*) that supports links to other documents, as well as graphics, audio, and video files. A computer user can navigate from one document to another simply by clicking on links that are available in the HTML documents. Not all Internet servers are part of the World Wide Web.

Z

Zone of proximal development. A central construct in Vygotsky's social development theory, problems that fall into the zone of proximal development are those that a learner is able to solve in collaboration with adults or peers but that are too difficult to solve alone. Vygotsky argued that having learners work together to solve problems in their common zone of proximal development is an important condition of cognitive development.

Appendix

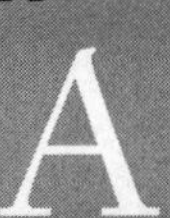

Sample Lesson Plan: Introducing Family Nursing

Lynne E. Young

RECOMMENDED STRATEGIES

1. On a flip chart, write the schedule for class and, prior to class, post it at the front of the classroom in a highly visible location. Refer to the flip chart when providing the overview of the lesson.
2. Keep to the schedule, especially with regard to the timing of the nutrition/coffee break.
3. Prepare the material for this class in Power Point presentation format to focus learners' attention on the exercises and content and to add to the aesthetics of the classroom.
4. This class is designed for class sizes of 40 to 90 participants.
5. It is recommended that the instructor walks around the class interacting with students during the reflective exercises, class discussions, and case study exercises to equalize power and to engage learners located a distance from the podium.

Schedule

9:00–9:10 Housekeeping/Overview of Lesson

9:10–9:30 Reflection #1

Individual Reflection

- Think of a time that you learned about health in your family:
  - What did you learn about?
  - Who taught you?
  - How did this person teach you?
  - Is this early learning evident in your life today?
- Note the responses to these questions on your note paper.

Pair/Share

- Share the response of one of the above questions with the person beside you.

9:30–9:40 Individuals volunteer to report back to the large group.
Instructor facilitates large group discussion.

9:40–10:00 Reflection #2

Individual Reflection

- What have you learned about health-related caring practices from your family?
  - What did you learn about?
  - Who taught you?
  - How did this person teach you?
  - Is this early learning evident in your life today?
- Note the responses to these questions on your note paper.

Note to readers: Be prepared for students to reveal poignant family stories. Prior to class anticipate how you will handle deeply emotional responses to these questions in this large group educational session.

Pair/Share

- Share the response of one question above with the person beside you.

10:00–10:10 Individuals volunteer to report back to large group.
Instructor facilitates large group discussion.
10:10–10:30 Nutrition/stretch break

Note to readers: The following material is presented in a traditional, teacher-centered style. Learners new to student-centered teaching respond well to having at least some aspect of class presented in this familiar way. Placing the instructor-led aspect of class after students reflect on their own experiences is consistent with constructivist pedagogical principles.

10:30–11:00 Instructor presentation.
Topics: Why family nursing?
Family nursing conceptualized as relational practice.

11:00–11:45 Case Study #1

Pair/Share

- You are a nurse in a health clinic. A middle-age man and his wife present to you.
- The man says that they came to the clinic because he is worried that his wife is depressed because she is in menopause.
- Turn to the person sitting next to you and quietly discuss what you will do.
- Note your plan of care.

Pairs volunteer to report back to large group.
Instructor facilitates large group discussion.

Try to bring out differences in opinion about the proposed plan of care within and among pairs. To do so, watch for cues in pairs during their interchanges that suggest that a particular pair is working out differences of opinion. Examining such differences in the classroom is enriching and challenges learners in a number of ways: to articulate their position; to present ideas clearly; to take a stand on a particular position; and to engage with opinions that may differ from their own. As Wheeler, a leading complexity theorist, remarked: "Progress in science [ideas/thinking] owes more to the clash of ideas than the steady accumulation of facts" (Davies, 2004, p. 3).

Case Study #2
Pair/Share

- You are a community nurse on a visit to a family suspected of child abuse. You walk into the home and see a 4-year-old child clinging to her mother.
- The social worker notes that there must be no abuse because the child is close to the mother. You observe many bruises on the child's arms.
- With the person sitting next to you, quietly discuss what you will do.
- Note your plan of care.

Pairs volunteer to report back to large group.
Instructor facilitates large group discussion.

11:45–11:55 Summarize main points.
Go over the instructions for learning activities/assignments for the upcoming week.

11:55–12:00 Evaluation of lesson.

Each student is asked to respond to the following questions on a piece of paper that is submitted anonymously to the instructor at the end of class:

1. What activity in today's lesson best supported your learning about family nursing? Why?
2. What activity in class did not support your learning about family nursing? Why?
3. What suggestions do you have for the instructor for improving this class?

References

Davies, P. (2004). John Archibald Wheeler and the clash of ideas. In J. D. Barrow, P. C. Davies, & C. L. Harper, Jr. (Eds.). *Science and ultimate reality: Quantum theory, cosmology, and complexity* (pp.3–26). Cambridge, UK: Cambridge University Press

Appendix

B Sample Course Outline

Lynne E. Young

NURSING 493—COMPLEX HEALTH CHALLENGES: ACUTE CARE SETTINGS

Course Description

This course provides opportunities for students to strengthen their knowledge about, and theoretical understandings of, nursing practice related to complex health challenges that present in acute care settings. Students explore and critique nurses' roles in practice and related issues/concepts specific to caring for individuals and families.

Ends-in-View

A warm welcome to N493, Complex Health Challenges: Acute Care Settings. The overall objective of this course is to facilitate your integration of core content of the BSN curriculum in preparation for your final clinical practice experiences. To this end, the course is designed to:

1. Provide students with opportunities to identify gaps in clinical knowledge.
2. Provide students with opportunities to develop skills with accessing resources to address knowledge gaps.
3. Provide students with opportunities to use case stories to develop new understandings.
4. Provide students with opportunities to use published research and other scholarly materials to inform clinical decision making.
5. Provide students with opportunities to develop group process skills, including group facilitation.
6. Provide students with opportunities develop teaching/presentation skills.

Process

Student-centered learning is the pedagogy used in this course, which is an approach consistent with the patient/client-centered focus of the University of Victoria Nursing Curriculum and health promoting nursing practice. Thus, there will be minimal teacher-centered instruction, with learning occurring primarily through individual learning activities and small and large group discussions.

This student-centered approach is designed to shift the focus of learning from the teacher to you, the learner; a shift that will enhance your capacity for professional nursing practice and develop skills for lifelong learning. Story-based learning, the model that guides learning in this course, evolved out of two student-centered methods of instruction, problem-based learning and case method teaching.

Problem-based learning. In the PBL approach, a case is presented to catalyze discussion and focus learning. Here, learners use a systematic process to identify learning issues and knowledge gaps, identify resources to address knowledge gaps, present newly evolving understandings to the tutor and other students, and to summarize succinctly in technical language "what is going on." The process is designed to develop professional knowledge and competencies (for example articulating complex concepts to peers) and skills for lifelong learning. PBL is used widely in medical education throughout the world and has been widely adopted in schools of nursing throughout the world.

Case method teaching. In case method teaching, the focus of learning is a case that simulates reality. Cases stimulate discussion and dialogue about practice problems and issues. Every case is open to "firing from all directions," main teaching/learning points that are embedded in the case are brought forward for discussion by the instructor during discussion.

Case method teaching precedes problem-based learning as a pedagogy. Case method teaching originated in the academic business community where leaders in the nonacademic business community pressured business schools **to prepare students to function in the real world.** Academics at Harvard responded by developing case method teaching. Academics in medicine, when faced with the same pressures from the community, adopted and adapted case method teaching naming their approach problem-based learning. Some nursing faculties have adopted PBL (e.g., McMaster University). With a view to moving away from the problem-orientation of PBL while retaining its strengths, Dr. Young, in consultation with students and faculty, adapted these approaches into what is called **story-based learning (SBL).** (See Chapter 8).

Story-based learning is a systematic approach to learning that allows students to gain skills with **problem-solving, information-seeking, and critical appraisal of a practice situation.** Using stories to focus learning provides students with an opportunity to **develop empathy for the lived experience of clients; expand knowledge of specific content areas**; and **integrate curriculum themes.**

EVALUATION OF LEARNING

	ASSIGNMENTS	MARK	DUE DATE
#1	Case study facilitation	15%	As per schedule
#2	Peer evaluations	10%	As per schedule
#3A	Case story for analysis	10%	October 9th
#3B	Individual case story for analysis	35%	November 27th
#4	Group presentations	30%	October 23rd, 30th, November 13th

Assignment # 1: Case Study Facilitation

As case study facilitator (CSF), your role will be to facilitate group work on a case story assigned by the instructor. In the role of facilitator, you will have an opportunity to further integrate your knowledge about, and skills with, group process acquired throughout the BSN program. As group facilitator, you will facilitate the task-related work of the group; guide students' acquisition of substantive knowledge by facilitating their use and sharing of resources; facilitate the morale component of the group; and stimulate critical analysis by posing questions. You will receive the case story that you will facilitate 1 week prior to your scheduled facilitation date. This will allow you to work up the case on your own using the story-based learning model as a guide prior to enacting your role as CSF.

Group facilitation will occur in **two** sequential classes. There will be time allotted during the first of these two classes for you to engage students in a discussion of the case; facilitate group members in identifying their learning issues and resources that might be used to address knowledge gaps; and, plan your group work. For example, during this first class, through a collaborative process that you facilitate, your group will decide who will be responsible for gathering information on particular aspects of the case story to bring back to the group. During the second class, time will be allotted for you to facilitate the group in the task of putting together a comprehensive analysis for presentation to the larger group.

EVALUATION OF CASE STORY FACILITATOR ROLE

Self-Evaluation (5%)

Reflection self-evaluation is a critical component of professional practice. While this course has been designed to provide you with an opportunity to exercise skills and qualities that you can build on in your professional life, it would not be complete without providing you with an opportunity for self-evaluation. In this assignment, you are asked to reflect then comment on how you developed your facilitation skills during this group facilitation exercise. In a one- to two-page (12 point, single-spaced) summary, reflect on your skill and knowledge development according to the criteria established for the role: (a) facilitating the task-related work of the group; (b) facilitating students' use and sharing of resources; (c) facilitating the morale component of the group; and (d) stimulating critical analysis by posing questions. Please provide examples. **Assign yourself a mark out of** 5.

Instructor Evaluation (5%)

You will receive a mark out of 5 from the instructor according to the criteria above: (a) facilitating the task-related work of the group; (b) facilitating students' use and sharing of resources; (c) facilitating the morale component of the group; and, (d) stimulating critical analysis by posing questions.

Peer Evaluation (5%)

You will receive a mark from your group members.

Assignment # 2: Peer Evaluations

You have an opportunity to evaluate the contributions of case story facilitators (CSF) on five different occasions. For each CSF peer evaluation submitted you will be assigned a mark out of 20. The mark out of 20 that you receive for submitted peer evaluations will derive from the following criteria for grading noted in this course outline. Roughly, excellent to exceptional peer evaluations will receive marks of 15 to 20 respectively; average work will receive a mark of 10 to 15; and barely adequate work will receive a mark of 0 to 10. The final mark for this assignment comprises 10% of the total mark for N493.

Assignment #3A: Case Story

(PART ONE OF A TWO-PART ASSIGNMENT)

Story writing is a creative endeavor, an opportunity to illustrate the innumerable factors that require a nurse's attention. The idea of writing stories that will then be analyzed is to provide you with a chance to express the layers of factors that impinge on real or imagined situations that have confronted or may confront you in professional practice. The **goal of writing a case story** is for you to expand your awareness of the myriad of factors influencing professional decision making.

You are asked to identify your knowledge gaps and select three from that list to focus your learning for this assignment. The three areas of focus must derive from a range of practice domains: e.g., physiological/clinical, family, social, psychological. Then, you are asked to write a case story from past experience **OR** your imagination that incorporates these aspects of practice. For example, if (a) orthopedic nursing, (b) family nursing, and (c) substance abuse are learning issues, you would write a case story that brings forward these three dimensions. Details of such a case that written into a story might be:

1. Jacque, 24-year-old suburban male.
2. Presented to ER with a fractured femur following MVA (motor vehicle accident).
3. AOB (Alcohol on breath) upon admission.
4. Jacque's partner/friend(?)Bob is sitting by Jacque's bed looking extremely anxious.

Recommended length for this assignment is 2 ½ to 3 ½ pages maximum, 1 to 2 pages for knowledge gaps and related knowledge categories; 1 page for the story; and 1 page for citations and Web search strategy.

Mark Allocation:

1. List of 3 knowledge gaps with explanation (3)
2. Story (4)
3. Citations for **research** articles that pertain to your topic with abstracts (2)
4. Literature search strategy (1)

Assignment #3B: Case Story

(PART TWO OF A TWO-PART ASSIGNMENT)

In this assignment, you will submit an edited version of the case story you prepared for Assignment 3A and an analysis of it. You will use the story-based learning model to guide the analysis. (See Chapter 8.)

This assignment is designed to provide you with an opportunity to integrate your knowledge of **pathophysiology, lab results, and biomedical procedures and treatments**, and **medications with your knowledge of nursing care.** Hence, assignments should address all of these aspects of a story.

Mark Allocation:
The assignment is evaluated according to the evaluation criteria for the course:

1. Edited case story (1)
2. What is going on here? (10)
3. What are the BIG questions? (4)
4. Referrals (3)
5. Nursing support (10)
6. Evaluation plan (5)
7. Reflection on learning (2)

Please submit a completed assignment of no more than 14 pages (single-spaced), using APA format for references. Charts, tables, or diagrams may be used to organize your work.

Individual case analyses will be copied and presented as a collection in a document that can be used by you as a clinical resource for your clinical practice experiences or as a study guide for RN exam preparation.

Assignment #4: Group Presentation of a Case Story

For this assignment, you will work with four to five other students to develop a story for analysis. The case story will be written so that the analysis addresses vital knowledge gaps of the larger group identified during the large group activity. The presentation of the case provides you with an opportunity to develop story writing skills; your capacity for case story analysis; your ability to work in a group; and, your teaching and presentation skills. **Each group has 45 minutes to present their work.**

The assignment is evaluated in two parts: a) the story and its analysis, and b) teaching/presentation. You are encouraged to use a student-centered pedagogy for this presentation. Peer evaluation will contribute to the overall mark assigned by the instructor. *Your group is encouraged to prepare a handout for the learners to facilitate learning as well as peer and instructor evaluation.*

Evaluation Criteria

1. Application of the story-based learning model (20%)

This assignment is designed to provide you with an opportunity to integrate your knowledge of **pathophysiology, lab results, diagnostic and biomedical procedures and**

treatments, and **medications with your knowledge of nursing care**. Hence, assignments should address all of these aspects of a story.

a. Case story (4)
b. What is going on here? (5)
c. What are the BIG questions? (2)
d. Referrals (2)
e. Nursing support & evaluation plan (5)
f. Reflection on learning (2)

2. Teaching/Presentation Skills (10%)

a. Clarity (3)
b. Supports learning (3)
c. Creative (2)
d. Professional (2)

Note: Please include your literature searches of the nursing data base (CINHAL) and other databases (PUBMED and WEBSPIR) with your assignment. It is expected that you will make it clear to the learners which sources you have used to fill identified knowledge gaps and/or to justify your nursing actions.

Assignment Submission Policy
Late assignments receive a deduction of one grade for each day beyond the due date (that is, if the assignment receives a B mark for content but is one day late, the final mark will be B-, two days C+, three days C, and so forth.). To avoid penalty, you may request an extension **in writing either on paper or by e-mail**. You must indicate a **new due date** when you submit a request for an extension. Failing to do so will result in a penalty.

Assignment Criteria
Thoroughness, thoughtfulness, creativity, ability to integrate core curriculum material (feminism, critical theory, and health promotion) wherever appropriate, demonstration of accountability and professionalism, level of competency with English grammar and spelling, and visual presentation of assignments with regards to typos and overall professional appearance comprise the grading criteria for this course. A hallmark of professionalism is that decisions are evidenced-based, hence, it is **expected** that students will draw on the scholarly and empirical literature to support the ideas presented in their work and that references are cited according to APA.

THANK YOU FOR YOUR CONTRIBUTIONS TO OTHERS' LEARNING.

Index

Page numbers followed by letters *b*, *f*, and *t* indicate boxes, figures, and tables, respectively.

D

Q

R

S

T